Atlas of Lymphoscintigraphy and Sentinel Node Mapping

Giuliano Mariani • Sergi Vidal-Sicart
Renato A. Valdés Olmos
Editors

Atlas of Lymphoscintigraphy and Sentinel Node Mapping

A Pictorial Case-Based Approach

Second edition

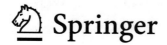 Springer

Editors
Giuliano Mariani
Regional Center of Nuclear Medicine
Department of Translational Research and
Advanced Technologies in Medicine and Surgery
University of Pisa
Pisa
Italy

Renato A. Valdés Olmos
Department of Radiology
Section of Nuclear Medicine and Interventional
Molecular Imaging Laboratory
Leiden University Medical Center
Leiden
The Netherlands

Sergi Vidal-Sicart
Nuclear Medicine Department
Hospital Clinic Barcelona
Barcelona
Catalonia
Spain

Institut d'Investigacions Biomèdiques
August Pi Sunyer (IDIBAPS)
Barcelona
Catalonia
Spain

ISBN 978-3-030-45298-8   ISBN 978-3-030-45296-4   (eBook)
https://doi.org/10.1007/978-3-030-45296-4

This Springer imprint is published by the registered company Springer Nature Switzerland AG
The registered company address is: Gewerbestrasse 11, 6330 Cham, Switzerland

Foreword

By providing invaluable morpho-functional imaging of the lymphatic system that would be very difficult to investigate otherwise, lymphoscintigraphy is currently the accepted standard of care in the differential diagnosis of lymphedema. Furthermore, in patients with a growing number of malignancies lymphoscintigraphy is used for sentinel lymph node (SLN) mapping, a procedure that constitutes one of the greatest success stories in contemporary surgical oncology, with a crucial role for accurate staging of a variety of solid tumors through an approach optimized to reduce surgical invasiveness as much as possible.

The second edition of the "Atlas of Lymphoscintigraphy and Sentinel Node Mapping: A Pictorial Case-Based Approach" provides an update on innovations related to this technique, using the same approach that has been the hallmark of success for the first publication.

This book is edited by Giuliano Mariani, Sergi Vidal-Sicart, and Renato A. Valdés Olmos (three distinguished specialists in the very intriguing field of radioguided surgery), and includes contributions from highly qualified international experts.

The atlas is structured into 16 well-established chapters and contains a huge number of very-high-quality illustrations, tables, and diagrams. This excellent book reviews all of the basic principles of lymphoscintigraphy and sentinel node biopsy (SLNB), and also provides a comprehensive overview of the technical procedural details. The practical aspects of the technique, from radiopharmacy and tracer administration to instrumentation and detection, as well as state-of-the-art applications, with excellent clinical cases, are described in an original and comprehensive fashion.

As stated by the editors, the aim of this book is to provide an in-depth description of this technology, to offer an extended guide with examples covering common clinical practice, and to deliver future perspectives and methodological improvements of this specific topic.

The final editorial outcome is a very exhaustive, fluent, and updated guide, enriched with explanatory images and tables that fulfill its ultimate goal to offer the best standard of health care received by our patients.

In conclusion, I highly recommend this excellent atlas not only to experts, but also to residents, clinicians, and everyone willing to approach the evolving clinical scenario in which lymphoscintigraphy and radioguided surgery are employed.

Vienna, Austria   Francesco Giammarile

Preface

Almost 30 years after the introduction of radioguided SLNB for staging purposes in melanoma and breast cancer, lymphoscintigraphy remains an essential component of the procedure. In fact, lymphoscintigraphy and radioguided surgery have transformed the paradigm of oncologic surgery from "open and see" to one of "see and open," providing to surgeons and nuclear physicians a helpful visual road map enabling to identify and remove SLNs or other adequately "labeled" lesions the operating room. In the evolution of nuclear medicine, this important role of lymphoscintigraphy for SLN mapping followed the original development of this imaging modality for applications aimed to identify causes of peripheral edema or for characterization of patients with intracavitary lymph effusions.

Especially since the first decade of this millennium, the use of lymphoscintigraphy has been extended to different malignancies, thus facilitating radioguided SLNB under the most sophisticated and/or complex anatomic conditions. The addition of single-photon emission computed tomography/computed tomography (SPECT/CT) to the imaging procedure has played an important role in this development. In fact, by combining the functional SPECT information with the anatomical CT findings, the resulting SPECT/CT images did evolve the abovementioned paradigm to a novel one, that is, "see, open, and recognize." The incorporation of the latter recognition function was based on the landmarks provided by SPECT/CT, which include information on the SLN location in relation to blood vessels, muscles, and other anatomical structures. The expertise accumulated with SPECT/CT has been crucial to expand the SLN procedure to other areas with particularly complex lymphatic drainage, such as the head and neck region and the pelvis. Based on this experience, regional staging in oral cavity cancers and in malignancies of the female and male reproductive systems is now becoming possible.

Although the indications for SLNB continue to evolve, in clinical practice the procedure continues to be of vital importance for regional lymph node staging. In classical applications such as melanoma and breast malignancies, the growing cancer risk stratification management occurring in recent years has led to the incorporation of new patient categories. Today in many cases with tumor-positive SLNs subsequent completion of regional lymph node dissection is no longer necessary—for example in patients with early breast cancer and favorable histology. Nevertheless, this process of selectivity in the clinical management of numerous patients has delineated an additional role for SLN mapping using lymphoscintigraphy and SPECT/CT. The accurate information of the modality is now being used also for surveillance of the lymph node stations at risk of metastatic dissemination by means of ultrasonography and other diagnostic imaging modalities including PET/CT. Furthermore, besides surgery, there is an increasing interest to apply lymphatic mapping in tailoring planning of other treatment alternatives, such as radiotherapy.

The structure of this new edition of this atlas book follows the previous one. However, the content of the chapters has been significantly upgraded and updated, incorporating state-of-the-art information with respect to clinical indications and technological advances. Chapters 1 and 2 include introductory elements and basic concepts concerning the anatomy, physiology, and pathophysiology of lymphatic circulation, whereas Chap. 3 presents the methodological aspects of lymphoscintigraphy, including radiopharmaceuticals and instrumentation.

From Chap. 4 onwards, the current contribution of lymphoscintigraphy for nononcologic lymphatic disorders as well as for SLN mapping related to staging in various malignancies is discussed by leading experts in the field.

The methodological approach using lymphoscintigraphy for the evaluation of edema of the extremities is extensively presented in Chap. 4, while in Chap. 5 the role of lymphoscintigraphy is discussed in relation to the differential diagnosis of peripheral edema and of intracavitary lymph effusion.

In Chap. 6 the concept of SLNB in relation to oncologic surgery is analyzed, and in Chap. 7 essential tools of radioguided SLNB concerning preoperative imaging (based on planar lymphoscintigraphy and SPECT/CT) are discussed in relation to guidance approaches using gamma probes, gamma cameras, and allied technologies in the operation room.

The role and criteria for interpretation of SPECT/CT in addition to planar lymphoscintigraphy are presented in Chap. 8. From Chap. 9 (breast cancer) to Chap. 16 (kidney and bladder cancer) the sequential chapters discuss the clinical impact of radioguided SLNB within the framework of a multidisciplinary approach in specific malignancies such as melanoma (Chap. 10), head and neck cancers (Chap. 11), lung cancer (Chap. 12), gastrointestinal cancers (Chap. 13), and cancers of the female (Chap. 14) and male (Chap. 15) reproductive systems.

All chapters of the book include an introductory section concerning pathophysiology of the specific diseases, as well as the current clinical indications for SLNB emphasizing the role of preoperative imaging including lymphoscintigraphy and SPECT/CT. The latter modalities are also discussed in the light of the dissemination routes for metastasis from primary tumors. Each chapter of the book is complemented by richly illustrated teaching cases, aimed to emphasize both the most commonly observed patterns and anatomic variants in lymphatic drainage as well as possible technical pitfalls.

For all chapters, specific learning objectives have been added together with key learning points for their different sections. These adjustments aim to facilitate the use of the atlas as a real textbook on lymphoscintigraphy in general and on SLN imaging and biopsy.

Initially conceived under the umbrella of the Italian Association of Nuclear Medicine, the first version of the book already crossed borders and this tendency has been reinforced in the current edition, by incorporating international experts in the field of radioguided surgery and lymphatic mapping as contributors. These specialists have collaborated in many cases with young colleagues to provide not only didactic but also high-quality pictorial examples and illustrations. Thanks to this confluence, a new generation is getting ready to carry the torch of the book initiative onwards.

We thank the support of Springer for making it possible to publish this book meeting the high technical levels required by an atlas.

Pisa, Italy   Giuliano Mariani
Barcelona, Spain   Sergi Vidal-Sicart
Leiden, The Netherlands   Renato A. Valdés Olmos

Acknowledgements

The editors and authors are indebted to colleagues from different groups who contributed additional teaching cases in some chapters of the book. Their contributions provide examples of how lymphoscintigraphy plays a practical role in patient management at critical points in the care of patients. The following is a list of these contributors:

Filippo Antonica
Giuseppe Rubini
    Center of Nuclear Medicine, University of Bari Medical School, Bari, Italy
Roberto Bartoletti
Marco Pagan
Girolamo Tartaglione
    Nuclear Medicine, Cristo Re Hospital, Rome, Italy
Antoni Bennássar
    Dermatology Department, Hospital Clinic Barcelona, Barcelona, Spain
Sebastian Casanueva
Carles Martí
    Maxillofacial Surgery Department, Hospital Clinic Barcelona, Barcelona, Spain
John Orozco
Erika Padilla-Morales
Núria Sánchez
Andrés Tapias
Agustí Toll
    Dermatology Department, Hospital Clinic Barcelona, Barcelona, Spain
    Nuclear Medicine Department, Hospital Clinic Barcelona, Barcelona, Catalonia, Spain
Paolo Carcoforo
Corrado Cittanti
Valentina de Cristofaro
Luciano Feggi
Stefano Panareo
Chiara Peterle
Ilaria Rambaldi
Virginia Rossetti
Ivan Santi
    Nuclear Medicine Unit, Department of Diagnostic Imaging and Laboratory Medicine, S. Anna University-Hospital of Ferrara, Ferrara, Italy
Joan Duch
    Nuclear Medicine Department, Hospital de la Santa Creu, Universitat Autònoma de Barcelona, Barcelona, Catalonia, Spain
Danilo Fortini
Alberto Fragano
Germano Perotti

Luca Zagaria
    Nuclear Medicine Unit, Fondazione Policlinico Universitario A. Gemelli IRCCS, Rome,
Italy
Luisa Locantore
    Nuclear Medicine Unit, University Hospital of Verona, Verona, Italy
José Luis Pallarés
    Department of General and Digestive Surgery, Hospital de la Santa Creu i Sant Pau,
Barcelona, Catalonia, Spain
Daphne D. D. Rietbergen
    Department of Radiology, Section of Nuclear Medicine, Leiden University Medical
Centre, Leiden, Netherlands

Contents

1   **Anatomy and Physiology of Lymphatic Circulation: Application to Lymphatic Mapping** 1
Omgo E. Nieweg, Pieter J. Tanis, and Stanley P. L. Leong

2   **Pathophysiology of Lymphatic Circulation in Different Disease Conditions** 7
Rossella Di Stefano, Giulia Dibello, Francesca Felice, and Paola A. Erba

3   **Methodological Aspects of Lymphatic Mapping: Radiopharmaceuticals, Multimodal Lymphatic Mapping Agents, Instrumentations** 21
Francesco Bartoli, Giuseppina Bisogni, Sara Vitali, Angela G. Cataldi,
Alberto Del Guerra, Giuliano Mariani, and Paola A. Erba

4   **Methodological Aspects of Lymphoscintigraphy: Bicompartmental Versus Monocompartmental Radiocolloid Administration** 53
Martina Sollini, Francesco Bartoli, Andrea Marciano, Roberta Zanca,
Giovanni D'Errico, Giuliano Mariani, and Paola A. Erba

5   **Lymphoscintigraphy for the Differential Diagnosis of Peripheral Edema and Intracavitary Lymph Effusion** 79
Martina Sollini, Roberto Boni, Andrea Marciano, Roberta Zanca,
Francesco Bartoli, and Paola A. Erba

6   **The Sentinel Lymph Node Concept** 143
Omgo E. Nieweg

7   **General Concepts on Radioguided Sentinel Lymph Node Biopsy: Preoperative Imaging, Intraoperative Gamma Probe Guidance, Intraoperative Imaging, Multimodality Imaging** 151
Federica Orsini, Federica Guidoccio, Sergi Vidal-Sicart,
Renato A. Valdés Olmos, and Giuliano Mariani

8   **SPECT/CT Image Generation and Criteria for Sentinel Lymph Node Mapping** 171
Renato A. Valdés Olmos and Sergi Vidal-Sicart

9   **Preoperative and Intraoperative Lymphatic Mapping for Radioguided Sentinel Lymph Node Biopsy in Breast Cancer** 185
Lenka M. Pereira Arias-Bouda, Sergi Vidal-Sicart,
and Renato A. Valdés Olmos

10   **Preoperative and Intraoperative Lymphatic Mapping for Radioguided Sentinel Lymph Node Biopsy in Cutaneous Melanoma** 219
Sergi Vidal-Sicart, Andrés Perissinotti, Daphne D. D. Rietbergen,
and Renato A. Valdés Olmos

11 **Preoperative and Intraoperative Lymphatic Mapping for Radioguided
    Sentinel Node Biopsy in Head and Neck Cancers** 261
    Renato A. Valdés Olmos, W. Martin C. Klop, and Maarten L. Donswijk

12 **Preoperative and Intraoperative Lymphatic Mapping for Radioguided
    Sentinel Node Biopsy in Non-small Cell Lung Cancer** 291
    Giuseppe Boni, Franca M. A. Melfi, Giampiero Manca, Federico Davini,
    and Giuliano Mariani

13 **Preoperative and Intraoperative Lymphatic Mapping for Sentinel Node
    Biopsy in Cancers of the Gastrointestinal Tract** 299
    Carmen Balagué and Irene Gomez

14 **Preoperative and Intraoperative Lymphatic Mapping for Radioguided
    Sentinel Node Biopsy in Cancers of the Female Reproductive System** 315
    Angela Collarino, Annalisa Zurru, and Sergi Vidal-Sicart

15 **Preoperative and Intraoperative Lymphatic Mapping for Radioguided
    Sentinel Node Biopsy in Cancers of the Male Reproductive System** 331
    Hielke Martijn de Vries, Joost M. Blok, Hans N. Veerman,
    Florian van Beurden, Henk G. van der Poel, Renato A. Valdés Olmos,
    and Oscar R. Brouwer

16 **Preoperative and Intraoperative Lymphatic Mapping for Radioguided
    Sentinel Lymph Node Biopsy in Kidney and Bladder Cancers** 357
    Axel Bex, Teele Kuusk, Oscar R. Brouwer, and Renato A. Valdés Olmos

Index...373

Anatomy and Physiology of Lymphatic Circulation: Application to Lymphatic Mapping

Omgo E. Nieweg, Pieter J. Tanis, and Stanley P. L. Leong

Contents

1.1 **Introduction** 2

1.2 **Physiology of Lymph Flow** 2

1.3 **Anatomy of the Lymphatic System** 2

1.4 **Lymphatics of the Breast** 3

1.5 **Lymphatics of the Skin** 3

1.6 **Visualisation of Lymphatics and New Developments** ... 5

References 5

Learning Objectives
- To learn the importance of the lymphatic system in oncology
- To learn how cancer cells enter the lymphatic system
- To understand how lymph is propelled through its vascular system
- To learn how radiolabelled proteins and colloids that are used for lymphoscintigraphy are accumulated and retained in lymph nodes
- To become familiar with the anatomy of the lymphatic system of the breast
- To gain knowledge on the various locations of sentinel lymph nodes (SLNs) in breast cancer patients
- To become familiar with the anatomy of the lymphatic system of the skin
- To understand that there are inter-individual but also intra-individual variations in lymphatic drainage routes from the skin
- To appreciate that these intra-individual variations in lymph drainage may have an inadvertent clinical consequence
- To appreciate that continuing research in the anatomy and physiology is increasing our understanding of the lymphatic system and has clinical implications
- To understand the concept of SLNs based on the anatomy and physiology of the lymphatic system

O. E. Nieweg (✉)
Department of Surgery, Melanoma Institute of Australia, Sydney, NSW, Australia

Faculty of Medicine and Health, The University of Sydney, Sydney, NSW, Australia

Department of Melanoma and Surgical Oncology, Royal Prince Alfred Hospital, Sydney, NSW, Australia
e-mail: omgo.nieweg@melanoma.org.au

P. J. Tanis
Department of Surgery, Amsterdam University Medical Centers, University of Amsterdam, Amsterdam, Noord-Holland, The Netherlands

S. P. L. Leong
Department of Surgery, California Pacific Medical Center and Research Institute, San Francisco, CA, USA

© Springer Nature Switzerland AG 2020
G. Mariani et al. (eds.), *Atlas of Lymphoscintigraphy and Sentinel Node Mapping*, https://doi.org/10.1007/978-3-030-45296-4_1

1.1 Introduction

The lymphatic system is a complex network of ducts and lymph nodes diffused throughout the human body, and exhibits considerable variation comparable to other anatomical structures such as the arterial or venous system. Excess of interstitial fluid originating from the blood is returned to the blood circulation via the lymphatic system. In contrast to the blood circulation, lymph flow is unidirectional away from the local tissues. Lymph is similar to blood plasma and contains immune cells as part of the defence against microorganisms. Furthermore, lymphatic capillaries in the intestinal villi absorb the fats and fat-soluble vitamins that give the lymph its milky appearance in this part of the lymphatic system.

The lymphatic system has become an important field of interest in oncology in the last few centuries. The system functions actually in two opposite manners in cancer. It defends the body against circulating cancer cells, but it also provides a route for dissemination and a site of cancer growth if the defence mechanism fails. The significant impact of lymphatic dissemination on staging, treatment and outcome of solid cancers has stimulated investigations aimed at gaining more insight into several aspects of the lymphatic system.

The aim of this chapter is not to provide a complete overview of lymphatic anatomy and physiology, but rather to point out some relevant topics for clinicians involved in lymphatic mapping of cancer and to outline recent developments and subjects for further research.

> **Key Learning Point**
> - The lymphatic system defends the body against circulating cancer cells, but it also provides a route for dissemination and a site of cancer proliferation.

1.2 Physiology of Lymph Flow

Lymph flow starts with absorption of interstitial fluid through the inter-endothelial junctions of the lymphatic capillaries, which function as valves [1]. Small particles up to 25 nm may enter the openings at this level, whereas larger particles are transported through the endothelium by pinocytosis. Lymphatic capillaries are kept open by collagen filaments attached to the surrounding connective tissue. The osmotic pressure gradient is also important for filling of lymphatic capillaries. Since the capillaries have no valves, the lymph fluid at this level may flow either way.

The next lymphatic structures are the collecting lymphatic vessels. These vessels contain bicuspid semilunar valves 2–3 mm apart, preventing backflow of the fluid [2]. There is active propulsion of lymph by longitudinal and circular layers of smooth muscle, which contract 10–15 times per minute. Lymphatic peristalsis is regulated by several delicate mechanisms [3, 4]. Because of the presence of valves, intermittent external pressure is another mechanism for unidirectional flow.

From the lymphatic collecting vessels, lymph flows into the marginal sinus of lymph nodes. From this subcapsular sinus, the fluid drains into medullary sinuses between the germinal centres, where it is filtered through the action of numerous phagocytic cells. The filtered lymph is collected in the hilum of the node where it drains into the efferent lymphatic vessel. Lymph nodes are important elements of the immune system. In addition to lymphocytes, lymph nodes contain macrophages, which are responsible for the phagocytosis of the radiolabelled proteins and colloids that are used for lymphoscintigraphy. Different types of relationships between lymph vessels and lymph nodes exist in which the germinal centres may be bypassed [5, 6]. A few large lymphatic trunks eventually return the body's daily production of 2–4 L of lymph back into the venous circulation at the junction of the internal jugular and subclavian veins [7].

> **Key Learning Point**
> - Phagocytosis by macrophages is responsible for the uptake of radiolabelled proteins and colloid radiopharmaceuticals that are used for lymphoscintigraphy.

1.3 Anatomy of the Lymphatic System

The lymphatic system consists of a network of lymph vessels and some 600 lymph nodes. The lymphatic systems of different tissues and organs are similar, although there are some specific features. Lymphatic capillaries are abundant in the skin and in other covering structures such as the periosteum and joint capsule. Rich lymphatic plexuses are also found underlying the mesothelium of the pleura, peritoneum and pericardium, and underneath the mucosa of the digestive, respiratory and genito-urinary tracts. Most solid organs like the liver, spleen, adrenal, kidney, prostate, testis, uterus and ovary have a superficial or subserous lymphatic plexus [8]. In contrast, deep lymphatics within the parenchyma have only been clearly demonstrated in the adrenal gland, kidney and ovary. Lymphatic capillaries are probably absent in the central nervous system, striated muscles, eyeball and internal ear. The collecting lymphatic vessels are present in nearly all vascularised tissues and are often situated adjacent to blood vessels. The interested reader is referred to the classic textbooks for an extensive description of the lymphatic system in the human body [8, 9]. The lymphatic systems of the breast and the skin are being studied most extensively in the era of sentinel lymph node biopsy (SLNB), and these will be described in more detail.

1.4 Lymphatics of the Breast

Although the lymphatic system of the breast was studied as early as at the end of the eighteenth century, research is still ongoing [10]. Current research is mainly focussed on unravelling the network of communicating small lymphatic vessels from both the skin and the underlying parenchyma in the different regions of the mammary gland. These vessels join into several collecting ducts that are connected to specific lymph nodes within the regional nodal fields. This broad anatomical concept originates from the numerous lymphatic drainage patterns that have been observed during lymphatic mapping of breast cancer over the last 25 years. These clinical observations do not concur with the simpler concepts proposed in the past. The best known of these historic descriptions originates from Sappey. He postulated centripetal lymph flow from the mammary ducts to a common subareolar plexus [11]. From this lymphatic plexus, a medial and a lateral collecting vessel were assumed to pass to the axilla. This system was suggested to have multiple anastomoses with a superficial system of dermal lymphatics from the greater mammary region that also drains to the axilla. Sappey and others, like Rouvière, denied the existence of the so-called posterior lymphatic network of the breast [12]. However, this posterior network does exist and was originally described at the end of the eighteenth century [6]. It

mainly drains to the internal mammary nodal chain and to interpectoral (Rotter) lymph nodes. Collecting lymphatic vessels from the deep breast tissue drain to these lymph nodes and may be encountered during mastectomy with SLNB (Fig. 1.1).

Several other sites that may harbour lymph nodes draining to the breast have subsequently been described. During SLNB, one may encounter supraclavicular lymph nodes, intercostal nodes, contralateral internal mammary chain nodes, intramammary nodes and paramammary (Gerota) nodes at the level of the inframammary fold (Fig. 1.2). There may even be a SLN in the contralateral axilla in nonphysiological circumstances [13–17]. Furthermore, lymph nodes in the axilla were divided into external mammary lymph nodes, scapular lymph nodes, central lymph nodes, axillary vein lymph nodes and subclavicular lymph nodes [9, 18]. Drainage patterns from each region of the breast have been quantified using lymphoscintigraphic data [19, 20]. Although the pattern of lymph drainage varies from person to person, it appears stable over time within an individual [21].

The anatomical relation between the lymphatic drainage of the breast and of the arm at the level of the axilla is of increasing interest in recent years [22]. A clinical application of combined lymphatic mapping of the arm and breast is axillary reverse lymphatic mapping [23]. The objective of this approach is to identify and subsequently spare lymphatic ducts and nodes essential for lymph drainage of the upper extremity during breast SLNB, in order to prevent lymphoedema. Initial results have shown that specific regions of the breast and arm may have a common SLN.

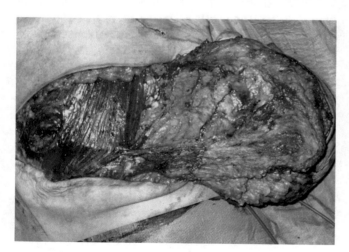

Fig. 1.1 A blue-stained lymphatic running from a tumour in the upper outer quadrant of the left breast along the posterior surface of the breast, through the pectoral muscle to the third intercostal space. This lymphatic was seen during mastectomy after removal of two axillary SLNs and of three internal mammary chain lymph nodes

> **Key Learning Points**
> - The communication between the lymphatic vessels of the skin and the underlying breast parenchyma is still the subject of research.
> - This posterior part of the breast mainly drains to the internal mammary chain and to interpectoral (Rotter) lymph nodes.
> - SLNs can be found at various locations in and around the breast.

1.5 Lymphatics of the Skin

The skin has a rich lymphatic network that mainly drains to lymph node fields in the groin, axilla and neck, but also to several less known lymph node locations. The SLN concept has contributed substantially to the present knowledge of lymphatic drainage of the skin. Clinical application of lym-

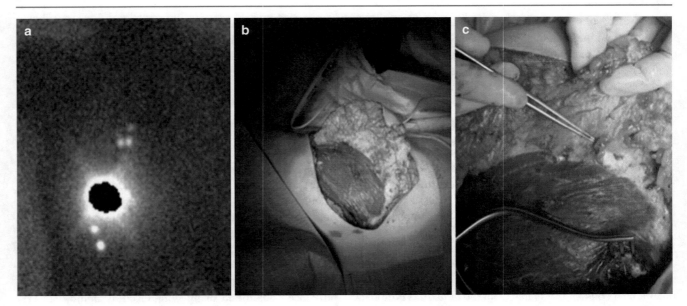

Fig. 1.2 (**a**) Lymphoscintigraphy using ^{99m}Tc-nanocolloid with direct drainage to paramammary lymph nodes at the level of the inframammary fold. (**b**) Overview and (**c**) detail: intraoperative identification of a paramammary lymph node with a tiny blue afferent lymphatic duct during mastectomy indicated by the tweezers; an internal mammary chain SLN was also retrieved

phatic mapping using blue dye started in the late 1980s in patients with melanoma, and this cancer is now one of the most frequent indications for the procedure—along with breast cancer. For many years, the prediction of lymphatic drainage from the truncal skin was based on Sappey's lines (midline and transverse at the level of the umbilicus) [11]. Recently, analysis of more than 5000 lymphoscintigrams at Melanoma Institute Australia has shown that drainage often crosses these lines, which results in a much greater zone of ambiguity than postulated by Sappey [24]. Several less common and unexpected lymphatic drainage routes have been described to lymph nodes in the epitrochlear fossa, popliteal fossa, triangular intermuscular space on the back and bicipital sulcus and subcutaneously in the flank or adjacent to the areola [25]. Studying lymphatic drainage in a canine torso, Suami and colleagues found perforating lymph vessels originating from the skin, penetrating the abdominal wall and directly draining into para-aortic lymph nodes [26]. This is now also seen in humans. Still, melanoma surgeons encounter SLNs in even stranger and more unexpected locations.

Similar to the axilla, the groin has also been subdivided into different zones [27]. The groin lymph nodes receive lymph from the lower extremity, the trunk and the external genitals. Lymphatic drainage patterns to the groin with corresponding first- and second-tier lymph nodes differ depending on the specific area of the skin [28, 29]. Collecting lymphatic vessels from the limb may also bypass the groin and directly drain into para-iliac or obturator lymph nodes in the pelvis. Miura and colleagues defined the great and small saphenous lymphatic vessels and a third deep lymphatic vessel ascending along the main three arteries of the lower leg with direct drainage to the external iliac lymph nodes [30].

Drainage from the upper part of the trunk and upper limb is rather complex, given the potential connections to lymphatic fields in the axilla, but also in the neck [31]. The neck has traditionally been subdivided into different lymph node levels to enable selective neck dissection for cancers from different skin areas. This relatively rough anatomical classification has been refined in the SLN era. Lymphatic mapping has revealed an almost inexhaustible variation in lymph drainage from the skin of the head and neck. Lymphatic drainage patterns may be even discordant over time in the head and neck, as demonstrated by serial repeat lymphoscintigraphy [32, 33]. These observations are probably related to physiological changes, technical shortcomings or close anatomical relationships in the head and neck region.

So, lymph flow from the skin varies from one person to another, but it is also variable within an individual. Various factors determine the lymph flow speed such as time of the day, physical activity, medication and hydration status of the patient. There is also intra-individual variation of the pattern of lymph flow. The same skin site may drain to different lymph nodes at various points in time [32]. This phenomenon may be responsible for false-negative SLN procedures.

Key Learning Point
- SLNs can be found in locations outside the major nodal fields.

1.6 Visualisation of Lymphatics and New Developments

The techniques that are used to visualise the lymphatic system, as well as the physiological conditions in which the studies are performed, have significant impact on the information that is gained. Anatomists often use cadavers, while surgeons and nuclear medicine physicians examine the lymphatic system under physiological conditions in living human beings. Differences in physiologic conditions or age may have contributed to conflicting anatomical theories. For example, studying the lymphatic anatomy of the mammary gland in pregnant women or in foetuses may yield results that differ from those found in elderly women [34, 35].

Nevertheless, the most important determinants for unravelling the lymph system anatomy are the type of tracer and the injection site. Anatomists used materials like air, oil, milk, Indian ink or mercury with subsequent macroscopic visualisation of the larger lymphatic vessels. This approach has several methodological limitations related to dilution of the tracer, accuracy of tissue dissection and size restrictions of what can be macroscopically identified.

Lymphangiographic studies using direct tracer administration into lymph vessels are intrinsically different from techniques based on injection into the interstitium of tissues of interest, with subsequent tracer uptake into the lymphatic capillaries. The latter approaches are considered to reflect more closely the actual clinical conditions, as they visualise the normal physiological mechanisms of lymph formation at the site of interest.

The introduction of radiopharmaceuticals for lymphatic mapping was an important step forward in the collection of knowledge of the anatomy of the lymphatic system, obviating the need for macroscopic visualisation. By using colloidal Gold-198 particles of about 5 nm in size, pioneers like Turner-Warwick, Hultborn and Vendrell-Torné were able to identify dominant and minor lymphatic drainage routes from different regions of the breast [36–38]. Suami et al. recently published anatomical cadaver studies based on techniques combining both approaches [39]. Very small lymph vessels were microscopically cannulated and injected with a radio-opaque contrast medium in both antegrade and retrograde directions. After the injections, radiographs were made of the whole specimen and parallel slices, followed by computerised image processing. Even three-dimensional images of the arrangement of lymphatic ducts could be obtained by using high-resolution computed tomographic lymphangiography [40].

In addition to vital dyes and radiocolloids, fluorescent tracers in the near-infrared spectrum are increasingly being used for lymphatic mapping. ^{99m}Tc-tilmanocept is a new radiopharmaceutical that was approved for clinical use in 2013. A strong advantage in its use is rapid clearance from the injection site [41]. It binds to mannose receptors to become internalised into macrophages. Parungo and colleagues used quantum dots and HAS 800 to study lymphatic drainage from the peritoneal cavity in rats [42]. These authors were able to identify primary drainage to the celiac, superior mesenteric and periportal lymph nodes, with rerouting directly to intrathoracic nodes via chest wall lymphatics after bowel resection. Using the same technique, they also demonstrated that the highest mediastinal lymph nodes of station I are the first-echelon nodes of the pleural space in rats and pigs [43]. By using two different quantum dots, two separate lymphatic drainage pathways could be simultaneously visualised in a two-colour image, as demonstrated by a Japanese group [44]. Such a technique enables further exploration of overlapping lymphatic drainage patterns. Indocyanine green fluorescence lymphography is increasingly being used in routine clinical practice of SLNB, but is also a promising method to increase our knowledge of physiology of the lymphatic system [45]. These new developments illustrate the continuing interest in the anatomy and physiology of the lymphatic system and the clinically relevant progress.

References

1. Schmid-Schonbein GW. Microlymphatics and lymph flow. Physiol Rev. 1990;70:987–1028.
2. Foster RS Jr. General anatomy of the lymphatic system. Surg Oncol Clin N Am. 1993;5:1–13.
3. Aukland K, Reed RK. Interstitial-lymphatic mechanisms in the control of extracellular fluid volume. Physiol Rev. 1993;73:1–78.
4. Olszewski WL, Engeset A. Lymphatic contractions. N Engl J Med. 1979;300:316.
5. Ludwig J. Ueber Kurschlusswege der Lymphbahnen und ihre Beziehungen zur lymphogen Krebsmetastasierung. Pathol Microbiol. 1962;25:329–34.
6. Tanis PJ, Nieweg OE, Valdés Olmos RA, et al. Anatomy and physiology of lymphatic drainage of the breast from the perspective of sentinel node biopsy. J Am Coll Surg. 2001;192:399–409.
7. Browse NL, Stewart G. Lymphoedema: pathophysiology and classification. J Cardiovasc Surg. 1985;26:91–106.
8. Gray H. The lymphatic system. In: Gray H, editor. Anatomy of the human body. Philadelphia: Lea and Febiger; 1918. p. 2000. www.bartleby.com/107/.
9. Haagensen CD. Lymphatics of the breast. In: Haagensen CD, Feind KR, Herter FP, Slanetz CA, Weinberg JA, editors. The lymphatics in cancer. Philadelphia: WB Saunders Company; 1972. p. 300–87.
10. Blumgart EI, Uren RF, Nielsen PM, et al. Lymphatic drainage and tumour prevalence in the breast: a statistical analysis of symmetry, gender and node field independence. J Anat. 2011;218:652–9.
11. Sappey PHC. Anatomie, physiologie, pathologie des vaisseaux lymphatiques considérés chez l'homme et les vertébrés. Paris; A Delahaye et E Lacrosnier; 1874.
12. Tanis PJ, van Rijk MC, Nieweg OE. The posterior lymphatic network of the breast rediscovered. J Surg Oncol. 2005;91:195–8.
13. Barranger E, Montravers F, Kerrou K, et al. Contralateral axillary sentinel lymph node drainage in breast cancer: a case report. J Surg Oncol. 2004;86:167–9.

14. Caplan I. Revision anatomique du système lymphatique de la glande mammaire (a propos de 200 cas). Bull Assoc Anat. 1975;59:121–37.

15. Perre CI, Hoefnagel CA, Kroon BBR, et al. Altered lymphatic drainage after lymphadenectomy or radiotherapy of the axilla in patients with breast cancer. Br J Surg. 1996;83:1258.

16. Tanis PJ, Nieweg OE, Valdés Olmos RA, et al. Impact of non-axillary sentinel node biopsy on staging and treatment of breast cancer patients. Br J Cancer. 2002;87:705–10.

17. Van der Ploeg IM, Oldenburg HS, Rutgers EJT, et al. Lymphatic drainage patterns from the treated breast. Ann Surg Oncol. 2010;17:1069–75.

18. Spratt JS. Anatomy of the breast. Major Probl Clin Surg. 1979;5:1–13.

19. Blumgart EI, Uren RF, Nielsen PM, et al. Predicting lymphatic drainage patterns and primary tumour location in patients with breast cancer. Breast Cancer Res Treat. 2011;130:699–705.

20. Estourgie SH, Nieweg OE, Valdés Olmos RA, et al. Lymphatic drainage patterns from the breast. Ann Surg. 2004;239:232–7.

21. Tanis PJ, Valdés Olmos RA, Muller SH, et al. Lymphatic mapping in patients with breast carcinoma: reproducibility of lymphoscintigraphic results. Radiology. 2003;228:546–51.

22. Pavlista D, Eliska O. Relationship between the lymphatic drainage of the breast and the upper extremity: a postmortem study. Ann Surg Oncol. 2012;19:3410–5.

23. Noguchi M. Axillary reverse mapping for breast cancer. Breast Cancer Res Treat. 2010;119:529–35.

24. Reynolds HM, Dunbar PR, Uren RF, et al. Three-dimensional visualisation of lymphatic drainage patterns in patients with cutaneous melanoma. Lancet Oncol. 2007;8:806–12.

25. Roozendaal GK, de Vries JD, van Poll D, et al. Sentinel nodes outside lymph node basins in patients with melanoma. Br J Surg. 2001;88:305–8.

26. Suami H, O'Neill JK, Pan WR, et al. Perforating lymph vessels in the canine torso: direct lymph pathway from skin to the deep lymphatics. Plast Reconstr Surg. 2008;121:31–6.

27. Daseler EH, Anson BJ, Reimann AF. Radical excision of the inguinal and iliac lymph glands; a study based upon 450 anatomical dissections and upon supportive clinical observations. Surg Gynecol Obstet. 1948;87:679–94.

28. Leijte JA, Valdés Olmos RA, Nieweg OE, et al. Anatomical mapping of lymphatic drainage in penile carcinoma with SPECT-CT: implications for the extent of inguinal lymph node dissection. Eur Urol. 2008;54:885–90.

29. Van der Ploeg IM, Kroon BBR, Valdés Olmos RA, et al. Evaluation of lymphatic drainage patterns to the groin and implications for the extent of groin dissection in melanoma patients. Ann Surg Oncol. 2009;16:2994–9.

30. Miura H, Ono S, Nagahata M, et al. Lymphoscintigraphy for sentinel lymph node mapping in Japanese patients with malignant skin neoplasms of the lower extremities: comparison with previously investigated Japanese lymphatic anatomy. Ann Nucl Med. 2010;24:601–8.

31. Veenstra HJ, Klop WM, Speijers MJ, et al. Lymphatic drainage patterns from melanomas on the shoulder or upper trunk to cervical lymph nodes and implications for the extent of neck dissection. Ann Surg Oncol. 2012;19:3906–12.

32. Kapteijn BA, Nieweg OE, Valdés Olmos RA, et al. Reproducibility of lymphoscintigraphy for lymphatic mapping in cutaneous melanoma. J Nucl Med. 1996;37:972–5.

33. Willis AI, Ridge JA. Discordant lymphatic drainage patterns revealed by serial lymphoscintigraphy in cutaneous head and neck malignancies. Head Neck. 2007;29:979–85.

34. Pan WR, Suami H, Taylor GI. Senile changes in human lymph nodes. Lymphat Res Biol. 2008;6:77–83.

35. Suami H, Pan WR, Taylor GI. Historical review of breast lymphatic studies. Clin Anat. 2009;22:531–56.

36. Hultborn A, Hulten L, Roos B, et al. Topography of lymph drainage from mammary gland and hand to axillary lymph nodes. Acta Radiol Ther Phys Biol. 1971;10:65–72.

37. Turner-Warwick RT. The lymphatics of the breast. Br J Surg. 1959;46:574–82.

38. Vendrell-Torne E, Setoain-Quinquer J, Domenech-Torne FM. Study of normal mammary lymphatic drainage using radioactive isotopes. J Nucl Med. 1972;13:801–5.

39. Suami H, Pan WR, Mann GB, et al. The lymphatic anatomy of the breast and its implications for sentinel lymph node biopsy: a human cadaver study. Ann Surg Oncol. 2008;15:863–71.

40. Pan WR, Rozen WM, Stella DL, et al. A three-dimensional analysis of the lymphatics of a bilateral breast specimen: a human cadaveric study. Clin Breast Cancer. 2009;9:86–91.

41. Wallace AM, Hoh CK, Ellner SJ, et al. Lymphoseek: a molecular imaging agent for melanoma sentinel lymph node mapping. Ann Surg Oncol. 2007;14:913–21.

42. Parungo CP, Soybel DI, Colson YL, et al. Lymphatic drainage of the peritoneal space: a pattern dependent on bowel lymphatics. Ann Surg Oncol. 2007;14:286–98.

43. Parungo CP, Colson YL, Kim SW, et al. Sentinel lymph node mapping of the pleural space. Chest. 2005;127:1799–804.

44. Hama Y, Koyama Y, Urano Y, et al. Simultaneous two-color spectral fluorescence lymphangiography with near infrared quantum dots to map two lymphatic flows from the breast and the upper extremity. Breast Cancer Res Treat. 2007;103:23–8.

45. Unno N, Nishiyama M, Suzuki M, et al. A novel method of measuring human lymphatic pumping using indocyanine green fluorescence lymphography. J Vasc Surg. 2010;52:946–52.

Pathophysiology of Lymphatic Circulation in Different Disease Conditions

Rossella Di Stefano, Giulia Dibello, Francesca Felice, and Paola A. Erba

Contents

2.1   **History** 7

2.2   **Physiology of the Lymphatic System** 8

2.3   **Lymphatic Circulation and Lipid Absorption** 9

2.4   **Pathophysiology of Lymph Drainage Failure** 10

2.5   **Lymphedema** 12

2.6   **Lymphatic Malignancies** 16

2.7   **Lymphangiothrombosis and Acute Lymphangitis** 16

2.8   **Pathophysiology of Lymphatic Circulation in Systemic Diseases** 16

2.9   **Concluding Remarks** 19

References 20

Learning Objectives
- To become familiar with the physiology and pathophysiology of lymphatic circulation
- To comprehend the causes and pathophysiology of lymphedema
- To learn about the newly discovered roles of lymphatic circulation in systemic diseases

R. Di Stefano (✉)
Cardiovascular Research Laboratory, Department of Surgical, Medical, Molecular and Critical Area, University of Pisa, Pisa, Italy

Section of Sport Medicine, Department of Clinical and Experimental Medicine, University of Pisa, Pisa, Italy
e-mail: rossella.distefano@unipi.it

G. Dibello · F. Felice
Cardiovascular Research Laboratory, Department of Surgical, Medical, Molecular and Critical Area, University of Pisa, Pisa, Italy

P. A. Erba
Regional Center of Nuclear Medicine, Department of Translational Research and Advanced Technologies in Medicine and Surgery, University of Pisa, Pisa, Italy

2.1 History

The first description of lymphatic vessels began in ancient Greece with Hippocrates (460–370 BC) and Aristotle (384–322 BC) who described vessels of the human body that may have been lymphatic vessels. More stringent reference to the lymphatic vessels came from Alexandria, where Erasistratus (ca. 304–250 BC) described milky arteries in the mesentery. Later, in the seventeenth century AD, Gaspare Aselli was the first physician/anatomist to document the functional lipid uptake and transport of lipid-rich meals in the white mesentery veins of dogs. The studies that followed Aselli's initial observations established that these vessels constituted a distinct vascular network that was separated but connected to the blood vascular system. The first gross anatomy of lymphatic vessels was definitely established at the beginning of the nineteenth century [1]. It was only at the end of the 1990s that investigators started to identify the receptor of vascular endothelial growth factor (VEGFR)-3 [2], the prosperous homeobox 1 (PROX1), the transcription factor [3], the membranes integral podoplanin glycoprotein (PDPN) [4], and hyaluronic receptor 1 of the lymphatic vessel (LYVE1) as specific lymphatic markers [5]. Subsequently, investigations

© Springer Nature Switzerland AG 2020
G. Mariani et al. (eds.), *Atlas of Lymphoscintigraphy and Sentinel Node Mapping*,
https://doi.org/10.1007/978-3-030-45296-4_2

in this field flourished through molecular genetic studies on embryo development, revealing more than 50 genes involved in the specific maturation of lymphatic vessels [6]. The lymphatic system was thus identified as an almost ubiquitous regulator of numerous physiological and pathological processes. Lymphatic vessels have been identified in organs which previously were thought not to exist, such as the eye, where they are involved in the regulation of intraocular pressure [7], or in the central nervous system, where they drain cerebral macromolecules and immune cells [8]. Moreover, pioneering studies have revealed lymph node lymphatic endothelial cells as antigen-presenting cells involved in the induction of peripheral immune tolerance [9]. These seminal findings have opened unexpected avenues for advancing knowledge on the lymphatic system in cardiovascular medicine [10].

Key Learning Points
- Recognition of the existence of lymphatic circulation has evolved slowly over the course of history, mainly because of the difficulties in visualizing the transparent vessels.
- We know now that lymphatic vessels are almost ubiquitous within different organs and show a remarkable heterogeneity, with different genes involved in development, reflecting their functional specialization.
- Unexpected advances in knowledge on the lymphatic system have recently emerged in cardiovascular medicine.

2.2   Physiology of the Lymphatic System

The lymphatic circulation should be considered as part of the peripheral cardiovascular system, as it interlinks closely with blood circulation both at its origins (the interstitial space) and at its final drainage point (the thoracic duct). To a large extent, the anatomy of lymphatic channels parallels that of the veins, and the two systems show many similarities in structure and function.

The lymphatic circulation includes the lymph, lymphatic vessels, lymph nodes (stations along the drainage route where fluid and cell exchange between blood and lymph occurs), and other lymphoid tissues, particularly the spleen and bone marrow. Through its own specialized cell, the lymphocyte, a close relationship exists between the peripheral lymphatic system, blood circulation, spleen, and liver (Fig. 2.1). Therefore, while lymph drainage has a predominant "plumbing" role, the lymphatic circulation does possess also important immunological roles.

The lymphatic vascular network consists of smaller blind-ended capillaries and larger collecting lymphatic vessels. The lymphatic capillaries are composed of a single layer of overlapping endothelial cells "oak leaf shaped" and lack a continuous basement membrane and pericytes. The distinctive oak leaf-shaped endothelial cells of initial lymphatics are loosely apposed with overlapping borders and linked each other by discontinuous, button-like junctions. Regions between buttons are open, so as to allow the entry of fluid and cells without repetitive formation and dissolution of intercellular junctions. These specific structures may function as primary lymphatic valves that prevent the tissue fluid taken up by lymphatic capillaries to be released back into the interstitial space (Fig. 2.2). Therefore, the lymphatic capillaries are highly permeable to interstitial fluid and macromolecules, such that, when the surrounding interstitial pressure changes, the lymphatics either expand and fill with lymph or contract and push lymph [12].

The capillaries drain into pre-collecting lymphatic vessels, which will merge into larger secondary collecting lymphatic vessels covered by smooth muscle cells, which provide contractile activity to assist lymph flow and possess a continuous basement membrane. Tissue fluid collected in the larger collecting lymphatics drains into the thoracic duct and is then returned to the blood circulation through lymphatic-venous connections at the junction of the jugular and subclavian veins.

At the distal capillaries, the systemic blood circulation loses about 2–4 L of fluid and about 100 g of protein into the interstitium per day. Normal physiology of lymphatics deals with draining from the tissue spaces these materials that cannot return to the bloodstream directly. Colloids, several types of cells (extravasated red cells, macrophages, lymphocytes, tumor cells, etc.), bacteria, and other microorganisms are channeled through the lymphatics, presumably as a protective mechanism to prevent noxious agents from directly entering the bloodstream. This is the reason why cellulitis and erysipelas can be a recurrent problem. Similarly, inorganic matters such as carbon and silica are removed by the lymphatics, as demonstrated by the black-stained pulmonary lymph nodes in coal miners.

Key Learning Points
- The lymphatic circulation should be considered as part of the peripheral cardiovascular system, as it interlinks closely with blood circulation.
- It consists of smaller blind-ended capillaries and larger collecting lymphatic vessels. The lymphatic capillaries are composed of a single layer of endothelial cells and lack a continuous basement membrane and pericytes, making them highly permeable to interstitial fluid and macromolecules.

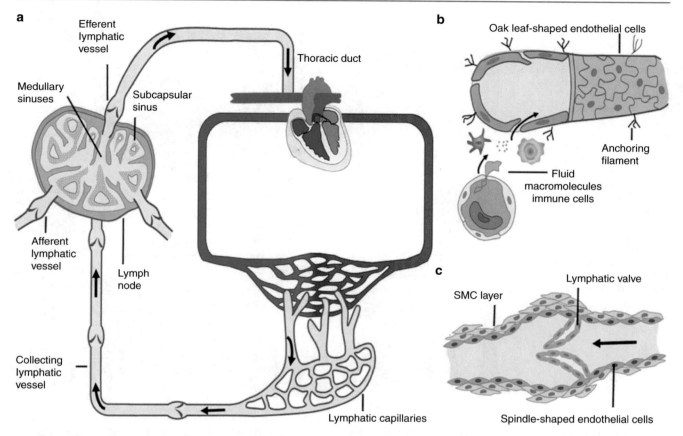

Fig. 2.1 Schematic representation of the vascular circulation (arterial system, *red*; venous system, *blue*) and of lymphatic circulation (*green*), and their interrelationship. (**a**) Net of lymphatic capillaries drains tissue fluid and macromolecules from tissues through major lymphatic vessels and lymph nodes. The lymph is driven into the venous system through the left subclavian and the right subclavian veins, respectively. (**b**) Interstitial fluid, macromolecules, and immune cells are collected by lymphatic capillaries. (**c**) Lymphatic collectors contain intraluminal valve and SMC layers that permit the unidirectional lymph flow (*reproduced with permission from* [11])

- Tissue fluid collected in the larger collecting lymphatics drains into the thoracic duct and is then returned to the blood circulation through lymphatic–vasculature connections at the junction of the jugular and subclavian veins.
- Normal physiology of lymphatic circulation involves a daily drainage of about 2–4 L of fluid and about 100 g of protein from the tissue spaces directly to the bloodstream.

2.3 Lymphatic Circulation and Lipid Absorption

Lymphatic circulation is essential for the adsorption of lipids from the intestine. The major products of lipid digestion (fatty acids and 2-monoglycerides) enter the enterocyte either by simple diffusion or via a specific fatty acid transporter protein in the membrane. Once inside the enterocyte, fatty acids and monoglycerides are transported into the endo-plasmic reticulum, where they are used to synthesize triglycerides. Beginning in the endoplasmic reticulum and continuing in the Golgi apparatus, triglycerides are packaged with cholesterol, lipoproteins, and other lipids into particles called chylomicrons. Transport of lipids into the circulation is different from what occurs with sugars and amino acids. In fact, instead of being adsorbed directly into capillary blood, chylomicrons are transported first into the lymphatic vessels that penetrate each intestinal villus.

Chylomicron-rich lymph then drains into the lymphatic system, which rapidly flows into blood. Blood-borne chylomicrons are rapidly disassembled and their constituent lipids utilized throughout the body. When large amounts of chylomicrons are being absorbed, lymph draining from the small intestine has a milky appearance, such that the mesenteric lymphatics are easy to see (first described as "venae alba et lacteae" or "white veins" by Aselli in the seventeenth century). Recent studies have shown that the lacteal is not simply acting as a passive duct; on the contrary, it is able to respond to autonomic nerve stimulation to the encircling smooth muscle cells and actively transport the absorbed lipid [13].

Fig. 2.2 Schematic representation of the lymphatic system. The lymphatic capillaries are composed of a single layer of overlapping endothelial cells and lack a continuous basement membrane. Collecting lymphatic vessels are provided with smooth muscle cells, a basement membrane, and luminal valves that prevent lymph backflow. The unique structure of capillary lymphatic vessels accounts for the uptake of interstitial fluid, macromolecules, cells, and lipids that filtrate continuously from the blood capillary network (*reproduced with permission from* [11])

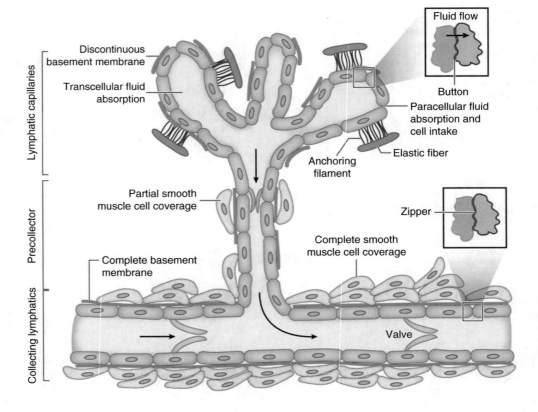

Compounds absorbed by the intestinal lymphatics drain via the cisterna chyli and the thoracic duct, thus entering systemic circulation at the junction of the left internal jugular vein with the left subclavian vein, thereby avoiding potential first-pass metabolism. Consequently, drug transport via the intestinal lymphatics may confer delivery advantages in terms of increased bioavailability and possibility of directing delivery to the lymphatic system.

Key Learning Points

- Lymphatic circulation is essential for the adsorption of lipids from the intestine.
- Instead of being adsorbed directly into capillary blood, the major products of lipid digestion, chylomicrons, are transported first into the lymphatic vessels that penetrate each intestinal villus.
- When large amounts of chylomicrons are being absorbed, lymph draining from the small intestine has a milky appearance.
- Compounds absorbed by the intestinal lymphatics drain via the cisterna chyli and the thoracic duct, into the systemic circulation at the junction of the left internal jugular vein with the left subclavian vein, thereby avoiding potential first-pass metabolism.
- Consequently, drug transport via the intestinal lymphatics may confer delivery advantages in terms of increased bioavailability and direct delivery.

2.4 Pathophysiology of Lymph Drainage Failure

Physiology of lymphatic circulation requires three intimately interconnected steps: (1) transport of prelymph across the interstitial space and into the initial lymphatics, (2) movement of lymph through the network of noncontractile initial lymphatics, and (3) active pumping of lymph through a series of contractile collecting trunks.

Under normal circumstances, water acts predominantly as a solvent or vehicle for the colloids, cells, and materials that can be drained only via the lymph route. Nevertheless, lymphatics also serve as an "overflow pipe" to drain excess interstitial fluid. This role of lymphatic circulation as "safety valve" against fluid overload involves the lymphatic system in every form of edema, although at variable degrees.

Edema is an excess of interstitial fluid, whose volume must increase by over 100% before edema becomes clinically detectable. Edema develops when the capillary filtration rate exceeds the lymphatic drainage rate for a sufficient period, a condition that results from an imbalance between capillary filtration and lymph drainage:

$$D_v / D_t = F_v - F_l$$

where D_v/D_t is the rate of swelling, F_v is the net capillary filtration rate, and F_l is the lymph flow.

Therefore, the pathogenesis of any edema involves either a high filtration rate or a low lymph flow, or a combination of the two factors. Elevation of capillary pressure is usually secondary to chronic elevation of venous pressure caused by heart failure, fluid overload, or deep vein thrombosis. On the other hand, reduced plasma colloid osmotic pressure (e.g., hypoproteinemia) raises the net filtration rate and lymph flow; changes in capillary permeability (e.g., inflammation) increase the escape of protein into the interstitium, and water follows osmotically. Impairment of lymph drainage results in the predominant accumulation of protein and water in the interstitial space, since lymph is the sole route for returning escaped protein to the plasma.

Most edemas arise from increased capillary filtration overwhelming lymph drainage; therefore, any edema incriminates the lymphatic system through its failure to keep up with demand. Edema is initially soft and pitting, and then hard, non-pitting, accompanied by skin thickening. Impairment of local immune response leads to recurrent skin infections, further insult to the tissue, and worsening of lymphedema.

2.4.1 Role of Leukotrienes and Inflammation in Lymphedema

Leukotrienes are a group of short-lived lipidic mediators produced primarily by pro-inflammatory immune cells, like macrophages, neutrophils, eosinophils, mast cells, and dendritic cells. In response to diverse immune and inflammatory stimuli, these lipid mediators elicit potent inflammatory responses through binding to, and activation of, their cognate G protein-coupled receptors.

Recent investigations have demonstrated the mechanistic role of the leukotriene B4 (LTB4) in the molecular pathogenesis of lymphedema. LTB4 is a strong chemoattractant and activator of leukocytes and one of the most potent lipid chemotactic factors for neutrophils. The biological function of LTB4 is mediated primarily by BLT1 or BLT2 receptors. When acting through the BLT1 receptor, LTB4 regulates migration and activity of cells of both innate and adaptive immunity and plays essential roles not only in physiological defense against infection, but also in the pathogenesis of a number of chronic diseases, such as obesity, insulin resistance, type 2 diabetes, and atherosclerosis.

It has consistently been observed that LTB_4 promotes lymphedema development, thereby involving tissue inflammation as the mechanistic platform for the development of acquired lymphedema. When the mechanisms that explain the impact of LTB_4 in acquired lymphatic vascular insufficiency have been explored, lower concentrations of LTB_4 were surprisingly demonstrated to have a prolymphangiogenic effect, thus suggesting a possible role for this eico-

sanoid in lymphatic repair at more physiological levels [14]. Higher concentrations of LTB_4 inhibit both VEGFR3 mRNA expression and VEGFR3 protein phosphorylation. Additionally, higher LTB_4 concentrations inhibit Notch signaling, a pathway known to be important for both lymphatic development and maintenance [11].

Such new knowledge constitutes the pathophysiologic basis for pilot studies that have demonstrated the benefit of anti-inflammatory therapy with ketoprofen in patients with lymphedema, favoring the restoration of a failing lymphatic circulation [15].

2.4.2 Aging of Lymphatic Vessels

Lymphatic-related diseases, such as lymphedema, are prevalent in the elderly. The aging process induces changes in structure and function of the lymphatic system. In the 1960s, the specific "varicose bulges" in muscular lymphatic vessels were observed to increase with age [16]. Muscle cell atrophy, elastic element destruction, and aneurysm-like formations were also found in aged lymphatic vessels. Aging-associated alterations in lymphatic contractility decrease pump efficiency, a mechanism that results in excessive retention of tissue fluid within the interstitial spaces. Reduced responsiveness to inflammatory stimuli in aged lymphatic vessels decreases the normal capacity to react against foreign organisms. High permeability is caused by the loss of glycocalyx and the dysfunction of junctional proteins. In addition, increased caspase-3 activity, dissociation of the VE-cadherin/catenin complex, and low expression of actin cytoskeleton that occur in aged blood vessels are present also in aged lymphatic vessels [17] (Fig. 2.3).

Knowledge of the aging-related diseases of lymphatic vessels is critical to our understanding of lymphatic vessel-related diseases.

Key Learning Points

- Impairment of lymph drainage results in accumulation of protein and water in the interstitial space, which corresponds clinically to lymphedema.
- Lymphedema becomes clinically detectable when excess of interstitial fluid increases by over 100%.
- It has recently been recognized that leukotrienes, lipidic mediators with potent pro-inflammatory properties, are involved in the pathogenesis of lymphedema.
- Aging decreases the efficiency of lymphatic contractility pump, thus contributing to abnormal retention of tissue fluid within the interstitial spaces.

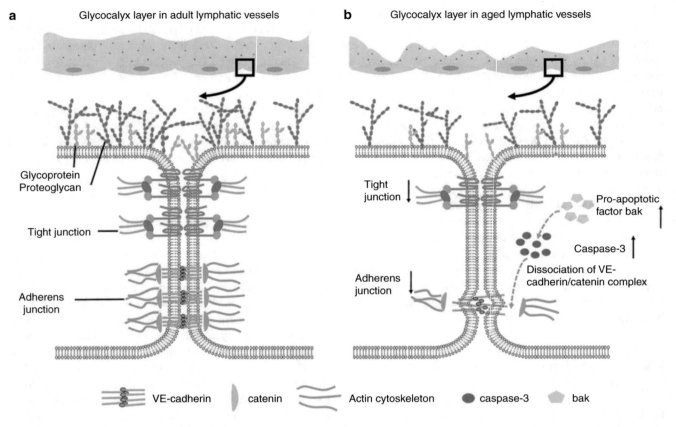

Fig. 2.3 Glycocalyx layer and intercellular junctions of lymphatic vessels in aging process. (**a**) Continuous glycocalyx in adult lymphatic vessels. (**b**) Discontinuous glycocalyx in aged lymphatic vessel. Increased pro-apoptotic factor back activates caspase-3 to disrupt the downstream protein β-catenin, which leads to decreased adherent junctions and impaired barrier function (*reproduced with permission from* [17])

2.5 Lymphedema

Lymphedema is an edema arising from a failure of lymph drainage, which can be induced by several causes (see Table 2.1). First, there may be an intrinsic abnormality of the lymph-conducting pathways. Such conditions are referred to as **primary lymphedema**, which means that no other identifiable causes can be found. Primary lymphedema occurs because of the imperfect development of the lymphatic vascular system in utero. It can be familial (as with Milroy's disease and Meige's syndrome), or genetic, such as those associated with Turner and Noonan syndromes or the congenital vascular Klippel-Trenaunay syndrome, where malformed lymphatics coexist with an aberrant venous system. Sporadic cases of primary lymphedema are more frequent than the familial or genetic associated forms.

The identification of mutant genes in primary hereditary human lymphedemas has defined some crucial pathways during lymphovascular development and lymphangiogenesis. In particular, lymphangiogenesis requires adequate expression of the C isoform of the vascular endothelial growth factor (VEGF) which binds to its receptors (VEGFR-2

Table 2.1 Mechanisms and causes of lymph drainage failure

Mechanism	Causes
Reduced lymph-conducting pathways	Aplasia-hypoplasia of the whole vessel
	Acquired obliteration of lymphatic lumen
Poorly functioning pathways	Failure of pump contractility
Obstructed pathways	Scar from lymphadenectomy, radiation therapy, or infection
Incompetent lymphatics with reflux	Megalymphatics
	Lymphatic hyperplasia

and VEGFR-3) under the control of the master regulator of lymphangiogenesis, the transcriptional factor Prox 1 [3]. VEGFR-3 is highly expressed on lymphatic endothelial cells. During the embryonic stage, VEGFR-3 acts as a receptor for both VEGF-C and VEGF-D, and its activation stimulates lymphatic vessel formation, thus representing the main molecular mechanism involved in the development and growth of the lymphatic system (Fig. 2.4).

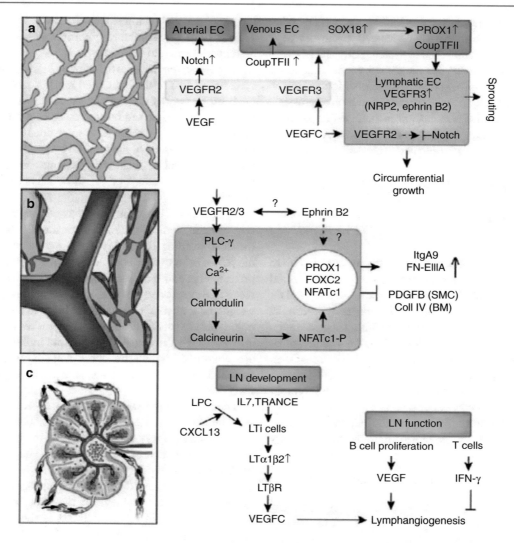

Fig. 2.4 Main molecular mechanisms involved in the development and growth of the lymphatic system. (**a**) Lymphatic capillaries derive from venous endothelial cells. After arteriovenous differentiation controlled by Notch and COUP-*TFII* transcription factors, Sox18 activates Prox1, which interacts with COUP-TFII and induces lymphatic endothelial differentiation, involving enhanced expression of VEGFR-3. VEGF-C then induces the sprouting of the LECs to generate new vessels. VEGF-C and VEGF can also increase the size of lymphatic vessels by stimulating circumferential growth. (**b**) Formation of lymphatic valves requires a calcium-induced signal via phospholipase C-g and calmodulin to calcineurin that dephosphorylates the NFATc1 transcription factor, which enters the nucleus and induces valve-specific genes in a complex with FoxC2 (T. Petrova, University of Lausanne, personal communication cited in [18]). VEGFR-2, VEGFR-3, and ephrin B2 are upstream regulators of the pathways necessary for valve development. PDGF-B and collagen IV production is inhibited simultaneously. (**c**) In developing lymph nodes, lymphangiogenesis is first induced when IL-7

and TRANCE stimulate LTi cells that develop from lymphatic precursor cells under the influence of the chemokine CXCL13. The LTi cells produce LTα1β2, which activates VEGF-C expression via the LTb receptor in stromal organizer cells. In adult lymph nodes, B-cell proliferation stimulates VEGF-mediated lymphangiogenesis, whereas T-cell-derived cytokines restrict lymphangiogenesis by producing interferon-γ. *Notch* neurogenic locus notch homolog protein, *COUP-TFII* chicken of albumin upstream promoter transcription factor II, *Sox18* sex-determining region Y Box 18, *Prox1* prospero-related homeodomain transcript factor, *LEC* lymphatic endothelial cell, *VEGF* vascular endothelial growth factor, *NFATc1* nuclear factor of activated T cells, cytoplasmic, calcineurin-dependent 1, *FoxC2* forkhead box protein C2, *ItgA9* integrin a9, *PDGF-B* platelet-derived growth factor, *IL-7* interleukin-7, *TRANCE* tumor necrosis factor (ligand) superfamily, member 11, *CXCL13* chemokine (cys × cys motif) ligand 13, *LTα1β2* heterotrimeric lymphotoxin (α1β2) (*reproduced with permission from* [18])

An example of genetic primary lymphedema, the first to be identified, is provided by the Milroy's disease, which is characterized by early-onset congenital lymphedema. In this syndrome, heterozygous missense mutations in the FLT4 (VEGFR3) gene inactivate the kinase activity of VEGFR-3.

It is characterized by bilateral lower limb lymphedema, which is usually present at birth.

Another example, one of the most common primary lymphedemas, the lymphedema-distichiasis (LD) syndrome, is an autosomal dominant disorder with variable expression.

It is caused by mutations in the FOXC2 gene, which codes for FOXC2, a transcription factor involved in the development of the lymphatic and vascular system [19]. The LD syndrome is characterized by late childhood or pubertal onset lymphedema of the limbs, and by distichiasis (double row of eyelashes). While the latter is the most common expression of LD, venous insufficiency occurs in half of the patients. Other associations have been reported, including congenital heart disease, ptosis, cleft lip/palate, and spinal extradural cysts.

The currently known mutations of at least 19 different genes are involved in lymphatic development associated with primary lymphedema [20], the most frequent being GJC2, FOXC2, CCBE1, VEGFR-3, PTPN14, GATA2, and SOX18 (Table 2.2) [18].

Although genetic molecular investigation contributes to provide proper genetic counseling for parents of an affected child with congenital lymphedema, they cannot explain those forms presenting later in life (*lymphedema tarda*). In these cases, the latent period before swelling suggests that a failure of growth or regeneration following a damage or injury might be the real cause underlying edema, rather than an abnormal development of lymphatics since birth.

In **secondary lymphedemas**, damage to the lymph-conducting pathways may occur secondary to any number of causes originating primarily outside the lymphatic system. Secondary lymphedema is more common than primary lymphedema, as it can result from a wide variety of causes, such as the post-thrombotic syndrome, surgical or radiation therapy, trauma, and infections.

In chronic venous insufficiency, as in the post-thrombotic syndrome, most of the interstitial fluid is unable to return to the heart by way of the obstructed veins. Therefore, the volume of fluid transported by the lower extremity lymphatics increases to compensate for the venous occlusion. This safety valve function of the lymph vessels continues until the lymphatic valvular mechanism becomes insufficient; then, reflux occurs, swelling of the limb increases, and ulcers develop.

Lymphedema frequently coexists with lipedema, a condition affecting only women. Lipedema is a bilateral, symmetrical swelling of the lower extremities extending from the pelvic brim to the ankles. Histologically, its hallmark is a gross increase in the subcutaneous fat layer, only limited to the areas mentioned above. The patient may be normal in weight, or even thin in the upper half of the body, but grossly obese from the pelvic brim down. Lymph vessels in lipedema are coiled, the prelymphatic canals and initial lymph vessels are abnormal, lymph transport velocity is reduced, and lymphedema involves both lower extremities (including the feet).

The most common **secondary upper-arm lymphedema** is to be expected after axillary lymph node dissection for breast cancer surgery, and/or radiation therapy in the upper arm. The incidence of breast cancer-related lymphedema, however, ranges widely between 6 and 70%; it may be a common underreported morbidity, considering the relation between lymphatic drainage of the upper extremity (UE) and of the breast in the caudal part of the axilla. Sentinel lymph node (SLN) groups for the UE and breast share connections in 24% of cases, which could explain lymphedema after surgery if damaged [21]. Lymphedema is generally localized at the arm on the side of breast surgery, and patients with a high peripheral blood vascular filtration rate seem to be predisposed to this complication [22, 23]. GJC2 (CX47) mutations are associated with a predisposition toward the development of postmastectomy lymphedema [24]. A clear relationship between the number of lymph nodes removed and the risk of lymphedema has not been definitely established, and clinical trials are focusing on the reduction of axillary lymph node dissections, even in the presence of a positive SLN [25].

The most common cancers in which treatments cause **secondary lower limb lymphedema** are melanoma, sarcoma, and pelvic tumors (including cervix, uterus, and prostate); it is noteworthy that pelvic cancers and infiltrating sarcomas can present with lymphedema, probably as failure of lymphatics to regenerate and re-anastomose satisfactorily through scarred or irradiated tissue secondary to cancer treatment.

Table 2.2 Gene abnormalities identified in different lymphedema syndromes

Gene	Disease name	Clinical manifestation
FLT4 (VEGFR-3)	Hereditary lymphedema IA (AD)	Congenital lymphedema
GJC2	Hereditary lymphedema IC (AD)	Lymphedema of the extremities, onset at <15 years of age
FOXC2	Lymphedema-distichiasis syndrome	Lymphedema of mainly lower limbs, triple row of eyelashes, varicose veins
CCBE1	Hennekam lymphangiectasia-lymphedema syndrome (AR)	Lymphedema of the extremities, intestinal lymphangiectasias, mental retardation
SOX18	Hypotrichosis-lymphedema-telangiectasia syndrome (AD)	Lymphedema, alopecia, telangiectasia
PTPN14	Lymphedema-choanal Atresia syndrome (AR)	Lymphedema of lower limbs in children, lack of nasal airways
GATA2	Emberger syndrome (AD)	Lymphedema of lower extremities and genitalia, immune dysfunction, cutaneous warts, deafness

AD autosomal dominant, *AR* autosomal recessive
Adapted from [18]

Trauma of the lymphatic channels (either from elective surgery or by accident) has to be extensive in order to induce lymphedema. Indeed, the experimental reproduction of lymphedema is extremely difficult, owing to the highly efficient regenerative powers of lymphatics.

Parasitic lymphedema is the most common cause of lymphedema worldwide. It is caused by the microfilariae of *Wuchereria bancrofti* and *Brugia malayi*, which can be transmitted to humans by different mosquito species. When these microfilariae reach the lymph vessels, they develop into adult worms; the resulting inflammation and fibrosis cause progressively increasing lymphatic obstruction. Elephantiasis is the end result of repeated infections, developing over many years.

Another tropical form of lymphedema is podoconiosis (endemic nonfilarial elephantiasis), a noninfectious geochemical disease of the lower limb lymphatic vessels evolving from chronic barefoot exposure to red-clay soil originating from volcanic rock. The hypothesis is that mineral particles in red-clay soils are absorbed through the skin of the foot and phagocytized by macrophages in the lymphatic system of the lower limbs, thus causing an inflammatory reaction in the lymphatic vessels resulting in fibrosis and vessel obstruction [26].

As common remark, all chronic limb lymphedemas cause functional impairment, disfiguration of the limb, and severe psychological damage.

Intracavitary lymphedema is the accumulation of chyle in the peritoneal cavity. Chyle can be defined as "milky lymph" which flows from the lacteals of the gut through the cisterna chyli and then through the thoracic duct. Chylous ascites occurs after abdominal surgeries or neoplastic infiltration of the abdominal lymphatic structures, as well as following traumas, lymphatic dysplasia, intraperitoneal lymphatic fistula within the framework of congenital defects of the lymphatic system, rupture of the lymphatic cyst, as well as an infectious and inflammatory process in lymph nodes. Ascitic fluid with triglyceride levels greater than 110 mg/dL is diagnostic of chylous ascites; total protein content varies usually from 1.4 to 6.4 g/dL, with a mean of 3.7 g/dL.

Chylothorax is a form of lipid pleural effusion characterized by the presence of chyle in the pleural space, which can be the result of obstruction or disruption of the thoracic duct, or one of its major tributaries. A triglyceride concentration >110 mg/dL is virtually diagnostic, but the presence of chylomicrons confirms the diagnosis. However, chylothorax defined by these criteria represents a heterogeneous group of clinical entities. The presence of chylomicrons or triglyceride levels >110 mg/dL in a pleural effusion should be considered evidence of chyle leakage of indeterminate clinical significance. In the case of an acute or chronic chylothorax due to possible injury of the thoracic duct injury, this evaluation is crucial, as surgical ligation of the thoracic duct is often entertained. In contrast, a cholesterol-rich effusion is typically the result of long-standing pleurisy with elevated cholesterol levels in the pleural space; most cases of cholesterol pleural effusions are attributed to tuberculous or to rheumatoid pleurisy. Distinguishing between a chylothorax and a cholesterol effusion is critical. A chylothorax develops after injury or obstruction of the thoracic duct, leading to leakage of chyle into the pleural space, and is characterized by an increased triglyceride concentration and by the presence of chylomicrons. In contrast, a cholesterol effusion is a long-standing effusion associated with an elevated cholesterol concentration (usually greater than 250 mg/dL) and with a thick pleural rind; this condition represents a form of lung entrapment. The accumulation of chyle in the pericardial space, or chylopericardium, occurs most frequently after trauma, and cardiac and thoracic surgery, or in association with tumors, tuberculosis, or lymphangiomatosis. When its precise cause cannot be identified, it is called primary or idiopathic chylopericardium, a quite rare clinical condition. Etiology can be primary or the result of various clinical situations, particularly trauma (thoracic duct lesions), neoplasms (primary such as lymphangioma or through invasion of the lymphatic system by other neoplasms), and filaria infection. Primary forms are the result of malformation of the intestinal lymph circulation and its relationship with the systemic circulation, resulting in megalymphatics that develop fistulas following even minimal trauma, and that can be located at atypical sites in the body.

Key Learning Points

- The cardinal manifestation of lymphatic dysfunction is lymphedema.
- Primary lymphedemas have been identified in hereditary diseases associated with specific genetic defects.
- Secondary lymphedemas occur secondarily to any causes originating primarily outside the lymphatic system.
- Secondary lymphedemas are more common than primary lymphedemas; the post-thrombotic syndrome, surgical or radiation therapy, trauma, infections, and neoplasms are the most frequent etiologies.
- Intracavitary lymphedema may occur because of accumulation of lymph in the peritoneal cavity, as well as in the pleural or in the pericardial space.

2.6   Lymphatic Malignancies

Solid tumors can originate in the lymphatic tissues. Lymphangiosarcoma, a malignant tumor of unknown molecular pathogenesis, causes primary or secondary lymphedema. Lymphangio-leiomyomatosis is a tumor characterized by the infiltration of abnormal smooth-like cells through the pulmonary interstitium, perivascular spaces, and lymphatics of young females, and it leads to lymphatic disruption and final respiratory failure. Kaposi's sarcoma is an angiogenic tumor of lymphatic endothelial cells (LECs). The lymphatic vessels also provide a route for tumor cells to metastasize, and the lymph node microenvironment may select tumor cells with increased metastatic potential.

Key Learning Points
- Tumors can originate in the lymphatic tissues.
- Most frequently, the lymphatic circulation serves as the primary route for the metastatic spread of tumor cells to regional lymph nodes.
- Propagation to lymph nodes is one of the main prognostic factors in patients with solid epithelial cancers: after reaching the SLNs, tumor cells will spread into distant lymph nodes and other organs.
- On the other hand, direct hematogenous metastatic spread can occur independently from metastatic spread through the lymphatic system.

2.7   Lymphangiothrombosis and Acute Lymphangitis

Obliterative processes consequent to lymphangiothrombosis or recurrent lymphangitis might occur in the same way as for veins, since lymph can clot in the same way as blood; unfortunately, there is no clinical investigation for ascertaining the presence of lymph thrombosis.

Lymphangitis, an inflammation of the lymphatic collectors, is clinically evident as a red streak up the limb corresponding to the inflamed vessels. Edema is often an accompanying feature. Infection is generally limited to the lymph nodes, and lymphadenitis may give rise to painful swelling in the groin or axilla (depending on the site of infection). Lymphangitis can be recurrent. When lymphatic insufficiency exists and the local system fails in its host defense duty, recurrent infection can occur, presenting clinically as recurrent erysipelas.

Erysipelas is a skin infection that is usually caused by β-hemolytic group A streptococci. After having had erysipelas in an extremity, a significant percentage of patients develops persistent swelling or suffers from recurrent erysipelas.

Although persistent swelling after erysipelas is most likely caused by secondary lymphedema, a study [27] proved that patients presenting with a first episode of erysipelas often have signs at lymphoscintigraphy of preexisting lymphatic impairment in the other, clinically non-affected, leg. This means that subclinical lymphatic dysfunction of both legs may be an important predisposing factor. Therefore, treatment of erysipelas should focus not only on the infection, but also on the lymphological aspects; in this regard, long-term treatment for lymphedema is essential in order to prevent recurrence of erysipelas and aggravation of the preexisting lymphatic impairment.

Based on the clinical experience that lymphangitis or cellulitis is not always followed by the development of lymphedema, it can be speculated that lymphedema is the result of vulnerable lymphatics with preexisting lymphatic insufficiency, although proving which came first—the cellulitis or the lymphatic insufficiency—is still difficult.

Key Learning Points
- There are no clinical investigations for ascertaining the presence of lymph thrombosis.
- Lymphangitis, an inflammation of the lymphatic collectors, is clinically evident as a red streak up the limb; edema is often an accompanying feature, and lymphangitis can recur.
- Erysipelas is a skin infection usually caused by β-hemolytic group A streptococci.
- Subclinical lymphatic dysfunction may be an important predisposing factor for erysipelas.
- Therefore, treatment of erysipelas should focus not only on the infection per se, but also on the lymphatic components of the clinical problem.
- This includes long-term treatment of lymphedema in order to prevent recurrence of erysipelas and further worsening of the preexisting lymphatic impairment.

2.8   Pathophysiology of Lymphatic Circulation in Systemic Diseases

The new emerging concept of lymphangiogenesis strongly emphasizes the contribution of lymphatic circulation to the initiation, maintenance, natural history, or therapeutic approach to a broad array of systemic diseases, including obesity, atherosclerosis, and cardiovascular diseases.

2.8.1   Obesity

Abnormality in the pathophysiologic regulation of lymphatic circulation might be involved in the pathogenesis of obesity.

The link between lymphatic function and adipose biology has recently been recognized [28]. Lymph nodes and collecting lymphatic vessels are usually embedded in visceral or subcutaneous fat, thus suggesting a relationship between lymphatic vessels and adipose metabolism. Additionally, ectopic growth of adipose tissue is observed in edematous regions of patients suffering from chronic lymphedema. In rats, chronic inflammation of the peripheral lymph nodes increases the number of adipocytes surrounding the nodes. Moreover, increased deposition of subcutaneous fat in edematous regions has been described in lymphedema-carrying Chy-mice with heterozygous inactivating mutation in VEGFR3, thus supporting the hypothesis that the lymph is adipogenic. Indeed, mice with heterozygous Prox1-inactivating mutation were found to have leaky lymphatic vessels and to develop obesity and inflammation resembling late-onset obesity in humans [29]. Prox1 heterozygous mice constitute the first in vivo model of lymphatic mediated obesity, where the leading cause of the obese phenotype is the abnormal lymph leakage due to disruption in lymphatic vascular integrity, particularly of the mesenteric lymphatic vessels; leaking of lymph exerts a potent adipogenic stimulus, although the exact factor responsible for such stimulus is presently still unknown.

Obese adipose tissue expansion is an inflammatory process that results in dysregulated lipolysis, increased circulating lipids, ectopic lipid deposition, and systemic insulin resistance. Lymphatic vessels provide a route of fluid, macromolecule, and immune cell clearance, and lymphangiogenesis increases this capability. Indeed, inflammation-associated lymphangiogenesis is critical in resolving acute and chronic inflammation, but it is largely absent in obese adipose tissue. Enhancing adipose tissue lymphangiogenesis could, therefore, improve metabolism in obesity. Furthermore, an improvement in obesity metabolism enhances lymphangiogenesis of adipose tissue. This hypothesis has recently been proved in transgenic mice with inducible expression of vascular endothelial growth factor (VEGF)-D under a tissue-specific lymphangiogenesis tightly controlled during obesity high-fat diets of 16 weeks. VEGF-D adipose overexpression induced de novo lymphangiogenesis in murine adipose tissue. When increasing VEGF-D signaling and lymphangiogenesis specifically in adipose tissue, the immune accumulation associated with obesity is reduced and the metabolic response is favored [30].

2.8.2 Arterial Hypertension

In animal models of hypertension it has been observed that extrarenal control of sodium balance and blood pressure can reside in the glycosaminoglycans, macrophages, and lymphatic vessels of the skin. Sodium ions in the skin interstitium can be stored in an osmotically inactive form bound to glycosaminoglycans that can provide an actively regulated interstitial Na^+ exchange mechanism that participates in volume and blood pressure homeostasis [22]. Na^+ magnetic resonance imaging of human body sodium distribution demonstrates that sodium is primarily accumulated in the skin and muscles [31]. In a recent clinical investigation [32] of skin biopsies in 91 patients (both hypertensive and with normal blood pressure) who had elective surgery with abdominal skin incision, the content of Na^+ and water, accumulation of macrophages (CD68), and density of lymphatic vessels (D2-40) and blood vessels (CD31) were calculated in the specimens of abdominal skin together with plasma NT-proANP, vascular endothelial growth factor (VEGF)-C, and VEGF-D concentrations. In the hypertensive group, the skin expression of CD68 and the serum concentration of VEGF-C were different than in the group with normal blood pressure. The results of this investigation suggest that cutaneous accumulation of Na^+ is associated with the presence of hypertension and is also correlated with the presence of CD68 macrophages and with decreased prevailing levels of VEGF-C, thus implying that the lymphatic system contributes significantly to this cascade of events leading to hypertension. These human observations suggest that further exploration of the lymphatic contribution to the pathogenesis and maintenance of hypertension might lead to novel interventions directed at the prevention and treatment of this highly morbid condition.

2.8.3 Atherosclerosis

Atherosclerosis is a chronic inflammatory disease of the arterial wall that develops silently over decades, evolving to fatty streaks characterized mainly by macrophages loaded with cholesterol esters. Continuous recruitment of monocytes into plaques drives the progression of this chronic inflammatory condition, sustained at least in part by the deposition of cholesterol crystals and immunity against cholesterol-associated apolipoproteins.

Although the link between cholesterol and inflammation that drives disease progression is not completely understood, it is established that removal of cholesterol from the arterial wall constitutes a step toward regression of atherosclerosis.

The presence of lymphatics in the arterial wall was described more than 100 years ago [33]. The presence of lymphatic vessels in the adventitia of arteries adjacent to small blood vessels, the *vasa vasorum*, that are expanded in atherosclerotic plaques, suggests that lymphatic vessels have a role in the development of atherosclerotic plaques [34]. Recently the existence of lymphatic vessels has been demonstrated in the adventitia as well as in intraplaque regions of human carotid endarterectomy specimens [35].

It is speculated that the lymphatic circulation could provide a protective pathway for lipid and inflammatory cell efflux from the arterial wall, thus counteracting the development of atherosclerotic plaques. The multistep process of cholesterol mobilization from extravascular tissues to biliary and non-biliary excretion is termed reverse cholesterol transport (RCT). Cholesterol removal from macrophage stores involves hydrolysis, mobilization, and efflux of cholesterol esters to lipoprotein acceptors such as apoAI, which results in the formation of HDL. HDL leaves the interstitial tissue and is transported through the bloodstream into the liver for disposal as biliary cholesterol and bile salts, or to the intestinal wall for trans-intestinal cholesterol efflux.

Although the initial and final steps of RCT have been well characterized, it was only recently shown that HDL primarily uses lymphatic vessels in the efflux from the interstitium to the bloodstream. Indeed, experimental evidences showed that induction of lymphangiogenesis by the administration of VEGF-C into the footpad improved lymphatic function, decreased footpad cholesterol content, and improved RCT in *ApoE−/−* mice [36]. In contrast, surgical disruption of collecting lymphatic vessels in the popliteal area reduced RCT from the footpad by as much as 80%. In another study, surgical ablation of lymphatic vessels in the tail also blocked RCT. In Chy-mice, which selectively lack dermal lymphatic vessels, RCT from the rear footpad was impaired by ≤77% [36].

The relevance of lymphatic RCT in atherosclerotic plaque is a surprising finding, and it would be important to determine why HDL prefers lymphatic vessels instead of the postcapillary venous system to exit the interstitial space.

Overall, animal models indicate that RCT is critically dependent on lymphatic vessels, and that the venous system is not enough to sustain RCT. Furthermore, inducing lymphangiogenesis could constitute a strategy to enhance RCT. This could be especially important in the case of hypercholesterolemia and obesity, conditions that were shown to directly impair lymphatic vessel function.

Despite extensive investigations, it remains to be assessed whether inducing intimal or adventitial lymphangiogenesis could enhance RCT and reverse atherosclerosis in patients with cardiovascular disease [37].

2.8.4 Myocardial Infarction

The presence of lymphatic vessels in the arterial wall and their role in atherosclerosis have stimulated investigations on whether lymphangiogenesis might improve myocardial function, particularly in the infarcted or dilated heart, where wall tension is grossly elevated [35].

Following myocardial infarction, cardiac lymphatic vessels undergo a profound lymphangiogenic response; in experimental settings in mice, ectopic VEGFC stimulation augments the lymphangiogenic response resulting in a transient improvement in post-myocardial infarction (MI) cardiac function. Therefore, inducing lymphangiogenesis could provide a pathway for inflammatory cell efflux to tip the balance in favor of wound healing within the injured adult heart. Despite the endogenous cardiac lymphangiogenic response post-MI, the remodeling and dysfunction of collecting ducts contribute to the development of chronic myocardial edema and inflammation—aggravating cardiac fibrosis and dysfunction. Therefore, therapeutic lymphangiogenesis may be a promising new approach for the treatment of cardiovascular diseases [38]. The roles of lymphatic vessels in MI and atherosclerosis are summarized in Fig. 2.5.

Key Learning Points
- Current knowledge leads to speculation that lymphatic circulation is involved in the pathogenesis of cardiovascular diseases, including obesity, hypertension, atherosclerosis, and myocardial infarction.
- Expansion of the adipose tissue in obesity is an inflammatory process that results in dysregulated lipolysis, increased circulating lipids, ectopic lipid deposition, and systemic insulin resistance.
- Lymphangiogenesis is critical in resolving acute and chronic inflammation, but it is largely absent in the adipose tissue of obese subjects; enhanced adipose tissue lymphangiogenesis could, therefore, improve metabolism in obesity.
- The presence of lymphatic vessels in the adventitia of arteries adjacent to *vasa vasorum* (that are expanded in atherosclerotic plaques) and the presence of lymphatic vessels inside human carotid endarterectomy specimens suggest that lymphatic vessels have some role in the development of atherosclerotic plaques.
- Cholesterol mobilization from extravascular tissues to biliary and non-biliary excretion, termed reverse cholesterol transport (RCT), is critically dependent on lymphatic vessels, and the venous system is not sufficient to sustain RCT. The relevance of lymphatic RCT is a surprising finding.
- Cardiac lymphatic circulation might improve myocardial function, particularly in the infarcted or dilated heart.
- Despite extensive investigations, it remains to be assessed whether inducing intimal or adventitial lymphangiogenesis could enhance RCT and thus reverse atherosclerosis in patients with cardiovascular disease.
- Therapeutic lymphangiogenesis might constitute a promising new approach for treating cardiovascular diseases.

Fig. 2.5 Role of lymphatic vessels in cholesterol metabolism, atherosclerosis, and myocardial infarction. (**a**) Epicardial lymphatic vessels stained for VEGFR3 and LYVE1. (**b**) Schematic overview of the heart with myocardial infarction caused by the occlusion of the atherosclerotic coronary artery. (**c**) Cross section of an atherosclerotic coronary artery and an adventitial lymphatic vessel. (**d**) Hypothetical model for the role of lymphatic vessels in high-density lipoprotein (HDL)-mediated cholesterol removal from atherosclerotic plaques (*adapted from* [10])

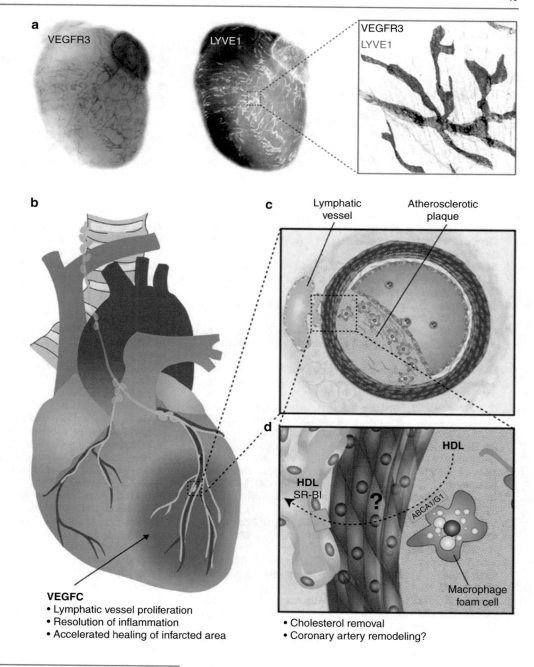

2.9 Concluding Remarks

The cardinal manifestation of lymphatic malfunction is lymphedema. Overall data from the last decade, however, indicate that lymphatic circulation is critically involved also in the pathogenesis of cardiovascular disease, including hypercholesterolemia, atherosclerosis, and obesity.

The concept that inflammation promotes lymphedema has opened new pharmacological strategies and therapeutic targets. Enhanced insights into the interplay between inflammation and pathological tissue remodeling are required to pave new therapeutic avenues in lymphedema and in other forms of lymphatic disorders.

The venous system is not sufficient by itself to sustain the multistep process of cholesterol mobilization from extravascular tissues to biliary and non-biliary excretion, termed reverse cholesterol transport. In this regard, the lymphatics play an important role, and promoting lymphangiogenesis could constitute a novel strategy to enhance reverse cholesterol transport.

Despite extensive investigations suggesting that therapeutic lymphangiogenesis may be a promising new approach for the treatment of cardiovascular diseases, it still remains to be assessed whether inducing intimal or adventitial lymphangiogenesis could enhance RCT and thus reverse atherosclerosis in patients with cardiovascular disease.

Acknowledgements This chapter is a revision of the original chapter written by R. Di Stefano, P. A. Erba, and G. D'Errico in the previous edition of the book.

References

1. Lord RS. The white veins: conceptual difficulties in the history of the lymphatics. Med Hist. 1968;12:174–84.
2. Kukk E, Lymboussaki A, Taira S, et al. VEGF-C receptor binding and pattern of expression with VEGFR-3 suggests a role in lymphatic vascular development. Development. 1996;122:3829–37.
3. Wigle JT, Oliver G. Prox1 function is required for the development of the murine lymphatic system. Cell. 1999;98:769–78.
4. Breiteneder-Geleff S, Soleiman A, Kowalski H, et al. Angiosarcomas express mixed endothelial phenotypes of blood and lymphatic capillaries: podoplanin as a specific marker for lymphatic endothelium. Am J Pathol. 1999;154:385–94.
5. Banerji S, Ni J, Wang SX, et al. LYVE-1, a new homologue of the CD44 glycoprotein, is a lymph-specific receptor for hyaluronan. J Cell Biol. 1999;144:789–801.
6. Yang Y, Oliver G. Development of the mammalian lymphatic vasculature. J Clin Invest. 2014;124:888–97.
7. Thomson BR, Heinen S, Jeansson M, et al. A lymphatic defect causes ocular hypertension and glaucoma in mice. J Clin Invest. 2014;124:4320–4.
8. Louveau A, Smirnov I, Keyes TJ, et al. Structural and functional features of central nervous system lymphatic vessels. Nature. 2015;523:337–41.
9. Cohen JN, Guidi CJ, Tewalt EF, et al. Lymph node-resident lymphatic endothelial cells mediate peripheral tolerance via Aire-independent direct antigen presentation. J Exp Med. 2010;207:681–8.
10. Aspelund A, Robciuc MR, Karaman S, et al. Lymphatic system in cardiovascular medicine. Circ Res. 2016;118:515–30.
11. Jiang X, Nicolls MR, Tian W, et al. Lymphatic dysfunction, Leukotrienes, and lymphedema. Annu Rev Physiol. 2018;80:49–70.
12. Brown P. Lymphatic system: unlocking the drains. Nature. 2005;436:456–8.
13. Choe K, Jang JY, Park I, et al. Intravital imaging of intestinal lacteals unveils lipid drainage through contractility. J Clin Invest. 2015;125:4042–52.
14. Tian W, Rockson SG, Jiang X, et al. Leukotriene B4 antagonism ameliorates experimental lymphedema. Sci Transl Med. 2017;9:eaal3920.
15. Rockson SG, Tian W, Jiang X, et al. Pilot studies demonstrate the potential benefits of antiinflammatory therapy in human lymphedema. JCI Insight. 2018;3.
16. Zerbino DD. [Senile changes in the outflow lymphatic vessels]. Arkh Anat Gistol Embriol. 1960;39:37–42.
17. Shang T, Liang J, Kapron CM, et al. Pathophysiology of aged lymphatic vessels. Aging (Albany NY). 2019;11:6602–13.
18. Alitalo K. The lymphatic vasculature in disease. Nat Med. 2011;17:1371–80.
19. Sutkowska E, Gil J, Stembalska A, et al. Novel mutation in the FOXC2 gene in three generations of a family with lymphoedema-distichiasis syndrome. Gene. 2012;498:96–9.
20. Brouillard P, Boon L, Vikkula M. Genetics of lymphatic anomalies. J Clin Invest. 2014;124:898–904.
21. Pavlista D, Eliska O. Relationship between the lymphatic drainage of the breast and the upper extremity: a postmortem study. Ann Surg Oncol. 2012;19:3410–5.
22. McLaughlin SA. Lymphedema: separating fact from fiction. Oncology (Williston Park). 2012;26:242–9.
23. Stanton AW, Modi S, Mellor RH, et al. Recent advances in breast cancer-related lymphedema of the arm: lymphatic pump failure and predisposing factors. Lymphat Res Biol. 2009;7:29–45.
24. Finegold DN, Baty CJ, Knickelbein KZ, et al. Connexin 47 mutations increase risk for secondary lymphedema following breast cancer treatment. Clin Cancer Res. 2012;18:2382–90.
25. Wojcinski S, Nuengsri S, Hillemanns P, et al. Axillary dissection in primary breast cancer: variations of the surgical technique and influence on morbidity. Cancer Manag Res. 2012;4:121–7.
26. Tekola Ayele F, Adeyemo A, Finan C, et al. HLA class II locus and susceptibility to podoconiosis. N Engl J Med. 2012;366:1200–8.
27. Damstra RJ, van Steensel MA, Boomsma JH, et al. Erysipelas as a sign of subclinical primary lymphoedema: a prospective quantitative scintigraphic study of 40 patients with unilateral erysipelas of the leg. Br J Dermatol. 2008;158:1210–5.
28. Harvey NL. The link between lymphatic function and adipose biology. Ann N Y Acad Sci. 2008;1131:82–8.
29. Harvey NL, Srinivasan RS, Dillard ME, et al. Lymphatic vascular defects promoted by Prox1 haploinsufficiency cause adult-onset obesity. Nat Genet. 2005;37:1072–81.
30. Chakraborty A, Barajas S, Lammoglia GM, et al. Vascular endothelial growth factor-D (VEGF-D) overexpression and lymphatic expansion in murine adipose tissue improves metabolism in obesity. Am J Pathol. 2019;189:924–39.
31. Kopp C, Linz P, Dahlmann A, et al. ^{23}Na magnetic resonance imaging-determined tissue sodium in healthy subjects and hypertensive patients. Hypertension. 2013;61:635–40.
32. Chachaj A, Pula B, Chabowski M, et al. Role of the lymphatic system in the pathogenesis of hypertension in humans. Lymphat Res Biol. 2018;16:140–6.
33. Hoggan G, Hoggan FE. The lymphatics of the walls of the larger blood-vessels and lymphatics. J Anat Physiol. 1882;17:1–23.
34. Nakano T, Nakashima Y, Yonemitsu Y, et al. Angiogenesis and lymphangiogenesis and expression of lymphangiogenic factors in the atherosclerotic intima of human coronary arteries. Hum Pathol. 2005;36:330–40.
35. Kutkut I, Meens MJ, McKee TA, et al. Lymphatic vessels: an emerging actor in atherosclerotic plaque development. Eur J Clin Invest. 2015;45:100–8.
36. Martel C, Li W, Fulp B, et al. Lymphatic vasculature mediates macrophage reverse cholesterol transport in mice. J Clin Invest. 2013;123:1571–9.
37. Csanyi G, Singla B. Arterial lymphatics in atherosclerosis: old questions, new insights, and remaining challenges. J Clin Med. 2019;8(4). pii: E495. https://doi.org/10.3390/jcm8040495.
38. Henri O, Pouehe C, Houssari M, et al. Selective stimulation of cardiac lymphangiogenesis reduces myocardial edema and fibrosis leading to improved cardiac function following myocardial infarction. Circulation. 2016;133:1484–97; discussion 1497.

Methodological Aspects of Lymphatic Mapping: Radiopharmaceuticals, Multimodal Lymphatic Mapping Agents, Instrumentations

3

Francesco Bartoli, Giuseppina Bisogni, Sara Vitali, Angela G. Cataldi, Alberto Del Guerra, Giuliano Mariani, and Paola A. Erba

Contents

3.1   **Introduction** 21

3.2   **Radiopharmaceuticals for Lymphatic Mapping** 22

3.3   **Iodine-Based CT Contrast Agents for Lymphatic Mapping** 27

3.4   **MR, MRL, and PET/MRI Contrast Agents for Lymphatic Mapping** 29

3.5   **Contrast-Enhanced Ultrasound Imaging for Lymphatic Mapping** 33

3.6   **Optical Imaging Agents for Lymphatic Mapping** 34

3.7   **Multimodal Tracers for Lymphatic Mapping** 36

3.8   **Instrumentations for Lymphatic Mapping** 39

3.9   **Near-Infrared (NIR) Imaging for Lymphatic Mapping** 44

References 46

Learning Objectives
- To describe the radiopharmaceuticals; iodine-based CT contrast agents; contrast agents for MR, MRL, and PET/MRI; contrast-enhanced ultrasound imaging; optical imaging agents; and multimodal tracers
- To understand the basic concepts behind the radiopharmaceuticals and instrumentations used for lymphoscintigraphy and radioguided surgery
- To outline the most recent advances in radiopharmaceuticals and instrumentations
- To explain the working principles of handheld gamma probes and their most significant parameters, including sensitivity, spatial resolution, energy resolution, and signal-to-noise ratio
- To review the available handheld gamma probes and portable imaging devices and their clinical implementation
- To describe the basic concepts and the equipment for the use of indocyanine green fluorescence technique in surgery

F. Bartoli · S. Vitali · A. G. Cataldi · G. Mariani · P. A. Erba (✉)
Regional Center of Nuclear Medicine, Department of Translational Research and Advanced Technologies in Medicine and Surgery, University of Pisa, Pisa, Italy
e-mail: paola.erba@unipi.it

G. Bisogni · A. Del Guerra
"Enrico Fermi" Department of Physics, University of Pisa, Pisa, Italy

3.1   Introduction

Exploration of lymphatic circulation with radiopharmaceuticals constitutes one of the earliest applications of nuclear medicine, dating back to the early 1950s and steadily growing throughout the 1960s. A potent impetus to further growth in the clinical applications of lymphoscintigraphy derived from the introduction of agents for lymphatic mapping labeled with technetium-99m (^{99m}Tc). Up until the early 1990s, the predominant applications of lymphoscintigraphy were for assessing lymphatic circulation in patients with peripheral edema (to discriminate edema caused by insufficiency of venous drainage from edema caused by insufficiency of lymphatic drainage) and for assessing the lymph node tumor status in patients with cancer (based on absent lymph node visualization along a certain lymphatic basin in case of massive lymph node metastasis).

Starting in 1992–1993, a real revolution occurred with the use of lymphoscintigraphy for sentinel lymph node (SLN) mapping, initially in patients with cutaneous melanoma or with breast cancer, but soon expanding to include a variety of other solid epithelial cancers. SLN mapping combined with radioguided sentinel lymph node biopsy (SLNB) currently constitutes *the* standard of care for patients with melanoma, breast cancer, penile cancer, head and neck squamous cell cancers, and gynecological malignancies (primarily vulvar cancer and cervical cancer), while numerous clinical trials for validation of this approach are under way in patients with prostate cancer and, among others, cancers of the gastrointestinal tract. Thus, SLN mapping is by far the most common application worldwide of lymphoscintigraphy. On the other hand, peripheral lymphoscintigraphy in patients with edema or with intracavitary effusions maintains a well-established role in the clinical workup of these conditions—whereas the original use of lymphoscintigraphy per se for assessing the tumor status of lymph nodes in patients with cancers has completely vanished.

Advances in the design of novel radiopharmaceuticals for lymphatic mapping have gone in parallel with technological advances in instrumentations, both for external imaging and for intraoperative use during radioguided surgery. Technological advances also favor the development of hybrid imaging agents with multiple signatures (radioactive, optical, X-ray, or MR contrast) to take maximum advantage from the synergistic combination of different agents with different biological and physical properties—to the final best clinical benefit to patients.

This chapter reviews the status of the art of lymphatic mapping with regard to both the imaging agents employed and the instrumentations used for these investigations.

3.2 Radiopharmaceuticals for Lymphatic Mapping

3.2.1 Radiocolloids and Other Agents for SLN Mapping

Deposition of radioactive colloids in regional lymph nodes (LNs) was first observed by Walker after subcutaneous injec-

tion of colloidal gold (^{198}Au) [1]. Since a significant fraction of the activity remained at the injection site after subcutaneous administration of colloidal ^{198}Au (a radionuclide with a significant component of beta decay), radiation burden at the injection site limited the activity that could be safely administered. This led to search for agents with more favorable physical characteristics.

^{198}Au was soon replaced with particulate materials labeled with the most widely employed radionuclide for routine diagnostic procedures, i.e., ^{99m}Tc ($T_{1/2}$ = 6 h, exclusive 140 keV gamma radiation, available locally through a generator). The agents developed to this purpose include, among others, ^{99m}Tc-sulfur colloids, ^{99m}Tc-rhenium sulfide, ^{99m}Tc-nano- and micro-aggregated albumin, and ^{99m}Tc-antimony sulfide [2–14]. Neither ^{99m}Tc-antimony sulfide nor ^{99m}Tc-human serum albumin is currently commercially available in the United States. ^{99m}Tc-albumin nanocolloid (Nanocoll®) and ^{99m}Tc-rhenium sulfide colloids are used in Europe [15–18]. Filtered ^{99m}Tc-sulfur colloid (to limit particle size to about <200 nm or about <100 nm—depending on the pore size of the Millipore filter used) is one of the most commonly employed radiopharmaceuticals for lymphoscintigraphy in the United States. In addition, other radiocolloids such as ^{99m}Tc-stannous phytate [3], denatured ^{99m}Tc-collagen colloid, and ^{99m}Tc-stannous fluoride can be used. ^{99m}Tc-labeled Dextran 70, a sucrose polymer of high molecule weight, is another radiopharmaceutical option that can be used for SLN detection [19]; although it is not a true colloid, this compound behaves in a similar fashion as radiocolloids following interstitial injection. Table 3.1 lists the main features of radiopharmaceuticals that have been employed for lymphoscintigraphy, while Figs. 3.1 and 3.2 show the considerable variability in particle size among different preparations.

Generally, the labeling procedure consists of the adsorption of ^{99m}Tc on the particle's surface at nonspecific sites. Colloid quantity, and hence the available adsorption surface,

Table 3.1 Colloidal radiotracers and their particle size (modified from Bergqvist et al. [5])

Radiocolloid	Particle size	References
^{198}Au-colloid	5 nm; 9–15 nm	[4, 20]
^{99m}Tc-rhenium colloid (TCK-1)	10–40 nm; 50–500 nm	[14, 21]
^{99m}Tc-rhenium colloid (TCK-17)	50–200 nm; 45 nm; 3–15 nm	[14, 22]
^{99m}Tc-antimony sulfur colloid	2–15 nm; 40 nm	[14, 23]
^{99m}Tc-sulfur colloid (unfiltered)	100–1000 nm	[24]
^{99m}Tc-sulfur colloid (filtered)	38 nm (mean)	[25]
^{99m}Tc-stannous sulfur colloid	20–60 nm	[26]
^{99m}Tc-albumin nanocolloid (Nanocoll)	<80 nm	[27]
^{99m}Tc-microaggregated albumin (Microlite)	10 nm	[14]

must be used in large excess. In other cases, the labeling procedure is carried out as a coprecipitation process of ^{99m}Tc (Fig. 3.3).

Many factors influence transport of molecules from the interstitium to the lymphatic vessels. Since solutes must interact and cross over with components of the extracellular matrix to enter the lymphatic circulation, extracellular matrix composition and solute properties have significant influence on their ability to move through the interstitium into the lymphatics [28]. The most important properties of molecules in this regard are weight, size, shape, and charge [29–31].

Although molecules are transported both by convection and by diffusion, their size has a major impact on which mechanism predominates [32, 33]. Small molecules are primarily transported by diffusion, which is a slow process over longer distances. The slower transport of the largest molecules is explained by mechanical interaction with the extracellular matrix components, a mechanism that slows down movements of the molecules.

Uptake and retention of radiocolloids in lymph nodes greatly depend on the fact that they undergo phagocytosis once they have entered into the lymphatic circulation and are transported to the lymph nodes. The lymph node is a highly complex structure that contains lymphocytes, plasma cells, and macrophages in a collagen sheath. One fraction of the colloid remains inside the lymph node, where phagocytosis by macrophages occurs. The remaining portion, especially the smaller size fraction, proceeds through the efferent lymph vessels toward the next lymph node(s).

Colloids enter and exit the lymphatic circulation with different speeds depending on their sizes. Their migration through the lymphatic system is also inversely related to particle size. Particles smaller than a few nanometers usually leak into blood capillaries, whereas larger particles (up to about 100 nm) can enter the lymphatic capillaries and be transported to lymph nodes, where phagocytosis takes place [34]. Very small particles (<30 nm) migrate rapidly, with a

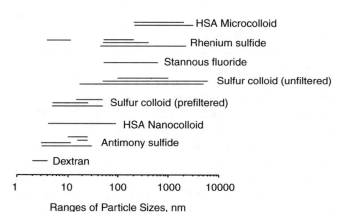

Fig. 3.1 Schematic representation of the ranges of particle sizes in nm in the main radiopharmaceuticals employed for lymphoscintigraphy. *HSA* human serum albumin

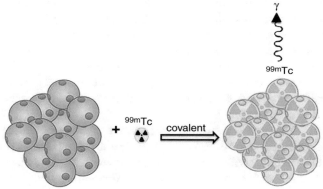

Fig. 3.3 Radiolabeling of nanocolloids with ^{99m}Tc (*reproduced with permission from Buckle T, van Leeuwen AC, Chin PT, Janssen H, Muller SH, Jonkers J, et al. A self-assembled multimodal complex for combined pre- and intraoperative imaging of the SLN. Nanotechnology. 2010;21(35):355101*)

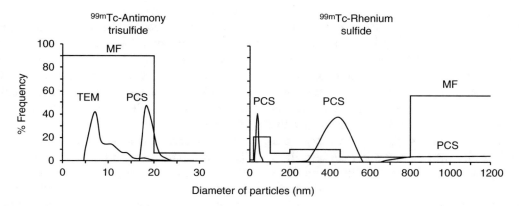

Fig. 3.2 Comparison of transmission electron microscopy (TEM), photon correlation spectroscopy (PCS), and membrane filtration (MF) to characterize size distribution of ^{99m}Tc-antimony trisulfide colloid and ^{99m}Tc-rhenium sulfide colloid (*adapted from Tsopelas C. Particle size analysis of ^{99m}Tc-labeled and unlabeled antimony trisulfide and rhenium sulfide colloids intended for lymphoscintigraphic application. J Nucl Med. 2001;42:460–466*)

small proportion remaining in the first lymph node encountered, therefore resulting in the visualization of additional nodes along the same lymphatic path. Larger particles (>100 nm) are trapped in the interstitial compartment for a relatively long period of time [12]. The fraction of tracer that is phagocytized locally or in lymph nodes increases with increasing size [35]. The smaller the molecule, the less convection influences its transport. Convection of dextrans of similar form, shape, and charge has been found to be significantly faster at a molecular weight of 71 kDa than lighter (3 and 40 kDa) and heavier (2 MDa) dextrans [36]. Albumin is convected three times slower than dextran of similar weight (71 kDa), thus suggesting that both the shape and the uneven distribution of charges in the albumin molecule have a relevant impact on its ability to move through the extracellular matrix.

Thus, similar size molecules can vary in their transport properties. In particular, negatively charged dextrans convect faster than neutrally charged dextran of similar size and shape, demonstrating that negatively charged molecules move more easily through the extracellular matrix. This feature is explained by the fixed negative charge of the glycosaminoglycans in the extracellular matrix. The repelling forces between the negatively charged molecules and the negatively charged extracellular matrix components might reduce mechanical interaction, and thus lower the resistance against convection.

Differences in surface characteristics of the colloids may account for differences in lymph node uptakes [31]. Early studies with liposomes have shown that specific surface properties (such as charge, hydrophobicity, and presence of targeting ligands) can influence both the rate of particle drainage from a subcutaneous injection site and the distribution within the lymphatic system. In rats, for instance, small, negatively charged liposomes localize in lymph nodes more effectively than positively charged vesicles when administered subcutaneously into the dorsal surface of the footpad [37].

These considerations are the main determinants for the selection of the suitable molecules both for peripheral lymphoscintigraphy and for SLN mapping. In fact, when peripheral lymphoscintigraphy is performed to assess and quantify tracer retention in local lymph nodes, the radiopharmaceutical should be characterized by high retention in the lymph nodes, i.e., should have a molecular size that promotes phagocytosis. Conversely, if depot washout techniques are used, smaller tracers that mimic in vivo transport of plasma proteins in the lymphatics (with faster interstitial and lymphatic transport and less local retention) are needed to produce faster and more reliable clearance data [38].

In the case of SLN mapping, the use of small particle size may cause problems to the surgeon in distinguishing between the true SLNs and other radioactive sites. The use of large particles reduces considerably the number of lymph nodes detected along a certain lymphatic pathway. It has been estimated that for a colloid size between 20 and 1000 nm, an average 1.3 lymph nodes are detected, whereas particles with size less than 80 nm show an average 1.7 lymph nodes [39–44]. However, the trend of larger molecules to remain at the injection site and their failure to enter in the lymphatic system may result in delayed or even no visualization of lymph nodes [45]. Therefore, the optimal colloidal size for lymphoscintigraphy is believed to be at least 80 nm and ideally around 200 nm [46].

There are significant advantages of using filtered ^{99m}Tc-sulfur colloid, including its low cost, excellent safety profile, and demonstrated clinical value. Nevertheless, this agent has several disadvantages, including minimal absorption from the injection site (typically <5% is absorbed), especially following subcutaneous administration, whereas intradermal administration is associated with faster absorption and visualization of the cutaneous lymphatics often within 1 min after radiocolloid injection. Even in the absence of beta radiation, the conversion electrons from ^{99m}Tc result in a radiation dose of 1–5 rads/injection site (depending on the volume of the injectate and activity administered).

The slow transit into the lymphatic system requires prolonged imaging times. Furthermore, the unpredictable nature of the absorption and transit can make it very difficult to reliably calculate tracer disappearance rates. ^{99m}Tc-sulfur colloid also requires an acidic pH to retain its stability, which often causes the patient to experience burning pain at the injection site [38]. The large particle size of ^{99m}Tc-sulfur colloid (30–1000 nm) [25] contributes to the minimal absorption and slow transit. An attempt to circumvent these difficulties led to the evaluation of filtered sulfur colloid for lymphoscintigraphy [25]. Utilization of a 0.1 μm filter yielded sulfur colloid with a stable particle size <50 nm. The properties of this filtered colloid are similar to those of antimony trisulfide colloid.

Albumin nanocolloid (Nanocoll®) has a reproducible colloid size distribution (95% of the particles being <80 nm) and ease of labeling. Its rapid clearance from the injection site makes it suitable for quantitative studies, and injections are reportedly painless. Thus, ^{99m}Tc-albumin nanocolloid may be more suitable for quantitative studies than ^{99m}Tc-sulfur colloid.

In addition to radiocolloids, a novel tracer with a retention mechanism in lymph nodes different from that of colloidal particles has recently been approved, both in the United States and in Europe, specifically for SLN mapping. ^{99m}Tc-mannosyl-DTPA-dextran (or ^{99m}Tc-tilmanocept, available commercially as Lymphoseek®) is a small-sized macromolecule with an average diameter equivalent to about 7.1 nm, which consists of a dextran backbone with multiple units of DTPA and of mannose covalently conjugated with the dextran backbone. The DTPA molecules serve for labeling with ^{99m}Tc, while the mannose residues determine the binding of ^{99m}Tc-tilmanocept to CD206 mannose receptors that are abundantly expressed on the surface of macrophages lining the lymph node sinusoid spaces. Advantages of ^{99m}Tc-tilmanocept versus the radiocolloid tracers commonly employed for SLN mapping include faster clearance from the site of interstitial injection (due to the small size of the agent), and higher retention in the SLN (due to an avid, specific ligand-receptor binding mechanism, which minimizes further migration of the agent to higher tier lymph nodes along the same lymphatic drainage pathway) [47].

Radioactive nanocolloids can also be used for PET, for example nanocolloidal albumin labeled with zirconium-89 (^{89}Zr, with physical decay half-life of 78 h) (Table 3.2) [48]. For the synthesis of this radiopharmaceutical, the precursor from the kit for labeling colloidal HSA with ^{99m}Tc was premodified with *p*-isothiocyanatobenzyl-desferrioxamine B (Df-Bz-NCS) and labeled with ^{89}Zr (Fig. 3.4).

To obtain Df-Bz-NCS-nanocolloidal albumin, polysorbate-citrate buffer (950 µL, pH 6.5) is added to the vial of nanocolloidal albumin (0.5 mg) followed by 45 µL of 0.1 M Na_2CO_3 to reach pH 9, and 167 nmol of Df-Bz-NCS in 20 µL of dimethyl sulfoxide (in 4–5 µL steps). After 30-min incubation at 37 °C, nonconjugated Df-Bz-NCS is removed by size-exclusion chromatography using a PD10 column and

polysorbate-citrate buffer at pH 6.5 as the eluent. Then, 200 µL of ^{89}Zr-oxalate (20–25 MBq) is added to a wobbling reaction vial followed by 90 µL of 2 M Na_2CO_3. After 3 min, the following solutions are added: 300 µL of 0.5 M N-(2-hydroxyethyl)piperazine-N9-(2-ethanesulfonic acid) buffer, pH 7.0; 710 µL of Df-Bz-NCS-nanocolloidal albumin (0.18 mg); and 700 µL of 0.5 M N-(2-hydroxyethyl) piperazine-N9-(2-ethanesulfonic acid) buffer, pH 7.0. The solution is incubated for 60 min at room temperature and then reaction mixture is purified through a PD10 column (eluent: polysorbate-citrate buffer, pH 6.5). No differences were observed between ^{89}Zr- and ^{99m}Tc-nanocolloidal albumin regarding particle size and uptake in the regional lymph nodes, thus indicating that coupling with ^{89}Zr does not alter the physic-chemical properties of nanocolloidal albumin.

3.2.2 Injected Volume and Activity for Lymphatic Mapping

The effects of varying concentrations of the particles and the influence of injected volume and activity parameters on the outcome of lymphoscintigraphy are still unclear. Bourgeois has investigated the effect of variable concentration (0.02 mg versus 0.2 mg) and volume (0.2 mL versus 1.0 mL) of ^{99m}Tc-HSA nanocolloids injected subcutaneously in the foot on lymph node uptake after 1 h during peripheral lymphoscintigraphy. He found that inguinal activity was highest using the highest quantity in the lowest volume [51].

Improvement in the SLN identification rate from 83 to 94% has been demonstrated with a 50% increase of injected activity [52]. Regarding volume of the injectate, because of the non-physiologic increase in interstitial pressure the administration of a large volume of injectate may lead to drainage toward both homoregional non-SLNs and to additional drainage regions [53].

Table 3.2 Radiopharmaceuticals for PET imaging of the lymphatic pathways

Radiotracer	Half-life	Ref
^{89}Zr-albumin nanocolloid (Nanocoll)	78.4 h	[48]
^{68}Ga-NEB	67 min	[49]
[^{18}F]AlF-NEB	110 min	[50]

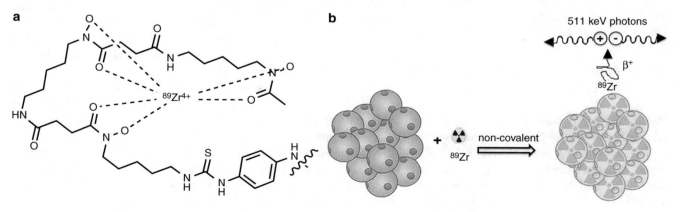

Fig. 3.4 Radiolabeling of compounds for lymphatic mapping with different positron-emitting radionuclides. (**a**) Df-Bz-NCS complex with ^{89}Zr^{4+}. (**b**) Radiolabeling of modified nanocolloids with ^{89}Zr

3.2.3 Factors Affecting Radiocolloid Uptake During Lymphatic Mapping

Mechanical massage over the radiocolloid injection site enhances the uptake and weakens the inverse correlation between particle size and speed of lymphatic drainage. Besides the influence of particle surface properties on radiocolloid uptake [31], an increase in venous pressure decreases concentration of macromolecules and leukocytes in the lymph [54]. Particle uptake by the lymphatic system is also temperature dependent. In this regard, protein transport across the canine lymphatic endothelium is enhanced with increasing temperature [55]. In addition to temperature, the pH of lymph or interstitial fluid may also alter lymph or particle uptake/transport. The colloid osmotic pressure of body fluids increases as pH increases (2.1 mmHg per pH-unit) [56]. Whether pH differences in interstitial or lymphatic fluid affect particle uptake in vivo, however, remains to be investigated.

Studies on prenodal collecting lymphatics of the lower extremities have shown that exercise indeed increases lymph flow [57, 58]. The type and intensity of the exercise have an important effect on the lymphatic function, and therefore on the outcome of a lymphoscintigraphic examination (see Chap. 4 for specific stress protocols).

Key Learning Points
- Following the pioneer studies on lymphatic circulation performed with colloidal ^{198}Au, the most widely employed agents for lymphatic mapping are colloidal particles labeled with ^{99m}Tc.
- The feasibility of lymphatic mapping with ^{18}F or ^{89}Zr labeling is also being explored.
- Injected volume and activity affect migration of the lymphatic mapping agents from the site of interstitial administration and their migration through the lymphatic circulation.
- Other physicochemical and biological factors affect radiocolloid uptake.

3.2.4 Other PET Radiopharmaceuticals for Lymphatic Mapping

PET lymphography has been investigated with intradermal administration of [^{18}F]FDG for combined diagnostic and intraoperative visualization of LNs [59]. Within 30 min after tracer injection, lymphatic vessels and LNs can be clearly revealed by PET in an animal modal. However, the clinical application of [^{18}F]FDG PET lymphography is challenged by the fast migration of the small molecules into blood circulation and it has never been translated into humans.

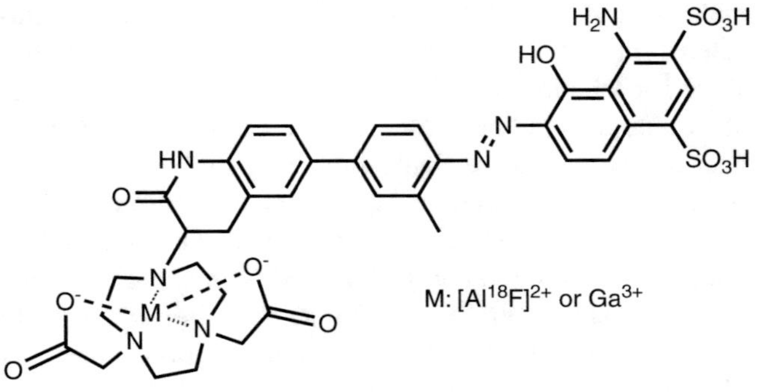

Fig. 3.5 Structure of ^{68}Ga-NEB or Al^{18}F-NEB

Recent developments of PET radiopharmaceuticals (Table 3.2) include a truncated form of the azo dye Evans blue (EB) after conjugation via a 1,4,7-triazacyclononane-N,N′,N″-triacetic acid (NOTA) linker (NEB) [60] labeled with either fluorine-18 by the formation of [^{18}F]aluminum fluoride complex ([^{18}F]AlF-NEB) or gallium-68 (^{68}Ga-NEB) (Fig. 3.5). The EB dye has high affinity for serum albumin and has been used clinically to determine blood volume [61]. Although recently discontinued in clinical practice, EB is still used as a sensitive marker of protein leakage from the vascular lumen in a variety of tissues during inflammation and traumatic injury [62]. After intravenous injection, [^{18}F]AlF-NEB complexed with serum albumin quickly, and thus most of the radioactivity remained in the blood circulation. [^{18}F]AlF-NEB has been successfully applied to evaluate cardiac function in a myocardial infarction model and vascular permeability in inflammatory and tumor models [50]; more recent studies have investigated [^{18}F]AlF-NEB along with the EB dye for lymphatic imaging after interstitial injection. ^{68}Ga-NEB synthesis consists of a mixture of ^{68}Ga freshly eluted from a ^{68}Ge/^{68}Ga generator using HCl 0.05 M and mixed with NaOAc 0.4 M to adjust pH to 4.5, to a vial containing the NEB, shaking, and incubation in a heating block at 95 °C for 10 min. Then, the product requires a passage through a C18 cartridge, elution with 2 mL of 80% ethanol/water, dilution in sterile saline solution, and filtration on a 0.22 μm aseptic filtration membrane. Quality control is performed with HPLC or ITLC, using $CH_3OH:NH_4OAc$ (v/v 1:1) as eluent [50].

After a mean injected dose of 139.5 ± 10.36 MBq (3.77 ± 0.28 mCi), PET images acquired at 30 min after intravenous administration showed cardiac ventricles, major arteries, and veins. The liver, spleen, and kidneys are also visible, with relatively low activity, whereas the bladder showed high activity, increasing over time. Although the blood vessels in the brain showed high radioactivity, the normal brain tissue had negligible accumulation of ^{68}Ga-NEB, indicating that the tracer does not cross the blood–brain barrier. The mean absorbed radiation doses based on multiple-

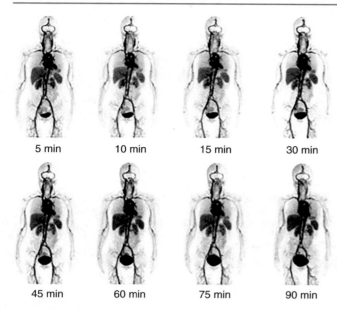

| 5 min | 10 min | 15 min | 30 min |
| 45 min | 60 min | 75 min | 90 min |

Fig. 3.6 Multiple-time-point whole-body maximum-intensity-projection PET images of a healthy woman at 5, 10, 15, 30, 45, 60, 75, and 90 min after intravenous administration of ⁶⁸Ga-NEB (*reproduced with permission from ref:* [63])

time-point PET revealed that the organs receiving relatively high doses were the kidneys, liver, spleen, and heart wall. The bladder wall also received high exposure due to renal excretion of the radioactivity (0.0683 ± 0.0090 mSv/MBq). The whole-body absorbed dose was 0.0151 ± 0.0001 mSv/MBq, with an effective dose of 0.0179 ± 0.0003 mSv/MBq. Upon PET/CT imaging, the LNs and lymphatic vessels as well as other desired tissues can be visualized, as shown in Fig. 3.6 [63].

After local administration, NEB forms a complex with albumin in the interstitial fluid and travels through the lymphatic system. Therefore, for the study of patients with lymphedema subcutaneous injection can be performed (see Chap. 4 for specific protocols).

Key Learning Points
- Newer perspectives for PET imaging of lymphatic circulation are based on the use of new radiopharmaceuticals including a truncated form of the azo dye Evans blue (EB) to be labeled with ⁶⁸Ga or ¹⁸F, after conjugation via a 1,4,7-triazacyclononane-N,N′,N″-triacetic acid (NOTA) linker (NEB).
- The synthesis of ⁶⁸Ga-NEB and [¹⁸F]AlF-NEB has been validated.
- Initial studies describe the biodistribution of NEB derivates in animal models as well as in humans, as evaluated by PET imaging.

3.3 Iodine-Based CT Contrast Agents for Lymphatic Mapping

In order to achieve higher levels of X-ray attenuation than those observed for biological tissue, elements of higher atomic number (Z) are incorporated into the contrast agent molecule. Iodine (Z = 53; M = 127) has historically been the atom of choice for CT imaging applications [64]. Sodium and lithium iodide were among the first water-soluble imaging agents. However, due to the associated toxicity at the iodine concentrations necessary for imaging they are not suitable for most clinical applications. Consequently, covalently bound iodine provides a better option in contrast media design.

Small-molecule iodinated contrast agents can be classified into two main categories: the "ionic" and "nonionic" molecules. Most ionic iodinated contrast agents studied to date are negatively charged species. Although widely used in the clinical routine, these ionic iodinated imaging agents possess several inherent disadvantages compared to nonionic contrast media.

Currently used contrast media exhibit high water solubility, low binding to biological receptors, low toxicity, and high bio-tolerability. A number of such contrast agents (both ionic and nonionic, and mono- and two-ring structures) are approved for medical use and clinically used worldwide (Table 3.3 and Fig. 3.7).

After i.v. injection, a contrast medium travels to the right heart, the pulmonary circulation, and the left heart before reaching the central arterial system. Contrast medium rapidly redistributes from the vascular to the interstitial spaces of the organs. Since iodinated contrast media consist of relatively small molecules that are highly diffusible, the transport of contrast media is predominantly "flow limited" and far less "diffusion limited." In a flow-limited process, the delivery of contrast medium through the circulatory system to an organ is a crucial determinant of contrast enhancement [65]. Well-perfused organs such as the kidney, the spleen, and the liver show high contrast enhancement during the initial circulation (first pass) of contrast medium to the organs. Contrast material-enhanced blood recirculates (normal recirculation may range in 15–40 s) and may contribute to the overall pattern of contrast enhancement achieved at CT imaging acquisition. For relatively long i.v. infusions, recir-

Table 3.3 Some common commercially available small-molecule iodinated contrast agents and their indicated clinical uses [64]

Common name	Commercial name	Manufacturer
Iohexol	Omnipaque™	GE Healthcare
Iopromide	Ultravist™	Bayer Healthcare
Iodixanol	Visipaque™	GE Healthcare
Ioxaglate	Hexabrix™	Mallinckrodt Imaging
Iothalamate	Cysto-Conray II™	Mallinckrodt Imaging
Iopamidol	Isovue™	Bracco Imaging

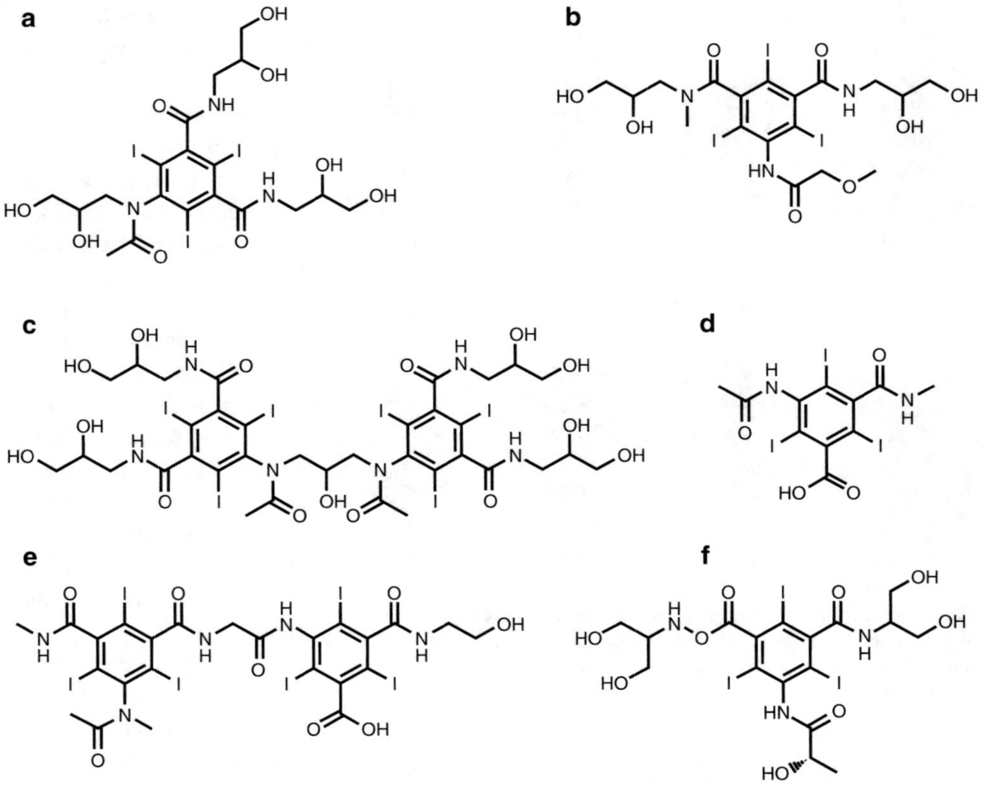

Fig. 3.7 Common iodinated contrast agents: (**a**) iohexol; (**b**) iopromide; (**c**) iodixanol; (**d**) ioxaglate; (**e**) iothalamate; (**f**) iopamidol

culation can even occur during the infusion of the contrast material [66].

Contrast enhancement at CT is affected by numerous interacting factors: patient (i.e., patient body size, cardiovascular circulation time, age, sex, venous access, renal function, hepatic disease), type and modality of contrast medium administration (i.e., duration of injection, injection rate, shape of injection bolus shape, contrast medium volume, concentration, physicochemical properties, use of a saline flush), and CT scanning. Contrast medium pharmacokinetics and contrast enhancement are determined solely by the patient and contrast medium factors and are independent from the CT scanning technique. Nevertheless, CT scanning factors play a critical role by allowing us to acquire contrast-enhanced images at a specific time point of contrast enhancement.

While current clinically approved small-molecule iodinated CT contrast agents offer safety and imaging efficacy, they do suffer from several drawbacks, which prevent them from being used for all applications:

- Nonspecific biodistribution.
- As small-molecular-weight molecules, they tend to undergo rapid renal clearance.
- High osmolality and/or high viscosity of the contrast media formulations can lead to renal toxicity [67–69] and/or adverse physiological effects [70–72].
- High "per-dose" concentrations are required.

- High rates of extravasation and equilibration between intravascular and extravascular compartments at the capillary level often make it difficult to obtain meaningful and clear CT images [73–75].

Contrast agents can access the lymphatic system by three different routes: intravenous, intralymphatic (direct lymphatic injection), or interstitial. Contrast agents for direct intralymphatic injection are not being developed due to the inherent difficulties in finding and cannulating the lymphatic vessels. Thus, the newer contrast agents tend to follow the other two routes. Methods developed for cancer imaging may well have application in other diseases affecting the lymphatics.

An iodized oil-in-water emulsion in which lipiodol was emulsified by a surfactant mixture (Tween 80 as the main surfactant and TPGS, Kollidon 12 PF, or Span 85 as the co-surfactant) was investigated in a preclinical study, showing that all the three types of emulsions formulated with different co-surfactants exhibited similar mean particle sizes (approximately 120–130 nm), and they were all effectively taken up in the targeted lymph node without significant differences in the mean values of peak Hounsfield units (HU), time to peak HU, and sustained enhancement duration. Lymph nodes showed peak enhancement 4–8 h after injection with sustained contrast enhancement, which means that the time window for CT can be expanded, in comparison with CT lymphography, using iopamidol. In addition, the compound was completely eliminated on delayed CT imaging, in contrast with lipiodol. CT lymphography using lipiodol showed continuously increased attenuation values even after 1 week [76].

In dogs, at lower injection volumes (0.1–0.5 mL), uptake of contrast material in target lymph nodes appeared incomplete, although the node was still well visualized. When larger volumes (2–4 mL) of contrast material were injected, marked opacification of target nodes occurred with good definition of lymph node margins. The dose response to iodinated particles injected subcutaneously or submucosally is predictable in terms of total iodine uptake and as measured by attenuation (HU) or iodine concentration in normal lymph nodes. Within the imaging time range evaluated, peak enhancement of lymph nodes appears to occur between 12 and 24 h after injection of contrast material. In cancerous lymph nodes, although nodes with greater than 25% tumor replacement were larger and had a higher total iodine uptake per node, node opacification (as expressed in HU or milligrams of iodine per cubic centimeter of lymph node tissue) was less than that in normal nodes and in lymph nodes with 25% or less tumor replacement. In addition, characteristic architectural alterations, including changes in the cortex, medulla, and cortico-medullary junction that resulted from the presence of tumor deposits, were useful in distinguishing between normal and cancerous lymph nodes [77]. In patients with breast cancer, 2 mL of iopamidol was administered into the two skin areas (the border between the upper medial and lateral quadrants, and the border between the lower medial and quadrants) overlying the left mammary gland, dividing the volume equally to identity SLNs. The exact mechanism(s) of iopamidol uptake and transport in the lymphatic system is still unknown. This agent appears to penetrate easily into the lymphatics through the clefts in the terminal lymphangioles of the interstitial space, as with other water-soluble, low-molecular-weight solutes. The relatively long duration of the nodal enhancement may be related to slow transit and sequestration of iopamidol in the lymph node sinusoid spaces.

Key Learning Points
- Iodine-based CT contrast agents can be classified into two main categories: the "ionic" molecules and the "nonionic" molecules.
- Biodistribution of iodinated contrast agents varies according to various factors that affect their binding to plasma proteins and/or to other endogenous compounds.
- High-viscosity iodinated contrast agents are being investigated as to their ability to explore the lymphatic structures and circulation.
- There are well-known drawbacks in the use of iodinated contrast media that should always be considered before administration to patients.

3.4 MR, MRL, and PET/MRI Contrast Agents for Lymphatic Mapping

The MRI signal arises from the excitation of low-energy nuclear spins, which occur in a permanent magnetic field by applying radiofrequency pulses followed by measurement of the spin relaxation processes (i.e., T1 recovery or T2 decay). Different chemical environments as well as water concentration result in different signal strengths and therefore provide contrast between fat, tissue, and bones. Paramagnetic compounds can be used to enhance the contrast of MR images by promoting relaxation of water near the compound. MRI contrast agents are classified as either T1 (i.e., positive) or T2 (i.e., negative).

The contrast agents in clinical use are low-molecular-weight Gd^{3+}-based complexes (0.5–1 kDa) with one molecule of water in the inner sphere [78] and relaxivity ranging from 3 to 5 mM/s at 1.5 or 3 T (clinical magnetic fields).

The macromolecular contrast agent albumin–gadolinium diethylenetriamine penta-acetic acid (albumin-Gd-DTPA) consists of human serum albumin to which paramagnetic properties are conferred by covalent binding from 9 to 18 Gd-DTPA-chelates per protein molecule. Whereas Gd-DTPA distributes from the intravascular to the extravascular space and is rapidly cleared from the body through renal excretion [79], making it unfavorable as a blood pool agent, albumin-Gd-DTPA shows high relaxivity and remains largely confined to intravascular spaces [80, 81]. This compound has been used to quantify delivery, transport rates, and volumes of macromolecular fluid flow through the interstitial-lymphatic continuum in tumors [82].

Intracutaneous injection of extracellular, paramagnetic contrast agents has recently been proposed for identifying abnormal lymphatic pathways by MR lymphography (MRL) [83–85]. These agents include Gd-labeled dendrimers [86, 87], macrocyclic Gd complexes [83], and Gd-labeled dextran [88] (Table 3.4 and Fig. 3.8).

Table 3.4 Main features of Gd-based contrast agents with potential use of MR lymphography

Contrast agent	Enhancement and physicochemical effect	References
Gd-DOTA	Positive-ionic-macrocyclic	[78, 89]
Gd-DTPA	Positive-ionic-linear	[78, 90]
Gd-DTPA-BMA	Positive-ionic-linear	[91]
Gd-HP-DO3A	Positive-ionic-macrocyclic	[92]
Gd-DTPA-BMEA	Positive-ionic-linear	[93]
Gd-DO3A-butrol	Positive-ionic-macrocyclic	[78]
Gd-BOPTA	Positive-ionic-linear	[78]

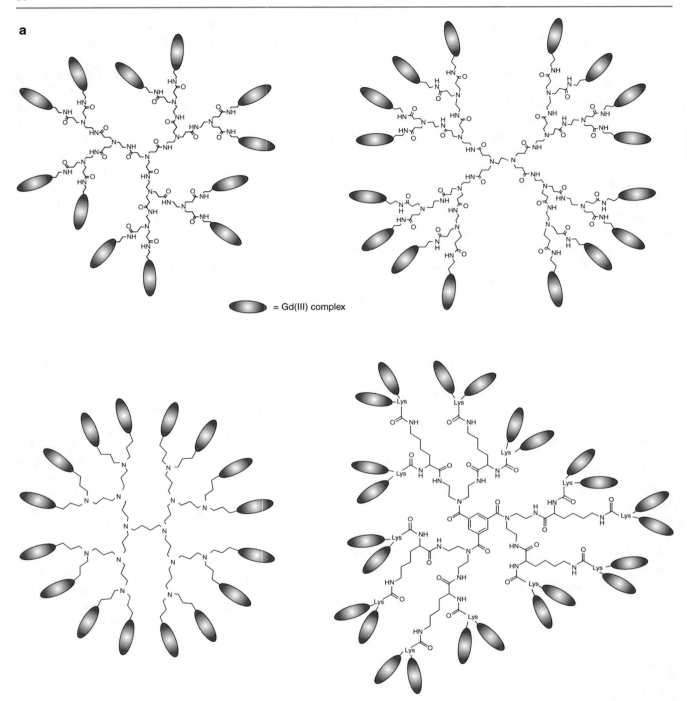

= Gd(III) complex

Fig. 3.8 Most common Gd complexes used as MRI contrast-enhancement agents. (**a**) Gd-labeled dendrimers. (**b**) Macrocyclic Gd complexes. (**c**) Gd-labeled dextran (*reproduced with permission from ref.* [78])

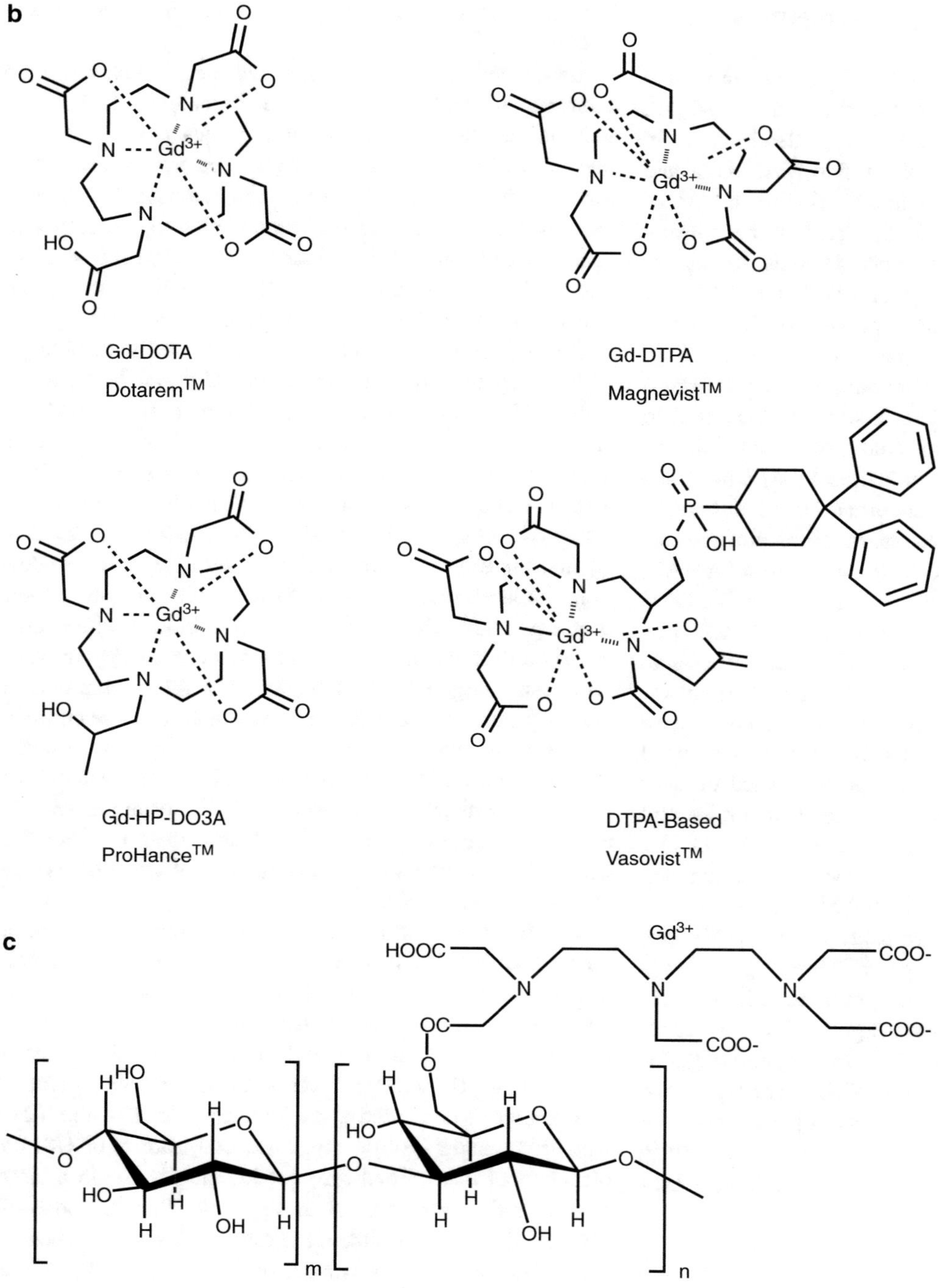

b

Gd-DOTA

Dotarem™

Gd-DTPA

Magnevist™

Gd-HP-DO3A

ProHance™

DTPA-Based

Vasovist™

c

Fig. 3.8 (continued)

3.4.1 Dendrimers for Lymphatic Mapping

This definition identifies a family of synthetic monodispersed polymers that can be produced at predefined and chemically identical sizes. Two forms of dendrimers are commercially available: poly-amidoamine (PAMAM) and diaminobutane-core poly-propylimine (DAB or PPI). Different generations (sizes) of dendrimers have been investigated as MRL macromolecular contrast agents. Kobayashi et al. used interstitially injected generation-6 (G6) PAMAM dendrimers to image the lymphatic system and SLNs in normal mice and in mice with xenografted breast tumors [94]. G6 was injected directly into the mammary gland or peritumorally, and three-dimensional reconstruction was used to aid anatomical localization. The same group used a similar contrast agent in a mouse lymphoma model [95]. They were able to differentiate normal and abnormal lymphatics and to distinguish intralymphatic from extra-lymphatic disease. Kobayashi et al. also compared MRL with either PAMAM dendrimers of different generations or less hydrophilic DAB generations in murine models [86]. PAMAM-G8 was retained in the fine lymphatic vessels without major leakage, thus resulting in excellent imaging of the lymphatic channels. However, PAMAM-G4 provided a better contrast of lymph nodes that were close to the liver, due to a reduced background signal. DAB dendrimers are expected to clear more rapidly from the circulation due to their uptake and excretion by the liver and kidneys. Indeed, DAB-G5 was cleared more rapidly from the lymphatic vessels, but retained in the lymph nodes. Therefore, PAMAM dendrimers may perform better for imaging the lymphatics, while DAB dendrimers are more optimal for lymph node imaging.

Another interesting advance in lymph node imaging is the use of dual-modality contrast agents. Talanov et al. synthesized a PAMAM G6 dendrimer conjugated to gadolinium for MRL and to the cyanine derivative Cy5.5 for optical imaging [96]. The agent was injected into the mammary fat pad of mice and SLNs were successfully imaged on MRI, followed by similarly successful optical imaging.

3.4.2 Superparamagnetic Iron Oxide Particles (SPIONs and USPIOs) for Lymphatic Mapping

Superparamagnetic iron oxide nanoparticles (SPIONs) [97] are single-domain magnetic iron oxide particles with hydrodynamic diameters ranging from single nanometers to >100 nm [98–100]. SPIONs are typically classified into three categories based on their hydrodynamic diameter: (1) oral (large) SPIONs at 300 nm–3.5 μm, (2) standard (regular) SPION (SSPIO) nanoparticles at 50–150 nm, and (3) ultrasmall SPIO (USPIOs) nanoparticles less than 50 nm [99, 100].

Larger SPIONs exhibit higher nonspecific uptake by the mononuclear phagocyte system or reticuloendothelial system than smaller USPIOs, which indicates a higher percentage of passive uptake of larger particles for tissues rich in macrophages, such as the liver, spleen, lymph nodes, or bone marrow [99]. Faster biodegradation rates in the liver and spleen have been recently reported for monodisperse 5 nm iron oxide cores in comparison with 15 and 30 nm iron oxide cores coated with the same coating molecules [101].

SPIONs can be monodisperse and coated with biologically compatible ligands, are chemically and biologically stable [102], and are generally nontoxic in vivo [103]. However, commercially available SPION contrast agents are composed of polydisperse inorganic cores ranging from ~16 to ~200 nm. Generally, large SPIONs function as T2 contrast agents, whereas small SPIOs have limited T2 activity and therefore are potential T1 contrast agents. In addition, the large size of existing SPIONs [104] prevents their efficient renal clearance after i.v. administration, thus greatly differing from GBCA as to their clearance pathways. As a result, large HD SPIONs predominantly accumulate in the body [105] and can cause a persistent negative contrast over several weeks or months, which prevents repeated imaging studies and limits the clinical management of patients. Furthermore, current SPION formulations are almost quantitatively metabolized and absorbed into the iron pool, thus potentially causing clinical side effects due to iron overload [105].

USPIOs are macromolecular MR contrast agents with a long serum half-life that can be utilized for systemic lymph node imaging. Following intravenous injection, they are phagocytosed by circulating macrophages and transported to the lymph nodes. Clustering of the iron oxide particles within these phagocytic cells produces local field inhomogeneities and results in decreased signal intensity on T2- and T2*-weighted images [106]. The pharmacodynamics of USPIO dictates that the optimal time for imaging is 24–36 h after administration. Anzai et al. have shown that the dose of USPIO administered affects the degree of signal reduction [107]. They injected dose ranges of 0.3–1.7 mg Fe/kg in five healthy volunteers. The 1.7 dose produced the greatest signal decrease on T2*-weighted imaging. Further studies have suggested that a higher dose of 2.6 mg Fe/kg performs even better. However, the higher concentrations of iron within the lymph node may mask small intranodal tumor cell foci [108]. The translation of these macromolecules into clinical application is restricted by delayed renal clearance and uptake into the reticuloendothelial system. Furthermore, interstitial MRL with commercially available extracellular Gd chelates is markedly limited by nonspecific distribution. In fact, the contrast agents circulate and then freely distribute in the extracellular space. Extracellular fluid agents are mainly eliminated by renal excretion. Gadolinium enters the liver through the hepatic artery and portal vein, and is freely redistributed into the interstitial space. In contrast to iodine molecules, which are imaged by CT, the effect of gadolinium is assessed by MR imaging rather than by imaging the molecule itself. Gadolinium exhibits an amplification effect, because several adjacent water protons surrounding a gadolinium atom are relaxed.

Despite the promise of MMCMs for use in MRL, USPIOs are the only agents that have been investigated in humans. Iron oxide-based contrast agents seem ideally suited to lymph node imaging when used for staging purposes. However, for SLN mapping, interstitial injection of Gd-based macromolecules, such as dendrimers, seems to be a superior choice.

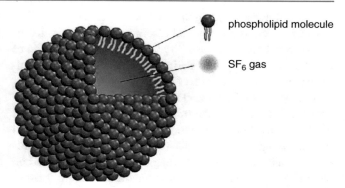

Fig. 3.9 General structure of microbubbles (*reproduced with permission from ref* [117])

Key Learning Points
- Contrast agents for MR imaging, MR lymphography, and PET/MRI are described in this section.
- Gadolinium contrast agents for MRI include Gd-labeled dendrimers, macrocyclic Gd complexes, and Gd-labeled dextran.
- The use and biodistribution of superparamagnetic iron nanoparticles as MR contrast agents are described in this section.

3.5 Contrast-Enhanced Ultrasound Imaging for Lymphatic Mapping

Contrast-enhanced ultrasound (CEUS) using microbubbles has been widely used both in preclinical experiments and in the clinical setting [109–116]. Microbubbles are gas-filled particles with an average diameter of several micrometers (Fig. 3.9). Microbubbles larger than red blood cells (RBCs) would be trapped in the capillaries, and submicron-size microbubbles scatter ultrasound poorly and have insufficient stability. During ultrasonography, the energy pulses generated by the transducer array cause rapid variations of pressure (up to several megapascals) in tissues. Therefore, microbubbles in blood undergo volume oscillations at clinical diagnostic ultrasound imaging frequencies (1–15 MHz). Microbubbles vibrate, resonate, and re-emit sound, and resulting backscatter ultrasound signal is detected. The re-emitted ultrasound contains signal at harmonic frequencies [118]. Sensitive microbubble detection relies on the ability of the imaging system to differentiate bubble backscatter signal from tissue background. Modern ultrasound imaging techniques can depict individual bubbles with particle mass less than 1 pg [119]; hence the required mass of ultrasound

contrast material is low, comparable with the dose of some nuclear medicine agents. For clinical enhancement of the blood pool, a microbubble contrast aqueous dispersion volume of 0.1–5 mL (concentration ≈109 bubbles/mL) is routinely injected or infused i.v.

Once administered i.v., micron-size bubbles circulate in the bloodstream for minutes [120]. The bubble clearance mechanism is different from clearance of other types of microparticles and nanoparticles, in that gas is cleared through gas exchange via expiration by the lungs. For example, within 6 min after i.v. administration of perflutren (Optison), 99.9% of C_3F_8 is exhaled. Residual microbubble shell material and some intact bubbles are cleared by phagocytosis (the rate of this process depends on the bubble shell material and PEG coat) [121]. The major sites for microbubble accumulation are the liver (Kupffer cells) and spleen (macrophages) [122, 123].

Ultrasound contrast agents are generally considered safe, since serious adverse events have been reported very rarely [124]. In 2007, the U.S. Food and Drug Administration (FDA) introduced a "black box" warning for microbubble use owing to the risk of serious cardiopulmonary reactions in some patients. The warning was later relaxed because it was recognized that the rate of adverse reactions of microbubbles is comparable to or lower than that of other types of contrast agents [125], and use of microbubbles does not affect mortality in an undesired way [126].

In preclinical studies, microbubbles have been shown to accumulate in SLNs but not in second-tier lymph nodes, probably due to the avidity of macrophages for the shell material [127, 128]. In a pilot clinical trial, patients with breast cancer received a periareolar intradermal injection of microbubbles preoperatively, lymphatic channels were visualized immediately by ultrasonography, and putative axillary SLNs were identified. The sensitivity of SLN detection in this study was 89% [129]. Similar to MRI, differentiation of benign and malignant lymph nodes can be achieved with CEUS because of the different accumulation of microbubbles in normal and metastatic LNs [130]. Several limitations of CEUS prevent broad application of this technique for SLN mapping, such as poor spatial resolution, slow migration of the microbubble, inaccessibility to ultrasound exploration of the thorax and deep retroperitoneum, as well as its dependence on operator experience [131].

Photoacoustic imaging (PAI) is a hybrid imaging modality based on the detection of the ultrasonic waves generated by pulse laser-induced transient thermoelastic expansion within biological tissues [132–135]. In combination with different contrast agents including methylene blue, carbon nanotubes, gold nanocages, gold nanorods, and gold nanobeacons [136–139], PAI showed potential for improved detection of metastases in preclinical models. However, no clinical application has been reported so far, possibly due to the lack of bedside imaging system. In addition, the still limited signal penetration and challenges in control of the surgical field with conductive gel currently constitute serious drawbacks of this imaging technique.

> **Key Learning Points**
> - Microbubbles used for contrast-enhanced ultrasound imaging are described in this section.
> - The biodistribution of microbubbles used for contrast-enhanced ultrasound imaging is described in this section.
> - Microbubbles for contrast-enhanced ultrasound imaging are being employed in preclinical and clinical trials as lymphatic mapping agents.

3.6 Optical Imaging Agents for Lymphatic Mapping

Optical imaging is a rapidly advancing branch of medical imaging. The method does not imply radiation exposure, although the main advantage of optical imaging lies in its high resolution and its ability to image at a molecular level.

Substances that absorb light energy change to an unstable excitation state from the ground state and then revert back to the ground state after energy transition. This energy transition includes vibrational energy, heat energy, and light energy (fluorescence). A substance that selectively absorbs light of a certain wavelength is called a chromophore. When it emits fluorescence after absorption of excitation light, it is called a fluorophore. In most cases, fluorescent light has lower energy and a longer wavelength than the excitation light, since fluorophores release a certain amount of energy in the form of vibrational relaxation before photoemission. Some fluorophores can be administered into the body to act as a kind of imaging contrast medium; these fluorophores are called exogenous fluoro-

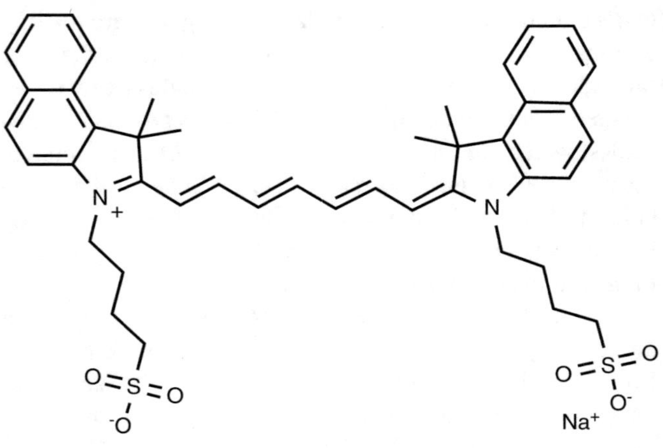

Fig. 3.10 Chemical structure of indocyanine green (ICG)

phores. The body intrinsically emits fluorescence, as many components of the body exhibit weak fluorescence (autofluorescence); these components are called endogenous fluorophores. Organic fluorophores include fluoresceins, rhodamines, and most cyanines. Among the many kinds of fluorophores, fluorescence tracers for biological application are limited to biomolecules that emit near-infrared (NIR) spectrum wavelengths to minimize autofluorescence and improve signal-to-background ratios. Hemoglobin, muscle, and fat are least absorbent in this light range, thus allowing deeper tissue penetration of photons [140].

Currently, the U.S. FDA-approved fluorescent contrasts include only fluorescein and indocyanine green (ICG) (Fig. 3.10). Newer organic fluorophores, including sulfonated indocyanine dyes (e.g., Cy 7), sulfonated carbocyanine dyes (e.g., Alexa Fluor 750), and sulfonated rhodamine dye (e.g., Alexa Fluor 633), are synthetic fluorescent dyes with better optical characteristics and are more photostable and brighter than the preexisting original dyes [141]. Fluorescent probes are safe and they can be conjugated to antibodies, peptides, or proteins as optimal lymphatic tracers due to their small size. Since the conjugations of fluorophore and macromolecules may have a toxicity profile different from its original components separately, their toxicity must be validated before clinical application. Furthermore, the optimal fluorescent signals are still insufficient to provide adequate image quality as compared to inorganic fluorophores, although their fluorescence is more intense than fluorescein or ICG. The main disadvantage remains the poor depth sensitivity of the technique, since penetration beyond 1–2 cm is currently unrealistic; this factor mainly limits its use to animal studies or to human applications that require only superficial imaging (e.g., SLN imaging).

ICG is an amphiphilic, tricarbocyanine iodide dye (mass = 751.4 Da) that is reconstituted in aqueous solution of pH 6.5 for intravenous injection. ICG was introduced as a blood pool agent to measure cardiac output and was granted FDA approval in 1959 [142]. Intravascularly, the compound binds to plasma proteins that confine most of the bolus to the intravascular space until hepatic uptake and excretion into bile (with clearance rate of 18–24% per minute by the liver) [143]. The plasma proteins, notably serum albumin and α- and β-lipoproteins, bind to the lipophilic component of ICG by the hydrophobic regions of the proteins [144]. This interaction does not alter the protein structure but produces a nontoxic interface and decreases extravasation of the dye [145]. Plasma proteins compete with the tendency of the dye to aggregate in the blood; protein binding leads to the formation of ICG monomers from aggregates in an attempt to establish equilibrium [145]. Of the injected ICG, 98% is bound to plasma proteins while the remaining 2% is free in the serum. Free ICG is then excreted into the bile by glutathione S-transferase, while bound ICG remains within the intravascular space for a longer period [146].

While occupying the intravascular space, the continuing decomposition reaction of ICG releases singlet oxygen molecules that bind to the breakdown products and thermally decompose into carbonyl compounds of low toxicity. Since the singlet oxygen remains within the ICG system, the dye has an LD_{50} (50% lethal dose) of 50–80 mg/kg. With a standard dose of less than 2 mg/kg, ICG is virtually nontoxic, provided that the patient does not suffer from allergy to iodide. The quick clearance rate allows the dye to be used for multiple injections during a procedure, thus being advantageous over other similar substances such as the clinical dye bromsulfthalein [147]. In general, ICG is regarded as safe; however, caution should be adopted in patients with renal failure [148]. Although ICG appears dark green under natural light, it appears more fluorescent than green once injected into the human body in amounts <20 mg [149]. The molecule is generally excited between 750 and 800 nm, and fluorescence is viewed around the maximum peak of 832 nm [143].

Although ICG interacts with plasma proteins, its tendency toward aggregation must be considered to set appropriate parameters for its application. For intravenous injection, water is the desired solvent as the sulfate group of ICG promotes its solubility, while saline solution promotes aggregation of the molecule. The concentration of the dye must be kept below 15 mg/L in the body when used for fluorescent studies, because at higher concentrations it begins to aggregate as a result of van der Waals attractions [144]. In addition to aggregation properties, ICG is relatively unstable before injection and is weakly fluorescent compared with alternative agents. The aqueous solution for injection has limited stability, especially when exposed to light, and must be used within 6–10 h after dilution [143]. As a result, ICG is produced and distributed as a powder for medical applications to reduce its decomposition before use.

Recent advances of nanotechnology have led to the development of quantum dots (QDs). A QD is a nano-sized crystal composed of semiconductor materials (Fig. 3.11). When QDs absorb enough light energy to cause an electron to leave the valence band and to enter the conduction band, an electron-hole pair is produced. During the recombination process between the electron and the hole, light is emitted [19, 28]. The emission wavelength is closely associated with both the composition and size of the QD. As a consequence, the wavelength is dependent on the particle size when the material that makes up QDs is the same. Therefore, by changing the size of QDs, various emission wavelengths can be simultaneously produced by a single-excitation light pulse, a property which enables multiplexed biological imaging. Advantages of QD over conventional fluorophores include a wider excitation range, a sharp and nearly symmetrical emission peak, higher quantum yields, greater penetration depth, longer photostability, and resistance to photobleaching (due to their inorganic composition) [151, 152].

An in vivo multicolor lymphatic imaging technique with QD has been successfully employed in animal models [153]. Kim et al. used type II QD, coated with polydentate phosphine to allow solubility and serum stability in mouse and pig models [154]. A 400 pm concentration of quantum dots was injected intradermally for SLN imaging. This method of SLN lymphog-

Fig. 3.11 Schematic representation of the structure and chemico-physical properties of a quantum dot (QD) (*reproduced with permission from ref* [150])

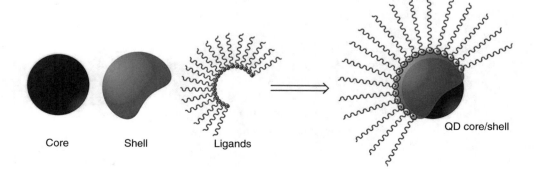

Core   Shell   Ligands   QD core/shell

raphy was then shown to be equivalent to the traditional "blue dye" method, showing lymph nodes up to 1 cm deep, along with the lymphatic vessels. This technique may also allow more accurate fluorescence analysis of SLNB specimens.

A critical limitation of QD technology is its potential toxicity, since many of the current-generation QDs are based on a cadmium-selenium core. However, newer, more biocompatible high-yield fluorescent nanoparticles are being developed [155]. The size of QDs makes them ideal candidates for imaging the lymphatic system following interstitial injection. Hama et al. have shown the ability of fluorescence lymphangiography using two NIR QDs with different emission spectra to visualize two separate lymphatic flows that drain into a common nodal basin [153]. Two QDs with emission peaks of 705 and 800 nm were injected simultaneously into the mouse mammary fat pad and the middle phalanx of the upper extremity, respectively. The lymphatics were successfully imaged as they drained into the axillary lymph nodes. This technique could offer SLN detection while concurrently predicting the likelihood, or potential avoidance, of lymphedema following subsequent treatment. Padera et al. have demonstrated the use of multiphoton laser scanning microscopy (MPLSM) to obtain images of deep lymphatic vessels [156]. MPLSM uses a solid-state laser to produce photons in pulses, and a computer-controlled scanning mirror for detection. The light produced is in the infrared spectrum; thus the photons are of a longer wavelength than confocal laser scanning microscopes, and are, therefore, less damaging to tissues and able to achieve greater depth penetration. Padera et al. showed an increased ability to quantify lymphatic size and were able to accurately calculate the density of angiogenic vessels. Leu et al. have shown the reliability of optical imaging techniques in humans. They compared 16 patients with systemic sclerosis with 16 age-matched controls. Imaging of the fingers demonstrated evidence of lymphatic microangiopathy in the affected skin of systemic sclerosis patients [157]. The advances summarized above, along with the development of newer biocompatible fluorescent markers, might in the future allow optical techniques to be more widely used in patients.

Key Learning Points
- Indocyanine green (ICG) and quantum dots (QD) are used as optical imaging agents.
- Upon intravenous administration, ICG interacts with plasma proteins in a variety of ways.
- Upon interstitial administration, ICG can be used for optical guidance during lymphatic mapping for SLNB.
- The physicochemical properties of quantum dots and their applications for lymphatic mapping are described in this section.

3.7 Multimodal Tracers for Lymphatic Mapping

The recent development of nanotechnology has enabled to produce new multimodality functional imaging probes. PET/optical dual-functional imaging probes are imaging agents which combine both a PET tracer and fluorescent tracer, allowing the convenient use of the combined system with single injection [158]. Fluorescence and gamma-emitting agents can also be conjugated for preoperative imaging and for intraoperative guidance [149]. In fact, the radionuclide provides deep-tissue imaging of the whole body, while optical imaging enables a longitudinal study even after radionuclide decay. Moreover, optical and PET or SPECT imaging can be cross-validated with dual-function probes, since replacing isotopes with fluorescent markers may affect the biodistribution of a tracer [159]. For example, Evans blue (EB), a dye molecule binding with plasma proteins, has been labeled with ^{99m}Tc (^{99m}Tc-EB, Fig. 3.12) for SLN mapping. ^{99m}Tc-EB combines both radioactive and optical signals and can be administered as a single injection for SLN identification [160]. A hybrid fluorescent-radioactive tracer has also been applied for SLN mapping by mixing ICG with ^{99m}Tc-labeled albumin nanocolloid (Fig. 3.13) [161]. The lymphatic drainage pattern of ICG/^{99m}Tc-nanocolloid is identical to that of ^{99m}Tc-nanocolloid in the clinical setting and all preoperatively identified SLNs could be localized using combined radio- and fluorescence guidance intraoperatively.

Similarly, NIR/MR dual probes for lymphatic imaging have also been developed [162]. With these probes, both NIR and MR imaging can be obtained following a single injection. Most of the PET/MR and SPECT/MR bimodal imaging probes are nanoparticles or nano-sized structures, because it is difficult for small molecules to carry two or more imaging reporters and even targeting groups as a single entity due to their limited loading capacity (Table 3.5). The advantage of nano-sized structures is that they allow for carrying multimodal imaging reporters and targeting biomolecules. Approaches for the development of novel multimodal PET/SPECT-MR probes are mainly through surface modifications, by conjugating an MR imaging reporter such as paramagnetic Gd^{3+} or superparamagnetic iron oxides (SPIOs),

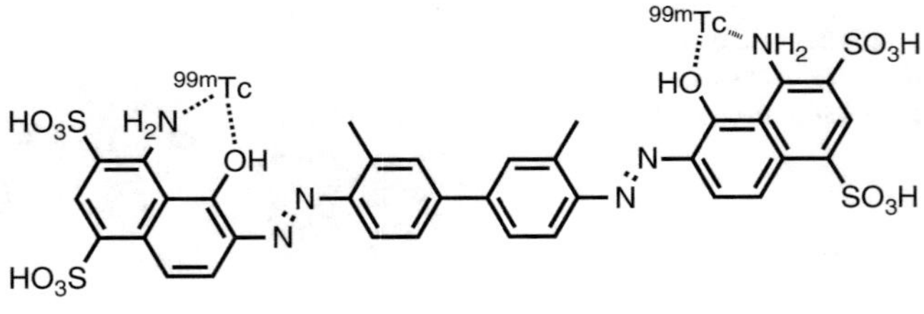

Fig. 3.12 Chemical structure of ^{99m}Tc-labeled Evans blue (^{99m}Tc-EB), with two ^{99m}Tc atoms conjugated with a single EB molecule

Fig. 3.13 Schematic process of ICG conjugation with ^{99m}Tc-albumin nanocolloid. γ denotes radiation emitted from the radionuclide ^{99m}Tc, while λ denotes frequency of lights exciting ICG and, in turn, emitted by ICG (*reproduced with permission from ref* [89]: *Buckle T, van Leeuwen AC, Chin PT, Janssen H, Muller SH, Jonkers J, et al. A self-assembled multimodal complex for combined pre- and intraoperative imaging of the SLN. Nanotechnology. 2010;21(35):355101*)

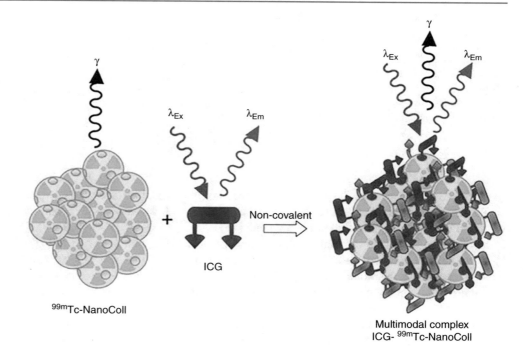

^{99m}Tc-NanoColl

ICG

Non-covalent

Multimodal complex
ICG- ^{99m}Tc-NanoColl

Table 3.5 Bimodal agents for imaging lymph nodes (LNs), including SLN mapping

Probe	PET or SPECT reporter	MR reporter	Applications	References
^{124}I-SA-MnMEIO	^{124}I	MnFe$_2$O$_4$	Axillary and brachial LNs imaging	[163]
^{68}Ga-NOTA-IO-Man	^{68}Ga	SPIO	LN imaging	[164]
^{64}Cu-DTCBP-SPION	^{64}Cu	SPION	LN mapping	[165]
^{99m}Tc-SPIONs	^{99m}Tc	SPION	SLN mapping	[166]
^{69}Ge-SPION	^{69}Ge	SPION	SLN mapping	[167]
^{89}Zr-ferumoxytol	^{89}Zr	Ferumoxytol	SLN mapping	[168]

and by incorporating a PET/SPECT radionuclide together with other functionalities.

SPIOs with a composition of MnFe$_2$O$_4$ (MnMEIO) coated with serum albumin were used to radiolabel the protein with ^{124}I (^{124}I-SA-MnMEIO) as a bimodal imaging probe to image SLNs in vivo [163]. ^{124}I-SA-MnMEIO can be directly radiolabeled by conjugation of ^{124}I with the ortho position of tyrosine residue in albumin using Iodo-Beads. The ^{124}I ion from Iodo-Beads in solution will be oxidized to form a reactive ^{124}ICl species, which reacts with the ortho position of tyrosine. Two different LNs, brachial and axillary LNs, could be clearly identified and localized with PET/MR fusion imaging; however, axillary LN was unambiguously spotted when MRI single modality was used only due to its location far

from the injection site compared with brachial LN. A dual-PET/MR imaging probe, ^{68}Ga-NOTA-IO-MAN, was synthesized using a new methodology for targeting LNs [164]. A different strategy was developed to radiolabel clinically approved SPIOs such as Endorem/Feridex. A bifunctional chelator dithiocarbamate bisphosphonate (DTCBP) was conjugated with Endorem with high affinity for both the metallic radionuclide ^{64}Cu and dextran-coated SPIO nanoparticles to facilitate the radiolabeling in high yields, providing a highly stable bimodal probe both in vitro and in vivo [165]. PET/MR imaging studies confirmed the dual probe's potential for imaging SLN in a non-tumor model. SPIOs radiolabeled with ^{99m}Tc were reported as a dual-SPECT/MR probes feasible for imaging SLNs [166]. Both SPECT and MR images showed the accumulation of ^{99m}Tc-SPIONs in LNs after subcutaneous injection in rats. The high uptake of ^{99m}Tc-SPIONs found in SLN from biodistribution studies indicated that ^{99m}Tc-SPIONs could have future applications in breast cancer and malignant melanoma. Inspired by the technology that the parent ^{68}Ge radionuclide in the ^{68}Ge/^{68}Ga generator is bound to metal oxide TiO$_2$, the SPIONs were labeled with ^{69}Ge in the absence of a chelator, as a PET/MR probe. Incorporating PET radionuclides such as ^{69}Ge and ^{59}Fe into SPIOs without a chelator during the nanoparticle synthesis is one of the new synthetic approaches to generating multimodal nanoparticles. For example, a dual-PET/MR probe ^{69}Ge-SPION@PEG was prepared by incorporating ^{69}Ge, which was generated by ^{69}Ga(p,n)^{69}Ge from a cyclotron, into SPIOs for SLN imaging. The hydrophilic coating poly(acrylic acid) (PAA) of SPION was PEGylated to increase the in vivo stability. Uptake of ^{69}Ge-SPION@PEG

Table 3.6 Trimodal agents for imaging lymph nodes (LNs), including SLNs

Probe	PET (SPECT) reporter	MR reporter	Third imaging reporter	Applications	References
^{124}I-TCL-SPIONs	^{124}I	SPION	^{124}I Cherenkov radiation as optical	SLN imaging	[169]
^{68}Ga-SPION	^{68}Ga	SPION	^{68}Ga Cherenkov optical	SLN imaging	[170]
^{68}Ga[MNPSiO2(NIR797)]	^{68}Ga	CoFe2O4	NIR797 fluorescence	SLN imaging	[171]
^{64}Cu-DOTA-MSN-Gd-DTTA-FTIC	^{64}Cu	Gd-DTTA	FTIC fluorescence	SLN mapping and tumor metastases	[172]
^{64}Cu-ZW800-Gd3-MSN	^{64}Cu	Gd3-MSN	ZW800 fluorescence	SLNs	[173]

in normal BALB/c mice in the popliteal LN from in vivo PET images and contrast enhancement in MR images demonstrated its possible application in LN mapping [167].

Another PET/MRI multimodal nanoparticle, ^{89}Zr-ferumoxytol, has been tested in preclinical disease models, the results demonstrating that the particles can be used for high-resolution tomographic studies of lymphatic drainage [168].

Even more complex, trimodal imaging has emerged as a novel imaging strategy for translational research, which combines three different modalities together such as PET/SPECT-MR-Optical to provide complementary information and achieve synergistic advantages over any single modality alone (Table 3.6). The main challenge of trimodal imaging lies in developing an efficient platform that incorporates various imaging modality reporters without disturbing each other while maintaining the entity intact.

A very interesting approach for the preparation of a PET/MR/optical trimodal imaging probe is based on ^{124}I conjugation with SPIO nanoparticles. Clearly, the trimodal nanoparticles are characterized by the long physical emission half-life of ^{124}I (4.2 days). Their emission of high-energy positron decay with a β^+ mean energy of 819 keV led to strong Cherenkov radiation as an optical imaging reporter in which no fluorescent dye is needed, unlike in the case of previously described trimodal imaging reporter probes. SPION with cross-linked polymer coating layers containing PEG (TCL-SPION) was selected as an MR imaging reporter [169]. Consistent results were also found in the ex vivo optical and micro-PET images of the dissected LNs. Similar to ^{124}I, ^{68}Ga enables Cherenkov radiation that can be used as an optical imaging reporter [170] MNP-SiO$_2$(NIR797), a magnetic silica nanoparticle encapsulating the NIRF dye in a silica shell, was reported as a trimodal PET-MR-NIRF probe for in vivo SLN imaging in mice. Nanoparticles with particle size of 45 ± 6 nm were selected for SLN mapping, as they were optimal for entering the lymphatic vessels and retaining in the capillary vessels within the lymphatics. The trimodal tracer was injected into the forepaw of mice for SLN mapping using PET, MR, and NIRF. When 100 µg of ^{68}Ga-MNPSiO$_2$(NIR797) was subcutaneously injected, PET images of axillary and brachial LNs and clear signals of NIRF in axillary and brachial

LNs could be obtained; however, MR imaging of axillary LNs was possible only at doses higher than 200 µg of ^{68}Ga-MNPSiO$_2$(NIR797) [171]. When radiolabeling with [^{18}F]fluoride or ^{64}Cu/^{99m}Tc-bisphosphonate (BP) conjugates to Fe$_3$O$_4$@NaYF4 core/shell nanoparticles with different cation dopants in the shell or core, the inorganic core-shell nanoparticles were applied as trimodal probes for SLN imaging. In vivo LN imaging studies showed obvious advantages of combining different imaging modalities. When combined with highly sensitive PET, but not MRI alone, the in vivo imaging studies offered improved presurgical mapping of iliac and popliteal LN locations and provided more details to interpret SLN imaging that are relevant to the pathology of LNs and tumor metastasis in humans. Fluorescence could offer additional information of anatomical and functional changes during surgery and subsequently during pathological examination of excised tissues [172]. A mesoporous silica-based triple-modal imaging nanoprobe (MSN-probe) possesses the long-term imaging ability to track tumor metastatic SLNs. In this system, three imaging tags including the NIR dye ZW800, T1 contrast agent Gd^{3+}, and positron-emitting radionuclide ^{64}Cu were integrated into MSNs by different conjugation strategies. Due to their high stability and long intracellular retention time, signals from tumor draining SLNs are detectable up to 3 weeks. These examples demonstrate the advantages of using a PET/SPECT-MR bimodal probe for SLN mapping, which can be used to further evaluate the metastatic status of a tumor [173].

Key Learning Points

- Hybrid multimodal agents include ^{99m}Tc-Evans blue, ICG conjugated with ^{99m}Tc-albumin nanocolloid, Gd^{3+}, or superparamagnetic iron oxides (SPIOs) by incorporating a PET/SPECT radionuclide with its associated functionalities, such as ^{124}I-SA-MnMEIO, ^{68}Ga-NOTA-IO-MAN, ^{99m}Tc-SPIONs, ^{69}Ge-SPION@PEG, ^{89}Zr-ferumoxytol, MNP-SiO2(NIR797), ^{68}Ga-MNPSiO2(NIR797), and ^{64}Cu- or ^{99m}Tc-bisphosphonate conjugates to Fe3O4@NaYF4 core/shell nanoparticles.

3.8 Instrumentations for Lymphatic Mapping

Conventional SLN mapping is based on the combined use of blue dye and lymphoscintigraphy, or on lymphoscintigraphy alone, with the perspective of using PET/CT or PET/MR imaging sometimes in the future [174]. To increase the performance of the SLN procedure over conventional imaging with large field-of-view gamma cameras, intraoperative portable gamma cameras have recently been developed to obtain preoperative imaging of the SLN. The following sections provide a review of the available intraoperative probes and portable imaging devices, their working principle, and clinical implementation.

3.8.1 Intraoperative Probes for Radioguided Surgery

The working principle of the intraoperative probes for SLN detection (also called gamma probes) is the conversion of the 140 keV photons emitted by ^{99m}Tc into electrons by photoelectric effect or Compton scattering and the production of a signal processed by a custom readout electronics [175]. Indeed, most commercially available handheld gamma detection probes are generally designed for detecting radioisotopes of gamma-ray energies in the low-energy emission range (up to 150 keV) and medium-energy emission range (150–400 keV), which enable to detect radioisotopes such as ^{99m}Tc (140 keV), ^{111}In (171 keV and 247 keV), ^{123}I (159 keV), and ^{125}I (35 keV).

The intraoperative probes for SLN detection can be divided into two main categories: the first one includes probes based on scintillation detectors (both crystal and plastic types), while the second group includes the semiconductor-based probes [176–184]. The typical configuration for intraoperative probes, both for scintillator or semiconductor, is shown in Fig. 3.14.

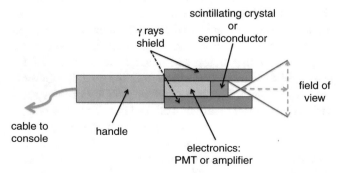

Fig. 3.14 General design of a handheld intraoperative gamma probe for intraoperative search of the target tissue (SLN or tumor) to be resected during surgery, with schematic representation of its main components

The most significant parameters defining the performances of gamma probes are (1) overall sensitivity (efficiency), (2) spatial resolution (radial and lateral), (3) energy resolution, and (4) signal-to-noise ratio.

Sensitivity is the detected count rate per unit of activity and it is determined at the tip of the probe. Radial resolution is the width of the measurement cone where the radiation is detected at a defined distance. With a wider cone, background signal may overcome the signal generated at the target source. With a narrower cone, background is reduced and detection of the target source is more accurate. Lateral spatial resolution is the capability to accurately localize the position of a target source and to separate two adjacent sources. Energy resolution is the capacity of the gamma detection system to discriminate between radiations of different energies. This property is essential to distinguish between two simultaneously administered radionuclides that have different energies and to discriminate scattered from primary photons. The latter property relates to the ability of the probe to discriminate the signal from the target with respect to the noise represented by the background radiation within the surrounding tissue.

The scintillator absorbs the radiation and emits a number of visible photons proportional to the energy absorbed; in turn, visible light is measured by using a photon detector, usually a photomultiplier (PMT). The crystals used for scintillator detector probes include thallium-activated sodium iodide (NaI[Tl]), thallium-activated cesium iodide (CsI[Tl]), cerium-activated lutetium orthosilicate (LSO[Ce]), bismuth germanate (BGO), and cerium-doped gadolinium orthosilicate (GSO[Ce]).

The high penetration power of gamma rays means that background events could come from parts of the patient outside the target volume of interest. Although a fraction of these events is attenuated within the patient body, in order to further reduce the background the gamma probes are equipped with a shield (material such as lead, tungsten, gold, or platinum), and collimators (designed with different lengths and apertures for different field of views, FOV) that prevent attenuated radiation from nontarget locations (i.e., scattered radiation) from accessing the detector head and thus producing spurious counts. Side- and back-shielding can be important when there is a localized radiation source (the injection site of the ^{99m}Tc-labeled agent for radioguided SLNB) in close proximity with the target (the SLN). Collimation of the detector head results in better spatial resolution and higher signal-to-noise ratio as compared to radiation emitted from surrounding tissues. However, when collimation is too pronounced it reduces sensitivity of the probes, by decreasing the detection aperture and lengthening the distance to the actual source position. Furthermore, a thicker shielding or a longer collimator is needed when detecting higher energy gammas, but this increases the overall weight and size of the gamma probe.

The final elements in the system are the electronics and the readout. Since the scintillator detector provides a signal proportional to the deposited energy, it is possible to make spectroscopy and to set the sensitive energy range of the probe to select the desired gamma energy and eliminate part of the scattered radiation. The count rate of the probe is then fed to a ratemeter, which also drives an audio output. An increase in loudness or frequency indicates to the surgeon proximity of the probe to the target tissue.

Semiconductors are a valid alternative to scintillators as detector material for the intraoperative probes. When radiation is absorbed in a solid-state detector, ionization occurs by promoting electrons out of the valence band to the conduction band where electrons can flow in the crystal lattice. When the electron moves to the conduction band, a positive charge (hole) in the lattice is created which is free to move in the valence band. If an electric field is applied across the sensitive volume of the detector, the excess of charge (both electrons and holes) is collected by the opposite electrodes, thus providing a signal which is proportional to the energy released in the detector. Crystalline materials that are used in such detectors are cadmium telluride (CdTe), cadmium zinc telluride (CdZnTe), and mercuric iodide (HgI_2).

Scintillation-based detection systems present both pros and cons with respect to semiconductor-based systems. On the one hand, scintillator-based detectors have a higher sensitivity (because of the higher density and atomic number they are better suited for medium-to-high gamma energy detection), but a poorer energy resolution and scatter rejection due to the indirect mechanism of the radiation detection (the primary gamma converts in the scintillator, then the light should be conveyed to the PMT, and the signal finally converted from optical to electrical). Furthermore, scintillation-based detectors tend to have a much bulkier probe head profile and weight. On the other hand, semiconductor-based probes are direct detectors (the energy released in the material by radiation is directly converted into a charge signal) and thus they have a higher energy resolution and scatter rejection capability. Likewise, semiconductor-based probes tend to have a much more compact probe head design; they can be manufactured in small size and they can have a very thin entrance window that enables to count low-energy beta and gamma rays.

To improve SLN localization using a gamma probe during surgery, a novel technological possibility is the so-called freehand SPECT device that combines a positioning system attached to the conventional gamma probe with a tracking system on the patient's body and permits virtual reconstruction of the position of a radioactive source in a 3-D environment. In particular, the system combines acoustic signals with 3-D imaging for the localization of areas with focal radioactivity accumulation in the operating room. The system consists of a spatial localization system and two tracking targets that are fixed on the gamma probe and on the patient,

respectively [185]. The localization system consists of an optical camera and an infrared localization device. The 3-D images generated with the freehand SPECT probe are visualized on the screen. The images can be displayed in real time so that information on the depth of a lymph node (or of other radiolabeled target tissue of interest, e.g., a hyperfunctioning parathyroid adenoma upon administration of ^{99m}Tc-sestamibi) is available (Fig. 3.15).

After the development of PET lymphoscintigraphy techniques (described in Chap. 4), handheld gamma detection probes specifically designed for detecting the high-energy 511 keV photon emissions generated by the electron-positron annihilation process, characteristic of radionuclides such as ^{18}F or ^{68}Ga, have recently become available. These probes have been designated as "PET" probes. The overall weight and size of these probes are generally dependent on the thickness of side- and back-shielding (typically in lead, tungsten, gold, or platinum) and the length of the collimator [186]. To improve the current "PET" probe design (increase of side/back-shielding, or collimation length, or crystal diameter/thickness) without resulting in configurations that are too large in size, too heavy, and of greater cost, novel "PET" probe designs are being developed in which the efficacy is not dependent upon side- and back-shielding, collimation, or crystal diameter/thickness. Examples of such probes are secondary K-alpha X-ray fluorescence [187, 188], active electronic collimation [188], and other crystal geometry designs using multiple small crystals with specific novel geometric configurations for optimizing and maximizing background rejection capabilities [188].

Many commercial intraoperative gamma probes are available; an example of a gamma probe with its console (control unit) is presented in Fig. 3.16 [189].

Several factors determine the choice of a particular intraoperative probe. From the point of view of the surgeon, there are many desirable design features of detection probe systems that are important [175, 182]. Gamma probes for radioguided SLNB require high spatial resolution to allow for a more precise localization of small lymph nodes.

Other features such as the shape, weight, and ergonomical design of an intraoperative probe are critical. The audible signal and digital display of the detector control unit are also important for providing critical output information to the surgeon, enabling quick and accurate localization of the radionuclide without distraction from the overall activity in the surgical field. Flexibility and adaptability of the system are also functional to different clinical issues, such as removable side-shielding, interchangeable collimators, interchangeable detector probes, and user-adjustable energy windows for different radionuclides. Finally, the recent development of handheld self-contained gamma detection probes based on wireless Bluetooth technology eliminates the need for cables that normally connect the probe to the control unit [190, 191].

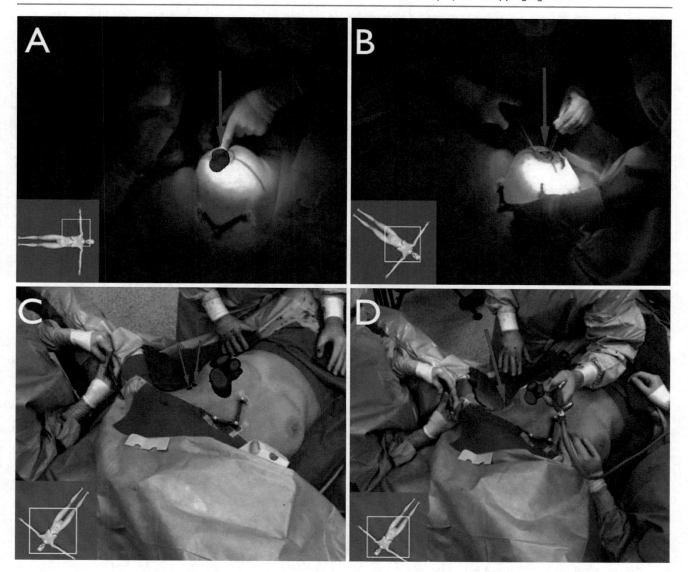

Fig. 3.15 Freehand SPECT device used for radioguided surgery in a patient with non-palpable breast cancer. (**a**) Overlay of freehand SPECT 3-D image on the video display shows high retention of radiocolloid at the intratumoral injection site. (**b**) After tumor removal, the absence of radioactivity accumulation in the surgical field confirms complete excision of the tumor. (**c, d**) A similar approach is used to guide the surgeon for complete removal of SLNs (red arrows) (*reproduced with permission from ref* [185])

Key Learning Points

- Main kinds of handheld gamma probes for intraoperative use during radioguided surgery have been developed, depending on specific clinical use.
- Gamma probes for SLN detection can be divided into two categories: probes based on scintillation detectors (both crystal and plastic types) and probes based on semiconductor detectors.
- The physical principles most commonly used in gamma probes are the scintillation in an organic or inorganic material, and the production of electron-hole pairs in a semiconductor.
- Different materials are used for either scintillation or semiconductor gamma probes.
- Compact, ergonomical, flexible gamma probes for radioguided biopsy of the SLN with high spatial resolution have been developed.

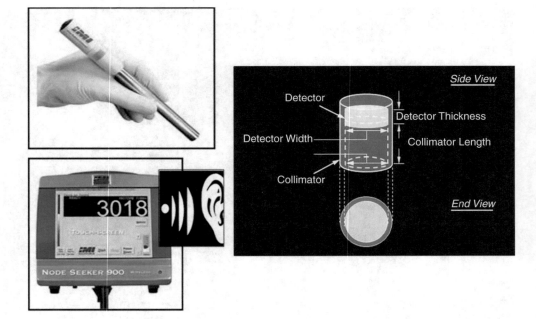

Fig. 3.16 Commercial gamma probe (upper left panel), with diagram of the detector's structure (right panel), and control unit (lower left panel)

3.8.2 Portable Gamma Cameras for Lymphatic Mapping

Although non-imaging intraoperative probes are still the standard equipment for detection of the radiolabeled tissue in the operating room, they cannot provide further details on source configuration. The exact localization of a source can only be performed if the tip is under direct contact with the tissue after the surgical incision.

In this regard, intraoperative real-time imaging with portable gamma cameras provides an overview of all radioactive hot spots in the whole surgical field [180, 192]. For instance, its position can be adjusted to also show SLNs near the injection area, which can easily be overlooked by using the non-imaging probe. Discriminating a SLN from an upper-tier node is based on the amount of counts simultaneously recorded with the camera, which can be correlated to the preoperative scintigraphic images. The gamma camera can also be used in conjunction with the gamma probes.

Imaging devices must meet several requirements to be employed for the intraoperative use. Among them are a portable and stable design, no delay between image acquisition and display (real-time imaging), and possibility for continuous monitoring, spatial orientation on screen, real-time quantification, and display of the counts recorded. Finally, they should also have an adequate spatial resolution, sensitivity, and field of view.

Examples of such cameras are shown in Fig. 3.17. While the first devices were quite heavy and bulky handheld devices, new-generation portable gamma cameras are lighter and/or equipped with stable support systems.

Among the instruments available on the market, we mention only few that implement these requirements with different approaches in the radiation detector. One of the most widely used devices is the Sentinella S102 (from Oncovision, Valencia, Spain) [193] that is equipped with a CsI(NA) continuous scintillating crystal readout by PSPMTs and different collimators (pinhole collimators, 2.5 and 4 mm in diameters, and divergent) (Fig. 3.17a). The pinhole collimator enables visualization of the whole surgical filed depending on the distance between the camera and the source. The field of view is 4 × 4 cm at 3 cm from the source, and 20 × 20 cm at 15 cm from the source. This device has been integrated in a mobile and ergonomic support that is easily adjustable. The imaging head is located on one arm that allows positioning on the specific area. Another approach is based on the use of the CZT as radiation detector. For instance in the Anzai eZ-SCOPE Handheld Gamma Camera [194], the detector is made of a single tile of CdZnTe, patterned in an array of 16 × 16 pixels at a pitch of 2 mm. The head is equipped with a series on interchangeable parallel-hole collimators to achieve different performances in terms of spatial resolution and/or sensitivity. The field of view is 3.2 × 3.2 cm and weight is 800 g (Fig. 3.17b).

A further development of the intraoperative gamma camera is the LumaGEM from Gamma Medica Ideas [195]. It is based on the CZT pixel technology and was originally developed for breast gamma imaging. The field of view is 13 × 13 cm and the intrinsic spatial resolution is 2 mm. This camera is also equipped with exchangeable parallel hole collimator and it is integrated in a work-stand articulated arm.

Recent technological advances lead to speculate that, in the near future, the PMT-based systems will be

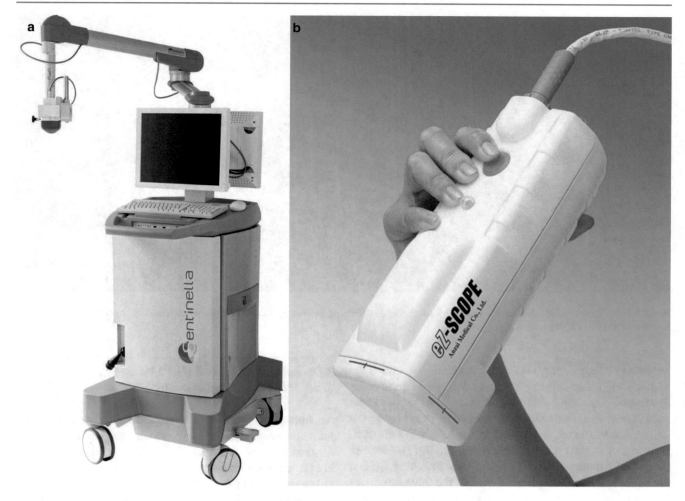

Fig. 3.17 Examples of portable gamma cameras for intraoperative use: (**a**) Recent-generation portable gamma camera with improved ergonomical details and adequate support system for intraoperative use (model Sentinella S102, manufactured by Oncovision, Valencia, Spain). (**b**) Portable gamma camera with a weight <1 kg but without support system (eZ-Scope, manufactured by Anzai Medical, Tokyo, Japan)

replaced with cameras based on scintillators coupled with solid-state photodetectors. In these systems the photodetector will be an array of photodiodes (more likely silicon photomultipliers, the so-called SiPM) coupled to a slab or a matrix of crystals designed to be coupled one to one to the photosensors [196]. In such a way, the thickness of the detector (including crystal, photodiodes, and electronics) coupled to a shallow collimator could be less than 5 cm, so that it would be compact enough to be brought into a surgery room as an intraoperative imaging probe.

Most beta probes commercially available are non-imaging systems and therefore suffer from the lack of ancillary information of the tissue area to be explored. A novel, handheld digital imaging beta probe (IBP), suitable for use during surgery in conjunction with beta-emitting radiopharmaceuticals such as [18F]FDG, for real-time imaging of a surveyed area with higher spatial resolution and sensitivity, lower sensitivity to background radiation, and greater ease of operation than existing instruments, is shown in Fig. 3.18 [197]. This is a visual mapping device to locate and confirm excision of [18F]FDG-avid primary tumors and metastases. The proposed handheld IBP includes a 140 μm thick microstructured CsI:Tl film optically coupled to a highly sensitive electron-multiplying charge-coupled device (EMCCD) via a flexible fiber-optic (FO) conduit. The microcolumnar structure of the CsI:Tl scintillator minimizes the spread of scintillation light to typically less than 100 μm, and allows for the detection of beta radiation with high spatial resolution. The EMCCD is a back-thinned, thermoelectrically cooled (−35 °C), 512×512-pixel CCD optically bonded to a 1:1 fiber-optic (FO) window. The EMCCD has 16×16 μm pixels, and an effective imaging area of approximately 8.2×8.2 mm. The

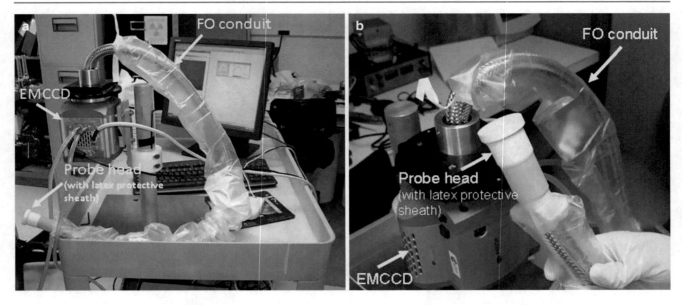

Fig. 3.18 (**a**) Prototype of the handheld Imaging Beta Probe™ (IBP™). (**b**) Close-up view of the probe head, covered by a latex sheath (*reproduced with permission from ref.* [197])

advantage of the EMCCD is that it internally amplifies the signal with a user-selectable gain and minimizes the noise associated with the CCD readout amplifier by the same gain factor. In order to increase its active imaging area, a 2:1 or 3:1 FO taper is coupled to the IBP's FO conduit, resulting in an effective imaging area of 16.4 × 16.4 mm or 24.6 × 24.6 mm, respectively. An index matching fluid is used for the optical coupling of each of the three interfaces between the FO faceplate, 3:1 FO taper, FO bundle, and EMCCD. A 24 μm thick aluminum foil (negligible attenuation of β-radiation) is placed in front of a CsI(Tl) film to shield the IBP from ambient light. Due to its high density and high average atomic number the CsI:Tl film, while only ~140 μm thick, completely absorbed and enabled the detection of every incident beta particle, while being highly insensitive to gamma background. Furthermore, the high light output of CsI(Tl) (56,000 ph/MeV) and high sensitivity of the EMCCD photodetector increased overall IBP sensitivity and effectiveness.

> **Key Learning Points**
> • Handheld gamma probes for radioguided surgery have been developed for a wide variety of applications and are commercially available.
> • With the development of PET lymphoscintigraphy techniques, dedicated "PET" probes specifically designed for detecting resultant high-energy 511 keV gamma emissions have become available.

3.9 Near-Infrared (NIR) Imaging for Lymphatic Mapping

An impressive surge of interest has recently occurred for fluorescence-guided surgery, which has led to a steady demand for new commercial fluorescence imaging devices. For the greatest clinical impact, an imaging system must provide a solution to the immediate clinical goal with important new information that affects the patient outcome in a way that seamlessly blends into current clinical workflow. There are several new fluorescence imagers that have been cleared for commercial use by the 510(k) process at the U.S. FDA for open-surgical use with ICG (Table 3.6) [198].

Near-infrared (NIR) imaging using for example ICG has been developed for functional imaging of location and patency of vascular structures in neuro-, ophthalmologic, and vascular surgeries since the 1980s. The wavelength of NIR light is approximately 700–1000 nm. This range is the least absorbed by blood or water; thus, this "optical window" has been regarded as the best wavelength of imaging to provide the deepest penetration of the signal. Subsequently, ICG NIR imaging has been applied to various procedures in general surgery, providing functional information of the perfusion of the organs, visualization of the biliary tract and hepatic tumors, and margins of the anatomic segments of the liver. NIR imaging systems are composed of excitation light sources and special filters and cameras optimized for the NIR wavelength of light. ICG is excited at 700–800 nm, and the emitted maximal signal is 800–840 nm [199, 200]. For ICG fluorescent imaging (FI), the fluorescent dye ICG is intravenously administered through a peripheral venous line and the tissue in the region of interest is illuminated with near-infrared light at a wavelength of 785 nm with a total output of 80 mW in a field of view of 10 cm in diameter (1 mW/cm²) operating at a distance of approximately 20 cm above the tissue. The fluorescence emission of the excited dye is detected by an infrared-sensitive charge-coupled device (CCD) camera system. The camera is equipped with a band-pass filter for the selective transmission of light at the emission maximum of ICG (830 nm) (Fig. 3.19). The fluorescent imaging images are then displayed and recorded in real time on a computer monitor. The laser has an excellent safety profile for both patient and operating staff. Because of

the low power density of the emitted laser energy, there is no tissue warming. Although ICG-FI has turned to be a more and more common technique to evaluate intraoperative organ perfusion, only few studies tried to quantitatively validate the technique for visceral perfusion assessment [201].

Figure 3.20 and Table 3.7 summarize the current leading fluorescence guidance systems. The PerkinElmer Solaris, Curadel ResVet LabFlare, and SurgVision Explorer Air are not 510(k) cleared for human use, while the others are for ICG procedures. All of them can image ICG in surgical trials, with differing levels of sensitivity and with different features [198].

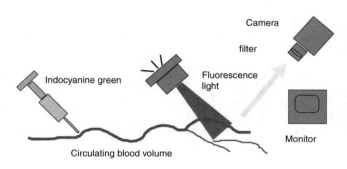

Fig. 3.19 Indocyanine green fluorescent imaging (IDG-FI): After intravenous injection, the region of interest is illuminated with near-infrared light (785 nm). The fluorescence emission of the excited dye is detected by an infrared-sensitive charge-coupled device camera system (dynamic range 54 dB) equipped with a band-pass filter for the selective transmission of light at the emission maximum of ICG (830 nm) (*reproduced with permission from ref. [201]*)

> **Key Learning Points**
> - With the recent development of fluorescence-guided surgery, new fluorescence imaging devices have become commercially available.
> - Among near-infrared techniques, indocyanine green fluorescence is the most commonly used for functional imaging of vascular structures in neuro-, ophthalmologic, and vascular surgeries.

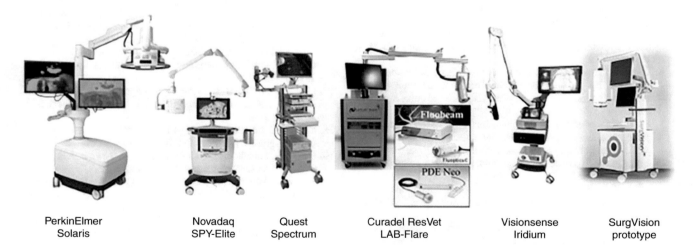

| PerkinElmer Solaris | Novadaq SPY-Elite | Quest Spectrum | Curadel ResVet LAB-Flare | Visionsense Iridium | SurgVision prototype |

Fig. 3.20 Current leading fluorescence-based guidance systems. From left to right: Solaris™ Open-Air Fluorescence Imaging System (printed with permission, 2015–2016 PerkinElmer, Inc., all rights reserved); NOVADAQ Spy-Elite™ (copyright 2016 Novadaq Technologies Inc.); Quest Spectrum™ (copyright Quest Medical Imaging); Fluobeam®, Hamamatsu PDE-Neo™ (copyright 2016 Fluoptics); Lab-FLARE® Model R1 (copyright CURADEL); Visionsense Iridium™ (copyright Visionsense); SurgVision Explorer Air prototype (image courtesy of SurgVision) (*reproduced with permission from ref. [24]: DSouza AV, Lin H, Henderson ER, Samkoe KS, Pogue BW. Review of fluorescence guided surgery systems: identification of key performance capabilities beyond indocyanine green imaging. J Biomed Opt. 2016;21(8):80901*)

Table 3.7 ICG fluorescence imaging systems approved through FDA clearance based on the 510(k) process, after demonstration of the device being safe and effective, with substantial equivalence to a predicate device [198]

Company	Fluorescence imaging system	Year approved/510(k) cleared	FDA 510(k) number	Indication approved for
Novadaq Technologies, Inc.	SPY imaging system	2005	K042961	Blood flow
Novadaq Technologies, Inc.	SPY imaging system SP2000	2007	K063345	Tissue perfusion and transfer circulation in free flaps, plastic, and reconstructive surgery
Novadaq Technologies, Inc.	SPY fluorescent imaging system SP2001	2008	K073088	510(k) with SPY SP2000
Novadaq Technologies, Inc.	SPY fluorescent imaging system SP2001	2008	K073130	510(k) for modified device
Novadaq Technologies, Inc.	SPY intraoperative imaging system	2011	K100371	Additional gastrointestinal imaging
Hamamatsu Photonics K.K.	PDE photodynamic eye	2012	K110480	510(k) with SPY K063345 and K073130
Hamamatsu Photonics K.K.	PDE Neo	2014	K133719	510(k) with PDE K110480 for modified device
Fluoptics	Fluobeam 800 clinical imaging device	2014	K132475	510(k) with PDE
Quest Medical Imaging	Artemis light engine	2015	K141164	510(k) with Karl Storz and Olympus Winter
Quest Medical	Artemis handheld imaging system	2015	K143474	510(k) with PDE and Fluobeam 800
VisionSense Ltd.	VS3-IR-MMS system	2015	K150018	510(k) with SPY 063345

References

1. Walker LA. Localization of radioactive colloids in lymph nodes. J Lab Clin Med. 1950;36:440–9.
2. Segal AW, Gregoriadis G, Black CD. Liposomes as vehicles for the local release of drugs. Clin Sci Mol Med. 1975;49:99–106.
3. Ikeda I, Inoue O, Kurata K. New preparation method for ^{99m}Tc-phytate. J Nucl Med. 1976;17:389–93.
4. Strand SE, Persson BR. Quantitative lymphoscintigraphy I: basic concepts for optimal uptake of radiocolloids in the parasternal lymph nodes of rabbits. J Nucl Med. 1979;20:1038–46.
5. Bergqvist L, Strand SE, Persson BR. Particle sizing and biokinetics of interstitial lymphoscintigraphic agents. Semin Nucl Med. 1983;13:9–19.
6. Turner JH. Post-traumatic avascular necrosis of the femoral head predicted by preoperative technetium-99m antimony-colloid scan. An experimental and clinical study. J Bone Joint Surg Am. 1983;65:786–96.
7. Patel HM, Boodle KM, Vaughan-Jones R. Assessment of the potential uses of liposomes for lymphoscintigraphy and lymphatic drug delivery. Failure of 99m-technetium marker to represent intact liposomes in lymph nodes. Biochim Biophys Acta. 1984;801:76–86.
8. Patel HM, Russell NJ. Liposomes: from membrane model to therapeutic applications. Biochem Soc Trans. 1988;16:909–10.
9. Strand SE, Bergqvist L. Radiolabeled colloids and macromolecules in the lymphatic system. Crit Rev Ther Drug Carrier Syst. 1989;6:211–38.
10. Allen TM, Hansen CB, Guo LS. Subcutaneous administration of liposomes: a comparison with the intravenous and intraperitoneal routes of injection. Biochim Biophys Acta. 1993;1150:9–16.
11. Moghimi SM, Davis SS. Innovations in avoiding particle clearance from blood by Kupffer cells: cause for reflection. Crit Rev Ther Drug Carrier Syst. 1994;11:31–59.
12. Moghimi SM, Rajabi-Siahboomi R. Advanced colloid-based systems for efficient delivery of drugs and diagnostic agents to the lymphatic tissues. Prog Biophys Mol Biol. 1996;65:221–49.
13. Ikomi F, Hanna GK, Schmid-Schönbein GW. Mechanism of colloidal particle uptake into the lymphatic system: basic study with percutaneous lymphography. Radiology. 1995;196:107–13.
14. Sherman AI, Ter-Pogossian M. Lymph-node concentration of radioactive colloidal gold following interstitial injection. Cancer. 1953;6:1238–40.
15. Pecking A, Firmin F, Rain JD, et al. Lymphoedema of the upper limb following surgery or radiotherapy. Investigation by indirect radioactive lymphography. Nouv Press Med. 1980;9:3349–51.
16. Bräutigam P, Vanscheidt W, Földi E, et al. The importance of the subfascial lymphatics in the diagnosis of lower limb edema: investigations with semiquantitative lymphoscintigraphy. Angiology. 1993;44:464–70.
17. Mostbeck A, Partsch H. Isotope lymphography—possibilities and limits in evaluation of lymph transport. Wien Med Wochenschr. 1999;149:87–91.
18. Partsch H. Practical aspects of indirect lymphography and lymphoscintigraphy. Lymphat Res Biol. 2003;1:71–3; discussion 3–4.
19. Henze E, Schelbert HR, Collins JD, et al. Lymphoscintigraphy with Tc-99m-labeled dextran. J Nucl Med. 1982;23:923–9.
20. Kazem I, Antoniades J, Brady LW, et al. Clinical evaluation of lymph node scanning utilizing colloidal gold 198. Radiology. 1968;90:905–11.
21. Nagai K, Ito Y, Otsuka N, et al. Clinical usefullness on accumulation of ^{99m}Tc-rhenium colloid in lymph nodes. Radioisotopes. 1980;29:549–51.
22. Nagai K, Ito Y, Otsuka N, et al. Deposition of small ^{99m}Tc-labelled colloids in bone marrow and lymph nodes. Eur J Nucl Med. 1982;7:66–70.
23. Warbick A, Ege GN, Henkelman RM, et al. An evaluation of radiocolloid sizing techniques. J Nucl Med. 1977;18:827–34.

24. Davis MA, Jones AG, Trindade H. A rapid and accurate method for sizing radiocolloids. J Nucl Med. 1974;15:923–8.
25. Hung JC, Wiseman GA, Wahner HW, et al. Filtered technetium-99m-sulfur colloid evaluated for lymphoscintigraphy. J Nucl Med. 1995;36:1895–901.
26. Kleinhans E, Baumeister RG, Hahn D, et al. Evaluation of transport kinetics in lymphoscintigraphy: follow-up study in patients with transplanted lymphatic vessels. Eur J Nucl Med. 1985;10:349–52.
27. Gommans GM, Gommans E, van der Zant FM, et al. ^{99m}Tc Nanocoll: a radiopharmaceutical for sentinel node localisation in breast cancer—in vitro and in vivo results. Appl Radiat Isot. 2009;67:1550–8.
28. Swartz MA. The physiology of the lymphatic system. Adv Drug Deliv Rev. 2001;50:3–20.
29. Atkins HL, Hauser W, Richards P. Visualization of mediastinal lymph nodes after intraperitoneal administration of ^{99m}Tc-sulfur colloid. Nucl Med (Stuttg). 1970;9:275–8.
30. Frier M, Griffiths P, Ramsey A. The physical and chemical characteristics of sulphur colloids. Eur J Nucl Med. 1981;6:255–60.
31. Ikomi F, Hanna GK, Schmid-Schönbein GW. Size- and surface-dependent uptake of colloid particles into the lymphatic system. Lymphology. 1999;32:90–102.
32. Aukland K, Reed RK. Interstitial-lymphatic mechanisms in the control of extracellular fluid volume. Physiol Rev. 1993;73:1–78.
33. Swartz MA, Fleury ME. Interstitial flow and its effects in soft tissues. Annu Rev Biomed Eng. 2007;9:229–56.
34. Mariani G, Moresco L, Viale G, et al. Radioguided sentinel lymph node biopsy in breast cancer surgery. J Nucl Med. 2001;42:1198–215.
35. Weiss M, Gildehaus FJ, Brinkbäumer K, et al. Lymph kinetics with technetium-99m labeled radiopharmaceuticals. Animal studies. Nuklearmedizin. 2005;44:156–65.
36. Reddy ST, Berk DA, Jain RK, et al. A sensitive in vivo model for quantifying interstitial convective transport of injected macromolecules and nanoparticles. J Appl Physiol (1985). 2006;101:1162–9.
37. Mangat S, Patel HM. Lymph node localization of non-specific antibody-coated liposomes. Life Sci. 1985;36:1917–25.
38. Szuba A, Shin WS, Strauss HW, et al. The third circulation: radionuclide lymphoscintigraphy in the evaluation of lymphedema. J Nucl Med. 2003;44:43–57.
39. Paganelli G, De Cicco C, Cremonesi M, et al. Optimized sentinel node scintigraphy in breast cancer. Q J Nucl Med. 1998;42:49–53.
40. De Cicco C, Cremonesi M, Luini A, et al. Lymphoscintigraphy and radioguided biopsy of the sentinel axillary node in breast cancer. J Nucl Med. 1998;39:2080–4.
41. Wilhelm AJ, Mijnhout GS, Franssen EJ. Radiopharmaceuticals in sentinel lymph-node detection—An overview. Eur J Nucl Med. 1999;26:S36–42.
42. Noguchi M. Sentinel lymph node biopsy and breast cancer. Br J Surg. 2002;89:21–34.
43. Trifirò G, Viale G, Gentilini O, et al. Sentinel node detection in pre-operative axillary staging. Eur J Nucl Med Mol Imaging. 2004;31:S46–55.
44. Leidenius MH, Leppänen EA, Krogerus LA, et al. The impact of radiopharmaceutical particle size on the visualization and identification of sentinel nodes in breast cancer. Nucl Med Commun. 2004;25:233–8.
45. Nieweg OE, Jansen L, Valdés Olmos RA, et al. Lymphatic mapping and sentinel lymph node biopsy in breast cancer. Eur J Nucl Med. 1999;26:S11–6.
46. Chinol M, Paganelli G. Current status of commercial colloidal preparations for sentinel lymph node detection. Eur J Nucl Med. 1999;26:560.
47. Vera DR, Wallace AM, Hoh CK, et al. A synthetic macromolecule for sentinel node detection: ^{99m}Tc-DTPA-mannosyl-dextran. J Nucl Med. 2001;42:951–9.
48. Heuveling DA, Visser GW, Baclayon M, et al. ^{89}Zr-nanocolloidal albumin-based PET/CT lymphoscintigraphy for sentinel node detection in head and neck cancer: preclinical results. J Nucl Med. 2011;52:1580–4.
49. Hou G, Hou B, Jiang Y, et al. ^{68}Ga-NOTA-Evans blue TOF PET/MR lymphoscintigraphy evaluation of the severity of lower limb lymphedema. Clin Nucl Med. 2019;44:439–45.
50. Niu G, Lang L, Kiesewetter DO, et al. In vivo labeling of serum albumin for PET. J Nucl Med. 2014;55:1150–6.
51. Bourgeois P. Scintigraphic investigations of the lymphatic system: the influence of injected volume and quantity of labeled colloidal tracer. J Nucl Med. 2007;48:693–5.
52. Valdés-Olmos RA, Jansen L, Hoefnagel CA, et al. Evaluation of mammary lymphoscintigraphy by a single intratumoral injection for sentinel node identification. J Nucl Med. 2000;41:1500–6.
53. Werner JA, Dünne AA, Ramaswamy A, et al. Number and location of radiolabeled, intraoperatively identified sentinel nodes in 48 head and neck cancer patients with clinically staged N0 and N1 neck. Eur Arch Otorhinolaryngol. 2002;259:91–6.
54. Ikomi F, Hunt J, Hanna G, et al. Interstitial fluid, plasma protein, colloid, and leukocyte uptake into initial lymphatics. J Appl Physiol (1985). 1996;81:2060–7.
55. O'Morchoe CC, Jones WR, Jarosz HM, et al. Temperature dependence of protein transport across lymphatic endothelium in vitro. J Cell Biol. 1984;98:629–40.
56. Lund T, Wiig H, Reed RK, et al. A "new" mechanism for oedema generation: strongly negative interstitial fluid pressure causes rapid fluid flow into thermally injured skin. Acta Physiol Scand. 1987;129:433–5.
57. Engeset A, Sokolowski J, Olszewski WL. Variation in output of leukocytes and erythrocytes in human peripheral lymph during rest and activity. Lymphology. 1977;10:198–203.
58. Olszewski W, Engeset A, Jaeger PM, et al. Flow and composition of leg lymph in normal men during venous stasis, muscular activity and local hyperthermia. Acta Physiol Scand. 1977;99:149–55.
59. Thorek DL, Abou DS, Beattie BJ, et al. Positron lymphography: multimodal, high-resolution, dynamic mapping and resection of lymph nodes after intradermal injection of ^{18}F-FDG. J Nucl Med. 2012;53:1438–45.
60. Long X, Zhang J, Zhang D, et al. Microsurgery guided by sequential preoperative lymphography using ^{68}Ga-NEB PET and MRI in patients with lower-limb lymphedema. Eur J Nucl Med Mol Imaging. 2017;44:1501–10.
61. Gibson JG, Evans WA. Clinical studies of the blood volume I. Clinical application of a method employing the azo dye "Evans Blue" and the spectrophotometer. J Clin Invest. 1937;16:301–16.
62. Torabi M, Aquino SL, Harisinghani MG. Current concepts in lymph node imaging. J Nucl Med. 2004;45:1509–18.
63. Zhang J, Lang L, Zhu Z, et al. Clinical translation of an albumin-binding PET radiotracer ^{68}Ga-NEB. J Nucl Med. 2015;56:1609–14.
64. Lusic H, Grinstaff MW. X-ray-computed tomography contrast agents. Chem Rev. 2013;113:1641–66.
65. Bae KT, Heiken JP, Brink JA. Aortic and hepatic contrast medium enhancement at CT. Part I. Prediction with a computer model. Radiology. 1998;207:647–55.
66. Bae KT. Intravenous contrast medium administration and scan timing at CT: considerations and approaches. Radiology. 2010;256:32–61.
67. Riella MC. Nephrologists Sans Frontières: a Kidney Foundation—advancing research and helping patients meet their needs. Kidney Int. 2006;69:1285–7.

48 F. Bartoli et al.

68. Hizoh I, Haller C. Radiocontrast-induced renal tubular cell apoptosis: hypertonic versus oxidative stress. Invest Radiol. 2002;37:428–34.

69. Morcos SK, Thomsen HS, Webb JA. Contrast-media-induced nephrotoxicity: a consensus report. Contrast Media Safety Committee, European Society of Urogenital Radiology (ESUR). Eur Radiol. 1999;9:1602–13.

70. Jost G, Pietsch H, Lengsfeld P, et al. The impact of the viscosity and osmolality of iodine contrast agents on renal elimination. Invest Radiol. 2010;45:255–61.

71. Jost G, Pietsch H, Sommer J, et al. Retention of iodine and expression of biomarkers for renal damage in the kidney after application of iodinated contrast media in rats. Invest Radiol. 2009;44:114–23.

72. Pietsch H, Kies Sling F. Small animal imaging basics and practical guide. New York: Springer; 2011.

73. Mattrey RF, Aguirre DA. Advances in contrast media research. Acad Radiol. 2003;10:1450–60.

74. Hallouard F, Anton N, Choquet P, et al. Iodinated blood pool contrast media for preclinical X-ray imaging applications—A review. Biomaterials. 2010;31:6249–68.

75. Idé JM, Lancelot E, Pines E, et al. Prophylaxis of iodinated contrast media-induced nephropathy: a pharmacological point of view. Invest Radiol. 2004;39:155–70.

76. Chung YE, Hyung WJ, Kweon S, et al. Feasibility of interstitial CT lymphography using optimized iodized oil emulsion in rats. Invest Radiol. 2010;45:142–8.

77. Wisner ER, Katzberg RW, Griffey SM, et al. Characterization of normal and cancerous lymph nodes on indirect computed tomography lymphographic studies after interstitial injection of iodinated nanoparticles. Acad Radiol. 1996;3:S257–60.

78. Gries H. Extracellular MRI contrast agents based on gadolinium. In: Krause W, editor. Contrast agents I: magnetic resonance imaging. Berlin: Springer; 2002. p. 1–24.

79. Brasch RC, Weinmann HJ, Wesbey GE. Contrast-enhanced NMR imaging: animal studies using gadolinium-DTPA complex. AJR Am J Roentgenol. 1984;142:625–30.

80. Strich G, Hagan PL, Gerber KH, et al. Tissue distribution and magnetic resonance spin lattice relaxation effects of gadolinium-DTPA. Radiology. 1985;154:723–6.

81. Schmiedl U, Ogan M, Paajanen H, et al. Albumin labeled with Gd-DTPA as an intravascular, blood pool-enhancing agent for MR imaging: biodistribution and imaging studies. Radiology. 1987;162:205–10.

82. Pathak AP, Artemov D, Neeman M, et al. Lymph node metastasis in breast cancer xenografts is associated with increased regions of extravascular drain, lymphatic vessel area, and invasive phenotype. Cancer Res. 2006;66:5151–8.

83. Li C, Meng S, Yang X, et al. Sentinel lymph node detection using magnetic resonance lymphography with conventional gadolinium contrast agent in breast cancer: a preliminary clinical study. BMC Cancer. 2015;15:213.

84. Shiozawa M, Kobayashi S, Sato Y, et al. Magnetic resonance lymphography of sentinel lymph nodes in patients with breast cancer using superparamagnetic iron oxide: a feasibility study. Breast Cancer. 2014;21:394–401.

85. Tangoku A, Yamamoto S, Suga K, et al. Sentinel lymph node biopsy using computed tomography-lymphography in patients with breast cancer. Surgery. 2004;135:258–65.

86. Kobayashi H, Kawamoto S, Choyke PL, et al. Comparison of dendrimer-based macromolecular contrast agents for dynamic micro-magnetic resonance lymphangiography. Magn Reson Med. 2003;50:758–66.

87. Mounzer R, Shkarin P, Papademetris X, et al. Dynamic imaging of lymphatic vessels and lymph nodes using a bimodal nanoparticulate contrast agent. Lymphat Res Biol. 2007;5:151–8.

88. Cheng Z, Al Zaki A, Jones IW, et al. Stabilized porous liposomes with encapsulated Gd-labeled dextran as a highly efficient MRI contrast agent. Chem Commun (Camb). 2014;50:2502–4.

89. Ishiguchi T, Takahashi S. Safety of gadoterate meglumine (Gd-DOTA) as a contrast agent for magnetic resonance imaging. Drugs R&D. 2010;10:133–45.

90. Shimada M, Yoshikawa K, Suganuma T, et al. Interstitial magnetic resonance lymphography: comparative animal study of gadofluorine 8 and gadolinium diethylenetriamine-pentaacetic acid. J Comput Assist Tomogr. 2003;27:641–6.

91. Normann PT, Hals PA. In vivo stability and excretion of gadodiamide (GdDTPA-BMA), a hydrophilic gadolinium complex used as a contrast enhancing agent for magnetic resonance imaging. Eur J Drug Metab Pharmacokinet. 1995;20:307–13.

92. Cho SB, Lee AL, Chang HW, et al. Prospective multicenter study of the safety of gadoteridol in 6163 patients. J Magn Reson Imaging. 2020;51:861–8.

93. Baker JF, Kratz LC, Stevens GR, et al. Pharmacokinetics and safety of the MRI contrast agent gadoversetamide injection (OptiMARK) in healthy pediatric subjects. Invest Radiol. 2004;39:334–9.

94. Kobayashi H, Kawamoto S, Sakai Y, et al. Lymphatic drainage imaging of breast cancer in mice by micro-magnetic resonance lymphangiography using a nano-size paramagnetic contrast agent. J Natl Cancer Inst. 2004;96:703–8.

95. Kobayashi H, Kawamoto S, Brechbiel MW, et al. Detection of lymph node involvement in hematologic malignancies using micromagnetic resonance lymphangiography with a gadolinium-labeled dendrimer nanoparticle. Neoplasia. 2005;7:984–91.

96. Talanov VS, Regino CA, Kobayashi H, et al. Dendrimer-based nanoprobe for dual modality magnetic resonance and fluorescence imaging. Nano Lett. 2006;6:1459–63.

97. Ma X, Wang S, Hu L, et al. Imaging characteristics of USPIO nanoparticles (<5 nm) as MR contrast agent. Contrast Media Mol Imaging. 2019;2019:3687537.

98. Xiao YD, Paudel R, Liu J, et al. MRI contrast agents: classification and application (review). Int J Mol Med. 2016;38:1319–26.

99. Wang YX, Hussain SM, Krestin GP. Superparamagnetic iron oxide contrast agents: physicochemical characteristics and applications in MR imaging. Eur Radiol. 2001;11:2319–31.

100. Weissleder R. Molecular imaging: principles and practice. PMPH-USA: Raleigh; 2010.

101. Elias A, Tsourkas A. Imaging circulating cells and lymphoid tissues with iron oxide nanoparticles. Hematology Am Soc Hematol Educ Program. 2009;720–6.

102. Wei H, Bruns OT, Kaul MG, et al. Exceedingly small iron oxide nanoparticles as positive MRI contrast agents. Proc Natl Acad Sci U S A. 2017;114:2325–30.

103. McCarthy JR, Weissleder R. Multifunctional magnetic nanoparticles for targeted imaging and therapy. Adv Drug Deliv Rev. 2008;60:1241–51.

104. Ittrich H, Peldschus K, Raabe N, et al. Superparamagnetic iron oxide nanoparticles in biomedicine: applications and developments in diagnostics and therapy. Rofo. 2013;185:1149–66.

105. Weissleder R, Stark DD, Engelstad BL, et al. Superparamagnetic iron oxide: pharmacokinetics and toxicity. AJR Am J Roentgenol. 1989;152:167–73.

106. Bellin MF, Lebleu L, Meric JB. Evaluation of retroperitoneal and pelvic lymph node metastases with MRI and MR lymphangiography. Abdom Imaging. 2003;28:155–63.

107. Anzai Y, McLachlan S, Morris M, et al. Dextran-coated superparamagnetic iron oxide, an MR contrast agent for assessing lymph nodes in the head and neck. AJNR Am J Neuroradiol. 1994;15:87–94.

108. Hudgins PA, Anzai Y, Morris MR, et al. Ferumoxtran-10, a superparamagnetic iron oxide as a magnetic resonance enhancement agent for imaging lymph nodes: a phase 2 dose study. AJNR Am J Neuroradiol. 2002;23:649–56.

109. Dewitte H, Vanderperren K, Haers H, et al. Theranostic mRNA-loaded microbubbles in the lymphatics of dogs: implications for drug delivery. Theranostics. 2015;5:97–109.

110. Yoon YI, Kwon YS, Cho HS, et al. Ultrasound-mediated gene and drug delivery using a microbubble-liposome particle system. Theranostics. 2014;4:1133–44.

111. Jian J, Liu C, Gong Y, et al. India ink incorporated multifunctional phase-transition nanodroplets for photoacoustic/ultrasound dual-modality imaging and photoacoustic effect based tumor therapy. Theranostics. 2014;4:1026–38.

112. Fan CH, Lin WH, Ting CY, et al. Contrast-enhanced ultrasound imaging for the detection of focused ultrasound-induced blood-brain barrier opening. Theranostics. 2014;4:1014–25.

113. Liu HL, Fan CH, Ting CY, et al. Combining microbubbles and ultrasound for drug delivery to brain tumors: current progress and overview. Theranostics. 2014;4:432–44.

114. Vlaisavljevich E, Durmaz YY, Maxwell A, et al. Nanodroplet-mediated histotripsy for image-guided targeted ultrasound cell ablation. Theranostics. 2013;3:851–64.

115. Sirsi SR, Fung C, Garg S, et al. Lung surfactant microbubbles increase lipophilic drug payload for ultrasound-targeted delivery. Theranostics. 2013;3:409–19.

116. Streeter JE, Dayton PA. An in vivo evaluation of the effect of repeated administration and clearance of targeted contrast agents on molecular imaging signal enhancement. Theranostics. 2013;3:93–8.

117. Greis C. Ultrasound contrast agents as markers of vascularity and microcirculation. Clin Hemorheol Microcirc. 2009;43:1–9.

118. Stride E. Physical principles of microbubbles for ultrasound imaging and therapy. Cerebrovasc Dis. 2009;27:1–13.

119. Klibanov AL, Rasche PT, Hughes MS, et al. Detection of individual microbubbles of ultrasound contrast agents: imaging of free-floating and targeted bubbles. Invest Radiol. 2004;39:187–95.

120. Unnikrishnan S, Klibanov AL. Microbubbles as ultrasound contrast agents for molecular imaging: preparation and application. AJR Am J Roentgenol. 2012;199:292–9.

121. Bzyl J, Lederle W, Rix A, et al. Molecular and functional ultrasound imaging in differently aggressive breast cancer xenografts using two novel ultrasound contrast agents (BR55 and BR38). Eur Radiol. 2011;21:1988–95.

122. Walday P, Tolleshaug H, Gjøen T, et al. Biodistributions of air-filled albumin microspheres in rats and pigs. Biochem J. 1994;299:437–43.

123. Perkins AC, Frier M, Hindle AJ, et al. Human biodistribution of an ultrasound contrast agent (Quantison) by radiolabelling and gamma scintigraphy. Br J Radiol. 1997;70:603–11.

124. Jakobsen JA, Oyen R, Thomsen HS, et al. Members of Contrast Media Safety Committee of European Society of Urogenital Radiology (ESUR). Safety of ultrasound contrast agents. Eur Radiol. 2005;15:941–5.

125. Piscaglia F, Bolondi L. Italian Society for Ultrasound in Medicine and Biology (SIUMB) Study Group on Ultrasound Contrast Agents. The safety of Sonovue in abdominal applications: retrospective analysis of 23188 investigations. Ultrasound Med Biol. 2006;32:1369–75.

126. Main ML, Ryan AC, Davis TE, et al. Acute mortality in hospitalized patients undergoing echocardiography with and without an ultrasound contrast agent (multicenter registry results in 4,300,966 consecutive patients). Am J Cardiol. 2008;102:1742–6.

127. Lindner JR, Coggins MP, Kaul S, et al. Microbubble persistence in the microcirculation during ischemia/reperfusion and inflammation is caused by integrin- and complement-mediated adherence to activated leukocytes. Circulation. 2000;101:668–75.

128. Lurie DM, Seguin B, Schneider PD, et al. Contrast-assisted ultrasound for sentinel lymph node detection in spontaneously arising canine head and neck tumors. Invest Radiol. 2006;41:415–21.

129. Sever A, Jones S, Cox K, et al. Preoperative localization of sentinel lymph nodes using intradermal microbubbles and contrast-enhanced ultrasonography in patients with breast cancer. Br J Surg. 2009;96:1295–9.

130. Goldberg BB, Merton DA, Liu JB, et al. Sentinel lymph nodes in a swine model with melanoma: contrast-enhanced lymphatic US. Radiology. 2004;230:727–34.

131. Ravizzini G, Turkbey B, Barrett T, et al. Nanoparticles in sentinel lymph node mapping. Wiley Interdiscip Rev Nanomed Nanobiotechnol. 2009;1:610–23.

132. Wang LV, Hu S. Photoacoustic tomography: in vivo imaging from organelles to organs. Science. 2012;335:1458–62.

133. Mallidi S, Watanabe K, Timerman D, et al. Prediction of tumor recurrence and therapy monitoring using ultrasound-guided photoacoustic imaging. Theranostics. 2015;5:289–301.

134. Zhang R, Pan D, Cai X, et al. alpha$_v$beta$_3$-targeted copper nanoparticles incorporating an Sn 2 lipase-labile fumagillin prodrug for photoacoustic neovascular imaging and treatment. Theranostics. 2015;5:124–33.

135. Wilson KE, Bachawal SV, Tian L, et al. Multiparametric spectroscopic photoacoustic imaging of breast cancer development in a transgenic mouse model. Theranostics. 2014;4:1062–71.

136. Song KH, Stein EW, Margenthaler JA, et al. Noninvasive photoacoustic identification of sentinel lymph nodes containing methylene blue in vivo in a rat model. J Biomed Opt. 2008;13:054033.

137. De la Zerda A, Zavaleta C, Keren S, et al. Carbon nanotubes as photoacoustic molecular imaging agents in living mice. Nat Nanotechnol. 2008;3:557–62.

138. Kim JW, Galanzha EI, Shashkov EV, et al. Golden carbon nanotubes as multimodal photoacoustic and photothermal high-contrast molecular agents. Nat Nanotechnol. 2009;4:688–94.

139. Pan D, Pramanik M, Senpan A, et al. Near infrared photoacoustic detection of sentinel lymph nodes with gold nanobeacons. Biomaterials. 2010;31:4088–93.

140. Carrington C. Optical imaging sheds light on cancer's signature—regional blood flow and tissue oxygenization measures may permit earlier breast cancer detection. Diagnost Imag. www.diagnosticimaging.com. Accessed June 2004.

141. Berlier JE, Rothe A, Buller G, et al. Quantitative comparison of long-wavelength Alexa Fluor dyes to Cy dyes: fluorescence of the dyes and their bioconjugates. J Histochem Cytochem. 2003;51:1699–712.

142. Fox IJ, Brooker LG, Heseltine DW, et al. A tricarbocyanine dye for continuous recording of dilution curves in whole blood independent of variations in blood oxygen saturation. Proc Staff Meet Mayo Clin. 1957;32:478–84.

143. Alander JT, Kaartinen I, Laakso A, et al. A review of indocyanine green fluorescent imaging in surgery. Int J Biomed Imaging. 2012;2012:940585.

144. Landsman ML, Kwant G, Mook GA, et al. Light-absorbing properties, stability, and spectral stabilization of indocyanine green. J Appl Physiol. 1976;40:575–83.

145. Desmettre T, Devoiselle JM, Mordon S. Fluorescence properties and metabolic features of indocyanine green (ICG) as related to angiography. Surv Ophthalmol. 2000;45:15–27.

146. Engel E, Schraml R, Maisch T, et al. Light-induced decomposition of indocyanine green. Invest Ophthalmol Vis Sci. 2008;49:1777–83.

147. Rosenthal SM, White EC. Clinical application of the bromsulphalein test for hepatic function. J Am Med Assoc. 1925;84:1112–4.

148. Benya R, Quintana J, Brundage B. Adverse reactions to indocyanine green: a case report and a review of the literature. Catheter Cardiovasc Diagn. 1989;17:231–3.

149. Jung SY, Kim SK, Kim SW, et al. Comparison of sentinel lymph node biopsy guided by the multimodal method of indocyanine green fluorescence, radioisotope, and blue dye versus the radioisotope method in breast cancer: a randomized controlled trial. Ann Surg Oncol. 2014;21:1254–9.

150. Martínez Bonilla CA, Kouznetsov VV. "Green" quantum dots: basics, green synthesis, and nanotechnological applications. Green Nanotechnol. 2016:173–92. https://doi.org/10.5772/62327.

151. Chan WC, Maxwell DJ, Gao X, et al. Luminescent quantum dots for multiplexed biological detection and imaging. Curr Opin Biotechnol. 2002;13:40–6.

152. Alivisatos AP, Gu W, Larabell C. Quantum dots as cellular probes. Annu Rev Biomed Eng. 2005;7:55–76.

153. Hama Y, Koyama Y, Urano Y, et al. Simultaneous two-color spectral fluorescence lymphangiography with near infrared quantum dots to map two lymphatic flows from the breast and the upper extremity. Breast Cancer Res Treat. 2007;103:23–8.

154. Kim S, Lim YT, Soltesz EG, et al. Near-infrared fluorescent type II quantum dots for sentinel lymph node mapping. Nat Biotechnol. 2004;22:93–7.

155. Ow H, Larson DR, Srivastava M, et al. Bright and stable core-shell fluorescent silica nanoparticles. Nano Lett. 2005;5:113–7.

156. Padera TP, Stoll BR, So PT, et al. Conventional and high-speed intravital multiphoton laser scanning microscopy of microvasculature, lymphatics, and leukocyte-endothelial interactions. Mol Imaging. 2002;1:9–15.

157. Leu AJ, Gretener SB, Enderlin S, et al. Lymphatic microangiopathy of the skin in systemic sclerosis. Rheumatology (Oxford). 1999;38:221–7.

158. Seibold U, Wängler B, Schirrmacher R, et al. Bimodal imaging probes for combined PET and OI: recent developments and future directions for hybrid agent development. Biomed Res Int. 2014;2014:153741.

159. Culver J, Akers W, Achilefu S. Multimodality molecular imaging with combined optical and SPECT/PET modalities. J Nucl Med. 2008;49:169–72.

160. Tsopelas C, Bevington E, Kollias J, et al. ^{99m}Tc-Evans blue dye for mapping contiguous lymph node sequences and discriminating the sentinel lymph node in an ovine model. Ann Surg Oncol. 2006;13:692–700.

161. Brouwer OR, Buckle T, Vermeeren L, et al. Comparing the hybrid fluorescent-radioactive tracer indocyanine green-^{99m}Tc-nanocolloid with ^{99m}Tc-nanocolloid for sentinel node identification: a validation study using lymphoscintigraphy and SPECT/CT. J Nucl Med. 2012;53:1034–40.

162. Koyama Y, Talanov VS, Bernardo M, et al. A dendrimer-based nanosized contrast agent dual-labeled for magnetic resonance and optical fluorescence imaging to localize the sentinel lymph node in mice. J Magn Reson Imaging. 2007;25:866–71.

163. Choi JS, Park JC, Nah H, et al. A hybrid nanoparticle probe for dual-modality positron emission tomography and magnetic resonance imaging. Angew Chem Int Ed Engl. 2008;47:6259–62.

164. Yang BY, Moon SH, Seelam SR, et al. Development of a multimodal imaging probe by encapsulating iron oxide nanoparticles with functionalized amphiphiles for lymph node imaging. Nanomedicine (Lond). 2015;10:1899–910.

165. Torres Martin de Rosales R, Tavaré R, Paul RL, et al. Synthesis of 64Cu(II)-bis(dithiocarbamatebisphosphonate) and its conjugation with superparamagnetic iron oxide nanoparticles: in vivo evaluation as dual-modality PET-MRI agent. Angew Chem Int Ed Engl. 2011;50:5509–13.

166. Madru R, Kjellman P, Olsson F, et al. ^{99m}Tc-labeled superparamagnetic iron oxide nanoparticles for multimodality SPECT/MRI of sentinel lymph nodes. J Nucl Med. 2012;53:459–63.

167. Chakravarty R, Valdovinos HF, Chen F, et al. Intrinsically germanium-69-labeled iron oxide nanoparticles: synthesis and in-vivo dual-modality PET/MR imaging. Adv Mater. 2014;26:5119–23.

168. Thorek DL, Ulmert D, Diop NF, et al. Non-invasive mapping of deep-tissue lymph nodes in live animals using a multimodal PET/MRI nanoparticle. Nat Commun. 2014;5:3097.

169. Park JC, Yu MK, An GI, et al. Facile preparation of a hybrid nanoprobe for triple-modality optical/PET/MR imaging. Small. 2010;6:2863–8.

170. Madru R, Tran TA, Axelsson J, et al. ^{68}Ga-labeled superparamagnetic iron oxide nanoparticles (SPIONs) for multi-modality PET/MR/Cherenkov luminescence imaging of sentinel lymph nodes. Am J Nucl Med Mol Imaging. 2013;4:60–9.

171. Kim JS, Kim YH, Kim JH, et al. Development and in vivo imaging of a PET/MRI nanoprobe with enhanced NIR fluorescence by dye encapsulation. Nanomedicine (Lond). 2012;7:219–29.

172. Cui X, Mathe D, Kovács N, et al. Synthesis, characterization, and application of Core-Shell Co0.16Fe2.84O4@NaYF4(Yb, Er) and Fe3O4@NaYF4(Yb, Tm) nanoparticle as Trimodal (MRI, PET/SPECT, and optical) imaging agents. Bioconjug Chem. 2016;27:319–28.

173. Huang X, Zhang F, Lee S, et al. Long-term multimodal imaging of tumor draining sentinel lymph nodes using mesoporous silica-based nanoprobes. Biomaterials. 2012;33:4370–8.

174. Mathelin C, Piqueras I, Guyonnet JL. Development of technologies for sentinel lymph node biopsy in case of breast cancer. Gynecol Obstet Fertil. 2006;34:521–5.

175. Povoski SP, Neff RL, Mojzisik CM, et al. A comprehensive overview of radioguided surgery using gamma detection probe technology. World J Surg Oncol. 2009;7:11.

176. Woolfenden JM, Barber HB. Radiation detector probes for tumor localization using tumor-seeking radioactive tracers. AJR Am J Roentgenol. 1989;153:35–9.

177. Kwo DP, Barber HB, Barrett HH, et al. Comparison of NaI(T1), CdTe, and HgI2 surgical probes: effect of scatter compensation on probe performance. Med Phys. 1991;18:382–9.

178. Tiourina T, Arends B, Huysmans D, et al. Evaluation of surgical gamma probes for radioguided sentinel node localisation. Eur J Nucl Med. 1998;25:1224–31.

179. Schneebaum S, Even-Sapir E, Cohen M, et al. Clinical applications of gamma-detection probes—radioguided surgery. Eur J Nucl Med. 1999;26:S26–35.

180. Hoffman EJ, Tornai MP, Janecek M, et al. Intraoperative probes and imaging probes. Eur J Nucl Med. 1999;26:913–35.

181. Zanzonico P, Heller S. The intraoperative gamma probe: basic principles and choices available. Semin Nucl Med. 2000;30:33–48.

182. Mariani G, Vaiano A, Nibale O, et al. Is the "ideal" gamma-probe for intraoperative radioguided surgery conceivable? J Nucl Med. 2005;46:388–90.

183. Moffat FL. Targeting gold at the end of the rainbow: surgical gamma probes in the 21st century. J Surg Oncol. 2007;96:286–9.

184. Ricard M. Intraoperative detection of radiolabeled compounds using a hand held gamma probe. Nucl Instrum Method Phys Res A. 2001;458:26–33.

185. Guided intraoperative scintigraphic tumour targeting (GOSTT)—Implementing advanced hybrid molecular imaging and non-imaging probes for advanced cancer management. Vienna: IAEA Human Health Series; 2014.

186. Herrmann K, Nieweg OE, Povoski SP. Radioguided surgery. In: Current applications and innovative directions in clinical practice. Berlin: Springer; 2016.

187. Povoski SP, Chapman GJ, Murrey DA, et al. Intraoperative detection of ^{18}F-FDG-avid tissue sites using the increased probe counting efficiency of the K-alpha probe design and variance-based statistical analysis with the three-sigma criteria. BMC Cancer. 2013;13:98.

188. Povoski SP, Hall NC, Murrey DA, et al. Feasibility of a multimodal ^{18}F-FDG-directed lymph node surgical excisional biopsy approach for appropriate diagnostic tissue sampling in patients with suspected lymphoma. BMC Cancer. 2015;15:378.

189. Sarikaya I, Sarikaya A, Reba RC. Gamma probes and their use in tumor detection in colorectal cancer. Int Semin Surg Oncol. 2008;5:25.

190. RMD. Instruments Corp. https://www.surgeonschoice.net.au/Navigator_GPS_Manual.pdf. Accessed 10 Dec 2019.
191. Gamma Finder® II, W.O.M. World of Medicine AG. http://www.mesamedical.co.kr/new/DATA/mesa_hBUSINESS/7_mesa_hBUSINESS_FN04.pdf. Accessed 10 Dec 2019.
192. Bluetooth® Gamma Detection Probe, Neoprobe Corporation. http://www.hospiline.com.br/mammotome/documents/Products/Neoprobe/Model1100and1101OpsManualEngli.pdf. Accessed 10 Dec 2019.
193. Sentinella s-102. https://oncovision.com/sentinella/. Accessed 10 Dec 2019.
194. Anzai eZ-scope. http://www.nuclemed.be; https://www.accessdata.fda.gov/cdrh_docs/pdf9/K092471.pdf. Accessed 10 Dec 2019.
195. LumaGEM. http://www.cmr-naviscan.com/lumagem/. Accessed 10 Dec 2019.
196. Heckathorne E, Tiefer L, Daghighian F, et al. Evaluation of arrays of silicon photomultipliers for beta imaging. Nuclear Science Symposium Conference Record. 2008:1626–31.
197. Singh B, Stack BC, Thacker S, et al. A hand-held beta imaging probe for FDG. Ann Nucl Med. 2013;27:203–8.
198. DSouza AV, Lin H, Henderson ER, et al. Review of fluorescence guided surgery systems: identification of key performance capabilities beyond indocyanine green imaging. J Biomed Opt. 2016;21:80901.
199. Kim DW, Jeong B, Shin IH, et al. Sentinel node navigation surgery using near-infrared indocyanine green fluorescence in early gastric cancer. Surg Endosc. 2019;33:1235–43.
200. Kong SH, Bae SW, Suh YS, et al. Near-infrared fluorescence lymph node navigation using indocyanine green for gastric cancer surgery. J Minim Invasive Surg. 2018;21:95–105.
201. Duprée A, Rieß H, Detter C, et al. Utilization of indocyanine green fluorescent imaging (ICG-FI) for the assessment of microperfusion in vascular medicine. Innov Surg Sci. 2018;3:193–201.

Methodological Aspects of Lymphoscintigraphy: Bicompartmental Versus Monocompartmental Radiocolloid Administration

4

Martina Sollini, Francesco Bartoli, Andrea Marciano, Roberta Zanca, Giovanni D'Errico, Giuliano Mariani, and Paola A. Erba

Contents

4.1   **Introduction**.. 54

4.2   **Methodology of Lymphoscintigraphy**............................ 54

4.3   **Imaging for Lymphoscintigraphy**................................. 57

4.4   **Qualitative Visual Interpretation of Lymphoscintigraphy**....... 58

4.5   **Lymphoscintigraphy with Stress Test**........................... 59

4.6   **Quantitative Lymphoscintigraphy**................................ 59

4.7   **Virtual Reality for Preoperative Planning with Lymphoscintigraphy**....... 62

4.8   **PET/CT and PET/MR Lymphoscintigraphy**................... 63

4.9   **CT Imaging of Lymph Nodes and Lymphatic Circulation**...... 66

4.10 **Magnetic Resonance Imaging of Lymph Nodes and Lymphatic Circulation**...... 68

4.11 **Indocyanine Green Lymphography**............................... 72

References... 75

Learning Objectives
- Learn how to perform peripheral lymphoscintigraphy, including knowledge of injection procedures, acquisition protocols, and radiation dosimetry.
- Learn how to analyze lymphoscintigraphic images and to calculate semiquantitative parameters to be used in clinical practice for the differential diagnosis of edemas and for characterization of lymphedema.
- Learn how to perform, to analyze both visually and semiquantitatively, and to interpret PET/CT and PET/MR lymphoscintigraphy.
- Learn the basic concepts of CT imaging for lymph node assessment and for CT lymphography.
- Learn the basic concepts of MR imaging for lymph node assessment and for MR lymphography.
- Learn the basic concepts of indocyanine green lymphography.

M. Sollini
Department of Biomedical Sciences, Humanitas University, Milan, Italy

F. Bartoli · A. Marciano · R. Zanca · G. Mariani · P. A. Erba (✉)
Regional Center of Nuclear Medicine, Department of Translational Research and Advanced Technologies in Medicine and Surgery, University of Pisa, Pisa, Italy
e-mail: paola.erba@unipi.it

G. D'Errico
Department of Nuclear Medicine, Medical Research, Rome, Italy

G. Mariani et al. (eds.), *Atlas of Lymphoscintigraphy and Sentinel Node Mapping*,
https://doi.org/10.1007/978-3-030-45296-4_4

4.1   Introduction

Interstitial injection of radiolabeled compounds with sequential scanning imaging has been used to investigate the lymphatic system since the 1950s. This minimally invasive procedure, which simply requires intradermal or subcutaneous injection of a radiocolloid, has largely replaced the more invasive and technically difficult technique of lymphangiography [1, 2].

Despite the experience acquired over so many decades, protocols for performing lymphoscintigraphy are not yet standardized, and remarkable differences still persist among different centers. The main differences include important issues such as the type and site of injection, the use of dynamic and/or static acquisitions, and even the sequence of scintigraphic acquisitions. An additional crucial issue for performing lymphoscintigraphy is choice of the radiopharmaceutical, as discussed in detail in Chap. 3 of this book.

4.2   Methodology of Lymphoscintigraphy

Lymphoscintigraphy is based on the interstitial injection of a suitable radiopharmaceutical, a radiolabeled colloid where the size of the constituent particles is predefined within a certain range, so that they are too large to be removed by entering into the venous side of the blood capillaries, yet too small to be retained indefinitely at the injection site (as occurs for radiolabeled macroaggregates of human albumin); particles with such properties are in the range of 5–10 nm up to about 1000–2000 nm. After having been deposited in the extracellular fluid, these particles enter into the initial lymphatics by both direct passage through the inter-endothelial openings and vesicular transport through the endothelial cells [2, 3].

The interstitial route of administration is adequate for exploring lymphatic circulation because of some intrinsic features of lymphatic anatomy, and the fact that lymphatic vessels originate in the connective interstitium near the blood vessels. In the skin, the initial lymphatics are closely interconnected in a hexagonal pattern, through a set of precollectors, with deeper lymphatics in the dermis, where lymph fluid is transported in a centripetal fashion through collecting ducts and then to lymph nodes [3–5]. Therefore, exploration of the functional integrity of the lymphatic system begins with the demonstration of a normal transport of extracellular fluid, followed by evaluation of lymph flow along the lymphatic collectors until reaching the main thoracic lymph duct.

Fluid transport into the initial lymphatics occurs against a pressure gradient [3], since interstitial fluid pressure in the skin and subcutaneous tissue is slightly negative (-2 to -6 mm H_2O, or -0.15 to -0.44 mmHg) [6, 7], whereas the pressure in the lymphatic capillaries of the skin is positive [8]. The mechanisms allowing transport of particles against such pressure gradient include the presence of a suction force (generated through the contraction of the collecting lymphatics), coupled with the episodic increases in interstitial fluid pressure that are created during tissue movements [9]; active trans-endothelial transport [4] and phagocytosis followed by migration of macrophages into the lymphatic vessels also play a role [10]. Lymph flow progression in the collectors depends predominantly on lymphatic contraction [11].

The site of radiocolloid injection has a strong influence on the final results of lymphoscintigraphy. In fact, both the subcutaneous and the intradermal routes of injection are utilized in routine studies of superficial lymphatic circulation of the extremities. There is an ongoing debate as to which injection technique is best. Subcutaneous injection, recommended by many investigators [1, 12–14], has the advantage of negligible clearance of the radiocolloid through the blood vessels [1]. According to Mostbeck and Partsch, who compared subcutaneous and intramuscular injections of ^{99m}Tc-albumin nanocolloid, subcutaneous injection produced more reliable results, since it enabled to distinguish, using quantitative parameters, patients with lymphedema from healthy volunteers. Nevertheless, the intradermal injection route is still preferred by other authors [15–21].

However, it has been pointed out that the optimal route of injection may vary depending on the radiopharmaceutical employed, subcutaneous injection being optimal for the colloidal agents [22, 23]. Intradermal administration of non-colloidal agents (^{99m}Tc-human serum albumin, ^{99m}Tc-HSA) is associated with very rapid lymphatic transport, thus facilitating rapid evaluation and better quantification of lymphatic flow [19], although a non-negligible fraction of the radiopharmaceutical is removed from the injection site by way of the blood capillaries. Other colloidal or non-colloidal agents administered intradermally may not be as diagnostically reliable as ^{99m}Tc-HSA. However, comparison of intradermal and subcutaneous injections with ^{99m}Tc-HSA reveals better tracer kinetics after intradermal injection, and slow or no transport after subcutaneous injections [16].

Contrary to the superficial (or epifascial) routes of administration mentioned above (which results in visualization of the superficial lymphatic circulation), subfascial radiocolloid injection is utilized for exploring the deep lymphatic system of the extremities. This is normally achieved simply by injecting the radiocolloid intramuscularly.

When both epifascial and subfascial injections are performed sequentially, the procedure is called two-compartment lymphoscintigraphy. This approach is preferable for differentiating the possibly different mechanisms of extremity edema [23–25]. In fact, evaluating both the deep and the superficial circulation enhances the diagnostic accuracy of lymphoscintigraphy, as in this way it is possible to identify abnormalities of either the deep or the superficial lymphatic circulation.

In both phases of two-compartment lymphoscintigraphy, the radiocolloid is injected using a 25-gauge, 15 mm long needle, and administering a small volume of the radiocolloid suspension (0.2–0.3 mL) containing an activity of about 11–18 MBq. The procedure adopted in our center is described next.

For the deep lymphatic circulation of the lower extremities, we inject two aliquots of radiocolloid (7 MBq each) in 0.1 mL in the first and second inter-metatarsal space (identified by palpating the plants of both feet immediately proximal to the distal heads of the metatarsal bones, see Fig. 4.1) on each side, inserting the needle by about 12–13 mm to reach the inter-metatarsal

muscles below the deep fascia plantaris (Fig. 4.2). For the deep lymphatic circulation of the upper extremities, the radiocolloid (similar volume and activity as for the lower extremities) is injected in the second and in the third inter-metacarpal space (identified by palpating the palms of both hands the fossa in the inter-metacarpal space immediately proximal to the distal heads of the metacarpal bones, see Fig. 4.3) on each side, inserting the needle by about 10–12 mm to reach the inter-metacarpal muscles below the deep fascia palmaris (Fig. 4.4).

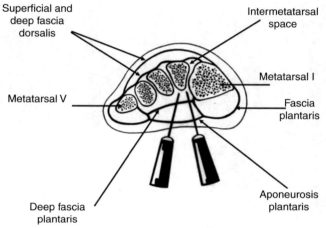

Fig. 4.1 Schematic representation of the technique of radiocolloid injection for deep lymphatic circulation of the lower extremities. Two aliquots are injected, respectively, in the first and in the second inter-metatarsal space that are identified by palpating the plants of both feet immediately proximal to the distal heads of the metatarsal bones

Fig. 4.3 Schematic representation of the technique of radiocolloid injection for the deep lymphatic circulation of the upper extremities. Two aliquots are injected, respectively, in the first and in the second inter-metacarpal space that are identified by palpating the palms of both hands immediately proximal to the distal heads of the metacarpal bones

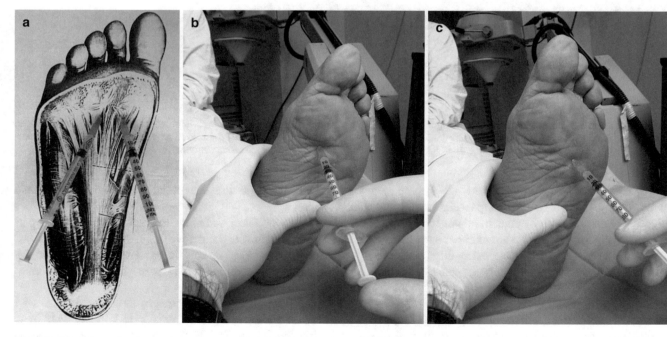

Fig. 4.2 (**a**) Schematic representation on anatomic drawing of the technique of radiocolloid injection for deep lymphatic circulation of the lower extremities. (**b, c**) Radiocolloid injection in the first (**b**) and in the second (**c**) inter-metatarsal space. The needle is inserted by about 12–13 mm, so to reach the inter-metatarsal muscles below the deep fascia plantaris

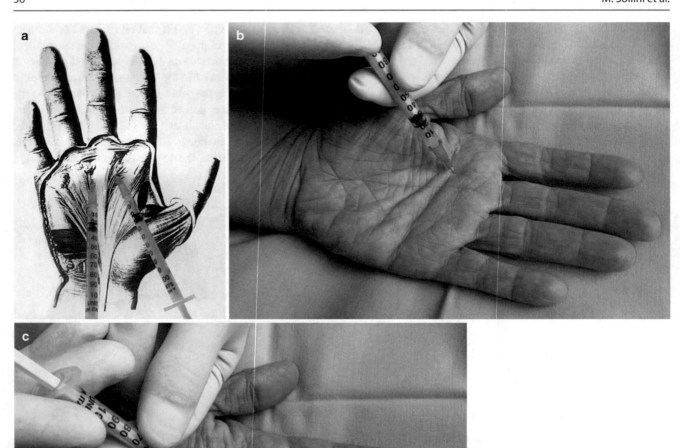

Fig. 4.4 (**a**) Schematic representation on anatomic drawing of the technique of radiocolloid injection for evaluating deep lymphatic circulation of the upper extremities. (**b**, **c**) Radiocolloid injection in the sec-ond (**b**) and in the third (**c**) inter-metacarpal space. The needle is inserted by about 10–12 mm, so as to reach the inter-metacarpal muscles below the deep fascia palmaris

For superficial lymphoscintigraphy, we prepare syringes in a similar manner as for deep lymphoscintigraphy, but with slightly higher radioactivity content (about 15–18 MBq). We inject two aliquots on the dorsum of either each foot or each hand (for the lower or the upper extremities, respectively), inserting the needle subdermally in sites corresponding approximately to the prior palmar injections, about 1–2 cm proximally to the interdigital web (Fig. 4.5).

We strongly recommend to not inject the radiocolloid directly into the interdigital web (as generally indicated by other authors), since this procedure may result in the visual-ization of either the superficial or the deep lymphatic systems.

Due to the faster and more complex pattern of the super-ficial lymphatic circulation, we prefer to perform full assess-ment of the deep lymphatic system first, followed by superficial lymphoscintigraphy as the last step of the com-bined procedure.

The injection sites are prepared by swabbing the area with either an iodine solution (especially in patients with frank lymphedema) or alcohol. Both limbs are always injected, using one side as a control for patients with unilateral lymphedema.

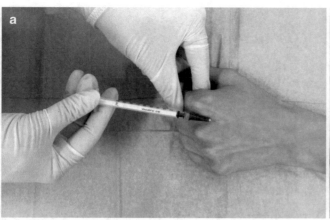 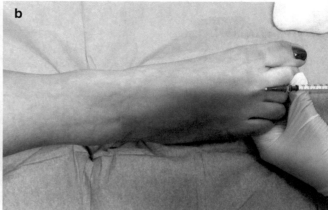

Fig. 4.5 For superficial lymphoscintigraphy we prepare syringes in a similar manner as for deep lymphoscintigraphy, but with slightly greater activity (about 15–18 MBq). The two aliquots are injected either on the dorsum of each foot (**a**) or in hand (**b**), inserting the needle subdermally in sites corresponding approximately to the previous palmar injections, about 1–2 cm proximal to the interdigital web

---

Key Learning Points
- Lymphoscintigraphy is based on the interstitial injection of radiolabeled colloids that drain from the injection site through the lymphatic pathway.
- Upon their interstitial administration, radiocolloids enter the initial lymphatics by both direct passage and vesicular transport.
- The interstitial route of administration is adequate for exploring lymphatic circulation.
- The site of radiocolloid injection has a strong influence on the final results of lymphoscintigraphy: both the subcutaneous and the intradermal routes of injection are utilized during routine studies of superficial lymphatic circulation of the extremities.
- Subfascial radiocolloid injection is utilized for exploring the deep lymphatic circulation of the extremities.
- When both epifascial and subfascial injections are performed sequentially, the procedure is called two-compartment lymphoscintigraphy.

4.3   Imaging for Lymphoscintigraphy

Images should be recorded with a dual-detector gamma camera, using high-resolution parallel-hole collimators, in both the spot-view mode and whole-body mode. Images should be recorded with a 20% window centered on the 140 keV photopeak of technetium-99m. Spot views can be acquired from feet to pelvis (for lower limbs) and from hands to axilla (including the chest, for upper limbs) for about 3–5 min, starting from the most distal to the most proximal portion of the limbs. Final spot views of the abdomen should also be acquired, to confirm passage of the radiocolloid to the systemic blood circulation within a physiological time window (as demonstrated by visualization of the liver and spleen), repeating the acquisitions up until 4–6 h post-administration in case of delayed radiocolloid drainage. After acquiring the spot images, a whole-body scan can be useful, from the distal feet until the abdomen for lower limbs, and from the hands to the chest and upper abdomen for upper limbs, using a scan speed of 12 cm/min.

Dynamic imaging is necessary if quantitation of lymphatic flow is planned (see below). SPECT or SPECT/CT is not generally required, but may be acquired if needed (Fig. 4.6) [26, 27].

For intracavitary lymph effusions, dual-phase lymphoscintigraphy is generally performed. In case of chylous ascites, subcutaneous injection in the interdigital space of both feet is preferred since the superficial circulation of the lower limbs accounts for the majority of lymph transport. During preparation for the exam, before radiocolloid injection, any external drainage line should be closed, whenever present. The gamma camera is generally positioned over the site of the effusion, and dynamic images are acquired from the time of radiocolloid injection until the evidence of radioactivity accumulation. Usually images are acquired for up to 8 h with sequential time points every approximately 30 min. During the second phase, a delayed image is acquired consisting of the acquisition of the region of interest in the same conditions as in the first phase, but with the drainage open. Although part of the radiopharmaceutical may be too large and can be trapped in the inguinal lymph nodes, the remaining part is sufficient to reach into the thoracic duct to demonstrate a possible lymphatic leak. Static images followed by SPECT and SPECT/CT acquisitions may complete the set of images, depending on the site of the intracavitary effusion [28, 29].

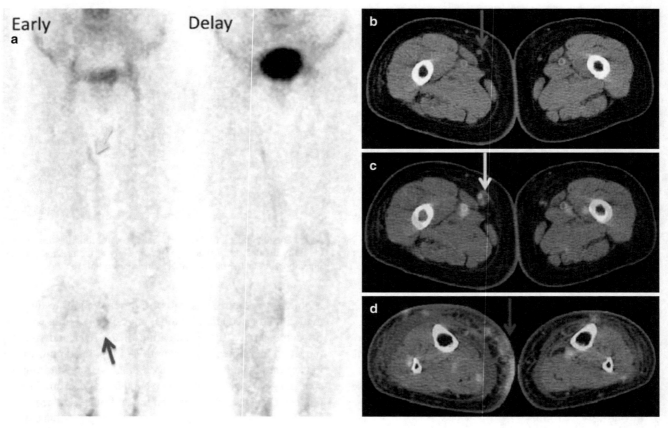

Fig. 4.6 Lymphoscintigraphy with ^{99m}Tc-nanocoll in an 81-year-old woman with bilateral lower limb lymphedema following surgery for uterine cervical cancer. The right lower limb, with more severe lymphedema, was considered as the affected side (ISL stage: II; LEL index: 338). (**a**) Both the early and delayed planar images show reduced/absent accumulation in inguinal lymph nodes. Although the planar images cannot discriminate the lymphatic vessel in the medial lower thigh from dermal backflow (red arrow in **a**), SPECT/CT images provide the correct information as dermal backflow (**d**, red arrow). Furthermore, whereas the planar images cannot determine whether the tubular accumulation in the medial thigh is lymphatic vessel or vein (yellow arrow in **a**), SPECT/CT showed vein to be the definitive answer (blue arrow in **b** and yellow arrow in **c**). Therefore, this case was classified as type 5 (*reproduced with permission from ref.* [26])

Scintigraphic acquisitions should be displayed with the intensity maximized, to depict the small fraction of radiocolloid that migrates from the injection site to the more proximal lymphatic stations.

Key Learning Points
- The protocol for lymphoscintigraphic imaging consists of spot views from feet to pelvis (for lower limbs) or from hands to axilla (including the chest, for upper limbs), and final spot views of the abdomen to confirm passage of the radiocolloid to the systemic blood circulation within a physiological time; a whole-body scan can also be useful.
- Dynamic imaging is necessary if quantitation of lymphatic flow is planned.
- For intracavitary lymph effusions, dual-phase lymphoscintigraphy is generally performed, consisting of static spot images followed by SPECT or preferably SPECT/CT imaging.

4.4 Qualitative Visual Interpretation of Lymphoscintigraphy

Qualitative lymphoscintigraphy is, in many cases, sufficient to establish a definite diagnosis [30]. However, there is still a lack of consensus on the criteria to be used for visual interpretation of lymphoscintigraphy, and expertise plays a critical role for diagnosis, particularly in case of borderline conditions [31].

A typical example of a normal two-compartment lymphoscintigraphy is shown in Fig. 4.7. Abnormal findings include asymmetrical visualization of lymphatic channels and collateral lymphatic channels, interrupted lymphatic vessels and lymph collection, asymmetrical or absent visualization of regional lymph nodes, and presence of "dermal flow" and/or "dermal back flow" [23–25].

For intracavitary lymph effusion, differences in radioactivity accumulated in all the images at the site of interest should be evaluated in order to define (a) normal pattern, when no significant differences in distribution of radiocolloids in all images until the 24th hour are detected;

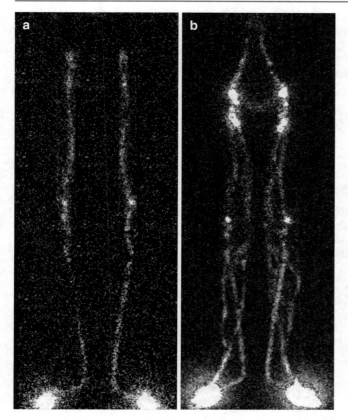

Fig. 4.7 Typical example of a normal pattern of two-compartment lymphoscintigraphy in lower limbs. (**a**) Step one of lymphoscintigraphy, obtained after deep injection as described in the text: symmetric migration of the radiocolloid along the vessels of the deep lymphatic circulation, with visualization of both the popliteal and the inguinal lymph nodes. (**b**) Step two of lymphoscintigraphy, obtained after subsequent radiocolloid injection in the subdermal space, as described in the text; in addition to the deep lymphatic vessels (still visualized by prior deep radiocolloid injection), the superficial lymphatic circulation is now visualized. The image represents therefore the sum of the two lymphatic systems, deep and superficial. From the superficial injection site a single lymphatic vessel originates on both sides, immediately dividing into two collaterals, one pointing symmetrically along the medial portion of the legs and thighs until the groin and the other pointing laterally; both vessels merge at the groins into the inguinal lymph nodes and continue in the main pelvic and abdominal lymphatic system

(b) positive test, in the presence of focal accumulation of radiocolloid that increases throughout the acquisitions until the end of the first stage; and (c) disappearance in the last acquisition at 24 h.

Key Learning Points
- Abnormal lymphoscintigraphic findings include asymmetrical visualization of lymphatic channels, development of collateral lymphatic channels, interrupted lymphatic vessels and lymph collection, asymmetrical or absent visualization of regional lymph nodes, and presence of "dermal flow" and/or "dermal back flow."

- For intracavitary lymph effusions, differences in radioactivity accumulated in all the images at the site of interest over time should be evaluated.

4.5   Lymphoscintigraphy with Stress Test

Lymphoscintigraphy can be performed by applying an intervention designed to augment lymphatic flow—such as changes in temperature, physical exertion, or administration of a pharmacologic agent. Although stress lymphoscintigraphy is recommended by most authors for its enhanced sensitivity and for its utility in the quantitation of lymphatic flow [23, 32], this approach is not universally employed [12, 14]. In the lower extremities, stress maneuvers include walking [33], standing [19], limb massage [20, 34], standardized treadmill exercise [22], and bicycle exercise [25]. In the upper extremities, the use of either repetitive squeezing of a rubber ball, a handgrip exercise device [35], or massage [20] has been proposed. Massage, exercise, and standing each enhances radiocolloid absorption from the injection site [19, 34, 36, 37]. Table 4.1 lists the different stress tests used by different authors.

Key Learning Points
- To augment lymphatic flow, lymphoscintigraphy can be performed by applying a "stress test" such as changes in temperature, physical exertion, or administration of a pharmacologic agent, massage, exercise, and standing/walking.

4.6   Quantitative Lymphoscintigraphy

Quantitation of lymphatic flow through lymphoscintigraphy has been proposed by many authors to enhance sensitivity of the technique in the diagnosis of lymphatic flow impairment [1]. According to the procedures employed, different quantitative parameters can be derived.

(a) *Transport Index (TI)* [35]: It is an overall parameter of transport kinetics ranging from 0 (normal) to 45 (pathological), designed by combining visual assessment of five criteria: (i) spatial radiocolloid distribution, (ii) temporal radiocolloid distribution, (iii) time of lymph node visualization, and (iv) graded visualization of lymph nodes and (v) graded visualization of lymphatic vessels. In a healthy extremity the TI should be <10. Following treatment, changes in this parameter are significantly correlated with volume changes of the extremities.

(b) *Transit Time (TT)*: It is the time it takes for the radiocolloid to reach the inguinal lymph nodes, and has

Table 4.1 Quantitative lymphoscintigraphy and stress tests in lymphedema: main clinical experience

Radiotracer	Route	ROIs	Imaging	Stress	Parameter	Author
[99m]Tc-nanocoll	sc	IS	10 × 6 s 120 × 60 s dynamic + static	1. Passive electric foot ergometer at 30 cycles/min for 2 h 2. Climb 150 steps	LN uptake % ID after (1) and (2) exercise	Weissleder et al. [1]
[99m]Tc-antimony trisulfide colloids	sc	LN	Dynamic		Modified TI index	Cambria et al. [13]
^{99m}Tc-HSA	id + sc	IS, LN	0–45 min dynamic, 0, 45, 90 min static	Walk	Clearance rate, LN uptake (time-activity curve)	Nawaz et al. [17]
[99m]Tc-nanocoll	sc, im	LN	15 min	15-min walking on horizontal treadmill 3.2 km/h	LN uptake % ID depth correction	Mostbeck et al. [22] Partsch et al. [23]
[99m]Tc-nanocoll	sc	LN	2 h	Bicycle 25 W	Lymph vessel uptake	Bräutigam et al. [25]
^{99m}Tc-HSA	sc	IS	10 min	3-h Walking	Clearance rate	Kataoka et al. [33]
[99m]Tc-nanocoll	sc	sc	0, 20 min, 2 h static	Flex and straighten feet 20 movements/min for 20 min	Transit time	Dabrowski et al. [38]
^{99m}Tc-HSA	sc	LN	Static + dynamic + static	Standardized treadmill walk (20 min) + walk at the brisk pace for 60 min	LN uptake at 2 h	Damstra et al. [39]
[99m]Tc-antimony trisulfide colloids	sc				LN uptake	Gloviczki et al. [40]
^{99m}Tc-HIG	sc	IS and LN	Dynamic + static up to 5.8 h	Squeezing a ball in hands simultaneously together with flexion at the elbow and pronation of the forearm (20 cycles/min)	Removal rate constant	Stanton et al. [41]
^{99m}Tc-HIG	id	LN, IS	0–2 h dynamic + static	None	Lymphatic transit time	Modi et al. [42]
[111]In/^{99m}Tc-HSA/HIgG	sc		3 h	30 fist clenchings	Clearance rate	Pain et al. [43]
[99m]Tc-nanocoll	sc	LN, liver	45, 150-min half-body images	None	Liver-to-lymph node ratio	Stamp et al. [44]
[99m]Tc-rhenium S	sc	IS	0–40 min	None	Colloid clearance	Pecking et al. [45, 46]
^{99m}Tc-HIG	id	IS	1 min; 5 × q 1 h	None	Clearance rate	Svensson et al. [47]
^{99m}Tc-HAS	im	IS	4 h	100 Submaximal contractions in 10 min	Clearance rate	Havas et al. [48]
[99m]Tc-antimony colloids	sc	IS	1 h	Bouts of arm cranking for 5 min at 0.6 Watts/kg or 75 contractions in 2.5 min at 50% MVC	Clearance rate	Lane et al. [49]
[99m]Tc-antimony colloids	sc	IS and LN	65 min	12 repeated sets of arm cranking for 2.5 min at 0.6 Watts/kg or 12 repeated sets of arm cranking for 2.5 min at 0.3 Watts/kg	Clearance rate	Lane et al. [50]
[99m]Tc-nanocoll	sc	IS, LN	0–30 min, dynamic 35 min + 3 h, static	Phase I no movement Phase II foot/toe movements for 5 min Phase III 1-h walking	Extraction % ID and LN uptake (time-activity curve with correction for decay and background)	Bourgeois [51]
[99m]Tc-nanocoll	id	IS, LN		Walk for 3 h	ROI analysis	Ketterings [52]
[99m]Tc-antimony colloids	sc		20–40 min, 1 h, 2 h	Normal walking 20 min	Clearance rate LN uptake % ID	Proby [53]

Table 4.1 (continued)

Radiotracer	Route	ROIs	Imaging	Stress	Parameter	Author
^{99m}Tc-HAS	id	LN	0–30 min	Standing 15 min	LN uptake (time-activity curve)	Suga [54]
^{99m}Tc-HIG, ^{99m}Tc-nanocoll	sc, id	IS	Dynamic intervals 10–171 min	None	Depot disappearance rate constant	O'Mahony et al. [55, 56]
^{99m}Tc-nanocoll	sc		0–100 Dynamic + static	Tip-toeing exercise in unison for 5 min Walk for 30 min	Extraction % ID and LN uptake (time-activity curve)	Bourgeois et al. [57]
^{99m}Tc-nanocoll	sc, id	IS, LN	0–100 min dynamic	None	LN % ID	Bourgeois et al. [58]
^{99m}Tc-nanocoll	sc	IS	Static	1. Massage + limb elevation 2. Walk/exercise 2 min	Tracer appearance time	Tartaglione et al. [59]
^{99m}Tc-HAS	sc	IS	0–25 min dynamic	Ergometric bicycle 75 w × 10 min	Wash rate constant	Jensen et al. [60]
^{99m}Tc-dextran	id	LS	0–30 min dynamic	Manual lymphatic therapy	Number of particles in ROI	De Godoy [37]

sc subcutaneous injection, *id* intradermal injection, *im* intramuscular injection, *IS* injection site, *LN* lymph node, *ID* injected dose

originally been proposed for use only in lower limb lymphoscintigraphy. When using large-size particle radiopharmaceutical as ^{99m}Tc-immunoglobulin, imaging up to 3 h is necessary, since the large particle sizes are drained slowly from the injection site to the lymph nodes. When using ^{99m}Tc-nanocolloids or filtered ^{99m}Tc-sulfur colloids, shorter acquisition times are adequate, with better quality images allowing easier interpretation [61, 62]. Although this parameter correlates with the severity of lymphatic dysfunction, a certain variability in TT estimation has been reported, suggesting that the information provided by the TT index should be employed in association with visual interpretation of the images for improved diagnostic accuracy [38].

(c) *Mean Transit Time (MTT)*: Time-activity curves from each injection site and each arm region are recorded. The input into the arm region is obtained as the (minus) time derivative of the injection site-activity curve. In the proposed model the arm-activity curve is considered to arise from the convolution of the retention function and the input function. The retention function is obtained by fitting the calculated arm-activity curve to the measured arm-activity curve. The MTT of activity passing through the arm is calculated as the time integral of the resulting retention function [63]. The average MTT of the lymphedema arm has been reported as 60.1 min (range 22–105 min) versus 5.4 min (range 1.2–8.7 min) in the contralateral, healthy arm.

(d) *Tracer Appearance Time (TAT)*: It is calculated as the time it takes for the radiocolloid to drain from the injection site to locoregional lymph nodes (normal value <10 min when using ^{99m}Tc-nanocoll and intradermal injection at the first interdigital space) [62]. By selecting an ilioinguinal node uptake of 9.7%, lymphedema could

be diagnosed with 86.8% sensitivity and 82.4% specificity [64].

When lymphatic dysfunction is bilateral, quantification of lymph node accumulation and clearance of activity from the injection site both become important parameters. It should be emphasized that these parameters are strongly influenced by the amount of exercise a patient can perform [65].

(e) *Transport Capacity (TC)*: It assesses the clearance of injected radioactivity, calculated as the ratio between the amount of activity transported from the depots to the groin lymph nodes over the first 2 h after injection and the injected activity; the normal reference limit is 15%. This parameter offers an objective measure of lymphatic function, capable of detecting reduced lymphatic drainage in the early stages, even before the appearance of clinical manifestations, or of qualitative changes in the lymphoscintigraphic pattern [1, 23, 25, 34, 39, 40, 66–69].

(f) *Removal Rate Constant (RRC)*: It represents local lymph flow per unit distribution volume of the flow marker; it is reduced by about 25% in the presence of lymphatic dysfunction involving a local impairment of lymphatic drainage [22, 41, 70].

(g) *Depot Activity Transported to Inguinal Lymph Nodes*: This modified method is employed in few protocols to estimate the depot clearance rate; by using attenuation correction, it takes into account the individual variation in tissue depth, in order to improve quantification of lymph node activity and to make this parameter more reliable [1, 23, 25, 42].

(h) *Lymphatic Drainage Efficiency (LDE)*: LDE is calculated as the percentage of injected activity (IIQ) in ilioinguinal nodes 150 min following subcutaneous foot web-space injection of ^{99m}Tc-nanocolloid and the percentage of activity leaving the injection depot by 150 min (k) as follows: LDE (%) = 100 (IIQ/k). IIQ, k, and LDE have been shown to be significantly lower in unilaterally normal compared with bilaterally normal limbs. LDE is lower in limbs displaying skin diversion and/or delay [71].

(i) *Uptake Index of the Left Inguinal (UIL) to the Right Inguinal Lymph Nodes (UIR)*: It provides the radioactivity ratio for inguinal nodes calculated in the whole-body images acquired at 2 h postinjection, and requires measurement of radioactivity at the injection site immediately after the administration to calculate the percentage of the radiocolloid administered into the left/right foot (WpL/WpR). Therefore, UIL/UIR is calculated as the percent fraction of count rate in the lymph nodes of the left/right inguinal region divided by the count rate over the total body × WpL/WpR [38]. Also the UIL/UIR ratio is used to identify lymphatic dysfunction; however, some variability in UIL/UIR determination has been reported, thus suggesting that also this quantitative parameter should be employed in association with visual interpretation of the images for improved diagnostic accuracy.

(j) *Washout Rate Constant (k) and Depot Half-Life* ($T_{1/2} = \ln 2/k$): These parameters of lymphatic function are calculated by linear regression analysis of the time-activity curve derived from images obtained over 20–25 min starting 40 min after injection of 10 MBq of ^{99m}Tc-HSA (30 min of rest + 10 min of ergometer bicycle at 75 W). The depot half-life is prolonged in case of lymphatic dysfunction (4.6 h versus 2.7 h in normal controls when using ^{99m}Tc-nanocoll); clearance of ^{99m}Tc-HSA is generally faster than clearance of ^{99m}Tc-nanocoll [22]. However, these parameters are influenced by the radiopharmaceutical injection technique, thus resulting to be somewhat unreliable to assess lymphatic dysfunction [31, 42, 43, 72–77].

(k) *Liver-to-Nodal Ratio (L/N Ratio)*: It is calculated based on regions of interest (ROIs) drawn, respectively, around the right lobe of the liver and around the ilioinguinal lymph nodes bilaterally in the anterior-view images acquired at 45 min and at 150 min postinjection; counts within the ROIs are corrected for background (ROIs on the same horizontal levels as the liver and lateral to the right edge of the ilioinguinal nodes, respectively). Normal values are 1.8 pixel^{-1} × 10^{-6} (range 1.3–5.5) at 45 min, and 2.5 pixel^{-1} × 10^{-6} (range 1.5–5) at 150 min. The 150-min L/N ratio is most frequently found to be abnormal in patients with lymphatic dysfunction, and is well correlated with the severity of lymphoscintigraphic abnormalities [44].

In patients with intracavitary lymph effusion, quantitative evaluation is performed assessing the ratio values (K) between the mean activity/per pixel detected (in all the sequential acquisitions) on ROIs integrated on the focal zone (suspected pathological area – "ROIp") and the mean activity/per pixel measured on a "nontarget area" = considered healthy area – "ROIh" located, as a rule, contralaterally. Accordingly, K is calculated as the ratio ROIp/ROIh. Therefore, a lymphoscintigraphy is defined as normal when stable K values are obtained throughout all of the images. On the contrary, increasing K values at sequential imaging times is consistent with the presence of intracavitary lymph effusion.

It should be noted that clearance values from the injection site may not allow, by themselves, to discriminate lymphedema from normal lymphatic function, as qualitative evaluation is invariably required [23].

> **Key Learning Points**
> - Quantitation of lymphatic flow through lymphoscintigraphy enhances sensitivity of the technique in the diagnosis of lymphatic flow impairment.
> - Different quantitative parameters can be derived depending on the procedure employed for lymphoscintigraphy.

4.7 Virtual Reality for Preoperative Planning with Lymphoscintigraphy

The conventional planar images of lymphoscintigraphy and SPECT/CT can be processed by dedicated software to visualize a 3D patient-specific model, thus creating a detailed 3D image of the anatomical structures. To this aim, the exact localization of the afferent lymphatic vessels is obtained by lymphoscintigraphy including SPECT/CT, which is of particular value because conventional planar imaging is not able to discriminate between lymph nodes and other structures, including lymphangiomas. The conversion of cross-sectional radiological images into 3D reconstruction and the generation of 3D visualization in virtual reality (Fig. 4.8) enable to visualize in 3D the lymphatic drainage pathways and the localization of the lymphatic malformation, but also to plan and perform the intervention without iatrogenic damage to the adjacent structures [78].

> **Key Learning Point**
> - Lymphoscintigraphy images can be processed by dedicated software to visualize a 3D patient-specific model, thus creating a detailed 3D image of the anatomical structures for surgical guidance.

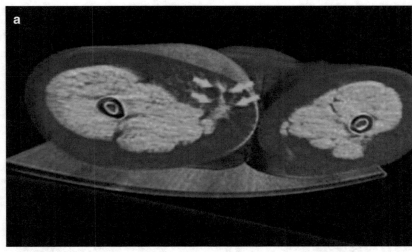
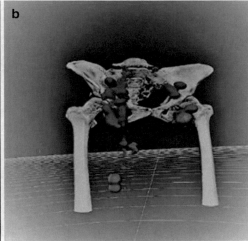

Fig. 4.8 (a) 3D reconstruction of a SPECT/CT acquisition of lympho-scintigraphy, based on the fusion of the CT images with the SPECT images and obtained by virtual reality software, showing the site of lymphatic malformation (green arrows). (b) 3D reconstructed hybrid image of the SPECT/CT acquisition obtained by virtual reality soft-ware, showing visualization of the lymphatic structures of the lower limbs. Note the extension of the malformation (conglomerate of tracer) from the region of the right thigh up to the abdominal cavity (*reproduced with permission from ref.* [78])

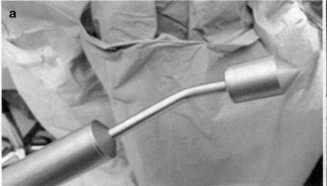
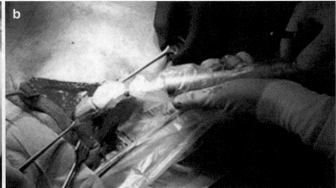

Fig. 4.9 (a) High-energy handheld probe based on the use of a five-crystal assembly in the detecting head for electronic collimation of the 511 keV annihilation photons. (b) Intraoperative use of the handheld high-energy probe (*reproduced with permission from ref.* [79])

4.8 PET/CT and PET/MR Lymphoscintigraphy

The intraoperative identification of sentinel lymph nodes (SLNs) using ^{89}Zr-nanocolloidal albumin consists of preoperative PET/TC imaging (Fig. 4.9) followed by intraoperative SLN detection using a handheld high-energy gamma probe. This has been achieved in patients with oral cavity carcinoma planned for surgical resection. The lymphoscintigraphy protocol consists of dynamic frames starting almost immediately after four peritumoral injections of ^{89}Zr-nanocolloidal albumin (average total activity of 5.9 ± 3.5 MBq). A high-energy handheld gamma probe designed to detect 511 keV photons can then be used for intraoperative SLN localization (Fig. 4.9).

Therefore, the combination of preoperative PET/CT imaging and intraoperative high-energy gamma probe allows optimal SLN detection [79].

In case of peripheral lymphoscintigraphy, local injection of ^{68}Ga-labeled NOTA-Evans blue (^{68}Ga-NEB) is performed using a small volume (about 0.5 mL) and an activity of 37 MBq/administration (Fig. 4.10). In patients with upper extremity swelling the site of injection is the subcutaneous tissue between the thumb and index finger of each hand. In case of lower limb lymphedema as well as in case of intra-cavitary lymphedema, ^{68}Ga-NEB is injected subcutaneously into the bilateral first web spaces of the feet (0.5 mL, 37 MBq/foot), followed by massage of the injection sites. The patients are also requested to walk after tracer injection [81].

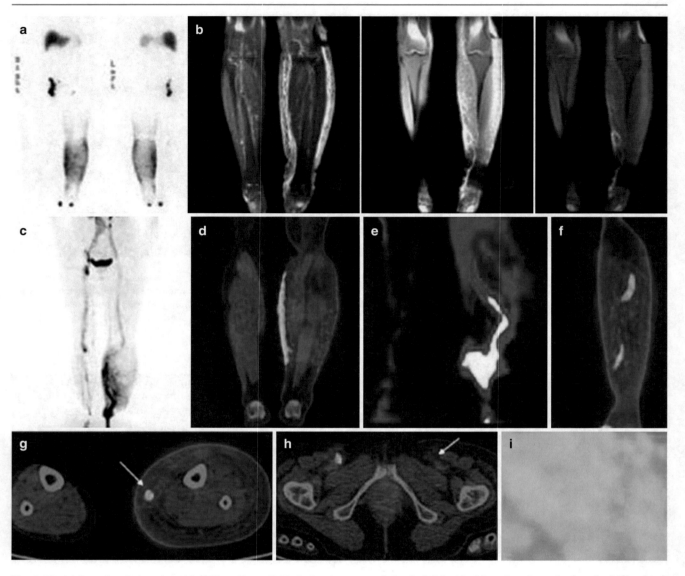

Fig. 4.10 (**a**) Lymphoscintigraphy with ^{99m}Tc-sulfur colloid obtained in a patient with severe edema of the left lower limb shows large and diffuse dermal backflow of the left lower limb, associated with absent tracer accumulation in left inguinal lymph nodes. (**b**) In the same patient, MR lymphangiography shows increased subcutaneous thickness and diffuse fibrosis of the left leg, as well as dilated and tortuous deep-seated lymphatic channels of the left medial calf (coronal images). PET/CT was acquired 60 min after interstitial injection of ^{68}Ga-NEB. The MIP image displayed in (**c**) shows severe and diffuse dermal backflow of the left leg, associated with reduced/absent tracer accumulation in left inguinal lymph nodes and a length of dilated and tortuous lymphatic channels of the left calf (as confirmed by fused PET/CT images shown in **d**, **e**, and **f**). Panels (**g**) and (**h**) display axial sections of the fused PET/CT images, respectively, at the leg level and at the inguinal level, the latter demonstrating reduced/absent visualization of inguinal lymph nodes. (**i**) Intraoperative ICG lymphangiography was unable to delineate lymphatic vessels, due to limited penetration depth of optical imaging and overall overgrowth of adipose tissue in stage III lymphedema (*reproduced with permission from ref.* [80])

4.8.1 PET/CT Imaging Protocol of Lymphatic Circulation

The ^{68}Ga-NEB PET/CT protocol consists of a whole-body acquisition at multiple time points after tracer injection. After low-dose CT scanning (120 kV, 35 mA, 3 mm layer, 512 × 512 matrix, 70 cm FOV), a whole-body PET acquisition is performed from the foot to the cervical area and covered by 7–9-bed positions (2 min/bed). At 60 and 90 min, the PET scan can be repeated (5–7-bed positions, 2 min/bed), covering from the foot ankle to the pubic symphysis. For those patients with suspected chylothorax, chyloperitoneum, or chyluria, the images are acquired 5–20 min after tracer injection. For those with lymphedema, longer intervals up to 1 h between tracer injection and image acquisition are recommended [82].

4.8.2 PET/MR Imaging Protocol of Lymphatic Circulation

In case of PET/MR, the imaging protocol consists of the acquisition of images 20 and 40 min after subcutaneous injections of ^{68}Ga-NEB into the first interdigital spaces of both feet (0.5 mL, 37 MBq/foot), by using an integrated PET/MR scanner (Fig. 4.11). The PET protocol consists of the acquisition of 3- or 4-bed positions, and the images are reconstructed with an ordered subset expectation maximizing algorithm (12 iterations, 28 subsets, Gaussian filter with FWHM of 6.0 mm) to a matrix of 192 × 192, with slice thickness of 2.94 mm. For each bed position, the MR protocol consists of axial T2-weighted imag-

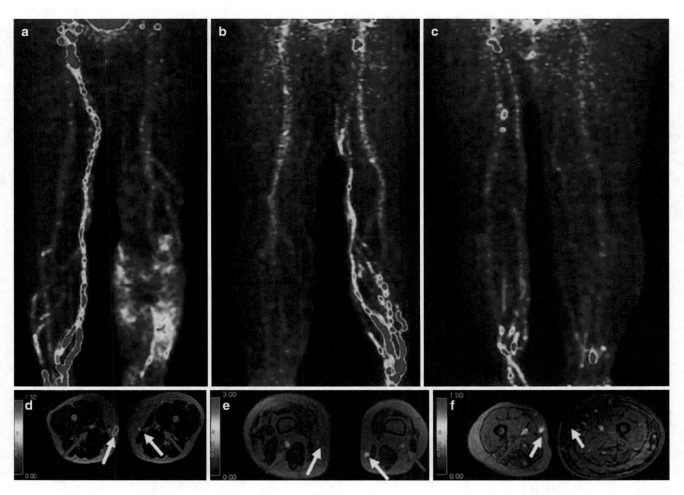

Fig. 4.11 ^{68}Ga-NEB TOF PET/MR lymphoscintigraphy patterns observed in three different cases (selected as representative examples of patients with minimal, moderate, and severe lower limb lymphedema, respectively) are displayed as the MIP images in (**a**), (**b**), and (**c**). The corresponding fused axial sections displayed in (**d**), (**e**), and (**f**) visualize well in each patient the deep lymphatic vessels (red arrows) and superficial lymphatic vessels (yellow arrows). (**a**) The PET MIP image at 20 min shows dermal backflow and reduced inguinal lymph node visualization on the affected left side. (**b**) The PET MIP image at 20 min shows dermal backflow and decreased inguinal lymph node visualiza-

tion on the right affected side. (**c**) The PET MIP image at 20 min shows dermal backflow and decreased inguinal lymph node visualization on the affected left side. (**d–f**): The corresponding fused axial PET/MR images show that ^{68}Ga-NEB accumulation in the superficial lymphatic vessels of the affected limb is less than that of the normal limb (yellow arrows). Instead, ^{68}Ga-NEB accumulation in the deep lymphatic vessels of the affected limb is equal to that of the normal limb (red arrows). It can also be noted that there is much more adipose fat deposition around the superficial than around the deep lymphatic vessels (*reproduced with permission from ref.* [82])

ing with a fast-recovery spin-echo (FSE) sequence, the iterative decomposition of water and fat with echo asymmetry and least-squares estimation (IDEAL) method to achieve better fat saturation, T1-weighted imaging with a FSE sequence, and IDEAL to obtain separated water, fat, and in-phase and out-of-phase images. After the first acquisition, the scanning can be repeated. Then, coronal MRI with large FOV is performed [82].

> **Key Learning Point**
> - PET/MR lymphoscintigraphy consists of the acquisition of images 20 and 40 min after subcutaneous injections of ^{68}Ga-NEB.

4.8.3 Imaging Interpretation of PET-Based Lymphoscintigraphy

Besides visual interpretation, several semiquantitative parameters can be used to assess the severity of lymphedema:

- Standardized uptake value (SUV) of superficial lymphatic vessels (SLV), denominated as SUV_{slv}
- SUV of deep lymphatic vessels (DVL), denominated as SUV_{dlv}
- Ratio of the two values above ($SUV_{slv/dlv}$)

To this aim, regions of interest (ROIs) for the middle of the crus, middle of the leg, and middle of the thigh are used to measure SUV_{svl} and SUV_{dvl}, set, respectively, as the average maximum SUV_{slv} and maximum SUV_{dlv} of these three regions. $SUV_{slv/dlv}$ is designed to assess the severity of lymphedema. The SUV is calculated based on the activity of ^{68}Ga-NEB and weight of the patient.

At PET/CT significant difference in the SUV_{slv} between the affected limbs and normal limbs was found in all subjects (affected limbs: 0.57 ± 0.32; normal limbs: 1.86 ± 1.43; $P < 0.05$), which was not found in the SUV_{dlv} (affected limbs: 0.64 ± 0.39; normal limbs: 0.63 ± 0.31; $P > 0.1$). The $SUV_{slv/dlv}$ ratio of the affected limbs showed also differences related to the severity of lymphedema [82]. Similarly, a significant difference in the SUV_{svl} between the affected limbs and normal limbs in all enrolled patients was found when using PET/MR, with a negative correlation between $SUV_{slv/dlv}$ and severity of lymphedema [82].

> **Key Learning Point**
> - PET/CT lymphoscintigraphy is interpreted visually or by calculating semiquantitative parameters such as the standardized uptake value (SUV) of superficial lymphatic vessels (SUV_{slv}), SUV of deep lymphatic vessels (SUV_{dlv}), and ratio of the two values above ($SUV_{slv/dlv}$).

4.9 CT Imaging of Lymph Nodes and Lymphatic Circulation

Most systemic imaging of the lymphatics is limited to the detection of enlarged lymph nodes on CT or MRI. Normal lymph nodes, despite the large flow of lymph through them, are tightly regulated in size. When they become infected or are the site of metastasis, they enlarge and become readily visible on CT and MRI, with secondary architectural changes often becoming apparent.

4.9.1 CT for Lymph Node Assessment

Traditionally, CT relies on size criteria to distinguish benign from metastatic lymph nodes; in particular, a maximum short-axis diameter >1 cm is considered malignant. The long axis of normal nodes is typically parallel to the lymphatic vessels. Characteristics of normal lymph nodes include horseshoe shape, a hilum containing central fat, smooth outline, and homogeneous CT density [83]. Moreover, they tend to be more elliptical than pathologic nodes. Pathologic nodes tend to be enlarged and irregular, and lose their central fat. However, micrometastases, particularly with breast cancer, are often found in lymph nodes with normal size and shape [84]. Further improvements in spatial resolution, cross-sectional imaging, and three-dimensional reconstructions may allow the assessment of additional morphological features of the nodal cortex and sinus to aid diagnosis. While these findings are useful in day-to-day clinical practice, they are inherently nonspecific. Small lymph nodes may contain microfoci of disease and not be enlarged or distorted in shape; conversely, enlarged nodes may simply be caused by hyperplasia rather than malignancy.

4.9.2 CT Lymphography (CT-LG)

Interstitially injected iopamidol-CT has been investigated for SLN identification in patients with cancer (Fig. 4.12). Suga et al. investigated the ability of thin-section, three-dimensional CT with iopamidol to correctly localize SLNs [86]. Seventeen patients with breast cancer underwent preoperative CT scanning after injection of iopamidol into peri-tumor and peri-areola areas. Perioperative blue-dye injections were performed for comparison. CT lymphography localized SLNs in all patients, and provided accurate anatomical mapping of SLNs and of connections to their afferent lymphatic vessels draining from the injection sites. The spatial resolution achieved may provide improved accuracy in guiding SLN biopsy (SLNB), but it does not provide real-time feedback to the surgeon. Minato et al. were also able to identify SLNs in 13/15 patients with breast cancer, either by enhancement of the lymphatic vessel draining into the SLN or by enhancement in the SLN itself, correlating well with blue-dye

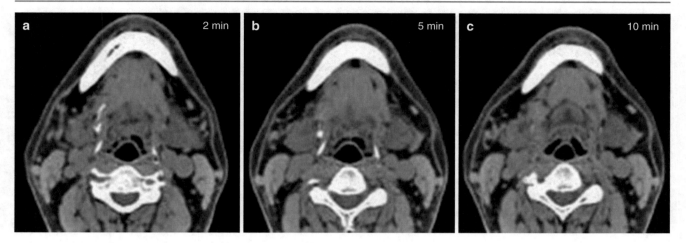

Fig. 4.12 Axial images from CT lymphography obtained after peritumoral injection of iopamidol in a patient with oral cancer. (**a**) SLN and lymphatic vessels visualized at 2 min postinjection. (**b**) Clear contrast enhancement of the SLN at 5 min postinjection, with disappearance of the lymphatic vessel. (**c**) Disappearance of both the SLN and lymphatic vessel at 10 min postinjection (*reproduced with permission from ref.* [85])

detection [87]. Suga et al. have also demonstrated CT-based detection of SLNs in esophageal cancer [88]. Using an endoscopic technique, they injected iopamidol peri-tumorally in nine esophageal cancer patients, prior to esophagectomy and regional lymph node dissection. Histology confirmed the high predictive value of SLNB guided by CT lymphography. A problem with iopamidol-based SLN imaging is that, due to its low molecular weight, this agent quickly opacifies and washes out of the lymph nodes. This creates a limited time window for scanning and/or surgery.

The interstitial CT-LG method described by Suga et al. [86, 89, 90] was also used for comprehensive high-definition 3D assessment of the lymphatic vessels of the extremities using multidetector-row CT (MDCT). Lymphoscintigraphy and indocyanine green (ICG) were used in the same patients as the gold standard imaging technique. A total of 0.8 mL of 1% Xylocaine® was injected subcutaneously into the first to fourth interdigital web space of the dorsum of the foot, using a 30-gauge needle, to reduce the pain. A total of 4 mL of iopamidol was then injected intradermally using a 24-gauge needle at the same sites. After iopamidol administration, the injection sites ware massaged gently for 10 min to facilitate migration of the contrast agent to the draining lymphatics. Thirty minutes after the administration of iopamidol, contiguous 1-mm-thick CT images were acquired from the tip of the foot to the groin area (120 kV and 250 mA, with a 50 cm field of view and a 512 × 512 matrix). Three-dimensional CT images can then be reconstructed using maximum intensity projection (MIP) and surface rendering techniques. In a study performed in patients with early-stage lymphedema, uptake of the contrast agent was limited to the dorsum of the foot and the leg, whereas the imaging results for the thigh were poor,

probably due to the slower flow of the contrast agent in lymphatic vessels, or alternatively the uptake of the contrast agent may be less in the lymphatic system compared to the radioisotope tracer used for lymphoscintigraphy. Considering the fact that lymph flows centrally over time, increasing the imaging time to 30 min or more and increasing the exercise load in addition to massaging the injected sites to increase the lymphatic flow may also be helpful. CT-LG provided high-resolution images of individual lymphatic vessels of the dorsum of the foot and leg, which have a typical diameter of 0.7–2.1 mm, which is a major advantage of CT-LG. In addition, the possibility of three-dimensional observation of deeper tissues might help in investigating the mechanism of dermal backflow: from collecting lymphatic vessels, several thinner lymphatic vessels branch out toward the dermis, transitioning to the dermal backflow.

> **Key Learning Points**
> - At CT imaging, lymph nodes with a maximum short-axis diameter >1 cm are considered malignant.
> - Pathologic/metastatic lymph nodes tend to be enlarged and irregular, and lose their central fat.
> - CT imaging following interstitial iopamidol injection has been investigated for SLN identification in patients with cancer.
> - The interstitial CT-LG method has also been used for comprehensive high-definition 3D assessment of the lymphatic vessels of the extremities using multidetector-row CT.

4.10 Magnetic Resonance Imaging of Lymph Nodes and Lymphatic Circulation

MRI has long been used in a manner similar to CT for lymph node staging. Unenhanced MR is equivalent to CT, since it relies predominantly on size criteria in order to distinguish benign from malignant lymph nodes. As with CT, there are a few morphological features that can aid the diagnosis of benign nodes, i.e., regular nodal outline, or homogenous signal intensity. However, absolute signal intensities of benign lymph nodes cannot be reliably distinguished from those of malignant lymph nodes on either T1- or T2-weighted images [91].

4.10.1 Dynamic Contrast-Enhanced MRI of Lymph Nodes

The technique of functional or dynamic contrast-enhanced MR imaging (DCE-MRI) is readily available in the clinical setting. DCE-MRI acquires serial images following the intravenous injection of a contrast agent, typically low-molecular-weight Gd-DTPA. Wash-in and washout curves can be derived from regions of interest (ROIs) for direct comparison, or pharmacokinetic models can be applied in order to derive permeability parameters. The resulting parameters reflect differences in blood flow and permeability and have been shown to correlate with the degree of angiogenesis within tumors. To this end, DCE-MRI may play a role in identifying malignant lymph nodes. Heiberg al., while performing DCE-MRI in patients with breast cancer, noticed that the DCE profiles of malignant nodes were similar to those of the primary cancer [92]. Murray et al. performed preoperative DCE-MRI in 47 women with newly diagnosed primary breast cancer [93]. Enhancement indices and nodal areas were correlated with the histopathology of excised nodes. Ten patients were found to have axillary metastases, and all of these patients had at least one lymph node with an enhancement index of >21%, with 100% sensitivity. However, specificity was only 56% due to frequent false-positive results, although more encouragingly a negative predictive value of 100% could be achieved. Kvistad et al. assessed 65 patients with more advanced, invasive breast cancer prior to treatment with surgery and axillary lymph node dissection [94]. Histology confirmed metastases in 24 patients. Using criteria based on changes in signal intensity, DCE-MRI correctly classified 57/65 patients (88% accuracy), yielding a sensitivity of 83% and specificity of 90%. Fischbein et al. used DCE-MRI to assess lymph nodes in 21 patients diagnosed with squamous cell carcinomas of the head and neck [95]. All patients underwent lymph node dissection; 68 lymph nodes were assessed and, unlike breast cancer, these malignant lymph nodes displayed significantly longer time to peak enhancement, reduced peak enhancement, decreased slope, and slower washout, compared with normal lymph nodes. This may reflect the typically necrotic nature of head and neck tumors and their draining lymph nodes.

4.10.2 Contrast-Enhanced Magnetic Resonance Lymphography

Preliminary reports on a novel technique of contrast-enhanced MR lymphography (MRL) are promising for the evaluation of chronic lymphedema. Compared to lymphoscintigraphy, MRL provides a noninvasive means to assess both the anatomy and functionality of the lymphatic system with a higher spatial and temporal resolution, with shorter time exam, and without the use of ionizing radiation. In addition, although lymphoscintigraphy and conventional fluoroscopic lymphangiography, being dynamic studies, allow real-time continuous evaluation of slow-flowing lymphatic channels, these techniques do not provide cross-sectional organ and soft-tissue detail. By contrast, MRL allows enhanced visualization of the lymphatic system with cross-sectional imaging and reveals a powerful diagnostic tool to evaluate lymphatic disease [96]. Furthermore, other MR exam components, such as 3D heavily T2-weighted and fat-suppressed sequences, enable the evaluation of subcutaneous soft tissues to delineate the presence, severity, and extent of lymphedema, as well as associated soft-tissue changes such as adipose tissue deposition and fibrosis [97].

A typical protocol used for an MRL exam consists of a 3D heavily T2-weighted sequence with spectral fat suppression to depict the severity and distribution of lymphedema, and a dynamic high-resolution fat-suppressed T1-weighted 3D spoiled gradient echo sequence before and after the injection of gadolinium-based contrast agent to image enhancement of lymphatic channels. In general, to emphasize the gadolinium-containing structures, such as lymphatic vessels, 3D maximum intensity projection (MIP) is performed to characterize and localize particular structures of interest on different image reconstructions [98, 99]. New MRL acquisition protocols have been proposed, consisting of a 3D isotropic T1-weighted fast spin-echo (FSE) or a 3D isotropic intermediate-weighted fast spin-echo. In patients with lymphedema, MRL using 3D T1-weighted FSE is suitable for preoperative planning and postoperative imaging of microsurgical lymphatic vessel reconstruction, as it provides better information regarding lymphatic vessels and their drainage. Therefore, this technique succeeds in visualizing the lymph vessel structures and lymphatic pathway in patients with lymphedema as compared to lymphangiography using the 3D intermediate-weighted FSE pulse sequence, which has the advantage of depicting lymph nodes in lymphedematous extremities [100]. Figures 4.13 and 4.14 show examples of direct contrast-enhanced magnetic resonance lymphangiography.

For contrast-enhanced MRL to identify an occult chylous leak, gadolinium contrast agent is injected into a main lymphatic vessel, and dynamic 3D T1-weighted MR imaging is acquired for 17 min, followed by high-resolution static 3D T1-weighted MR images acquired at 30 and 40 min after injection [101].

The MRL images are interpreted visually, adopting a qualitative analysis score [98, 103] to assess:

(a) The quality of drainage using a four-point scale:
 – Score 0, no drainage
 – Score 1, diffuse enhancement, interstitial
 – Score 2, partially diffuse enhancement, interstitial and vascular enhancement
 – Score 3, directed, vascular enhancement
(b) The delay of drainage:
 – Score 0, no drainage
 – Score 1, substantial delay with axillary/pelvic level >60 min for MR lymphangiography

– Score 2, slight delay: axillary/pelvic level >20 min for MR lymphangiography
– Score 3, no delay: lymph vessel enhancement in the first series of images, reaching axillary level <20 min for MR lymphangiography
(c) The depiction of lymph vessels which can be performed using either a three-point scale:
 – Score 0, no lymph vessels
 – Score 1, weak conspicuity
 – Score 2, strong conspicuity
 or a four-point scale:
 – Score 0, no lymph vessels
 – Score 1, poor conspicuity
 – Score 2, moderate conspicuity
 – Score 3, good conspicuity
(d) For enhancement of axillary/pelvic lymph nodes a three-point scale can be used:
 – Score 0, no lymph nodes
 – Score 1, moderate conspicuity
 – Score 2, good conspicuity

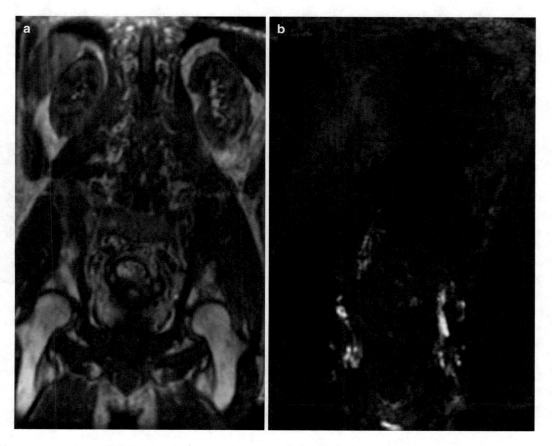

Fig. 4.13 Direct contrast-enhanced MR lymphangiography (DCMRL), performed in a patient with chylous leak by accessing the inguinal lymph nodes and then injecting gadolinium contrast into the lymphatic system. (**a**) Baseline coronal T1 image of the abdomen and pelvis obtained before gadolinium injection. (**b–d**) Coronal fat-suppressed T1 intranodal images after gadolinium injection demonstrate sequential opacification of the retroperitoneal lymphatic vessels (*reproduced with permission from ref.* [101])

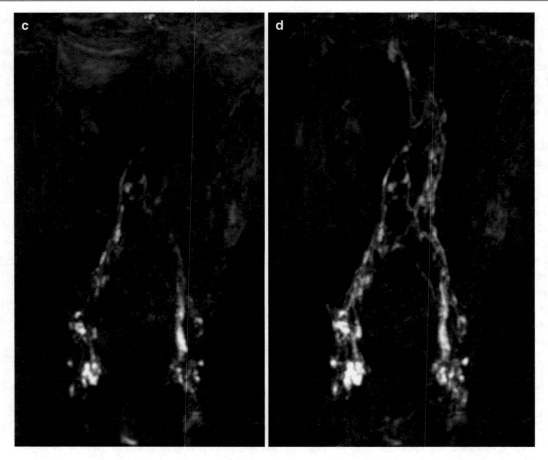

Fig. 4.13 (continued)

Anatomic levels up to which lymph vessel enhancement is visible can be evaluated based on a four-point scale:

- Upper arm:
    Level 0, hand
    Level 1, forearm
    Level 2, upper arm
    Level 3, axilla
- Lower limb:
    Level 0, feet
    Level 1, calf
    Level 2, thigh
    Level 3, pelvis

When contrast based on ultrasmall particles of iron oxide (USPIO) is used during MRI, the malignant cells, which cannot accumulate the contrast particles because they lack reticuloendothelial activity, retain their native MR signal, while normal lymph node tissue becomes darker. Therefore, in USPIO contrast-enhanced MRI, lymph nodes with tumor metastasis appear as relatively bright, compared with the "negative" contrast enhance-

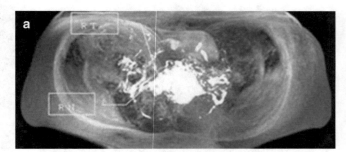

Fig. 4.14 Contrast-enhanced MR lymphography performed in a 38-year-old patient with cervical cancer (Ib1) by injecting gadodiamide into the cervical tissue. MR lymphography clearly shows the lymph nodes and lymphatic vessels. (**a**) MR lymphography in the axial view shows the lymph nodes and lymphatic vessels. The arrow marks the right cervical lymph nodes (R.N.), showing no abnormal increases and no filling defects. The other arrow displays the continuity of the right mall lymphatic channels (R.T.). (**b**) Sagittal view of MR lymphography. (**c**) Coronal view of MR lymphography, showing the lymph nodes and lymphatic vessels. Two arrows mark the left lymph nodes (L.N.), with no abnormal increase and no filling defects. The other arrow displays the continuity of the left small lymphatic channels (L.T.). The arrow marks the left lymph nodes (L.N.), clearly developed with no abnormal increase and no filling defect. The other arrow displays the continuity of the left small lymphatic channels (L.T.) (*reproduced with permission from ref.* [102])

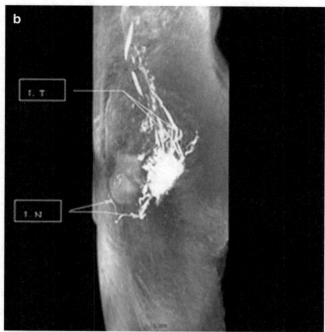

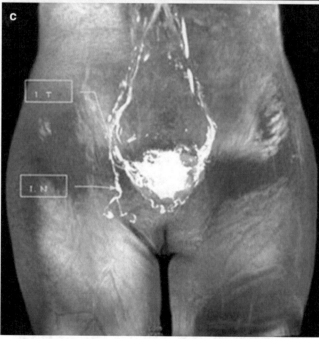

Fig. 4.14 (continued)

potential drawback of USPIO enhancement is with reactive lymph nodes, which may have low USPIO uptake because they predominantly contain lymphocytes, thus making it difficult to distinguish then versus metastatic nodes. USPIO-enhanced MRI can detect more normal lymph nodes than plain MRI alone. One major advantage of USPIO enhancement is that it visualizes normal lymph nodes throughout the body with a single injection, thus allowing multiple sites of disease to be evaluated. For interpretation purposes, it should be noted that the small amount of USPIO uptake by the liver, spleen, and bone marrow will also cause decreased signal intensity in these organs [106]. A number of studies have investigated USPIO-enhanced MRL as a means of detecting lymph node metastasis in patients. Anzai et al. [107] administered a low USPIO dose (1.7 mg Fe/kg body weight) to patients with head and neck cancers or with urological and pelvic cancers in whom lymph node metastasis was confirmed by histology; they reported 95% sensitivity with 84% specificity for the head and neck cancers, and 100% sensitivity with 80% specificity for urological and pelvic cancers, respectively [106]. The contrast agent was tolerated well, with no adverse side effects being reported when the agent was injected slowly, and metastatic lymph nodes were clearly detected. A phase III clinical study assessed the safety and efficacy of USPIO MRI in patients showing that USPIO-enhanced MRI was safe and effective and improved the diagnostic performance parameters, by increasing the positive predictive value by 20% and overall diagnostic accuracy by 14% [108].

DCE-MRI using macromolecular agents other than USPIO is at a relatively early stage of investigation, and the feasibility of MRL with Gd-containing liposomes in animal models has been demonstrated [109]. Good uptake was demonstrated in regional lymph nodes following subcutaneous injection, with the likely mechanism being trapping of the liposomes by macrophages. Misselwitz et al. used the macromolecular contrast medium Gadomer-17 to image the inguinal and iliac nodes in dogs following hind limb injection [110]. Enhancement was seen 15 min postinjection, but was maximal 60–90 min after injection, with signal enhancement increasing by as much as 450–960%, depending on the initial dose.

It is also possible to use MRI to image the lymphatic-convective transport in vivo. Pathak et al. selected two murine breast cancer lines with different degrees of invasiveness [111]. Using albumin-Gd-DTPA as a contrast agent, they were able to classify ROIs as "pooling" if the magnetic contrast concentration increased over time, or "draining" if it decreased relative to the early-phase images. The more invasive tumor line had a significantly higher number of "draining" voxels. Thus, the lymphatic drainage pattern correlates with the metastasis rate. Drainage may be affected by both "invasiveness" of the tumor and integrity of the extracellular

ment, or darkening, of lymph nodes not harboring metastasis (Fig. 4.15). However, this feature may be difficult to detect in cases of micrometastases, where there is sufficient normal tissue within the lymph node for USPIO uptake. Harisinghani et al. made this observation when investigating patients with pelvic malignancies, where a lymph node subsequently found to contain micrometastases produced a heterogeneous signal decrease on MRL [105]. Another

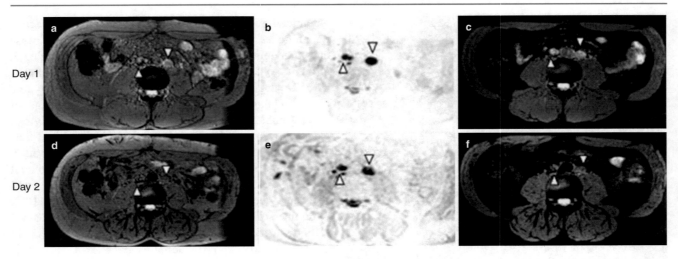

Fig. 4.15 Ferumoxytol-enhanced MR lymphography findings of metastatic lymph nodes. (**a–c**) Pre-administration of ferumoxytol; (**d–f**) 24 h post-administration. (**a, d**) T2∗ axial images; (**b, e**) diffusion-weighted images; (**c, f**) T2∗ spectral pre-saturation with inversion recovery (SPIR) images. These images refer to a 43-year-old man with Gleason 5+5 cancer, previously treated with radical prostatectomy and external beam radiotherapy. Enlarged para-aortic lymph nodes were seen (arrowheads). After administration of ferumoxytol, these lymph nodes retain their signal, indicating metastasis (*reproduced with permission from ref* [104])

matrix, which, if reduced, can facilitate passage of tumor cells, along with extracellular fluid.

Key Learning Points

- Similarly as CT, unenhanced MR imaging relies predominantly on size criteria to distinguish benign from malignant lymph nodes.
- Absolute signal intensities of benign lymph nodes cannot be reliably distinguished from those of malignant lymph nodes on either T1- or T2-weighted images.
- Contrast-enhanced MR lymphography (MRL) is promising for the evaluation of chronic lymphedema.
- A typical MRL protocol consists of a 3D heavily T2-weighted sequence with spectral fat suppression and a dynamic high-resolution fat-suppressed T1-weighted 3D spoiled gradient echo sequence, before and after the injection of gadolinium-based contrast agent to image enhancement of lymphatic channels.
- The MRL images are interpreted visually, adopting qualitative analysis scores including the quality of drainage, delay of drainage, and depiction/enhancement of lymph nodes.
- In USPIO MRI the malignant cells, which cannot accumulate the contrast particles because they lack reticuloendothelial activity, retain their native MR signal, while normal lymph node tissue becomes darker.
- It is also possible to use MRI to image the lymphatic-convective transport in vivo.

4.11 Indocyanine Green Lymphography

Indocyanine green (ICG) lymphography is becoming a popular alternate method for imaging the lymphatics. Several protocols can be used which share the intradermal/subcutaneous injection of ICG (0.2–0.3 mL) into the first web spaces of the feet (at the dorsum of the foot) or at the lateral border of the Achilles tendon when evaluating the lower limb. When investigating the upper limb, ICG is injected in the distal aspect of the upper limb at first and fourth web spaces and ulnar and radial volar wrist regions. Images can be acquired immediately after the injection or some time after injection, at rest or after exercise/massage using different equipment [112]. The fluorescence images are generally continuously observed on the monitor of a laptop computer. The video images of the lymphatic drainage are converted digitally into AVI- or MPEG2-formatted data and recorded on the hard disk of the computer. The movie files are later processed to select panoramic pictures that show the whole limb, by using specific software.

ICG lymphography was initially used for SLNB in patients with breast cancer [113]. When evaluating patients with edema, a normal ICG lymphography pattern is defined when superficial lymphatic vessels are visualized as linear paths from the injection sites to the superficial inguinal/axillary lymph nodes, except in regions with thick layers of fat, such as the thigh, where images cannot be clearly visualized. An abnormal ICG lymphography pattern is defined when lymphatic channels demonstrate retrograde lymphatic flow (dermal backflow pattern) and reduced or absent linear channel patterning (Figs. 4.16 and 4.17). Three dermal backflow patterns can be identi-

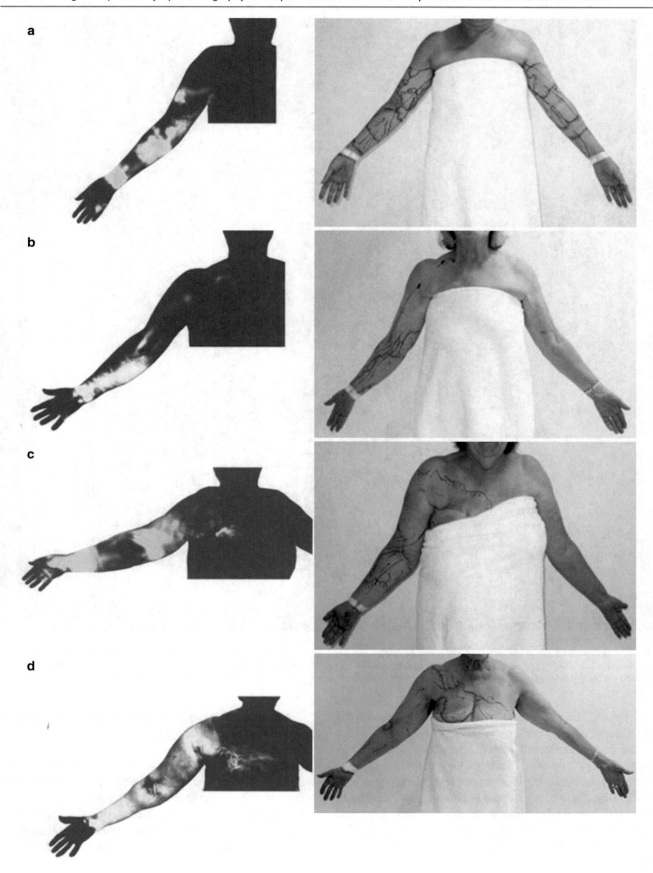

Fig. 4.16 Indocyanine green lymphography. Patterns of drainage pathway in ICG lymphography images (left) and tracing photos (right), showing lymphatic drainage toward the ipsilateral axilla (**a**), clavicular lymph nodes (**b**), parasternal lymph nodes (**c**), and contralateral axilla (**d**) (*reproduced with permission from ref.* [114])

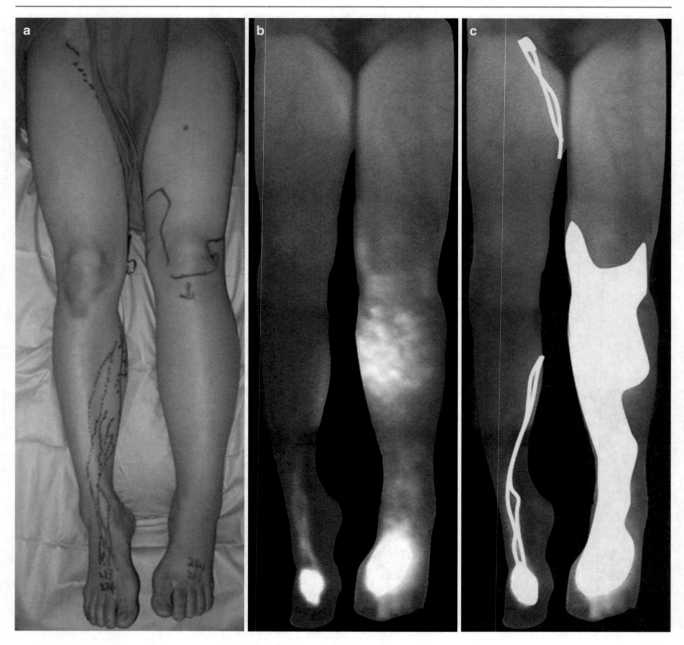

Fig. 4.17 Indocyanine green lymphography, showing an example of distal dermal backflow (DDB) pattern. (**a**) Left-leg primary lymphedema. (**b**) On indocyanine green lymphography, dermal backflow pattern is observed distal to the left knee (DDB pattern). Conversely, a linear pattern is observed in the whole right leg (normal pattern). (**c**) Enhanced lymphatics are yellow (*reproduced with permission from ref.* [115])

fied: splash, stardust, and diffuse, which correlate with the progression of lymphedema severity. These findings supported the generation of a novel anatomical lymphedema severity staging system, the dermal backflow staging system [116]. In addition, dermal backflow patterns can also be classified, according to their extension and visibility of enhanced lymphatics, into four sub-patterns: proximal dermal backflow (PDB), distal dermal backflow (DDB), less enhancement (LE), and no enhancement (NE) patterns.

For example, in lower limb lymphedema the PDB pattern can be summarized as follows:

- Dermal backflow pattern extending from the groin to the distal region, with linear pattern being observed distal to the extension of the dermal backflow patterns.
- DDB pattern, where the dermal backflow pattern is observed in the distal part of the lower extremity but not in the groin, and the remaining region show linear pattern or no enhanced images.

- LE pattern, where the linear pattern is observed only in the distal part of the lower extremity, and the remaining proximal part show no enhanced image; no dermal backflow pattern is observed.
- NE pattern, where no enhanced lymphatic image is observed other than at the injection sites; there is neither linear pattern nor dermal backflow pattern [115].

ICG lymphography can be employed for diagnosing lymphedema and for mapping lymphatic vessels prior to lympho-venous anastomosis surgery [112]. Indocyanine green lymphography can also be performed to obtain real-time fluorescent images of lymph flow to identify a chylous leak, allowing suture ligation, and thus repair of chylous fistulas in the chest and abdomen [117, 118]. In this case, ICG lymphography is performed by subcutaneous ICG injection into nearby lymph node regions, after which the chylous leak can be imaged intraoperatively with a near-infrared camera system.

Key Learning Points
- Indocyanine green (ICG) lymphography is becoming a popular alternate method for imaging the lymphatics.
- ICG lymphography was initially used for SLNB in patients with breast cancer, but can also be used for evaluation of patients with lymphedema.
- An abnormal ICG lymphography pattern is defined when lymphatic channels demonstrate retrograde lymphatic flow (dermal backflow pattern) and reduced or absent linear channel patterning.
- Four abnormal sub-patterns of ICG lymphography can be defined: proximal dermal backflow, distal dermal backflow, less enhancement, and no enhancement patterns, respectively.

References

1. Weissleder H, Weissleder R. Lymphedema: evaluation of qualitative and quantitative lymphoscintigraphy in 238 patients. Radiology. 1988;167:729–35.
2. Cornford ME, Oldendorf WH. Terminal endothelial cells of lymph capillaries as active transport structures involved in the formation of lymph in rat skin. Lymphology. 1993;26:67–78.
3. Szuba A, Rockson SG. Lymphedema: anatomy, physiology and pathogenesis. Vasc Med. 1997;2:321–6.
4. Ikomi F, Schmid-Schönbein GW. Lymph transport in the skin. Clin Dermatol. 1995;13:419–27.
5. Lubach D, Lüdemann W, Berens von Rautenfeld D. Recent findings on the angioarchitecture of the lymph vessel system of human skin. Br J Dermatol. 1996;135:733–7.
6. Adair TH, Vance GA, Montani JP, et al. Effect of skin concavity on subcutaneous tissue fluid pressure. Am J Phys. 1991;261: H349–53.
7. Aukland K, Reed RK. Interstitial-lymphatic mechanisms in the control of extracellular fluid volume. Physiol Rev. 1993;73:1–78.
8. Spiegel M, Vesti B, Shore A, et al. Pressure measurement in lymph capillaries of the human skin. Vasa Suppl. 1991;33:278.
9. Reddy NP, Patel K. A mathematical model of flow through the terminal lymphatics. Med Eng Phys. 1995;17:134–40.
10. Ikomi F, Hunt J, Hanna G, et al. Interstitial fluid, plasma protein, colloid, and leukocyte uptake into initial lymphatics. J Appl Physiol (1985). 1996;81:2060–7.
11. Olszewski WL, Jamal S, Manokaran G, et al. Bacteriologic studies of skin, tissue fluid, lymph, and lymph nodes in patients with filarial lymphedema. Am J Trop Med Hyg. 1997;57:7–15.
12. Pecking AP. Possibilities and restriction of isotopic lymphography for the assessment of therapeutic effects in lymphedema. Wien Med Wochenschr. 1999;149:105–6.
13. Cambria RA, Gloviczki P, Naessens JM, et al. Noninvasive evaluation of the lymphatic system with lymphoscintigraphy: a prospective, semiquantitative analysis in 386 extremities. J Vasc Surg. 1993;18:773–82.
14. Mortimer PS. Evaluation of lymphatic function: abnormal lymph drainage in venous disease. Int Angiol. 1995;14:32–5.
15. Ohtake E, Matsui K. Lymphoscintigraphy in patients with lymphedema. A new approach using intradermal injections of technetium-99m human serum albumin. Clin Nucl Med. 1986;11:474–8.
16. McNeill GC, Witte MH, Witte CL, et al. Whole-body lymphangioscintigraphy: preferred method for initial assessment of the peripheral lymphatic system. Radiology. 1989;172:495–502.
17. Nawaz MK, Hamad MM, Abdel-Dayem HM, et al. ^{99m}Tc human serum albumin lymphoscintigraphy in lymphedema of the lower extremities. Clin Nucl Med. 1990;15:794–9.
18. Nawaz MK, Hamad MM, Abdel-Dayem HM, et al. Lymphoscintigraphy in lymphedema of the lower limbs using ^{99m}Tc HSA. Angiology. 1992;43:147–54.
19. Suga K, Uchisako H, Nakanishi T, et al. Lymphoscintigraphic assessment of leg oedema following arterial reconstruction using a load produced by standing. Nucl Med Commun. 1991;12:907–17.
20. Williams WH, Witte CL, Witte MH, et al. Radionuclide lymphangioscintigraphy in the evaluation of peripheral lymphedema. Clin Nucl Med. 2000;25:451–64.
21. Miranda F, Perez MC, Castiglioni ML, et al. Effect of sequential intermittent pneumatic compression on both leg lymphedema volume and on lymph transport as semi-quantitatively evaluated by lymphoscintigraphy. Lymphology. 2001;34:135–41.
22. Mostbeck A, Partsch H. Isotope lymphography—possibilities and limits in evaluation of lymph transport. Wien Med Wochenschr. 1999;149:87–91.
23. Partsch H. Assessment of abnormal lymph drainage for the diagnosis of lymphedema by isotopic lymphangiography and by indirect lymphography. Clin Dermatol. 1995;13:445–50.
24. Bräutigam P, Földi E, Schaiper I, et al. Analysis of lymphatic drainage in various forms of leg edema using two compartment lymphoscintigraphy. Lymphology. 1998;31:43–55.
25. Bräutigam P, Vanscheidt W, Földi E, et al. The importance of the subfascial lymphatics in the diagnosis of lower limb edema: investigations with semiquantitative lymphoscintigraphy. Angiology. 1993;44:464–70.
26. Iimura T, Fukushima Y, Kumita S, et al. Estimating lymphodynamic conditions and lymphovenous anastomosis efficacy using ^{99m}Tc-phytate lymphoscintigraphy with SPECT-CT in patients with lower-limb lymphedema. Plast Reconstr Surg Glob Open. 2015;3:e404.

27. Baulieu F, Bourgeois P, Maruani A, et al. Contributions of SPECT/CT imaging to the lymphoscintigraphic investigations of the lower limb lymphedema. Lymphology. 2013;46:106–19.
28. Das J, Thambudorai R, Ray S. Lymphoscintigraphy combined with single-photon emission computed tomography-computed tomography (SPECT-CT): a very effective imaging approach for identification of the site of leak in postoperative chylothorax. Indian J Nucl Med. 2015;30:177–9.
29. Weiss M, Schwarz F, Wallmichrath J, et al. Chylothorax and chylous ascites. Clinical utility of planar scintigraphy and tomographic imaging with SPECT/CT. Nuklearmedizin. 2015;54:231–40.
30. Partsch H. Practical aspects of indirect lymphography and lymphoscintigraphy. Lymphat Res Biol. 2003;1:71–3; discussion 3–4.
31. Jensen MR, Simonsen L, Karlsmark T, et al. Lymphoedema of the lower extremities—background, pathophysiology and diagnostic considerations. Clin Physiol Funct Imaging. 2010;30:389–98.
32. Ogawa Y, Hayashi K. ^{99m}Tc-DTPA-HSA lymphoscintigraphy in lymphedema of the lower extremities: diagnostic significance of dynamic study and muscular exercise. Kaku Igaku. 1999;36:31–6.
33. Kataoka M, Kawamura M, Hamada K, et al. Quantitative lymphoscintigraphy using ^{99}Tc^m human serum albumin in patients with previously treated uterine cancer. Br J Radiol. 1991;64:1119–21.
34. Rijke AM, Croft BY, Johnson RA, et al. Lymphoscintigraphy and lymphedema of the lower extremities. J Nucl Med. 1990;31:990–8.
35. Kleinhans E, Baumeister RG, Hahn D, et al. Evaluation of transport kinetics in lymphoscintigraphy: follow-up study in patients with transplanted lymphatic vessels. Eur J Nucl Med. 1985;10:349–52.
36. Ikomi F, Hanna GK, Schmid-Schönbein GW. Mechanism of colloidal particle uptake into the lymphatic system: basic study with percutaneous lymphography. Radiology. 1995;196:107–13.
37. de Godoy JM, Santana KR, Godoy MF. Lymphoscintigraphic evaluation of manual lymphatic therapy: the Godoy & Godoy technique. Phlebology. 2015;30:39–44.
38. Dabrowski J, Merkert R, Kuśmierek J. Optimized lymphoscintigraphy and diagnostics of lymphatic oedema of the lower extremities. Nucl Med Rev Cent East Eur. 2008;11:26–9.
39. Damstra RJ, van Steensel MA, Boomsma JH, et al. Erysipelas as a sign of subclinical primary lymphoedema: a prospective quantitative scintigraphic study of 40 patients with unilateral erysipelas of the leg. Br J Dermatol. 2008;158:1210–5.
40. Gloviczki P, Calcagno D, Schirger A, et al. Noninvasive evaluation of the swollen extremity: experiences with 190 lymphoscintigraphic examinations. J Vasc Surg. 1989;9:683–9; discussion 90.
41. Stanton AW, Svensson WE, Mellor RH, et al. Differences in lymph drainage between swollen and non-swollen regions in arms with breast-cancer-related lymphoedema. Clin Sci (Lond). 2001;101:131–40.
42. Modi S, Stanton AW, Svensson WE, et al. Human lymphatic pumping measured in healthy and lymphoedematous arms by lymphatic congestion lymphoscintigraphy. J Physiol. 2007;583:271–85.
43. Pain SJ, Nicholas RS, Barber RW, et al. Quantification of lymphatic function for investigation of lymphedema: depot clearance and rate of appearance of soluble macromolecules in blood. J Nucl Med. 2002;43:318–24.
44. Stamp GF, Peters AM. Peripheral lymphovenous communication in lymphoedema. Nucl Med Commun. 2012;33:701–7.
45. Pecking AP. Evaluation by lymphoscintigraphy of the effect of a micronized flavonoid fraction (Daflon 500 mg) in the treatment of upper limb lymphedema. Int Angiol. 1995;14:39–43.
46. Pecking AP, Février B, Wargon C, et al. Efficacy of Daflon 500 mg in the treatment of lymphedema (secondary to conventional therapy of breast cancer). Angiology. 1997;48:93–8.
47. Svensson W, Glass DM, Bradley D, et al. Measurement of lymphatic function with technetium-99m-labelled polyclonal immunoglobulin. Eur J Nucl Med. 1999;26:504–10.
48. Havas E, Parviainen T, Vuorela J, et al. Lymph flow dynamics in exercising human skeletal muscle as detected by scintigraphy. J Physiol. 1997;504:233–9.
49. Lane K, Worsley D, McKenzie D. Lymphoscintigraphy to evaluate the effects of upper body dynamic exercise and handgrip exercise on radiopharmaceutical clearance from hands of healthy females. Lymphat Res Biol. 2005;3:16–24.
50. Lane K, Dolan L, Worsley D, et al. Lymphoscintigraphy to evaluate the effect of high versus low intensity upper body dynamic exercise on lymphatic function in healthy females. Lymphat Res Biol. 2006;4:159–65.
51. Bourgeois P, Munck D, Becker C. A three phase lymphoscintigraphic investigation protocol for the evaluation of lower limb edemas. Eur J Lymphology Relat Probl. 1997:10–21.
52. Ketterings C, Zeddeman S. Use of the C-scan in evaluation of peripheral lymphedema. Lymphology. 1997;30:49–62.
53. Proby CM, Gane JN, Joseph AE, et al. Investigation of the swollen limb with isotope lymphography. Br J Dermatol. 1990;123:29–37.
54. Suga K, Kume N, Matsunaga N, et al. Assessment of leg oedema by dynamic lymphoscintigraphy with intradermal injection of technetium-99m human serum albumin and load produced by standing. Eur J Nucl Med. 2001;28:294–303.
55. O'Mahony S, Rose SL, Chilvers AJ, et al. Finding an optimal method for imaging lymphatic vessels of the upper limb. Eur J Nucl Med Mol Imaging. 2004;31:555–63.
56. O'Mahony S, Solanki CK, Barber RW, et al. Imaging of lymphatic vessels in breast cancer-related lymphedema: intradermal versus subcutaneous injection of ^{99m}Tc-immunoglobulin. AJR Am J Roentgenol. 2006;186:1349–55.
57. Bourgeois P. Scintigraphic investigations of the lymphatic system: the influence of injected volume and quantity of labeled colloidal tracer. J Nucl Med. 2007;48:693–5.
58. Bourgeois P, Leduc O, Belgrado JP, et al. Scintigraphic investigations of the superficial lymphatic system: quantitative differences between intradermal and subcutaneous injections. Nucl Med Commun. 2009;30:270–4.
59. Tartaglione G, Pagan M, Morese R, et al. Intradermal lymphoscintigraphy at rest and after exercise: a new technique for the functional assessment of the lymphatic system in patients with lymphoedema. Nucl Med Commun. 2010;31:547–51.
60. Jensen MR, Simonsen L, Karlsmark T, et al. The washout rate of a subcutaneous ^{99m}Tc-HSA depot in lower extremity lymphoedema. Clin Physiol Funct Imaging. 2012;32:126–32.
61. Hung JC, Wiseman GA, Wahner HW, et al. Filtered technetium-99m-sulfur colloid evaluated for lymphoscintigraphy. J Nucl Med. 1995;36:1895–901.
62. Tartaglione G, Rubello D. The evolving methodology to perform limb lymphoscintigraphy: from rest to exercise acquisition protocol. Microvasc Res. 2010;80:540–4.
63. Hvidsten S, Toyserkani NM, Sørensen JA, et al. A scintigraphic method for quantitation of lymphatic function in arm lymphedema. Lymphat Res Biol. 2018;16:353–9.
64. Keramida G, Winterman N, Wroe E, et al. Importance of accurate ilio-inguinal quantification in lower extremity lymphoscintigraphy. Nucl Med Commun. 2017;38:209–14.
65. Kramer EL. Lymphoscintigraphy: defining a clinical role. Lymphat Res Biol. 2004;2:32–7.
66. Burnand KG, McGuinness CL, Lagattolla NR, et al. Value of isotope lymphography in the diagnosis of lymphoedema of the leg. Br J Surg. 2002;89:74–8.
67. Brorson H, Svensson H, Norrgren K, et al. Liposuction reduces arm lymphedema without significantly altering the already impaired lymph transport. Lymphology. 1998;31:156–72.
68. Carena M, Campini R, Zelaschi G, et al. Quantitative lymphoscintigraphy. Eur J Nucl Med. 1988;14:88–92.

69. Bourgeois P, Dargent JL, Larsimont D, et al. Lymphoscintigraphy in angiomyomatous hamartomas and primary lower limb lymphedema. Clin Nucl Med. 2009;34:405–9.
70. Noer I, Lassen NA. Evidence of active transport (filtration?) of plasma proteins across the capillary walls in muscle and subcutis. Acta Physiol Scand Suppl. 1979;463:105–10.
71. Keramida G, Wroe E, Winterman N, et al. Lymphatic drainage efficiency: a new parameter of lymphatic function. Acta Radiol. 2018;59:1097–101.
72. Stanton AW, Modi S, Bennett Britton TM, et al. Lymphatic drainage in the muscle and subcutis of the arm after breast cancer treatment. Breast Cancer Res Treat. 2009;117:549–57.
73. Stanton AW, Modi S, Mellor RH, et al. A quantitative lymphoscintigraphic evaluation of lymphatic function in the swollen hands of women with lymphoedema following breast cancer treatment. Clin Sci (Lond). 2006;110:553–61.
74. Pain SJ, Barber RW, Ballinger JR, et al. Side-to-side symmetry of radioprotein transfer from tissue space to systemic vasculature following subcutaneous injection in normal subjects and patients with breast cancer. Eur J Nucl Med Mol Imaging. 2003;30:657–61.
75. Pain SJ, Barber RW, Ballinger JR, et al. Local vascular access of radioprotein injected subcutaneously in healthy subjects and patients with breast cancer-related lymphedema. J Nucl Med. 2004;45:789–96.
76. Pain SJ, Barber RW, Ballinger JR, et al. Tissue-to-blood transport of radiolabelled immunoglobulin injected into the web spaces of the hands of normal subjects and patients with breast cancer-related lymphoedema. J Vasc Res. 2004;41:183–92.
77. Gothard L, Stanton A, MacLaren J, et al. Non-randomised phase II trial of hyperbaric oxygen therapy in patients with chronic arm lymphoedema and tissue fibrosis after radiotherapy for early breast cancer. Radiother Oncol. 2004;70:217–24.
78. Giacalone G, Yamamoto T, Belva F, et al. The application of virtual reality for preoperative planning of lymphovenous anastomosis in a patient with a complex lymphatic malformation. J Clin Med. 2019;8. pii: E371. https://doi.org/10.3390/jcm8030371.
79. Heuveling DA, Karagozoglu KH, Van Lingen A, et al. Feasibility of intraoperative detection of sentinel lymph nodes with 89-zirconium-labelled nanocolloidal albumin PET-CT and a handheld high-energy gamma probe. EJNMMI Res. 2018;8:15. https://doi.org/10.1186/s13550-018-0368-6.
80. Long X, Zhang J, Zhang D, et al. Microsurgery guided by sequential preoperative lymphography using 68Ga-NEB PET and MRI in patients with lower-limb lymphedema. Eur J Nucl Med Mol Imaging. 2017;44:1501–10.
81. Zhang J, Lang L, Zhu Z, et al. Clinical translation of an albumin-binding PET radiotracer 68Ga-NEB. J Nucl Med. 2015;56:1609–14.
82. Hou G, Hou B, Jiang Y, et al. 68Ga-NOTA-Evans Blue TOF PET/MR lymphoscintigraphy evaluation of the severity of lower limb lymphedema. Clin Nucl Med. 2019;44:439–45.
83. Luciani A, Itti E, Rahmouni A, et al. Lymph node imaging: basic principles. Eur J Radiol. 2006;58:338–44.
84. Cserni G. Metastases in axillary sentinel lymph nodes in breast cancer as detected by intensive histopathological work up. J Clin Pathol. 1999;52:922–4.
85. Sugiyama S, Iwai T, Izumi T, et al. CT lymphography for sentinel lymph node mapping of clinically N0 early oral cancer. Cancer Imaging. 2019;19:72. https://doi.org/10.1186/s40644-019-0258-9.
86. Suga K, Yuan Y, Okada M, et al. Breast sentinel lymph node mapping at CT lymphography with iopamidol: preliminary experience. Radiology. 2004;230:543–52.
87. Minato M, Hirose C, Sasa M, et al. 3-dimensional computed tomography lymphography-guided identification of sentinel lymph nodes in breast cancer patients using subcutaneous injection of nonionic contrast medium: a clinical trial. J Comput Assist Tomogr. 2004;28:46–51.
88. Suga K, Shimizu K, Kawakami Y, et al. Lymphatic drainage from esophagogastric tract: feasibility of endoscopic CT lymphography for direct visualization of pathways. Radiology. 2005;237:952–60.
89. Yamamoto S, Suga K, Maeda K, et al. Breast sentinel lymph node navigation with three-dimensional computed tomography-lymphography: a 12-year study. Breast Cancer. 2016;23:456–62.
90. Suga K, Yuan Y, Ueda K, et al. Computed tomography lymphography with intrapulmonary injection of iopamidol for sentinel lymph node localization. Invest Radiol. 2004;39:313–24.
91. Dooms GC, Hricak H, Moseley ME, et al. Characterization of lymphadenopathy by magnetic resonance relaxation times: preliminary results. Radiology. 1985;155:691–7.
92. Heiberg EV, Perman WH, Herrmann VM, et al. Dynamic sequential 3D gadolinium-enhanced MRI of the whole breast. Magn Reson Imaging. 1996;14:337–48.
93. Murray AD, Staff RT, Redpath TW, et al. Dynamic contrast enhanced MRI of the axilla in women with breast cancer: comparison with pathology of excised nodes. Br J Radiol. 2002;75:220–8.
94. Kvistad KA, Rydland J, Smethurst HB, et al. Axillary lymph node metastases in breast cancer: preoperative detection with dynamic contrast-enhanced MRI. Eur Radiol. 2000;10:1464–71.
95. Fischbein NJ, Noworolski SM, Henry RG, et al. Assessment of metastatic cervical adenopathy using dynamic contrast-enhanced MR imaging. AJNR Am J Neuroradiol. 2003;24:301–11.
96. Lohrmann C, Foeldi E, Speck O, et al. High-resolution MR lymphangiography in patients with primary and secondary lymphedema. AJR Am J Roentgenol. 2006;187:556–61.
97. Liu N, Zhang Y. Magnetic resonance lymphangiography for the study of lymphatic system in lymphedema. J Reconstr Microsurg. 2016;32:66–71.
98. Notohamiprodjo M, Weiss M, Baumeister RG, et al. MR lymphangiography at 3.0 T: correlation with lymphoscintigraphy. Radiology. 2012;264:78–87.
99. Lohrmann C, Felmerer G, Foeldi E, et al. MR lymphangiography for the assessment of the lymphatic system in patients undergoing microsurgical reconstructions of lymphatic vessels. Microvasc Res. 2008;76:42–5.
100. Jeon JY, Lee SH, Shin MJ, et al. Three-dimensional isotropic fast spin-echo MR lymphangiography of T1-weighted and intermediate-weighted pulse sequences in patients with lymphoedema. Clin Radiol. 2016;71:e56–63.
101. Kiang SC, Ahmed KA, Barnes S, et al. Direct contrast-enhanced magnetic resonance lymphangiography in the diagnosis of persistent occult chylous effusion leak after thoracic duct embolization. J Vasc Surg Venous Lymphat Disord. 2019;7:251–7.
102. Hong Y, Xiang L, Hu Y, et al. Interstitial magnetic resonance lymphography is an effective diagnostic tool for the detection of lymph node metastases in patients with cervical cancer. BMC Cancer. 2012;12:360. https://doi.org/10.1186/1471-2407-12-360.
103. Bae JS, Yoo RE, Choi SH, et al. Evaluation of lymphedema in upper extremities by MR lymphangiography: comparison with lymphoscintigraphy. Magn Reson Imaging. 2018;49:63–70.
104. Czarniecki M, Pesapane F, Wood BJ, et al. Ultra-small superparamagnetic iron oxide contrast agents for lymph node staging of high-risk prostate cancer. Transl Androl Urol. 2018;7:S453–S61.
105. Harisinghani MG, Saini S, Slater GJ, et al. MR imaging of pelvic lymph nodes in primary pelvic carcinoma with ultrasmall superparamagnetic iron oxide (Combidex): preliminary observations. J Magn Reson Imaging. 1997;7:161–3.
106. Bellin MF, Roy C, Kinkel K, et al. Lymph node metastases: safety and effectiveness of MR imaging with ultrasmall superparamagnetic iron oxide particles—initial clinical experience. Radiology. 1998;207:799–808.
107. Anzai Y, Blackwell KE, Hirschowitz SL, et al. Initial clinical experience with dextran-coated superparamagnetic iron oxide for detection of lymph node metastases in patients with head and neck cancer. Radiology. 1994;192:709–15.

108. Anzai Y, Piccoli CW, Outwater EK, et al. Evaluation of neck and body metastases to nodes with ferumoxtran 10-enhanced MR imaging: phase III safety and efficacy study. Radiology. 2003;228:777–88.

109. Fujimoto Y, Okuhata Y, Tyngi S, et al. Magnetic resonance lymphography of profundus lymph nodes with liposomal gadolinium-diethylenetriamine pentaacetic acid. Biol Pharm Bull. 2000;23:97–100.

110. Misselwitz B, Schmitt-Willich H, Michaelis M, et al. Interstitial magnetic resonance lymphography using a polymeric T1 contrast agent: initial experience with Gadomer-17. Invest Radiol. 2002;37:146–51.

111. Pathak AP, Artemov D, Neeman M, et al. Lymph node metastasis in breast cancer xenografts is associated with increased regions of extravascular drain, lymphatic vessel area, and invasive phenotype. Cancer Res. 2006;66:5151–8.

112. Akita S, Mitsukawa N, Kazama T, et al. Comparison of lymphoscintigraphy and indocyanine green lymphography for the diagnosis of extremity lymphoedema. J Plast Reconstr Aesthet Surg. 2013;66:792–8.

113. Kitai T, Inomoto T, Miwa M, et al. Fluorescence navigation with indocyanine green for detecting sentinel lymph nodes in breast cancer. Breast Cancer. 2005;12:211–5.

114. Suami H, Heydon-White A, Mackie H, et al. A new indocyanine green fluorescence lymphography protocol for identification of the lymphatic drainage pathway for patients with breast cancer-related lymphoedema. BMC Cancer. 2019;19:985. https://doi.org/10.1186/s12885-019-6192-1.

115. Yamamoto T, Yoshimatsu H, Narushima M, et al. Indocyanine green lymphography findings in primary leg lymphedema. Eur J Vasc Endovasc Surg. 2015;49:95–102.

116. Yamamoto T, Narushima M, Doi K, et al. Characteristic indocyanine green lymphography findings in lower extremity lymphedema: the generation of a novel lymphedema severity staging system using dermal backflow patterns. Plast Reconstr Surg. 2011;127:1979–86.

117. Kaburagi T, Takeuchi H, Oyama T, et al. Intraoperative fluorescence lymphography using indocyanine green in a patient with chylothorax after esophagectomy: report of a case. Surg Today. 2013;43:206–10.

118. Matsutani T, Hirakata A, Nomura T, et al. Transabdominal approach for chylorrhea after esophagectomy by using fluorescence navigation with indocyanine green. Case Rep Surg. 2014;2014:464017.

Lymphoscintigraphy for the Differential Diagnosis of Peripheral Edema and Intracavitary Lymph Effusion

Martina Sollini, Roberto Boni, Andrea Marciano, Roberta Zanca, Francesco Bartoli, and Paola A. Erba

Contents

5.1 Introduction 79

5.2 Differential Diagnosis 81

5.3 Diagnostic Characterization 82

5.4 Management of Lymphedema 85

5.5 Lymphoscintigraphy in the Management of Lymphedema 87

5.6 X-Ray Computed Tomography and Magnetic Resonance Imaging 92

5.7 Virtual Reality for Preoperative Planning 99

Clinical Cases 102

References 140

Learning Objectives
- Learn how lymphedema is defined in clinical practice, and classified and staged according to the International Society of Lymphology (ISL) guidelines and the Clinical, Etiologic, Anatomic, and Pathophysiologic approach in Lymphology (CEAP-L).
- Learn the conditions to be ruled out in the differential diagnosis of lymphedema.

- Learn the main therapeutic options for patients with lymphedema.
- Learn how to use properly different imaging modalities (such as bioimpedance spectroscopy, dual-energy X-ray absorptiometry, ultrasonography, venous Doppler ultrasound, conventional lymphoscintigraphy, PET/CT lymphoscintigraphy, magnetic resonance lymphography) for the diagnosis and management of patients with lymphedema.
- Learn how to integrate the information deriving from each imaging procedure for prognostic assessment and for treatment planning and evaluation.

M. Sollini
Department of Biomedical Sciences, Humanitas University, Milan, Italy

R. Boni
Nuclear Medicine Service, "Papa Giovanni XXIII" Hospital, Bergamo, Italy

A. Marciano · R. Zanca · F. Bartoli · P. A. Erba (✉)
Regional Center of Nuclear Medicine, Department of Translational Research and Advanced Technologies in Medicine and Surgery, University of Pisa, Pisa, Italy
e-mail: paola.erba@unipi.it

5.1 Introduction

Patients with lower extremity lymphedema present initially unilateral painless swelling that starts on the dorsal aspect of the foot, but eventually progresses to involve also the proximal portion of the limb. The edema is initially a pitting edema, but over time the subcutaneous tissue becomes fibrotic, resulting in non-pitting brawny edema. The edema

© Springer Nature Switzerland AG 2020
G. Mariani et al. (eds.), *Atlas of Lymphoscintigraphy and Sentinel Node Mapping*,
https://doi.org/10.1007/978-3-030-45296-4_5

can then spread circumferentially if treatment is not initiated, involving the skin which becomes hyperkeratotic, hyperpigmented, and papillomatous or verrucous, with increased skin turgor. The Kaposi-Stemmer sign, in which the examiner is unable to pinch a fold of skin at the base of the second toe on the dorsal aspect of the foot, indicates clinical lymphedema [1–3]. Ultimately, the skin is at risk for ulcerating and is the site of subsequent infection. Swelling associated with lymphedema results in a sensation of heaviness, discomfort, and impaired mobility of the limb. Angiosarcoma may develop in chronic lymphedematous limbs (Stewart-Treves syndrome), but is most commonly seen in the upper extremity following mastectomy with axillary lymph node dissection [4]. This condition is often referred to as lymphangiosarcoma, which is actually a misnomer, since the tumor is not derived from lymphatic vessels, but is rather derived from vascular endothelial cells within a condition of chronic lymphedema.

The International Society of Lymphology (ISL) has established a staging system for defining the severity of this disease. It is thus possible to identify the progression of the condition and the potential for successful treatment and improvement. This staging system, which applies only to the limbs (arms and legs), is based on the degree of swelling and on the condition of the skin and tissues. In the latest revision of the document for the evaluation and management of peripheral lymphedema [5] a four-stage scale for classification of a lymphedematous limb has been defined for conditions with increasing severities, as follows:

5.1.1 Stage 0 Lymphedema: Latent or Preclinical Stage

At this stage the patient is at risk of developing lymphedema; however, no swelling or other visible evidence of impaired lymph drainage is present. Stage 0 can be present for months, or years, before more severe signs appear. If specialized treatment is started at this stage, it may be possible to prevent the development of further stages of lymphedema.

5.1.2 Stage I Lymphedema

This condition indicates an early accumulation of interstitial fluid that is relatively high in protein content. There is visible swelling with protein-rich lymph. The swelling can be temporarily reduced by elevation of the limb; however, it soon reappears when the limb is returned to a normal position. The swollen tissues are soft, and pitting edema is present. Treatment should initiate as early as these clinical signs are detected, since waiting for the swelling to increase, or for an infection to develop, only makes the condition more

difficult to treat. Prompt treatment of this stage can often control the condition and may prevent it from becoming more severe.

5.1.3 Stage II Lymphedema

This stage denotes a further increase in swelling accompanied by concomitant tissue changes. Elevation of the limb will not reduce the swelling, and tissues become increasingly firm, due to fibrosis. Pressure against the limb produces only a slight pitting, or no pitting at all. The tissue changes at this stage increase the risks of even greater swelling, fibrosis, infections, and skin problems. Stage II lymphedema can usually be improved with intense treatment.

5.1.4 Stage III Lymphedema

Also known as *lymphostatic elephantiasis*, in this condition the tissue becomes extremely swollen and thickened, due to blockage of lymph flow and buildup of fluid in tissues. The tissues become increasingly fibrotic. Pressure does not produce any pitting. Normal elasticity is lost, and the skin hangs in folds and may change color. *Papillomas* and *hyperkeratosis* can develop. Changes in skin texture are disfiguring and can limit mobility. Infections become more common because of increased risks of ulcerations of the skin. These infections include fungal infections and open wounds that form within the skin folds. With intense therapy, stage III lymphedema can be improved and potentially be prevented from becoming even worse; however, it is rarely reversed to an earlier stage.

Within each stage, a functional severity assessment utilizes simple volume differences commonly determined using circumferential measurement (preferentially by flexible nonstretch tape) assessed as follows:

- Minimal (>5–<20% increase in limb volume), alternatively subdivided into
  - >5–10% as minimal
  - >10–<20% as mild
- Moderate (20–40% increase)
- Severe (>40% increase)

The above ISL stages only refer to the physical condition of the extremities. A more detailed and inclusive classification must be formulated according to improved understanding of the pathogenic mechanisms of lymphedema (e.g., nature and degree of lymphangiodysplasia, lymph flow perturbations, and nodal dysfunction as defined by anatomic features and physiologic imaging and testing), and underlying genetic disturbances, which are increasingly being elucidated. Recent publications combining both physical (phenotypic) findings with functional lymphatic imaging as well as those classifications which propose inclusion of disability grading, assessment of inflammation, and even immunohistochemical changes determined by biopsy of nodes/vessels may be forecasting the future evolution of staging. In addition, incorporation of genotypic information, expanded from what is available even in current screening, would further advance staging and classification of patients with peripheral (and other) lymphedema.

Factors such as extension, occurrence of erysipelas attacks, inflammation, and other descriptors or complications within their own individual severity determinations might also be included.

A new classification of limb lymphedema was proposed in 2009, inspired by the **C**linical, **E**tiologic, **A**natomic, and **P**athophysiologic (CEAP) classification for chronic venous insufficiency of the lower limbs. It adopts the acronym CEAP by adding the letter **L** (Lymphatic) to underline the aspect "lymphedema." This clinical classification is subdivided into five classes depending on the presence of clinical signs such as:

- The presence of lymphedema: 5-point scale:
  - No edema
  - Edema that disappears with night rest
  - Edema that persists after night rest
  - Fibrotic edema
  - Elephantiasis with skin lesions
- Extension of lymphedema:
  - Lower limbs:
      Foot, leg, thigh, genital, trunk
  - Upper limbs:
      Hand, forearm, arm, shoulder
- Presence of lymphangitis and/or leg ulcers
- Loss of functionality of the limb (grade of disability)

The etiological aspect considers two types of alterations of the lymphatic system: congenital and acquired. Pathophysiological conditions are subdivided into five groups: agenesia or hypoplasia, hyperplasia, reflux, overload, and obstruction. The CEAP-L classification was created to categorize patients with definite and objective marks (Table 5.1), to generate clinical reports with a common and

clear vocabulary, to stage the disease, to evaluate treatment, and to obtain epidemiological and statistical data [6]. Indeed, these authors found the application of the classification easy and highly reproducible in their experience.

Key Learning Points

- In patients with lower extremity lymphedema, clinical presentation progressively evolves from unilateral painless swelling on the dorsal aspect of the foot with pitting edema to circumferential involvement of the proximal portion of the limb; then to fibrosis of the subcutaneous tissue, non-pitting brawny edema, and skin changes that include hyperkeratosis and hyperpigmentation; and finally to papillomatous or verrucous skin, with increased skin turgor and increased risk for ulcers and subsequent infection.
- The Kaposi-Stemmer sign, in which the examiner is unable to pinch a fold of skin at the base of the second toe on the dorsal aspect of the foot, indicates clinical lymphedema.
- Angiosarcoma (Stewart-Treves syndrome) may develop in chronic lymphedematous limbs, as commonly seen in the upper extremity following mastectomy with axillary lymph node dissection.
- The ISL staging system applies only to the limbs and is based on the degree of swelling and on the condition of the skin and tissues. The current version is based on a three-stage scale for classification (from stage 0 to stage III); within each stage, a functional severity assessment (from minimal to severe) is used to assess the volume of the affected limb.
- The CEAP-L classification is subdivided into classes depending on the presence of clinical signs, such as presence and extension of lymphedema, presence of lymphangitis and/or leg ulcers, and loss of functionality of the limbs.
- The CEAP-L classification enables to categorize patients, generate clinical reports, stage the disease, evaluate treatment, and obtain epidemiological and statistical data.

Table 5.1 Clinical severity score [6]

1 point for each area of the limb involved
1 point for each limb involved
2 points for other areas involved (genitals, shoulders)
1–4 points according to the stage of edema
1 point symptomatic edema
1–3 points according to the stage of disability

5.2   Differential Diagnosis

Lymphedema should be considered whenever an edematous extremity without pain or inflammation is observed. Chronic venous insufficiency can be difficult to differentiate from early lymphedema because both exhibit pitting edema, and the skin changes typical of late-stage lymphedema are not present yet. Nevertheless, chronic venous insufficiency is often bilateral, rather than unilateral as is generally the case for lymphedema. Lymphoscintigraphy is often necessary to distinguish the two conditions, although such discrimination cannot always be made, since chronic venous insufficiency can actually lead to secondary lymphedema. Similarly, deep vein thrombosis can cause a postphlebitic syndrome, which can result in lipodermatosclerosis and chronic swelling of the limb [2, 3]. In nonfilarial regions of tropical Africa, Central America, and the Indian subcontinent, there is a condition that clinically presents in a similar fashion as filariasis, called podoconiosis, or nonfilarial elephantiasis. Moreover, in case of unilateral extremity lymphedema, especially in adults, solid tumors (primary and/or metastatic), lymphomas, and soft-tissue sarcomas, which may obstruct or invade more proximal lymphatics, must be considered.

Exclusion of general medical causes of lower extremity swelling should be a priority. These causes include, but are not limited to, renal failure, protein-losing nephropathy, hypoalbuminemia, congestive heart failure, pulmonary hypertension, drug-induced edema, obesity, and pregnancy [7]. Other conditions to consider in the differential diagnosis include lipedema (also known as lipomatosis of the leg), "armchair legs" (descriptive term that results from sitting in a chair all day and night with one's legs in a dependent position), and postoperative swelling.

Key Learning Points

- Chronic venous insufficiency is similar in presentation to early-stage lymphedema, but it is often bilateral rather than unilateral.
- Deep vein thrombosis can cause a postphlebitic syndrome, which can result in lipodermatosclerosis and chronic swelling of the limb.
- In nonfilarial regions of tropical Africa, Central America, and the Indian subcontinent, there is a condition that clinically presents in a similar fashion as filariasis, called podoconiosis.
- In case of unilateral limb lymphedema, especially in adults, solid tumors (primary and/or metastatic), lymphomas, and soft-tissue sarcomas must be considered.
- Lower extremity swelling could originate from general medical causes such as renal failure, protein-losing nephropathy, hypoalbuminemia, protein-losing enteropathy, congestive heart failure, pulmonary hypertension, drug-induced edema, obesity, and pregnancy.
- The diagnostic differential includes also lipedema and "armchair leg" edema.

5.3 Diagnostic Characterization

In 1976, Stemmer described the inability to pinch the skin of the proximal phalanx of the second or third toe in patients with lymphedema [8]. If the examiner is unable to grab the dorsal skin between his/her thumb and index finger, then the "Stemmer sign" is positive suggesting lymphedema [9]. However, the thickened skin and excess subcutaneous fibroadipose tissue with edema (as a consequence of inflammation, adipose deposition, and fibrosis) [10–12] might prevent the pinching of the dorsal skin of the extremity in patients with lymphedema. In contrast, other causes of swelling or limb overgrowth such as venous stasis, heart disease, liver failure, renal insufficiency, rheumatologic disease, lipedema, hemihypertrophy, posttraumatic swelling, and vascular anomalies do not result in enough inflammatory fibroadipose formation to prevent the pinching of the dorsal skin of the hand or foot. Furthermore, abnormalities in the body mass index (BMI) have been found to be associated with both false-negative and false-positive Stemmer signs. In particular, patients with lymphedema and a normal or reduced BMI could exhibit minimal swelling and a falsely negative sign, whereas obese patients without lymphedema could have a false-positive sign. On the other hand, obesity per se negatively affects lymphatic function by causing inflammation, fibrosis, and destruction of lymphatics [13–15]. The Stemmer sign has a sensitivity of 92% to predict lymphedema in patients who have the disease and a specificity of 57% to exclude lymphedema in patients who do not have the condition. A negative Stemmer sign does not rule out lymphedema, typically in patients with a normal BMI and stage I disease [16].

Objective measurement of limb swelling can be problematic. On the other hand, assessing size differences of the extremities and quantitative discrepancies between the unaffected and the affected limbs is critical, particularly in the early phases of lymphedema. Estimating differences in limb volume has been used as an indirect measure of changes in lymph fluid volume over time or with treatment, and is typically done through circumferential measurements, or through immersion techniques based on the measurement of volume displacement [17]. However, these methods are time consuming and somewhat operator dependent. Moreover, since these techniques measure only the overall volume of the limbs, possible differences in volume caused by left-right dominance, asymmetrical muscle atrophy, fibrous tissue deposition, or weight gain may incorrectly be attributed to fluid accumulation [18].

Bioimpedance spectroscopy (BIS) is a noninvasive procedure wherein an electrical current is passed through a body segment, and impedance to flow of the current is measured. This technique, which attempts to directly measure lymph

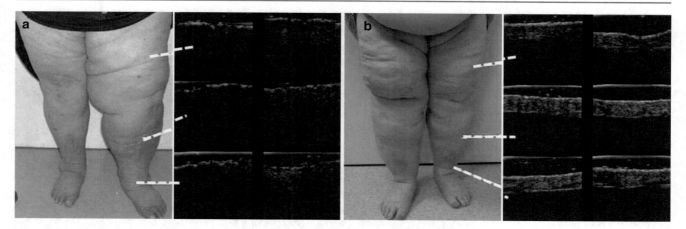

Fig. 5.1 Clinical appearance (left panel) and ultrasound pattern (right panel) in patients with lymphedema (**a**) or with lipedema (**b**). Increased volume of both lower limbs with predominant enlargement of the left is evident in the patient with lymphedema; the corresponding ultrasound examination indicates decreased echogenicity and increased thickness of the dermis. In the patient with lipedema increased lower limb volume is similarly evident, but with more pronounced symmetry; the corresponding ultrasound examination identifies normal echogenicity and thickness of the dermis, therefore confirming the diagnosis of lipedema versus lymphedema (*adapted from Naouri M* et al. [27])

fluid volume [19], is based on the principle that tissues such as fat and bone act as insulators, while electrolytic fluids conduct electricity; these features would make it possible to assess properties unique to lymphatic fluid, through measurement of the flow of current. BIS measures lymphedema based on the fact that low-frequency currents selectively pass through extracellular fluid compartments, whereas high-frequency currents pass through both the intra- and the extracellular fluids (the latter being selectively expanded in lymphedema) [20]. BIS analyzes both lymph fluid impedance and total fluid impedance [21], and impedance to current flow has been found to inversely correlate with fluid accumulation; therefore, reduced impedance values in an extremity indicate the presence of lymphedema.

Dual-energy X-ray absorptiometry (DEXA, or biphotonic absorptiometry) may help classify and define a lymphedematous limb but its greatest potential use may be to assess the chemical composition of limb swelling (especially increased fat deposition, which by its added weight can lead to muscle hypertrophy) [5].

A variety of other techniques have been described to measure limb edema, but most of them have not been validated or are either too complex or expensive for routine use [22, 23]. A practical difficulty in the clinical setting, even with validated techniques, is that extravascular fluid volume undergoes cyclic changes over days or weeks, and limb volume also has a pronounced circadian variation.

High-resolution cutaneous *ultrasonography* can be used to identify lymphedema, based on the presence of increased dermal thickness and decreased echogenicity as compared with lipedema and venous insufficiency [24]. In fact, in lymphedema loss of echogenicity of the skin and global and homogeneous dermal hypoechogenicity are observed, in contrast to the elective superficial dermis localization of

edema described in patients with venous insufficiency [25, 26]. These findings are caused by the accumulation of protein-rich exudative interstitial fluid in the skin and subcutaneous tissue; this fluid remains trapped at the production site because of its high protein content, whereas transudate edema caused by venous insufficiency is more mobile and accumulates in the superficial dermis only. However, in order to analyze dermal changes for identifying and quantifying dermal edema, the ultrasound device should operate at 20 MHz [27]. Figure 5.1 shows the clinical and ultrasound appearance for patients with lymphedema and with lipedema, respectively.

Whenever the clinical diagnosis of lymphedema is controversial, it can be either confirmed or ruled out with lymphoscintigraphy, which is considered the method of choice to evaluate the lymphatic pathways and their drainage pattern [28]. Direct lymphangiography using an iodine oil contrast agent capable of visualizing the lymphatics [29] (Fig. 5.2) is no longer routinely performed, because it can lead to life-threatening complications and is difficult to perform [31].

A venous Doppler ultrasound examination is often required to assess for deep venous thrombosis or venous disease, which can be associated with lymphedema. In fact, 20–30% of the patients with advanced chronic venous disease have associated lymphatic dysfunction, presumably due to secondary damage from overload, or from recurrent cellulitis [32].

If filariasis is suspected, one can perform a blood smear (collected at night) looking for the presence of microfilariae. Antigen testing by immunochromatographic card test (Binax) or enzyme-linked immunosorbent assay (TropBio) is more sensitive than microfilaria detection, irrespective of the time of the day blood is drawn [33].

Fig. 5.2 (**a**) Iodine oil lymphogram in a patient with chylous ascites, affected by AIDS-related peritoneal tuberculosis. Images obtained during the filling phase (right panel) show peritoneal extravasation of the contrast material. The site of leakage is seen immediately to the left of L4 (arrow). Images obtained during the storage phase (left panel) show extensive leakage in the form of oily droplets within the peritoneal cavity. (**b**) External genitalia lymphedema of parasitic origin: images obtained during the filling phase (left panel) show filling of the scrotum by left-sided lymphatic reflux; images obtained during the lymph node phase at 24 h (right panel) show accumulation of contrast material in the scrotum (arrowheads). The lymph nodes are normal. (**c**) Edema of the left leg caused by aplasia of the lymphatic vessels. The lymphogram obtained immediately after administration of the contrast agent shows no lymphatic vessels, associated with perivascular extravasation. Lymphatic drainage of the contrast material occurs mainly along the venous vessel sheaths (*adapted from Guermazi A* et al [30])

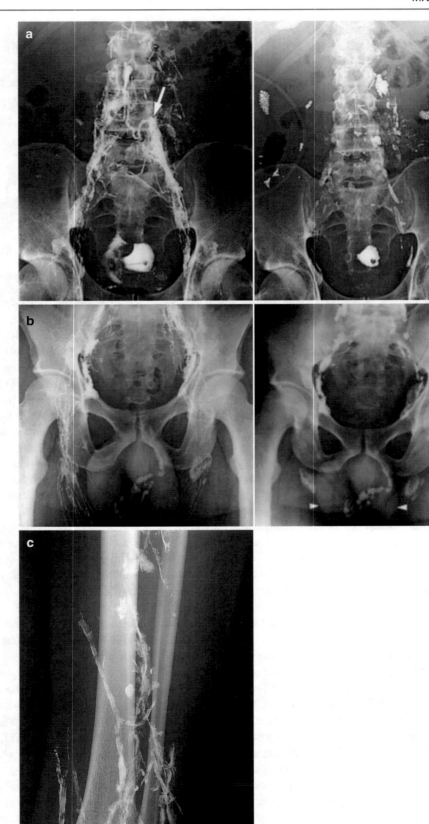

In addition to a thorough clinical history and physical examination, other diagnostic tests to rule out alternative causes of lower extremity edema include a complete metabolic profile, serum albumin, and urinalysis to screen for renal failure, hypoalbuminemia, and/or protein-losing enteropathy.

Key Learning Points

- The Stemmer sign has 92% sensitivity to predict lymphedema in patients who have the disease and 57% specificity to exclude lymphedema in patients without lymphedema.
- The body mass index (BMI) is associated with both false-negative and false-positive Stemmer signs, as a high BMI can lead to a false-positive while a low BMI can lead to a false-negative Stemmer sign.
- Circumferential measurements, or immersion techniques based on displacement, can be used to measure the limb volume.
- Reduced impedance values in an extremity are correlated with lymphedema.
- DEXA may be used to assess the chemical composition of limb swelling, especially increased fat deposition and muscle hypertrophy.
- Ultrasonography can rule out lipedema and venous insufficiency. In lymphedema a loss of echogenicity of the skin and a global and homogeneous dermal hypoechogenicity are observed, in contrast to the elective superficial dermis localization of edema described in venous insufficiency.
- A venous Doppler ultrasound examination is often needed to assess for deep venous thrombosis or venous disease, which can be associated with lymphedema.
- A blood smear or an antigen test can be performed to rule out filariasis.
- A complete metabolic profile, serum albumin, and urinalysis to screen for renal failure, hypoalbuminemia, and/or protein-losing enteropathy may be necessary for a complete differential diagnosis of lymphedema.

5.4 Management of Lymphedema

As a chronic and potentially disabling condition, lymphedema is associated with significant morbidity in terms of functional, cosmetic, and emotional consequences. Treatment efforts aim at minimizing the associated swelling, at restoring cosmesis and functionality of the limb, and at preventing potential complications associated with lymphedema, in particular infections such as cellulitis and lymphangitis. Treatments are lengthy and expensive, and involve a multi-disciplinary approach that can include rehabilitative therapy (elevation, exercise, compression devices, manual lymph drainage), skin care, and surgery [34, 35]. Therapy of peripheral lymphedema can be classified into conservative or nonoperative procedures and operative procedures.

Nonoperative treatment consists of physical therapy and adjuvants such as combined physical therapy and intermittent pneumatic pressure (or "pneumomassage"). Pneumomassage, thermal therapy, simple elevation (particularly by bed rest) of a lymphedematous limb, low-level laser therapy, and aquatic therapy/water-based exercise programs are the most common nonoperative procedures.

Drug therapies have so far been disappointing in the management of lymphedema. Although diuretic drugs are often prescribed, this therapy is actually not beneficial in lymphedema and should be employed only in patients with specific comorbidities or complications. Coumarin, a benzopyrone, has been reported to have some favorable effect on lymphedema, probably due to its mechanism of action that reduces vascular permeability, and thus capillary filtration. In addition, coumarin is thought to activate macrophage activity, which increases protein degradation, thus resulting in a reduction in fibrotic tissue. However, the clinical trials reported so far are generally of poor quality and long-term results of treatment of lymphedema with these agents are not available. Furthermore, some reports of hepatotoxicity have raised serious concern on their use [36]. Antibiotics should be administered for superimposed acute lymph stasis-related inflammations (cellulitis/lymphangitis or erysipelas) [5]. In case of lymphatic filariasis to eliminate microfilariae from the bloodstream, diethylcarbamazine, albendazole, or ivermectin is recommended [5]. Efficacy of boosting immunity by intra-arterial injection of autologous lymphocytes is unclear and requires independent, reproducible validation. Recent proposals for the use of anti-inflammatory drugs have not yet demonstrated efficacy and may face drawbacks if administered in the long term [5].

No special diet or restricted fluid intake has proved to be of therapeutic value for most uncomplicated peripheral lymphedemas. In breast cancer-related lymphedema and in obese patients, weight reduction has been shown to help. In chylous reflux syndromes a diet as low as possible or even free of long-chain triglycerides (absorbed via intestinal lacteals) and high in short- and medium-chain triglycerides is of benefit especially in children. Specific vitamin supplements may be needed in very low or no-fat diets. Some groups suggest diets with substances that may lower inflammation, but current clinical evidence is not sufficiently validated [5].

In complicated patients with lymphatic system overgrowth such as lymphangiodysplasia, specialized centers utilize pharmacotherapeutic options such as octreotide, OK-432, rapamycin, or other antiproliferative agents, in particular in newborns and children [5].

Surgical procedures aim to alleviate peripheral lymphedema by enhancing lymph return. When performed in advanced stages, surgery usually requires long-term combined physical therapy and/or other "pneumomassage" after the procedure to maintain edema reduction and ensure vascular/shunt patency.

Worldwide, surgical resection (in several forms) is the most widely used operative technique to reduce the bulk of lymphedema, in particularly in cases affecting the genitalia. Microsurgical procedures include (1) derivative methods such as lympho-venous anastomoses and (2) multiple lymphatic-venous anastomoses in a single surgical site with both the superficial and deep lymphatics. By these procedures a positive pressure gradient (lymphatic-venous) is created, thus evading the phenomenon of gravitational reflux without interrupting the distal peripheral superficial lymphatic pathways. Reconstructive methods are sophisticated techniques involving the use of a lymphatic collector (LLA) or an interposition vein segment (LVLA) to restore lymphatic continuity in lymphedema conditions due to a locally interrupted lymphatic system. Autologous lymph vessel transplantation mimics the normal physiology and has shown long-term patencies of more than 10 years. This procedure has generally been reserved to patients with unilateral peripheral lymphedema of the leg (due to the need for one healthy leg to harvest the graft), but it has also been utilized for bilateral upper extremity lymphedema where two healthy legs are available for harvesting lymphatic vessels [5].

Transplantation of superficial lymph nodes from an uninvolved area together with its vascular supply (vascularized lymph node transplantation) to the site of lymphadenectomy for cancer has been proposed both as a preventive and therapeutic approach to limb lymphedema. Liposuction (or suction-assisted lipectomy) using a variety of methods has been shown to completely reduce non-pitting, primarily non-fibrotic, extremity lymphedema due to excess fat deposition that has not responded to nonoperative therapy in both primary and secondary lymphedemas [5]. Surgical resection by "debulking" of excess skin and subcutaneous tissue of the lymphedematous limb can be associated with complications such as superficial lymphatic removal, significant scarring, risk of infection, and difficult wound healing. Debulking has been used mainly in the treatment of the most severe forms of fibrosclerotic lymphedema (elephantiasis) and in cases of advanced genital lymphedema. Caution should be exercised in removing enlarged lymph nodes or soft-tissue masses (e.g., lymphangiomas) in the affected extremity, as lymphedema may worsen thereafter [5].

The implantation of engineering/lymphatic tubes to transport lymph or engineered tubes/devices to promote new substitute lymphatic growth have not yet documented long-term value in large-scale studies, and these techniques are currently under controlled clinical investigation [5].

Omental transposition, enteromesenteric bridge operations, and implantation of threads to promote perilymphatic spaces (substitute lymphatics) have not shown long-term value and at the moment should not be considered as valid surgical options [5].

Key Learning Points

- Lymphedema is associated with significant morbidity including functional, cosmetic, and emotional consequences.
- Therapy is based on a multidisciplinary approach including rehabilitative therapy, skin care, and surgery.
- Nonoperative treatments consist of physical therapy and adjuvants.
- Medical treatments (diuretics, coumarin), diet, or restricted fluid intake is of limited value in patients with peripheral lymphedema.
- Surgical procedures aim to alleviate peripheral lymphedema by enhancing lymph return.
- Surgery usually requires long-term combined physical therapy and/or other "pneumomassage" treatments after the procedure.
- Surgical resection (in several forms) is the most widely used operative technique to reduce the bulk of lymphedema.
- Microsurgical procedures include (1) derivative methods such as lymphatic-venous anastomoses and (2) multiple lymphatic-venous anastomoses in a single surgical site with both the superficial and deep lymphatics.
- Sophisticated reconstructive techniques involve the use of a lymphatic collector or an interposition vein segment to restore lymphatic continuity.
- Liposuction has been shown to completely reduce non-pitting, primarily non-fibrotic, in patients with extremity lymphedema.
- Debulking has been used mainly in the treatment of the most severe forms of fibrosclerotic lymphedema (elephantiasis) and in cases of advanced genital lymphedema.
- The implantation of engineering/lymphatic tubes to transport lymph or engineered tubes/devices is currently under clinical investigation.
- Omental transposition, enteromesenteric bridge operations, and implantation of threads to promote perilymphatic spaces have not shown long-term value and at the moment should not be considered as valid surgical options.

5.5 Lymphoscintigraphy in the Management of Lymphedema

Qualitative and quantitative lymphoscintigraphy has been widely used for the differential diagnosis of lymphedema, for predicting the risk to develop lymphedema as well as for assessing the efficacy of physical and/or surgical treatments.

5.5.1 Lymphoscintigraphy for the Differential Diagnosis of Lymphedema

Lymphoscintigraphy has proved extremely useful for depicting the specific lymphatic abnormality and it has largely replaced conventional oil contrast lymphography for visualizing the lymphatic network. Although different protocols can be used (different radiotracers and administered activities, different injection volumes, intracutaneous versus subcutaneous or subfascial injections, one or more injections, different protocols of passive and active physical activity, varying imaging times, static and/or dynamic techniques—as discussed in detail in Chap. 4), the images, which can be easily repeated, offer remarkable insight into lymphatic structural abnormalities and (dys)function. Lymphoscintigraphy provides a functional assessment of lymphatic pumping, stasis, and obstruction that guides treatment and determines prognosis for expected outcome of treatment [37–40]. Lymphoscintigraphy is also employed to define the clinical characteristics, investigations, management, and outcomes of lymphedema in pediatric patients [41]. Purely qualitative analysis has been reported to be very accurate for confirming or excluding the diagnosis of lymphedema, with sensitivity as high as 92–96% and specificity as high as 100% [42]. Nevertheless, etiology of lymphedema is not invariably identified solely on the basis of lymphoscintigraphic images. In fact, despite the fact that patients with primary lymphedema tend to show a lack of lymphatic vessels and absent or delayed transport whereas those with secondary lymphedema tend to show obstruction with visualization of discrete lymphatic trunks and slow transport [43], primary lymphedema cannot be reliably differentiated from secondary lymphedema on the basis of lymphoscintigraphic findings alone [44].

For the lower limbs, a high positive association of popliteal lymph node uptake with the severity of lymphatic obstruction defined as appearance of dermal back flow was found in patients with both primary and secondary lymphedema [45, 46]. The duration of lymphedema was also longer in patients with dermal backflow and popliteal lymph nodes visualized during lymphoscintigraphy; both popliteal lymph node uptake and dermal backflow were important signs indicating longer disease duration and higher severity of lymphatic dysfunction [46]. In addition, a strong association between skin rerouting and popliteal lymph node visualization has been found; in particular, skin changes were detected in 38% of the patients with positive popliteal node uptake [45].

A recent study showed that transit time and dermal backflow at lymphoscintigraphy (found in about 97% of extremities by 45 min postinjection) did not predict clinical severity when adjusted for other clinical variables [47]. A subgroup analysis of a large study showed that false-negative lymphoscintigraphy occurs most likely in primary lymphedema with long duration of disease and infection history similar to patients with true-positive lymphoscintigraphy. However, repeated lymphoscintigraphies over time during follow-up showed appearance of lymphatic dysfunction consistent with lymphedema. Therefore, the results of this study suggest that patients with a high clinical suspicion of lymphedema and a normal lymphoscintigram are better treated conservatively, and that lymphoscintigraphy should be repeated in these cases [48].

Key Learning Points

- Qualitative and quantitative lymphoscintigraphy has been widely used for the differential diagnosis of lymphedema, for predicting the risk to develop lymphedema as well as for assessing the efficacy treatments, as it provides a functional assessment of lymphatic pumping, stasis, and obstruction in adults as well as in pediatric patients.
- Qualitative analysis of lymphoscintigraphy has 92–96% sensitivity and specificity close to 100% for the diagnosis of lymphedema.
- Primary lymphedema cannot be reliably differentiated from secondary lymphedema on the basis of lymphoscintigraphic examination alone.
- For the lower limbs, a high positive association of popliteal lymph node uptake with the dermal back flow was found in patients with both primary and secondary lymphedema.
- The duration of lymphedema is longer in patients with dermal back flow and popliteal lymph nodes visualized during lymphoscintigraphy.
- Patient with a high clinical suspicion of lymphedema and a normal lymphoscintigram are better treated conservatively; lymphoscintigraphy should be repeated in these cases to show the underlying lymphatic dysfunction.

5.5.1.1 Lymphoscintigraphy in Lipedema

In a recent study [49] in a prospective cohort study of women meeting the clinical criteria of lipedema, lymphoscintigraphy showed abnormal patterns in 47% of the patients, with no significant differences between the severity of lymphoscintigraphic abnormalities and clinical stage of lipedema. In addition, lymphoscintigraphic findings showed that patients with lipedema also presented impaired lymphatic transport assessed as transport index (TI) abnormalities. In addition, more severe lipedema may be associated with greater lymphatic transport abnormalities, with the mean TI being significantly greater for extremities with severe (stage 3/4) lipedema than those with mild or moderate (stage 1/2) lipedema (15.1 versus 9.7, $P = 0.049$). Mean difference in TI scores between each lower extremity for individual patients was 6.43 ($\pm$7.96 standard deviation) [50].

Key Learning Points
- Approximately 47% of patients with clinical lipedema have lymphoscintigraphic abnormalities indicating impaired lymphatic drainage.
- More severe lipedema may be associated with greater abnormalities in lymphatic transport.

5.5.1.2 Lymphoscintigraphy for Predicting the Risk to Develop Lymphedema

Lymphoscintigraphy can be used to predict the risk to develop lymphedema. In fact, in patients undergoing surgery for breast cancer, abnormalities of lymphatic drainage in postsurgical lymphoscintigraphy increases the risk of developing arm lymphedema [51–53]. It has also been shown that upper extremity lymphatic drainage after axillary lymph node dissection is not impaired in terms of lymphatic transport and/or venous function impairment after the axillary lymph node dissection procedure in comparison to the preoperative status. Qualitative analysis of lymphoscintigrams revealed most commonly disappearance of previously functioning lymph nodes and appearance of dermal backflow in subjects who developed lymphedema thereafter. Conversely, appearance of functioning lymph nodes in different locations after axillary lymph node dissection may indicate protection from development of upper extremity lymphedema [54]. In the postoperative period after breast surgery, a significant worsening of the degree of lymph node uptake and the velocity of lymph node visualization in the absence of dermal backflow and collateral circulation was observed, independently of postoperative complications or clinical characteristics [55]. On the contrary, the maximum lymphatic-pump pressure in the women who later developed breast cancer-related lymphedema was 1.7-fold higher than in those who did not develop lymphedema. Moreover, the rate of lymph tracer transport into the forearm was 2.2-fold greater in the women who later developed lymphedema [56]. Quantitative lymphoscintigraphy performed between 4 and 8 weeks after surgery to evaluate the lymphatic system in the early postoperative period, to be correlated with clinical results at the 1-year follow-up, revealed that the ratio of radiocolloid uptake rate of the affected to normal axilla and the ratio of radioactivity of the affected to normal axilla were significantly lower in the lymphedema group than in the non-lymphedema group. After adjusting the model for all significant variables (body mass index, N-stage, T-stage, type of surgery, and type of lymph node surgery), the ratio of radioactivity of the affected to normal axilla was associated with lymphedema (odds ratio = 0.14; 95% confidence interval, 0.04–0.46; $P = 0.001$) [57]. Similarly, functional lymphatic changes detected by lymphoscintigraphy after external beam radiation therapy can predict the development of arm lymphedema. Recently, lymphoscintigraphy including SPECT/CT of the axillary region has been employed to evaluate the impact of including, as target volumes in the radiation treatment plan, lymph nodes involved in arm drainage that could affect lymphedema [53]. This study demonstrated that radiation doses to these lymph nodes vary between zero and the full prescribed dose, therefore possibly affecting the development of lymphedema.

In patients with gynecological cancer-related lymphedema the prognostic assessment of qualitative lymphoscintigraphy before complex decompressive therapy showed that severity of dermal back flow, clinical stage, and therapy compliance are independent predictors of therapeutic response [58].

In patients undergoing surgery for melanoma of the trunk, primary prevention with microsurgical lympho-venous anastomosis prevented lymphedema after inguinal lymphadenectomy. In addition, lymphatic-venous multiple anastomoses proved to be successful for treating clinical lymphedema, particularly at the early stages [59]. Similar results have also been reported for patients with breast cancer [60, 61]. In addition, when lymphoscintigraphies performed in patients who underwent lymph node dissection (limited to the intra-abdominal lymph nodes) with or without radiotherapy for histologically confirmed ovarian, uterine, or prostate cancer were compared to lymphoscintigraphies obtained in patients with primary lower limb lymphedema, the appearance of lower limb lymphedema does not appear to be related to cancer treatment(s), but rather lower limb lymphedema may represent the development of a primary lymphatic disease that was latent prior to surgery [62].

The lack of visualization of inguinal lymph nodes predicted late postoperative leg edema also in patients with tibial fractures treated surgically [63].

Key Learning Points

- In patients undergoing surgery for breast cancer, lymphoscintigraphy shows disappearance of previously functional lymph nodes and appearance of dermal backflow in subjects who developed lymphedema, while appearance of functional lymph nodes in different locations after surgery indicates protection from the development of upper extremity lymphedema.
- Quantitative lymphoscintigraphy shows that the ratio of radioactivity of the affected to normal axilla is significantly lower in the lymphedema patients.
- Severity of dermal back flow, clinical stage, and therapy compliance are independent predictors of therapeutic response in patients with gynecological cancer-related lymphedema before complex decongestive therapy.
- In patients submitted to intra-abdominal lymph node dissection for histologically confirmed cancer, the appearance of lower limb lymphedema seems to be correlated with the development of a primary lymphatic disease that was latent prior to the therapeutic interventions.

5.5.1.3 Lymphoscintigraphy for Assessing the Efficacy of Physical and/or Surgical Treatments

Lymphoscintigraphy has been used in the assessment of interventional approaches in patients with lymphedema, including manual lymphatic massage [64–69], pneumatic compression [70–72], hyperthermia [73], pharmacologic therapies [74, 75], and surgery (both microsurgery [76–79] and vascularized lymph node transplantation [80]).

In women undergoing therapy for postmastectomy lymphedema, the degree of lymphatic function impairment prior to the treatment as assessed by lymphoscintigraphy correlates inversely with the outcome of manual lymphatic therapy [37]. Similarly, in patients with clinical stage I unilateral extremity lymphedema, lymphoscintigraphy can predict long-term response to multi-approach physical therapy. In this regard, the visualization of a main lymphatic vessel without collateral lymphatic vessels was the best predictor for a favorable response [81], as also was persisting lymph node visualization 4 h after radiocolloid administration [82].

In a recent study, the extent of dermal backflow (small extent/large extent), the level of lymphatic flow (trunk flow pattern/upper arm-restricted pattern/forearm-restricted pattern groups), and the visualization of lymph nodes (visualized/non-visualized) at lymphoscintigraphy were correlated with the change in the circumferential difference between the two sides of the body, the upper arm and forearm, with

the clinical outcome being variable in patients undergoing nonsurgical treatment. Upper arm edema was more significantly reduced after sympathetic ganglion block rather than after complex decongestive therapy in the small extent group, the forearm-restricted pattern group, and the non-visualized group. In the other groups, sympathetic ganglion block and complex decongestive therapy showed comparable therapeutic effects without statistical differences [83]. Lymphatic regeneration following both free-tissue [84] and lymphatic vessel transplantation [85] has also been assessed with lymphoscintigraphy. Additionally, lymphoscintigraphic classification of patients with secondary lymphedema correlates closely with the clinical stage scale and with findings at intraoperative examination during lymphatico-venous anastomosis [86]. In unilateral lymphedema, lymphoscintigraphic abnormalities of the contralateral limb may also be demonstrated in about 32% of patients [87]. The changes in clinical symptoms and the postoperative lymphoscintigraphic changes did not always correspond. However, there was a trend for the percentage of lymphoscintigraphic deterioration to be greater in the group with clinical deterioration [88].

An improvement of the transport index, well correlated with arm's volume reduction, was observed during long-term follow-up of patients with lymphedema treated with autologous lymph vessel transplantation, confirming that this procedure indeed improves lymph drainage [89, 90]. Similarly, postoperative lymphoscintigraphy showed improved lymphatic drainage in all cases of lymphedema submitted to a combined double-gastroepiploic vascularized lymph node transfer and a modified radical reduction with preservation of perforator vessels [80, 91].

The indications for lymphoscintigraphy can schematically be summarized as follows:

- Differential diagnosis of edema to distinguish venous from lymphatic etiology
- Assessment of pathways of lymphatic drainage
- Quantitation of lymph flow
- Identification of patients at high risk of developing lymphedema following axillary lymph node dissection
- Evaluation of the efficacy therapeutic interventions for lymphedema

Lymphoscintigraphy with ^{99m}Tc-sulfur colloid has recently been compared to the diagnostic performance of a new technique, PET/CT after interstitial injection of ^{68}Ga-labeled NOTA Blue Evans (^{68}Ga-NEB) [92]. This study showed that ^{68}Ga-NEB activity could be clearly observed in the lymphatic route on the PET/CT images from all the patients, showing consistent results in 8/13 cases; diagnostic images of ^{68}Ga-NEB PET/CT were obtained much faster than the conventional lymphoscintigraphic images. In the

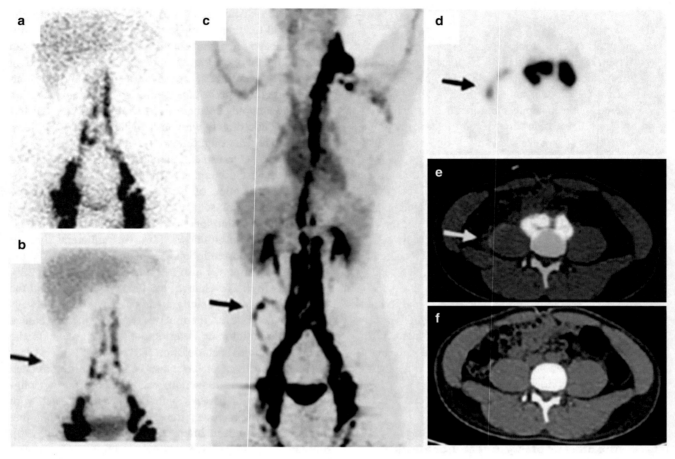

Fig. 5.3 A 17-year-old man (patient 4) with abdominal discomfort for more than 6 months. Chylous ascites was suspected, and nuclear medicine was consulted. 99mTc-sulfur colloid anterior image of the abdomen acquired 60 min after injection (**a**) was unremarkable. The image acquired 6 h after injection (**b**), however, revealed diffuse, mild radioactivity on the right side of the lower abdomen (arrow). In the 68Ga-NEB MIP image (**c**) acquired 5 min after tracer injection, clear linear activity (arrow) could be seen in the right abdomen. In transaxial PET (**d**), fusion (**e**), and CT (**f**) images, this activity (arrows) was located in the immediate anterolateral border of the right psoas muscle, indicating the site of the chyle leak. Intense activity in the inguinal, iliac, and paraspinal lymph nodes and thoracic duct was also better appreciated in 68Ga-NEB PET/CT images (*adapted from Zhang W et al.* [92])

remaining five cases, 68Ga-NEB PET/CT provided additional information in five patients (38.5% of the whole group under study). In particular, one patient had chyloperitoneum, two had chylothorax, and one had postsurgical limp swelling; 99mTc-sulfur colloid lymphoscintigraphy was unable to localize the site of chyle leak, whereas 68Ga-NEB PET/CT successfully identified the leak (Figs. 5.3, 5.4, and 5.5). In addition, in a young woman who had cystic lesions and pleural effusion, the site of chest abnormality was visualized on 68Ga-NEB PET/CT but not on 99mTc-sulfur colloid lymphoscintigraphy (Fig. 5.6). Therefore, this study suggests the feasibility of using of 68Ga-NEB PET/CT as an alternative to conventional lymphoscintigraphy in the evaluation of lymphatic disorders.

Key Learning Points
- Lymphoscintigraphy has been used to assess interventional approaches in patients with lymphedema, including manual lymphatic massage, pneumatic compression, hyperthermia, pharmacologic therapies, and surgery, both microsurgery and vascularized lymph node transplantation.
- In women undergoing therapy for postmastectomy lymphedema, the degree of lymphatic function impairment prior to the treatment as assessed by lymphoscintigraphy correlates inversely with the outcome of manual lymphatic therapy.

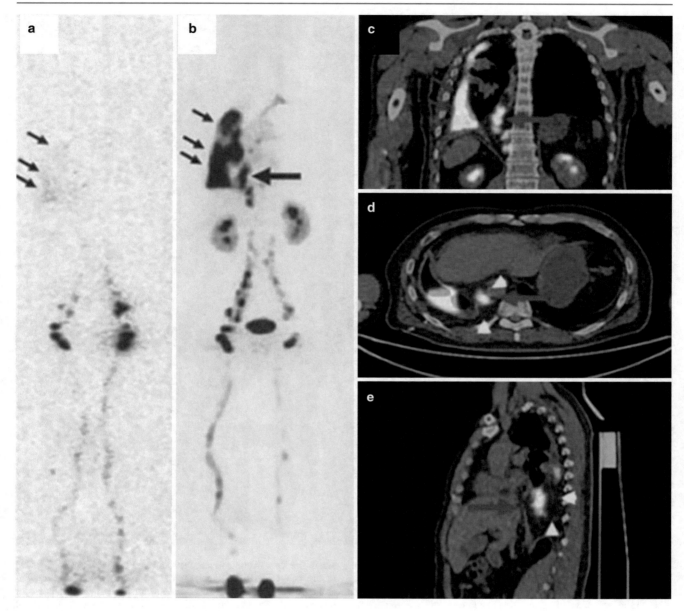

Fig. 5.4 A 43-year-old man with right-side persistent pleural effusion (patient 3). The patient had a remote history of motor vehicle accident. Laboratory examination of the fluid after thoracocentesis demonstrated chylothorax. ^{99m}Tc-sulfur colloid scintigraphy (**a**) revealed diffuse, mild activity in the right chest, consistent with the clinical findings of right chylothorax. However, the potential site of the chyle leak could not be identified. In comparison, ^{68}Ga-NEB PET/CT (**b**: MIP; **c**: coronal fusion; **d**: axial fusion; **e**: sagittal fusion) not only showed activity in the right-chest pleural effusion (small arrows), but also clearly revealed an additional vertically linear intense activity (large arrow) centered in the dilated thoracic duct and cisterna chyli with mild activity surrounding (arrowheads), consistent with the site of the leak (*adapted from Zhang W et al. [92]*)

- In patients with clinical stage I unilateral extremity lymphedema the visualization of a main lymphatic vessel without collateral lymphatic vessels at lymphoscintigraphy is the best predictor of long-term response to multi-approach physical therapy.

- ^{68}Ga-NEB PET/CT provides more information than lymphoscintigraphy with ^{99m}Tc-sulfur colloid, is faster than conventional lymphoscintigraphy, and is able to localize the site of the leak especially inside the thorax and abdomen.

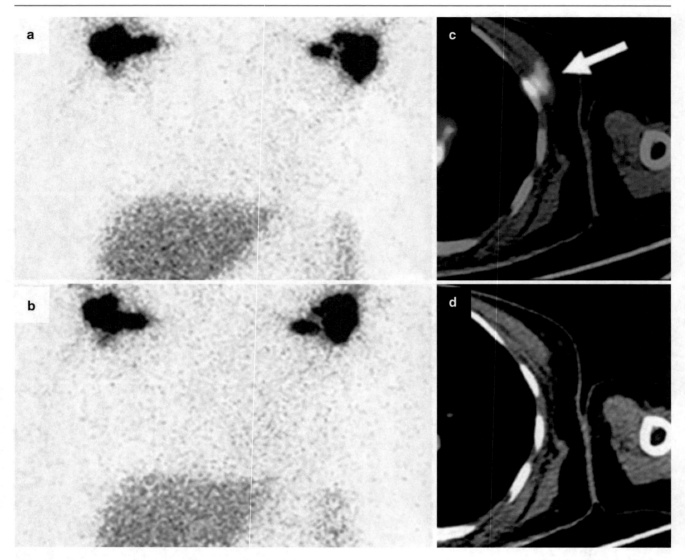

Fig. 5.5 Anterior ^{99m}Tc-sulfur colloid (SC) images were acquired at 2 h (**a**) and 6 h (**b**) after subcutaneous tracer injection between the thumb and index finger of the hands in a 44-year-old woman (patient 1) who had left-chest swelling and was status post-left mastectomy for breast cancer. The images revealed axillary lymph nodes bilaterally and minimally more tracer activity in the left chest without evidence of the site of the leak. In comparison, the transaxial images (**c**: fusion; **d**: CT) of the ^{68}Ga-NEB PET/CT acquired at 30 min after injection demonstrated a focal activity (arrow) underneath the left pectoralis major muscle, at the level of the left anterior fourth rib, indicating the site of the chyle leak (*adapted from Zhang W et al.* [92])

5.6 X-Ray Computed Tomography and Magnetic Resonance Imaging

X-ray computed tomography (CT) scanning or magnetic resonance imaging (MRI) of the lower extremities can detect in patients with lymphedema a "honeycomb" pattern of the subcutaneous tissue that is not characteristic of other types of edema. CT and MRI have been used to describe the morphologic changes due to the subcutaneous lipomatous hypertrophy [93–96].

CT-lymphography (CT-LG) was performed in patients with upper limb lymphedema [97]. Three-dimensional observation of deeper tissues at CT-LG has been used to help elucidating the mechanism of dermal backflow. According to the data obtained by Yamada et al. [98], lymphatic vessels that branch from collecting lymphatic vessels toward the dermis have an inner diameter wide enough to be confirmed with CT (Fig. 5.7). This was likely the observation of lymph flowing back to new or existing abnormal lymphatic vessels as it moves toward the dermis. From there, lymph flows back through capillary lymphatic vessels, leading to its storage in interstitial spaces (Fig. 5.8). It is unclear why such a phenomenon occurs there, but due to upstream blockage or increased internal pressure of lymphatic vessels, lymph appears to flow back from deeper areas to shallower areas, as if to escape [98].

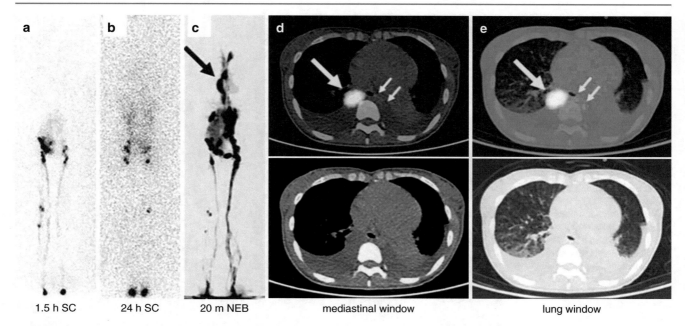

Fig. 5.6 A 25-year-old woman presented with shortness of breath for 3 months (patient 11). A diagnostic CT (images not shown) revealed many cystic structures in the chest, abdomen, and pelvis. In addition, bilateral pleural effusion was noted, which was subsequently shown as chylothorax. For this reason, lymphoscintigraphy was performed. The ^{99m}Tc-sulfur colloid (SC) images at 1.5 h (**a**) and 24 h (**b**) after injection in the feet both showed that the tracer reached abdomen/pelvis without much chest activity. However, in ^{68}Ga-NEB MIP PET image (**c**) acquired 20 min after tracer injection, there was clear, intense vertical activity (large arrow) in the thorax. In transaxial images (**d**: mediastinal window; **e**: lung window), the vertical activity was in an enlarged thoracic duct (large arrows). The chyle leak (small arrows) from the thoracic duct to the left chest was also noted. There were also many small cysts in both lungs (**e**) (*adapted from Zhang W* et al. [92])

Fig. 5.7 Three-dimensional imaging of lymphatic system. In the images (left: 3D reconstructed image, right: 1-mm-slice image), lymphatic vessels were clearly identified with higher contrast than surrounding tissues, and the diameters were measured (*adapted from Yamada K* et al. [98])

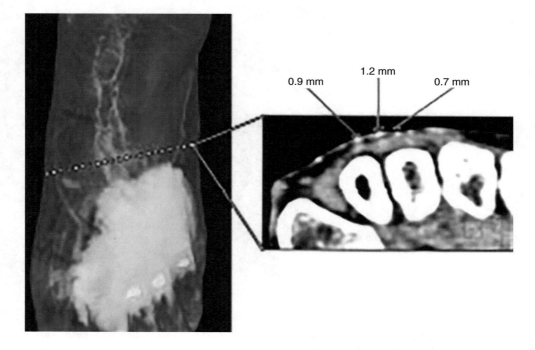

High-resolution magnetic resonance lymphangiography (MRL) following interstitial, intracutaneous injection of an extracellular, paramagnetic contrast agent has recently been proposed for identifying abnormal lymphatic pathways [99–101]. This technique, that has proved to be technically feasible in patients with primary or secondary lymphedema [63, 102, 103], visualizes the lymphatic vessels in a limb with lymph flow disturbances, but not the lymphatic vessels of a healthy limb. This is most probably due to the faster lymph flow speed in the healthy limb. Therefore, lymph circulation disorders should be suspected when contrast-enhanced lymphatic vessels are visualized with this test. Migration of the

Fig. 5.8 Detailed analysis of dermal backflow (DB) sites with CT-LG. Slice images (**a**, 1–4 from top to bottom) show some collecting lymphatic vessels (arrow) branching upward and medially toward the dermis (arrowhead), transitioning to the DB. In the representative high-contrast 3D image (**b**), lymphatic vessels were hidden under DB and could not be observed, but in the representative lower-contrast 3D image (**c**, where horizontal lines indicate the level of transaxial sections shown in ((**a**), lymphatic vessels that were previously hidden under the DB could now be recognized. Panel (**d**) is a schematic representation of DB: *C* Collector, *SLV*, small lymphatic vessel; *D*, dermis; *SF*, superficial fat layer; *DF*, deep fat layer; *DB* (blue area in the dermis), dermal backflow. (*Adapted from Yamada K* et al. [98])

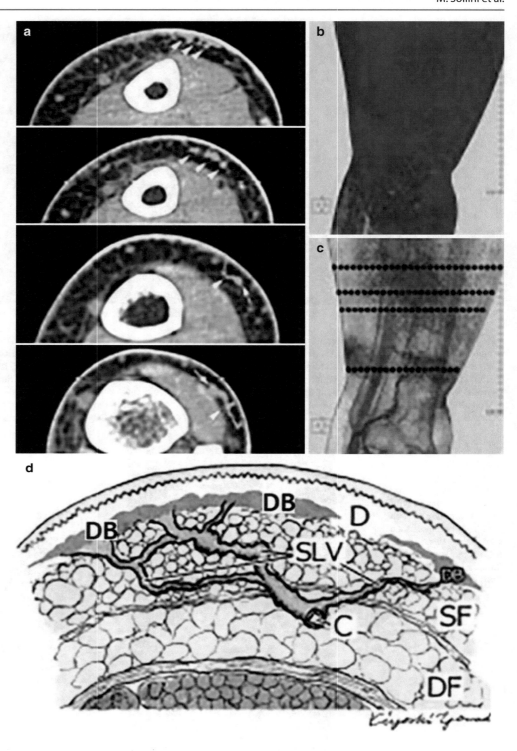

contrast agent by the draining lymphatic system to regional lymph nodes also allows real-time observation of the transport function of the lymphatic system and of the lymph nodes within a reasonable length of time. Furthermore, the specificity of absorption and transport of the contrast agent by the lymphatic system permits to visualize detailed morphologic changes of the lymphatic vessels and of the regional lymph nodes. Finally, quantitative assessment of abnormal lymph flow kinetics may be achieved by tracing the flow within the lymphatic vessels and comparing dynamic nodal enhancement and time-signal intensity curves between edematous and contralateral limbs. Figures 5.9 and 5.10, and 5.11 depict different MRL patterns in patients with lymphedema. However, it should be noted that MRL is still in an

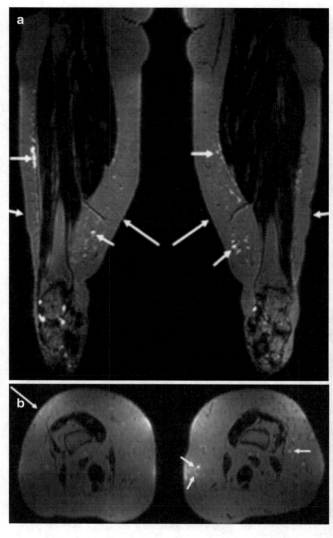

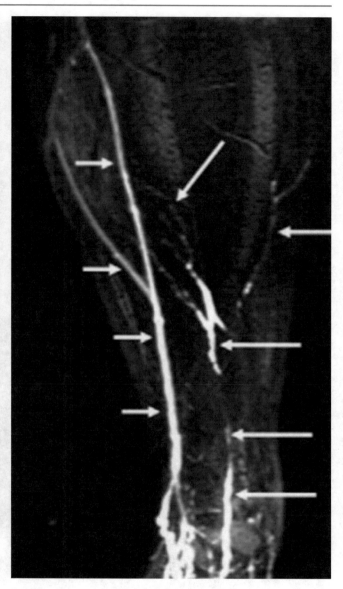

Fig. 5.9 Coronal (**a**) and axial heavily (**b**) T2-weighted 3D-TSE source images obtained in a patient with bilateral lipo-lymphedema of the lower extremities. The images show an increased layer of subcutaneous fat at the lower legs (upper panel, long arrows), subcutaneous regions of lymphedema (upper panel, short arrows), and severely enlarged layer of subcutaneous fat up to a diameter of 7.5 cm at the upper portion of both legs (lower panel, long arrows). Additionally, small areas of epifascial lymphedema are seen (short arrows in **b**) (*adapted from Lohrmann C et al.* [101])

Fig. 5.10 Frontal 3D spoiled gradient-echo MRL MIP image obtained 45 min after gadoteridol injection in a patient with bilateral lipedema, showing clearly enlarged lymphatic vessels that have a typical bead-like appearance up to a diameter of 2 mm at the level of the right lower leg (large arrows), indicating a subclinical status of lipo-lymphedema. High uptake of contrast material is evident in the lymphatic vessels at the right lower leg as well as in a vein (small arrow) (*adapted from Lohrmann C et al.* [101])

experimental validation phase, since the extravascular intracutaneous injection of contrast agents is an off-label use of such compounds. Side effects such as moderate necrosis, hemorrhage, and edema have been described. Furthermore, incorrect interstitial injection of the contrast agent may lead to severe venous contamination.

The first correlations between lymphoscintigraphic pattern as evaluated with ⁹⁹ᵐTc-nanocolloid (injected subcutaneously at the interdigital web) and MRL findings (3 Tesla system, gadopentetate dimeglumine, and mepivacaine injected intracutaneously in the first three interdigital spaces

of the forefoot) demonstrated clear concordance between the results of the two techniques, lymphoscintigraphy visualizing better the inguinal lymph nodes, and MR depicting the lymph vessels and morphology of lymph vessel abnormalities [30]. Figures 5.12 and 5.13 represent two examples of comparison between the two techniques in the same patient.

Further studies in upper extremity lymphedema [104] where MRL was performed before and after injection of a contrast agent by using a coronal T1-weighted 3D gradient-echo sequence with spectral fat saturation demonstrated higher spatial resolution and better depiction of lymph vessels with MRL than with lymphoscintigraphy. When MRL and lymphoscintigraphy are reported using a semiquantitative classification according to five patterns of lymphatic abnormalities (delay of drainage, drainage pattern, enhancement of lymph nodes, depiction of lymph vessels, anatomic levels), MRL lymphangiography showed sensitivities of 100% for all four categories, while lymphoscintigraphy yielded a sensitivity of 83.3% for delineation of lymph vessels and 100% for the other three categories. Specificity of MR lymphangiography was 85.7% for delay of drainage and 100% for other three categories, while lymphoscintigraphy showed specificity of 66.7% for pattern of lymphatic drainage and 100% for other three categories. Delay and pattern of drainage were the same in 83.3% and non-visualization of axillary LNs was indistinguishably noted in all patients on

both techniques. Anatomic level of enhanced lymph vessel was identical in 66.7% of the patients (Figs. 5.14 and 5.15). MR lymphangiography showed better performance for depiction of abnormal lymph vessels. MR lymphangiography and lymphoscintigraphy yielded similar results in all or most patients for evaluation of axillary lymph node enhancement and lymphatic drainage in upper extremity.

In another study [105], contrast-enhanced MRL was applied to the evaluation of the lower limb, providing superior anatomical and functional information, with high spatial resolution, in comparison to various techniques used in the diagnosis of lower limb lymphedema (i.e., lymphoscintigraphy, direct lymphography, unenhanced MR), and allowing more accurate diagnosis and classification of patients suffering from lymphoedema.

Another application of contrast-enhanced MRL is in the diagnosis of occult chylous leak after thoracic duct emboli-

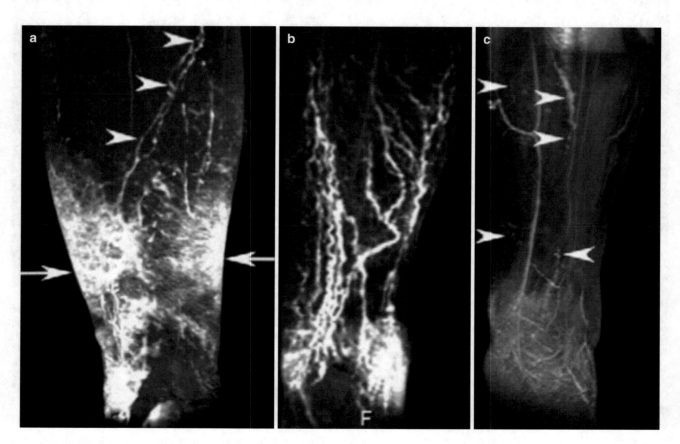

Fig. 5.11 Three-dimensional contrast MR lymphangiographies displaying various patterns of lymphatic drainage. (**a**) Increased skin lymphatic and dermal backflow in the medial and lateral region of lower leg (arrow), and dilated collectors in the upper part of leg (arrowhead). (**b**) Radially arranged dilated vessels in the lower leg of a patient with primary lymphedema. (**c**) Enhanced lymphatic vessels (arrowheads) distributed as a slender network over the lower extremity. (**d**) Bunches of extremely dilated and significantly enhanced lymphatic vessels (arrowheads) located in the medial and lateral portion of the thigh. (**e**) Single enhanced and dilated lymphatic vessel in a patient with primary lymphedema (arrowheads) with irregular outline in the leg. (**f**) Intensely enhanced dilated lymph vessel (arrowheads) with clear outline in the thigh (*adapted from Liu NF et al.* [102])

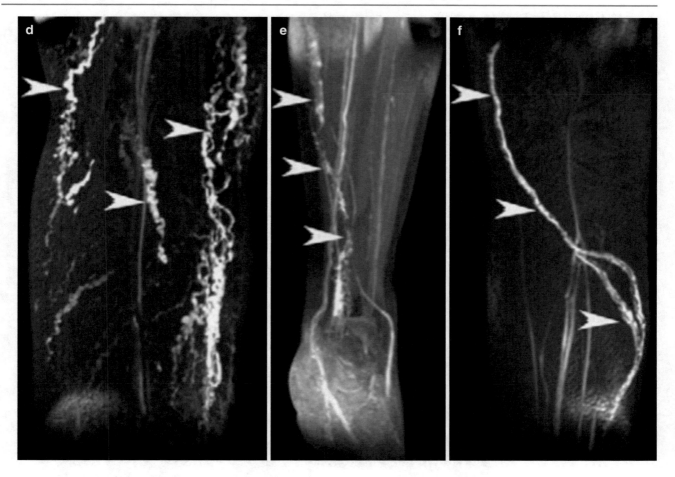

Fig. 5.11 (continued)

zation. In a case report [106] the direct contrast-enhanced MRL allowed the diagnosis of an occult chylous fluid leak from the right retroperitoneum into the right pleural space, after failure of both conventional lymphangiography and prophylactic TDE.

MRL has also been performed in combination with ^{68}Ga-NEB PET or as part of a PET/MR examination for visualizing morphologic and functional characteristics of lymphatic vessels, evaluating lymphedema, and guiding surgical intervention. Preoperative ^{68}Ga-NEB PET combined with MRL has been shown providing advantageous 3D images, higher temporal resolution, shorter time lapse before image acquisition after tracer injection, and more accurate pathological lymphatic vessel distribution with respect to traditional techniques (i.e., lymphoscintigraphy). This strategy has demonstrated significant advan-

tages in the evaluation of lymphedema severity, staging, and pathological location of lymph vessels to make individualized treatment plans [107]. Combined ^{68}Ga-NEB TOF-corrected PET/MR was used in patients with different clinical severity of unilateral lower limb lymphedema [108], with semiquantitative imaging assessment (ratio of the standardized uptake value (SUV) of superficial lymphatic vessel (SLV) versus SUV of deep lymphatic vessel (DVL) (SUVslv/dlv)). In this study, a significant difference in the SUVslv between the affected limbs and normal limbs in all subjects was found (not found in the SUVdlv) and the SUVslv/dlv of the affected limbs showed statistical differences within the groups with minimal, moderate, and severe lymphedema with a negative correlation, thus promising in evaluating bilateral lower limb lymphedema.

Fig. 5.12 Patient with stage II lymphedema of the right leg. (**a**) MRL image obtained with a 3.0 Tesla system after intracutaneous injection in the first three interdigital spaces of the forefoot of gadopentetate dimeglumine and mepivacaine. (**b**) Late-phase (2 h) lymphoscintigraphic images. In the right leg, diffuse lymphatic drainage (dashed arrow) and lymphangiectasia (solid white arrow) were detectable. MRL shows an early enhancing lymph node in the left groin (open arrow) and no contralateral iliac lymph node enhancement, thus suggesting delayed drainage in this leg. Lymphoscintigraphy clearly depicts diffuse drainage pattern (solid black arrow) and diminished right-sided inguinal lymph nodes. The radiocolloid was almost completely drained from the left leg at the time of acquisition, so that lymph vessels on this side were no longer visible (*adapted from Notohamiprodjo M et al. [63]*)

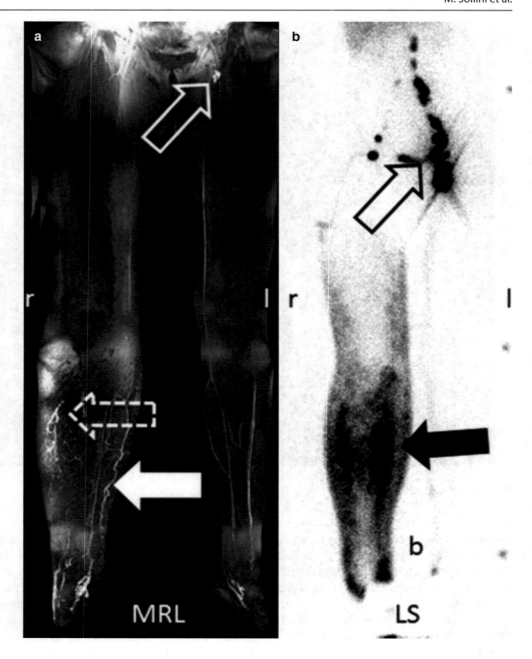

Key Learning Points

- Three-dimensional observation of deeper tissues at CT-LG has been used to help elucidating the mechanism of dermal backflow.
- MRL following interstitial, intracutaneous injection of an extracellular, paramagnetic contrast agent has proved to be technically feasible in patients with primary or secondary lymphedema, although it is still an experimental procedure.

- MRL allows real-time observation of the transport function of the lymphatic system and of the lymph nodes, depiction of detailed morphologic changes of the lymphatic vessels and of the regional lymph nodes, and quantitative assessment of abnormal lymph flow kinetics.
- MRL and lymphoscintigraphy have been compared in some studies.
- MRL has also been performed as part of ^{68}Ga-NEB PET/MR.

Fig. 5.13 Patient with stage II lymphedema of the left leg. (**a**) MRL image obtained with a 3.0 T MR system after injection of gadopentetate dimeglumine and mepivacaine in the first three interdigital spaces of the forefoot. (**b**) Late-phase (2 h) lymphoscintigraphic images. Lymphoscintigraphy shows that the pretibial lymph vessel is masked by the localized dermal backflow, whereas the lymph vessel is clearly visible in the MRL image. The marker position is indicated by "1" (*adapted from Notohamiprodjo M* et al. [63])

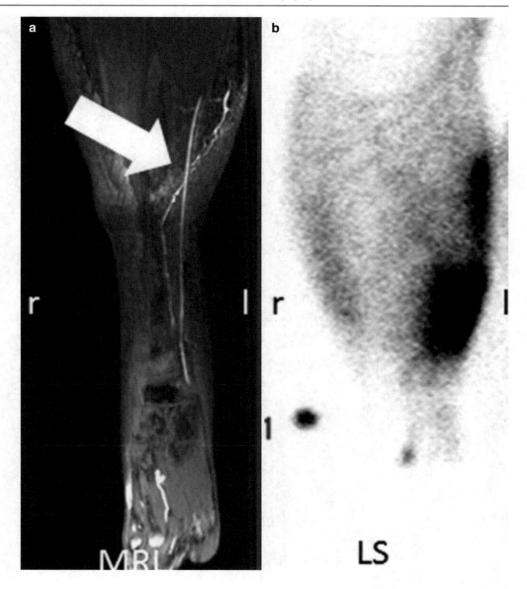

5.7 Virtual Reality for Preoperative Planning

Conventional images of lymphoscintigraphy and SPECT/CT processed by dedicated software to visualize this 3D patient-specific model, creating detailed 3D image of the anatomical structures, were used to plan lympho-venous anastomosis through virtual reality in a patient with a lymphatic malformation. The strategy of this intervention was to identify the lymphatics leaking into the malformation and to interrupt the inflow towards the lesion by redirecting the lymph toward the venous system. Localization of the lymphatic malformation was achieved without iat-

rogenic damage to the adjacent structures, an important goal, as previous resection was only temporarily successful, and scarring is a well-known complication of multi-stage surgery [109].

> **Key Learning Point**
> A personalized planning for lympho-venous anastomosis was performed in virtual reality elaborating the SPECT/CT images, resulting in a better localization of the leak and avoiding iatrogenic damage to the adjacent structures.

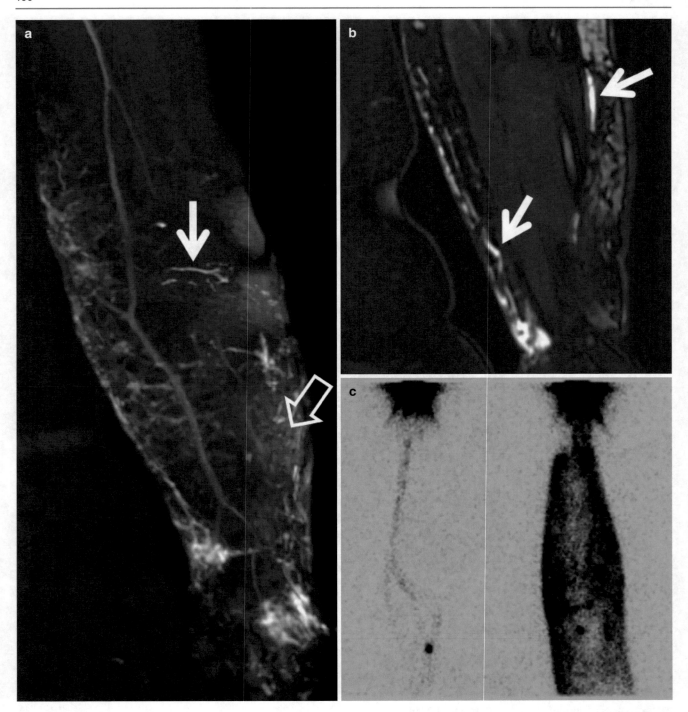

Fig. 5.14 Interstitial and vascular pattern of lymphatic drainage in a 48-year-old woman with stage II lymphedema of the left arm. (**a, b**) Beaded, dilated appearance of lymph vessels (lymphangiectasia) (solid arrow) and diffuse, interstitial enhancement (open arrow) around lymph vessels are visualized on maximum intensity projection images of MR lymphangiography 15 min after gadobutrol injection (**a**). The anatomical depth of lymph vessels (solid arrow) is demonstrated in coronal images (**b**). Lymphoscintigraphy image acquired 2 h after radiotracer injection shows diffuse lymphatic drainage at the left forearm (**c**) (*adapted from Bae JS* et al. [104])

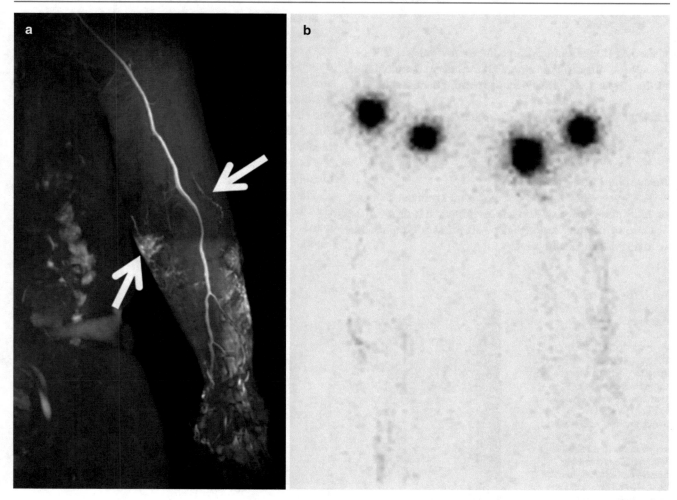

Fig. 5.15 Comparison of depiction of lymph vessels by MR lymphangiography and lymphoscintigraphy in a 55-year-old woman with stage II lymphedema. (**a**) MR lymphangiography clearly demonstrates beaded appearance of lymph vessels (white arrows) at the left elbow at both ulnar and radial sides. (**b**) Lymphoscintigraphy revealed only faint dotted line at the corresponding area (*adapted from Bae JS* et al. [104])

Clinical Cases

Case 5.1: Upper Limb Monocompartmental Lymphoscintigraphy in Stage III Primary Lymphedema of the Upper Left Arm Without Lymphadenomegaly

Luciano Feggi, Chiara Peterle, Corrado Cittanti, Valentina de Cristofaro, Stefano Panareo, Ilaria Rambaldi, Virginia Rossetti, and Ivan Santi

Background Clinical Case

A 45-year-old woman presented with spontaneous onset of mild non-pitting swelling in the upper left arm, in the absence of vascular lesions (stage III primary lymphedema with no lymphadenomegaly).

Anatomic location of edema: Left upper limb.
Lymphoscintigraphy

Lymphoscintigraphy was performed following administration of two aliquots of 2 mL containing 111 MBq ^{99m}Tc-albumin nanocolloid. Radiopharmaceutical injections were performed superficially in both hands (injection in first, second, third, and fourth interdigital spaces in each hand). A dual-detector SPECT gamma camera (E-cam Siemens Medical Solutions, Hoffman Estates, IL) equipped with low-energy high-resolution (LEHR) collimators was used to obtain planar images.

Planar images were acquired 5 min (early images) and 4 h (late images) after injection in anterior view (256 × 256 matrix, zoom factor 1.00, acquisition time 200 s for each view).

Fig. 5.16 Delayed drainage at the left upper limb in the early acquisitions and "dermal flow" in the 4-h acquisitions. A similar pattern is observed for lymph node uptake in the spot acquisitions over the thorax-upper abdomen: no lymph node uptake in the left axilla in the early acquisitions, however with some uptake in the delayed acquisitions (the left-side lymph nodes remaining always less evident than the contralateral lymph nodes). Based on the results of lymphoscintigraphy, the patient underwent combined therapy for lymphedema (pneumatic compression, wrapping of forearm, and massages)

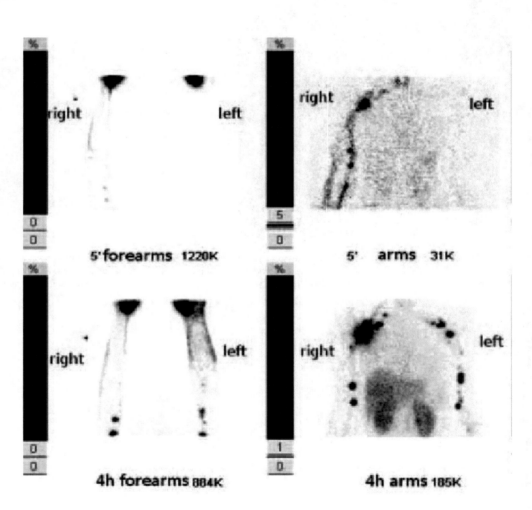

Case 5.2: Upper Limb Monocompartmental Lymphoscintigraphy in Non-pitting Edema of the Upper Left Limb in Patient with Rheumatoid Arthritis

Luciano Feggi, Chiara Peterle, Corrado Cittanti, Valentina de Cristofaro, Stefano Panareo, Ilaria Rambaldi, Virginia Rossetti, and Ivan Santi

Background Clinical Case

A 40-year-old woman with a history of rheumatoid arthritis and mild non-pitting edema in left upper limb (left hand and forearm) for 6 months.

Anatomic location of edema: Left upper limb.

Lymphoscintigraphy

Lymphoscintigraphy was performed following administration of two aliquots of 2 mL containing 74 MBq ^{99m}Tc-albumin nanocolloid. Radiopharmaceutical injections were performed superficially and bilaterally (injection in first, second, third, and fourth interdigital spaces in each hand). A dual-detector SPECT gamma camera (E-cam Siemens Medical Solutions, Hoffman Estates, IL) was used to obtain planar images. Time of acquisition after injection: 5 min after injections (early images): (a) hands and forearms (laid upon collimator); (b) arms and thorax; 4 h after injection (late images): (a) hands and forearms (laid upon collimator); (b) arms and thorax (256 × 256 matrix, zoom factor 1.00, acquisition time 200 s for each view).

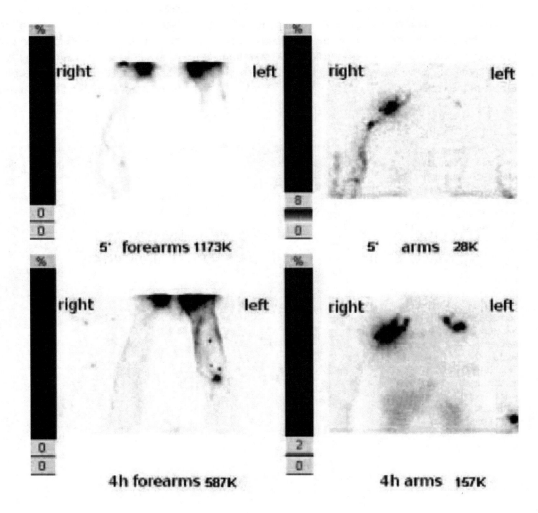

Fig. 5.17 Delayed drainage at left upper limb in the early acquisitions and "dermal flow" in the 4-h acquisitions. The pattern of lymphatic drainage is not totally normal also in the right arm, where no uptake in epitrochlear lymph nodes can be observed. No lymph node uptake in the left axilla at early imaging, with some uptake in the delayed acquisitions (but still much less intense than in the right axilla). Based on the results of lymphoscintigraphy, the patient underwent combined therapy for lymphedema (pneumatic compression, wrapping of forearm, and massages)

Case 5.3: Axillary Reverse-Mapping Lymphoscintigraphy in Breast Cancer Patient with Positive Sentinel Lymph Node (SLN) Before Lymphadenectomy

Luciano Feggi, Chiara Peterle, Corrado Cittanti, Valentina de Cristofaro, Stefano Panareo, Ilaria Rambaldi, Virginia Rossetti, Ivan Santi, and Paolo Carcoforo

Background Clinical Case

A 66-year-old woman underwent surgery for a left breast cancer finding positive SLN. Axillary dissection is necessary in patients with positive SLNs in breast cancer; in axillary basin lymph nodes may drain from either breast or arm; still, a lymph node which drains from both breast and arm is very rarely found, so the surgeon can spare a few nodes to preserve lymphatic arm drainage.

The ARM technique (axillary reverse mapping) allows to mark lymph nodes which drain from both hand and arm, so the surgeon can distinguish radioactive nodes (arm drainage) from "cold" ones (breast drainage) and remove only the breast-related ones.

Anatomic location of edema: No edema.
Lymphoscintigraphy

Lymphoscintigraphy was performed following administration of two aliquots of 0.4 mL containing 74 MBq ^{99m}Tc-albumin nanocolloid. Radiopharmaceutical injections were performed superficially and bilaterally (injection in first, second, third, and fourth interdigital spaces in each hand). A dual-detector SPECT gamma camera (E-cam Siemens Medical Solutions, Hoffman Estates, IL) equipped with low-energy high-resolution (LEHR) collimators was used to obtain planar images.

Time of acquisition after injection: (a) hands and forearms, 5 min after injection (laid upon collimator); (b) arms, 10 min after injection (anterior planar view); (c) axillary regions and thorax, 15 min after injection (anterior planar scan using cobalt wire as a landmark); (d) second acquisition only on axillary regions and thorax (anterior planar scan using cobalt wire as a landmark). Before late image of axillary regions and thorax, a radioguided occult lesion localization (ROLL) (after second nanocolloid intratumoral injection with ultrasound guidance) was performed to allow the surgeon to remove the breast primary tumor and left axillary nodes in one single time.

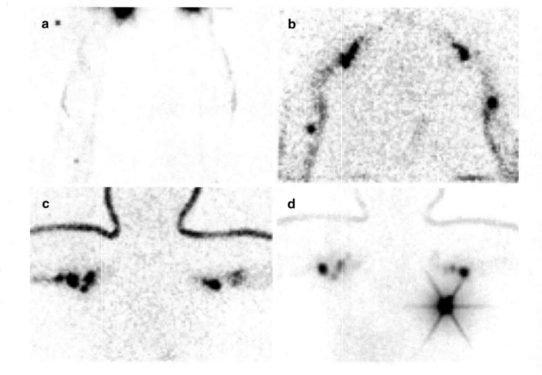

Fig. 5.18 Early acquisitions (**a**–**c**): normal lymphatic drainage in both upper limbs (mild delay in left upper limb early drainage; a month earlier, the patient underwent SLN removal in the left axillary basin). In *panel* (**d**) (late acquisition) the axillary reverse-mapping lymphoscintigraphy (ARM) is displayed, while the hottest focus in the left breast corresponds to intratumoral injection of ^{99m}Tc-albumin macroaggregates for ROLL. The lymph nodes that drain the upper limb, that accumulate the radiocolloid, will be spared during axillary dissection, thus decreasing the risk of secondary lymphedema possibly caused by axillary dissection

Case 5.4: Axillary Reverse-Mapping Lymphoscintigraphy in Breast Cancer Patient with Infiltrative Lobular Carcinoma and Positive SLN Before Lymphadenectomy

Luciano Feggi, Chiara Peterle, Corrado Cittanti, Valentina de Cristofaro, Stefano Panareo, Ilaria Rambaldi, Virginia Rossetti, Ivan Santi, and Paolo Carcoforo

Background Clinical Case

A 49-year-old woman with left breast cancer (infiltrative lobular carcinoma with positive SLN); we performed an ARM lymphoscintigraphy (axillary reverse-mapping lymphoscintigraphy), before the surgeon performed axillary dissection to spare lymph nodes that drain from hand and arm.

Anatomic location of edema: No edema.

Lymphoscintigraphy

Lymphoscintigraphy was performed following administration of two aliquots of 0.4 mL containing 74 MBq ^{99m}Tc-albumin nanocolloid. Radiopharmaceutical injections were performed superficially and bilaterally (injection in first, second, third, and fourth interdigital spaces in each hand). A dual-detector SPECT gamma camera (E-cam Siemens Medical Solutions, Hoffman Estates, IL) equipped with low-energy high-resolution (LEHR) collimators was used to obtain planar images.

Planar images were acquired in anterior view (256 × 256 matrix, zoom factor 1.00, acquisition time 200 s for each view).

Time of acquisition after injection: (a) hands and forearms, 5 min after injection (laid upon collimator); (b) arms, 10 min after injection (anterior planar scan); (c) axillary regions and thorax, 15 min after injection (anterior planar scan using cobalt wire as a landmark); (d) second acquisition only (late image) on axillary regions and thorax (anterior planar scan using cobalt wire as a landmark).

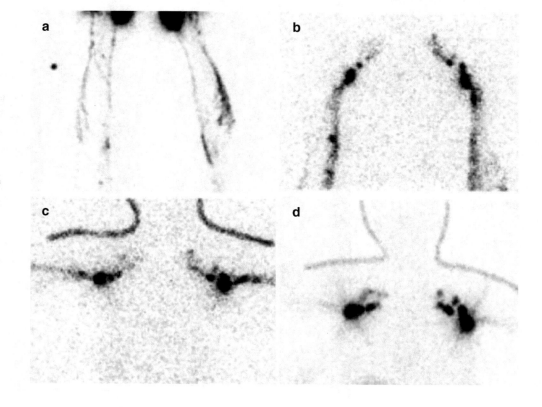

Fig. 5.19 Early images (**a–c**) show normal lymphatic drainage in both upper limbs (mild delay in left upper limb early drainage; 1 month earlier, the patient underwent SLN removal in the left axillary basin). *Panel* (**d**) is the late scan of axilla and thorax. The lymph nodes that drain the upper limb, that accumulate the radiocolloid, will be spared during axillary dissection, thus decreasing the severity of secondary lymphedema possibly caused by axillary dissection

Case 5.5: Lower Limb Monocompartmental Lymphoscintigraphy in Patient with Bilateral Swelling and Non-pitting Edema of the Lower Limbs

Luciano Feggi, Chiara Peterle, Corrado Cittanti, Valentina de Cristofaro, Stefano Panareo, Ilaria Rambaldi, Virginia Rossetti, and Ivan Santi

Background Clinical Case

A 62-year-old man with spontaneous onset of bilateral swelling and non-pitting edema in the lower limbs since 1 year.

Anatomic location of edema: Lower limbs.

Lymphoscintigraphy

Lymphoscintigraphy was performed following administration of two aliquots of 2 mL containing 111 MBq ^{99m}Tc-albumin nanocolloid. Radiopharmaceutical injections were performed superficially and bilaterally (injection in first, second, and fourth interdigital spaces and in the outer retromalleolar space in each foot). A dual-detector SPECT gamma camera (E-cam Siemens Medical Solutions, Hoffman Estates, IL) equipped with low-energy high-resolution (LEHR) collimators was used to obtain planar images. Planar images were acquired 10 min after radiopharmaceutical administration and walking exercise and 4 h, respectively, after injection (256 × 256 matrix, zoom factor 1.00, acquisition time 200 s for each view) in anterior planar scan from feet to abdominal region.

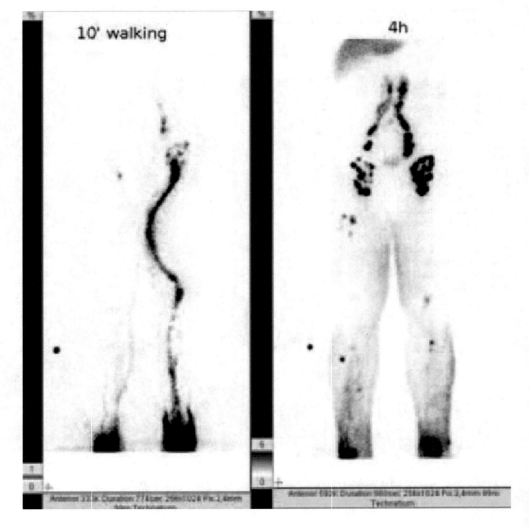

Fig. 5.20 Bilateral abnormal patterns of lymphatic drainage, as indicated by markedly delayed flow on the right side and mildly delayed flow on the left side in the early acquisition. The delayed acquisition shows the presence of bilateral "dermal backflow" with asymmetrical lymph node uptake (including an alternate pattern from the popliteal to the inguinal and to the lumbo-aortic lymph nodes). Based on the results of lymphoscintigraphy, the patient underwent combined therapy for lymphedema (pneumatic compression, wrapping of forearm, and massages)

Case 5.6: Lower Limb Bicompartmental Lymphoscintigraphy in Patient with Edema of the Left Lower Limb

Paola Anna Erba and Luisa Locantore

Background Clinical Case

A 47-year-old woman with edema of the left lower limb. Normal Doppler ultrasound. No family history of lymphedema.

Anatomic location of edema: Lower left limb.

Lymphoscintigraphy

For the deep lymphatic circulation (DLC): two aliquots of ^{99m}Tc-nanocolloid, 7 MBq each of injection in 0.1 mL in the first and second intermetatarsal space, identified by palpating the soles of both feet immediately proximal to the distal heads of the metatarsal bones on each side, inserting the needle by about 12–13 mm to reach the intermetatarsal muscles below the deep fascia plantaris. *For the superficial lymphatic circulation (SLC)*: three aliquots of about 10 MBq in 0.1 mL on the dorsum of each foot, inserting the needle subdermally in sites corresponding approximately to the prior palmar injections, about 1–2 cm proximally to the interdigital web. Spot and whole-body images were obtained from the distal feet up to the abdomen.

Spot images: 180 s/view, matrix 128 × 128, zoom 1.33

Whole-body images: matrix 128 × 1024, zoom 1, speed: 12 cm/min

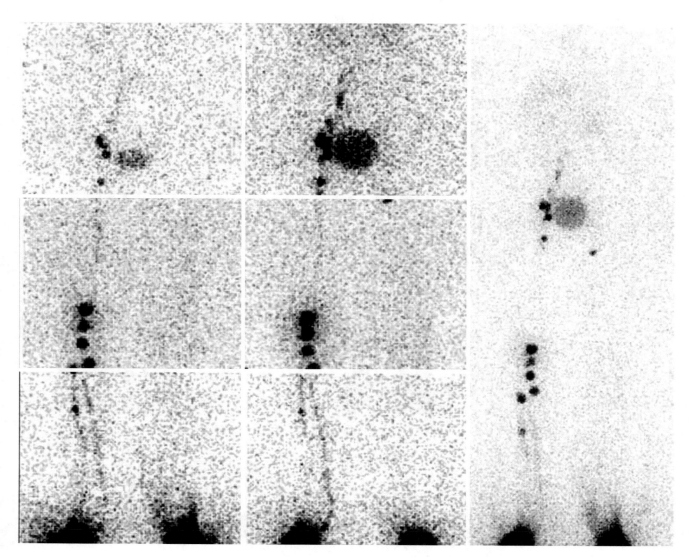

Figs. 5.21 and 5.22 Clear impairment of left lower lymph flow is evident in both the spot images (*Fig. 5.21*) and the whole-body image (*Fig. 5.22*), with minimal "dermal flow" at the distal medial portion of the left leg after radiocolloid injection for evaluating the DLC. No uptake can be seen in the left popliteal lymph nodes, while a single inguinal lymph node is detected after radiocolloid injection for the SLC. In addition, the DLC and SLC are simultaneously visualized at the right lower limb after radiocolloid injection for evaluating the DLC, indicating communication between the deep and the superficial lymphatic circulations. Multiple popliteal lymph nodes are detected on the right side, with normal pattern of the inguinal lymph nodes. Lumbo-aortic lymph nodes are faintly visualized, similarly as liver uptake

Case 5.7: Lower Limb Monocompartmental Lymphoscintigraphy in Patient with Bilateral Lower Limb Lymphedema

Giuseppe Rubini and Filippo Antonica

Background Clinical Case

A 32-year-old man with bilateral lower limb lymphedema. Clinicians suspected congenital dysplasia of the lower limb lymphatic vessels. Legs appeared edematous, size increased and the patient complained about fatigue and continuous pain even during sleep time. His daily actions were very limited.

Anatomic location of edema: Lower limbs.

Lymphoscintigraphy

Lymphoscintigraphy was performed following injections of two aliquots containing ^{99m}Tc-albumin nanocolloid, 37 MBq each of injection in 0.1 mL in the first and second intermetatarsal spaces. A dual-detector SPECT gamma camera (Millennium GE Healthcare, Milwaukee, WI) equipped with low-energy high-resolution (LEHR) collimators was used to obtain whole-body images after radiopharmaceutical injection. Whole-body planar images were acquired in anteroposterior projection, with a 256 × 1024 matrix and zoom factor 1.00 (speed: 12 cm/min) from the distal feet up to the abdomen.

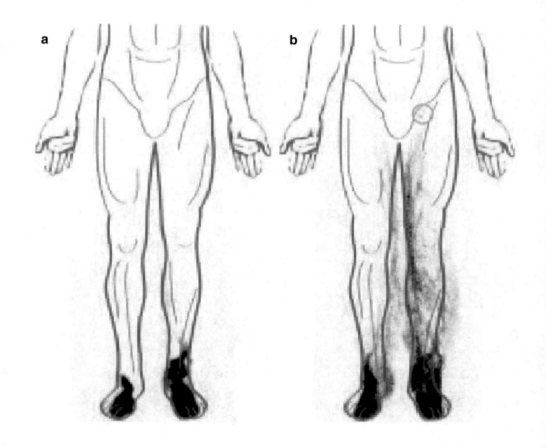

Fig. 5.23 Schematic representation of whole-body images in anterior view at 5–10, 30, 60, and 90 min (**a–d**, respectively) after radiocolloid injection and walking to stimulate lymphatic circulation. Radiocolloid drainage is delayed in both lower limbs, especially on the right side (no visualization of the groin lymph nodes in early scans). In later acquisitions, the right groin lymph nodes appear (*red circle*), delayed with respect to the right groin (*green circles*)

Fig. 5.23 (continued)

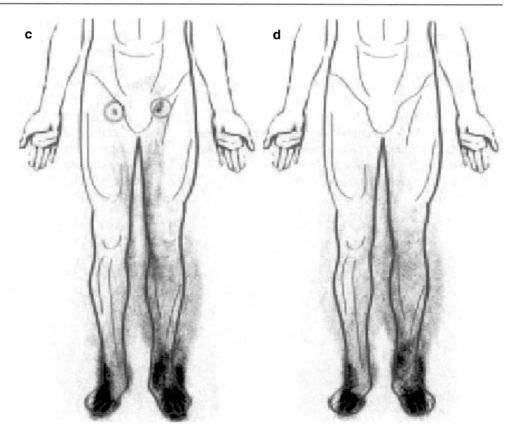

Case 5.8: Lower Limb Monocompartmental Lymphoscintigraphy in Patient Previously Submitted to Left Saphenectomy

Giuseppe Rubini and Filippo Antonica

Background Clinical Case

A 68-year-old woman previously submitted to saphenectomy of the left limb. Left limb appeared cold, size increased, and patient reported size increasing especially in the last year. Echo-color Doppler revealed decreased blood flow and tissue edema.

Anatomic location of edema: Lower limbs.
Lymphoscintigraphy

Lymphoscintigraphy was performed following injections of two 0.1 mL aliquots containing 36 MBq ^{99m}Tc-albumin nanocolloid, in the first and second intermetatarsal spaces. A dual-detector SPECT gamma camera (Millennium GE Healthcare, Milwaukee, WI) equipped with low-energy high-resolution (LEHR) collimators was used to obtain whole-body images after radiopharmaceutical injection. Whole-body planar images were acquired in anteroposterior projection, with a 256 × 1024 matrix and zoom factor 1.00 (speed: 12 cm/min) from the distal feet up to the abdomen.

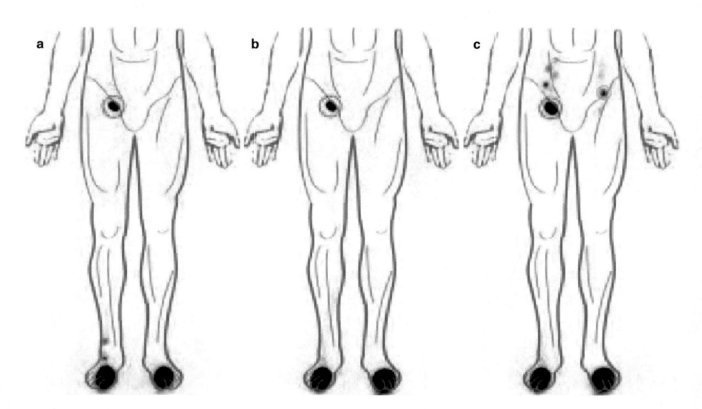

Fig. 5.24 Schematic representation of whole-body images in anterior view at 5–10, 30, and 60 min (**a–c**, respectively) after radiocolloid injection. Radiocolloid drainage is delayed in the left lower limb (no visualization of the groin lymph nodes in the early scans). In later acquisitions, the left groin lymph nodes appear (*green circle*). Radiocolloid drainage is normal in the right lower limb (*red* and *yellow circles*). These scintigraphic findings suggest secondary impairment of lymphatic drainage in the left lower limb

Case 5.9: Lower Limb Monocompartmental Lymphoscintigraphy in Patient with History of Lymphadenectomy of the Groin Basin for Melanoma

Giuseppe Rubini and Filippo Antonica

Background Clinical Case

Patient with a history of cutaneous melanoma of the right foot already surgically removed and submitted to lymphadenectomy of the groin basin due to groin SLN positivity for metastasis. The surgeon also removed pelvic lymph nodes to guarantee surgical radicality. Physical examination did not reveal any lymphadenopathy or lymphedema.

Anatomic location of edema: Lower limbs.

Lymphoscintigraphy

Lymphoscintigraphy was performed following injections of two 0.1 mL aliquots containing 36 MBq ^{99m}Tc-albumin nanocolloid, in the first and second intermetatarsal spaces. A dual-detector SPECT gamma camera (Millennium GE Healthcare, Milwaukee, WI) equipped with low-energy high-resolution (LEHR) collimators was used to obtain whole-body images after radiopharmaceutical injection. Whole-body planar images were acquired in anteroposterior projection, with a 256 × 1024 matrix and zoom factor 1.00 (speed: 12 cm/min) from the distal feet up to the abdomen.

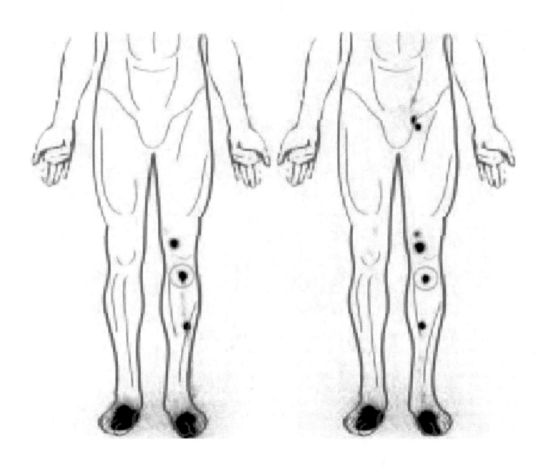

Fig. 5.25 Schematic representations of whole-body scans in anterior view, 5–10 min (*left panel*) and 30 min (*right panel*) after radiocolloid injection. Lymphatic drainage is delayed in the right lower limb (no visualization of the groin lymph nodes). Drainage is normal in the left lower limb, with normal visualization of the popliteal (*green circle*) and inguinal (*yellow circle*) lymph nodes

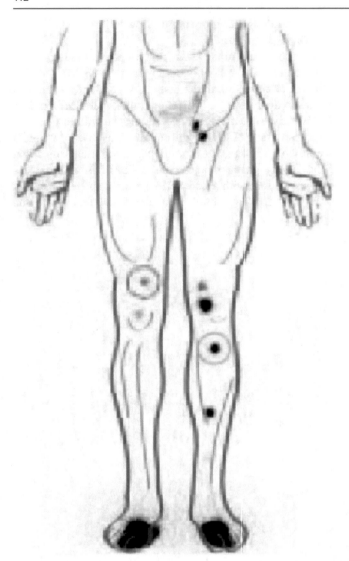

Fig. 5.26 Schematic representation of whole-body scans in anterior view 90 min after radiocolloid injection. In this delayed scan, the right popliteal lymph nodes appear (*red circle*), with faint visualization of the right groin lymph nodes. Radiocolloid drainage is normal in the left lower limb, with normal visualization of the popliteal (*green circle*) and inguinal (*yellow circle*) lymph nodes. These scintigraphic findings suggest secondary impairment of the lymphatic circulation in the right lower limb

Case 5.10: Postexercise Lower Limb Monocompartmental Lymphoscintigraphy in Patient with Bilateral Leg Edema

Luciano Feggi, Chiara Peterle, Corrado Cittanti, Valentina de Cristofaro, Stefano Panareo, Ilaria Rambaldi, Virginia Rossetti, and Ivan Santi

Background Clinical Case

A 50-year-old woman with previous hysterectomy due to uterine fibromatosis and multiple removals of lipomas of the legs underwent investigation, because of mild edema of the legs, more noticeable in the right one; ultrasound, performed before lymphoscintigraphy, showed saphenous–femoral vein junction incontinence with ectasia. Lymphadenomegaly was found in the right inguinal region.

Anatomic location of edema: Lower limbs (more evident in right one).

Lymphoscintigraphy

Lymphoscintigraphy was performed following administration of two doses of 2 mL containing 111 MBq ^{99m}Tc-albumin nanocolloid. Radiopharmaceutical injections were performed superficially and bilaterally (injection in first, second, and fourth interdigital spaces and in the outer retromalleolar space in each foot). A dual-detector SPECT gamma camera (E-cam Siemens Medical Solutions, Hoffman Estates, IL) equipped with low-energy high-resolution (LEHR) collimators was used to obtain planar images. Planar images were acquired 10 min (after radiopharmaceutical administration and walking exercise) and 4 h, respectively, after injection (256 × 256 matrix, zoom factor 1.00, acquisition time 200 s for each view) in anterior planar scans from feet to abdominal region.

Fig. 5.27 Near-normal visualization of bilateral lymphatic trunks and inguinal lymphatic basins both in the early and in the delayed (4 h) acquisitions. A single popliteal lymph node is visualized, only in the right lower limb (mild abnormality)

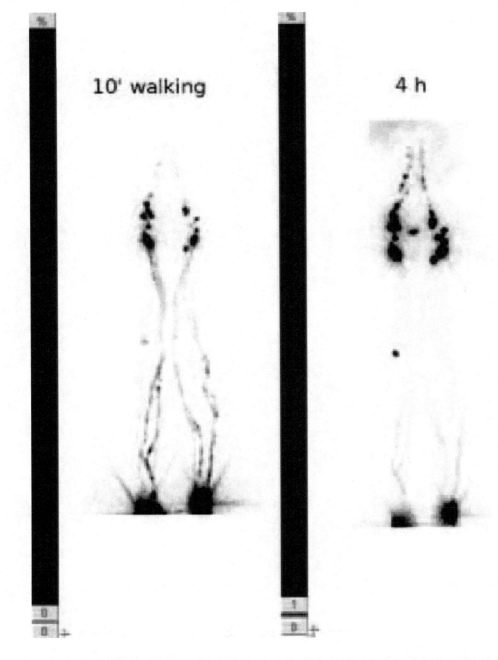

Case 5.11: Lower Limb Monocompartmental Lymphoscintigraphy at Rest and Postexercise with Semiquantitative Evaluation of the Tracer Appearance Time in Patient with Lymphedema of the Left Lower Limb Post-left Groin Lymphadenectomy

Girolamo Tartaglione, Roberto Bartoletti, and Marco Pagan

Background Clinical Case

A 45-year-old woman, with lymphedema of the left lower limb and history of cutaneous melanoma of the gluteus (pN1M0) and left groin lymph nodal dissection.

Anatomic location of edema: Lower limb.

Lymphoscintigraphy

All tight clothes and elastics were removed before tracer injection. Two aliquots of 0.3 mL containing 50 MBq ^{99m}Tc-albumin-nanocolloid were injected intradermally at the first interdigital area, on the top of the feet. Gentle massage was performed after injection in the area. Two scans were acquired starting immediately after injection (the first on the legs and the second on the thighs) following these parameters: planar static scan, preset time 5 min, matrix 128×128, 140 Kev $\pm$ 10%, and anterior and posterior views. A dual-head gamma camera (GE-Infinia) equipped with low-energy general-purpose (LEGP) collimators was used to provide increased sensitivity. If delayed or absent lymphatic drainage was perceived, then the patient was invited to perform 2 min of continuous isotonic exercise (walking). A postexercise static scan was acquired (128×128, 5 min) until the regional lymph nodes were visualized. The tracer appearance time (TAT, normal value less than 10 min) and lymph drainage patterns after exercise (see timeline) were evaluated.

Figs. 5.28 and 5.29 The scan at rest shows near-normal visualization of the main lymphatic vessels of the lower limbs, and a normal TAT, with a time-dependent increased accumulation of the radiocolloid in the left groin region. After exercise, radioactivity accumulation increases even further in the left groin region (lymphatic leakage). In this case exercise revealed a local failure of lymphatic drainage, which was helpful to develop a combined treatment approach

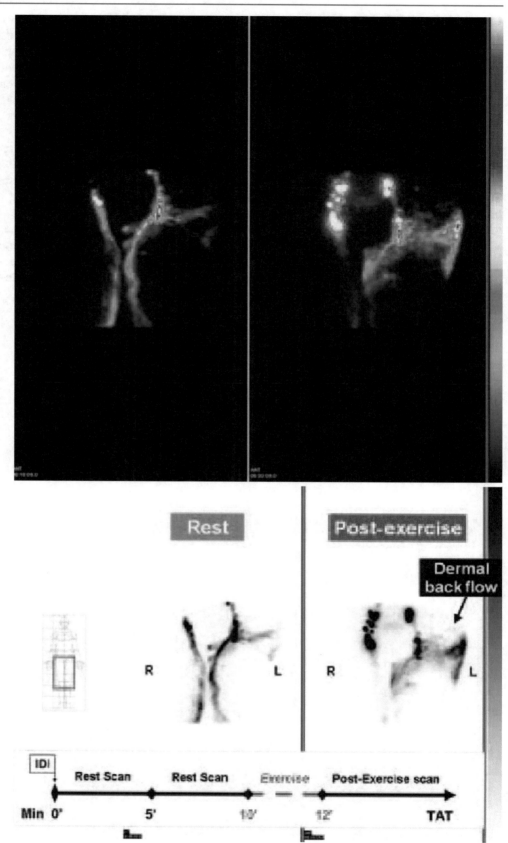

Case 5.12: Lower Limb Monocompartmental Lymphoscintigraphy at Rest and Postexercise with Semiquantitative Evaluation of the Tracer Appearance Time in Patient with Right Lower Limb Primary Lymphedema, Clinical Stage 3 According to Foeldi

Girolamo Tartaglione, Roberto Bartoletti, and Marco Pagan

Background Clinical Case

A 54-year-old woman, affected by a right lower limb primary lymphedema of clinical stage 3 according to Foeldi. The tissue at this stage is hard (fibrotic) and edema is non-pitting. The swelling is almost irreversible and the limb is very large and swollen.

Anatomic location of edema: Right lower limb.

Lymphoscintigraphy

All tight clothes and elastics were removed before tracer injection. Two aliquots of 0.3 mL containing 50 MBq ^{99m}Tc-albumin-nanocolloid were injected intradermally at the first interdigital area, on the top of the feet. Gentle massage was performed after injection in the area. Two scans were acquired starting immediately after injection (the first on the legs and the second on the thighs) following these parameters: planar static scan, preset time 5 min, matrix 128×128, 140 Kev $\pm$ 10%, and anterior and posterior views. A dual-head gamma camera (GE-Infinia) equipped with low-energy general-purpose (LEGP) collimators was used to provide increased sensitivity. If delayed or absent lymphatic drainage was perceived, then the patient was invited to perform 2 min of continuous isotonic exercise (walking). A postexercise static scan was acquired (128×128, 5 min) until the regional lymph nodes were visualized. The tracer appearance time (TAT, normal value less than 10 min) and lymph drainage patterns after exercise (see timeline) were evaluated.

Figs. 5.30 and 5.31 The scan at rest shows severely delayed lymphatic drainage on the right side, with visualization of a rich collateral circulation along the small saphena; no detectable lymph flow on the left side. After exercise, intense dermal backflow appears on the right side, while a normal lymph drainage can be observed on the left side. Dermal backflow is usually observed in case of severe obstruction of the main lymph pathway; when the pressure gradient increases over a certain threshold, it causes incompetence of the lymphatic vessel's valves, which causes inversion of lymph flow toward the dermis. In this patient, compression bandage therapy was ineffective, whereas a standard program of combined physical therapy yielded moderate clinical improvement

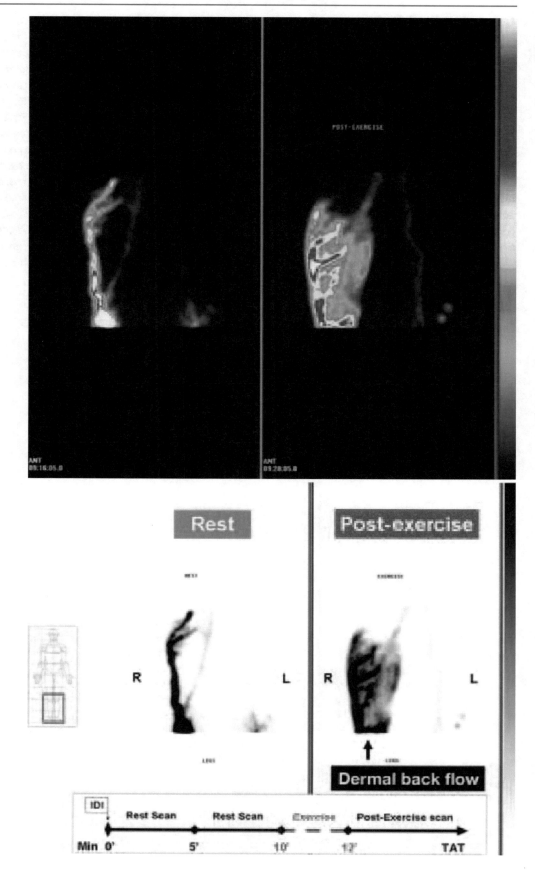

Case 5.13: Lower Limb Monocompartmental Lymphoscintigraphy at Rest and Postexercise with Semiquantitative Evaluation of the Tracer Appearance Time in Patient with Post-lymph Nodal Dissection Lymphedema of the Lower Limbs

Girolamo Tartaglione, Roberto Bartoletti, and Marco Pagan

Background Clinical Case

A 46-year-old man, affected by lymphedema of the lower limbs (clinical stage 2 according to Foeldi) secondary to bilateral groin lymph nodal dissection for cutaneous melanoma (7 years previously). The patient was treated in several centers with combined physical therapy programs, including a personalized program of exercise.

Anatomic location of edema: Lower limbs.

Lymphoscintigraphy

All tight clothes and elastics were removed before tracer injection. Two aliquots of 0.3 mL containing 50 MBq ^{99m}Tc-albumin-nanocolloid were injected intradermally at the first interdigital area, on the top of the feet. Gentle massage was performed after injection in the area. Two scans were acquired starting immediately after injection (the first on the legs and the second on the thighs) following these parameters: planar static scan, preset time 5 min, matrix 128 × 128, 140 Kev ± 10%, and anterior and posterior views. A dual-head gamma camera (GE-Infinia) equipped with low-energy general-purpose (LEGP) collimators was used to provide increased sensitivity. If delayed or absent lymphatic drainage was perceived, then the patient was invited to perform 2 min of continuous isotonic exercise (walking). A postexercise static scan was acquired (128 × 128, 5 min) until the regional lymph nodes were visualized. The tracer appearance time (TAT, normal value less than 10 min) and lymph drainage patterns after exercise were evaluated.

Figs. 5.32 and 5.33 The rest scan shows delayed lymph drainage in the left leg, with normal lymph drainage in the right leg. Exercise accelerated lymph drainage in the left leg. A second lymph drainage pathway was observed in the right leg, with unusual uptake of a popliteal lymph node. The scan demonstrates a shunt between the superficial and deep lymphatic system, as a compensatory mechanism in lymphedema of the right lower limb

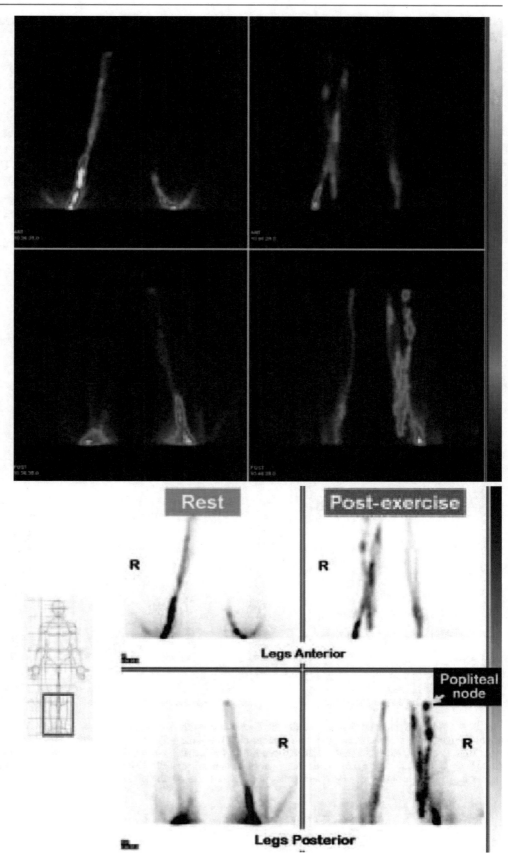

Case 5.14: Postexercise Lower Limb Monocompartmental Lymphoscintigraphy in Patient with Acute Edema of the Left Lower Limb and Painful Left Inguinal Lymphadenomegaly

Luciano Feggi, Chiara Peterle, Corrado Cittanti, Valentina de Cristofaro, Stefano Panareo, Ilaria Rambaldi, Virginia Rossetti, Ivan Santi, and Paolo Carcoforo

Background Clinical Case

A 77-year-old woman with pain and swelling of the left lower limb; ultrasound detected left inguinal lymphadenomegaly; after surgical removal, histological diagnosis was metastasis of neuroendocrine carcinoma (poorly differentiated), consistent with Merkel cell carcinoma metastasis (T2N1Mx). Her clinical presentation included edema of the left lower limb and pain; there was a left inguinal scar after surgical removal.

Anatomic location of edema: Left lower limb.

Lymphoscintigraphy

Lymphoscintigraphy was performed following administration of two aliquots of 2 mL containing 111 MBq ^{99m}Tc-albumin nanocolloid. Radiopharmaceutical injections were performed superficially and bilaterally (injection in first, second, and fourth interdigital spaces and in the outer retromalleolar space in each foot). A dual-detector SPECT gamma camera (E-cam Siemens Medical Solutions, Hoffman Estates, IL) equipped with low-energy high-resolution (LEHR) collimators was used to obtain planar images. Planar images were acquired 5 min and 4 h, respectively, after injection (256 × 256 matrix, zoom factor 1.00, acquisition time 200 s for each view) in anterior planar views of the feet and legs, thighs, and inguinal regions.

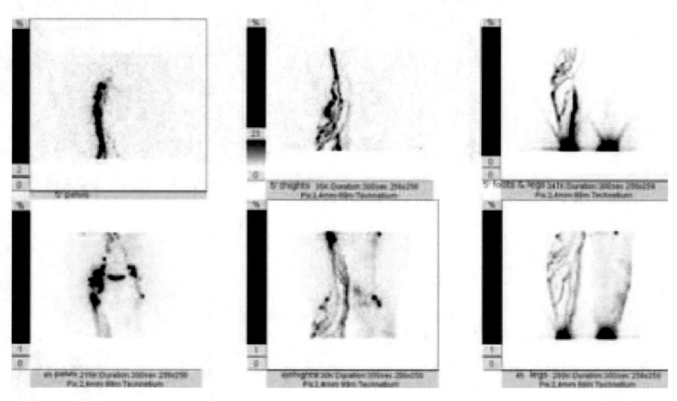

Fig. 5.34 Delayed lymphatic drainage of the left lower limb, with abnormal lymphatic function both in the early acquisition (only the right main lymphatic channel being visualized) and in the 4-h image (mild "dermal flow" in left leg). In the inguinal regions, asymmetrical radiocolloid uptake is observed in the lymph nodes (fewer nodes in left inguinal region). This pattern suggested involvement of the left inguinal lymph nodes causing abnormal drainage in the left lower limb. The patient therefore underwent further examinations, including a [18F] FDG PET/CT scan that visualized a primary tumor in the skin covering the left knee

Figs. 5.35 and 5.36 [18F] FDG PET/CT scan visualizing metastatic nodes in the left inguinal basin causing the abnormal lymphatic drainage in the left extremity

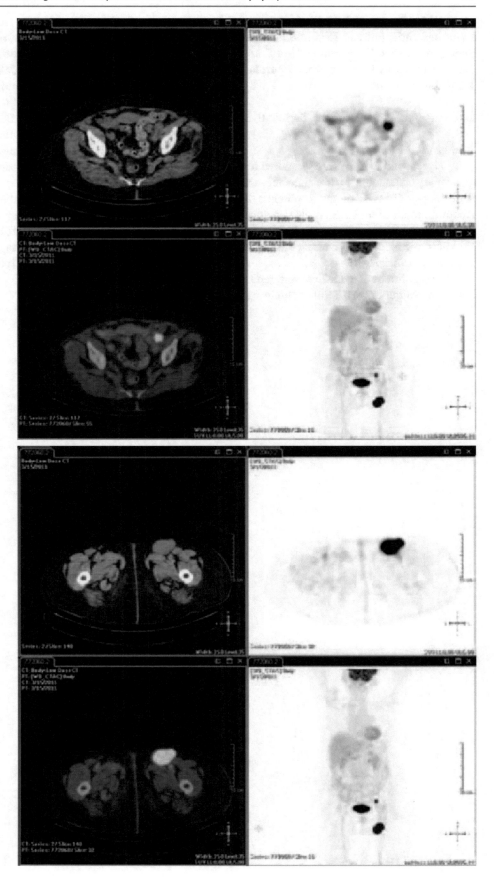

Case 5.15: Lower Limb Monocompartmental Lymphoscintigraphy at Rest and Postexercise with Semiquantitative Evaluation of the Tracer Appearance Time in Patient with Secondary Lymphedema of the Right Lower Limb

Girolamo Tartaglione, Roberto Bartoletti, and Marco Pagan

Background Clinical Case

A 71-year-old woman was submitted to surgical removal of primary melanoma of the right leg and sentinel lymph node biopsy (SLNB) of the popliteal lymph node (pN0). About 3 months after surgery she developed a lymphedema of right lower limb.

Anatomic location of edema: Right lower limb.

Lymphoscintigraphy

All tight clothes and elastics were removed before tracer injection. Aliquots of 0.3 mL containing 50 MBq ^{99m}Tc-albumin-nanocolloid were injected intradermally at the first interdigital area, on the top of the feet. Gentle massage was performed after injection in the area. Two scans were acquired starting immediately after injection (the first on the legs and the second on the thighs) following these parameters: planar static scan, preset time 5 min, matrix 128 × 128, 140 Kev ± 10%, and anterior and posterior views. A dual-head gamma camera (GE-Infinia) equipped with low-energy general-purpose (LEGP) collimators was used to provide increased sensitivity. If delayed or absent lymphatic drainage was perceived, then the patient was invited to perform 2 min of continuous isotonic exercise (walking). A postexercise static scan was acquired (128 × 128, 5 min) until the regional lymph nodes were visualized. The tracer appearance time (TAT, normal value less than 10 min) and lymph drainage patterns after exercise were evaluated.

Figs. 5.37 and 5.38 The scans at rest visualize three superficial collateral lymph channels of the right limb with normal visualization of lymph nodes in the right groin (TAT <10 min), and delayed lymph drainage of the left leg. Isotonic exercise accelerated lymph drainage toward the left groin's lymph nodes (TAT = 16 min), with a collateral lymph pathway and an area of radiocolloid collection in the middle third of the left leg. This test revealed a preexisting lymphatic disease of the lower limbs. A personalized program of combined physical therapy was based on the findings of lymphoscintigraphy

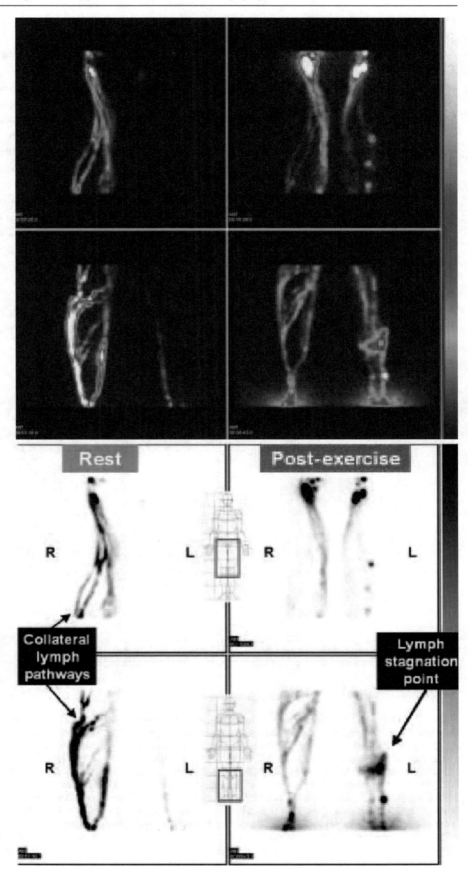

Case 5.16: Lower Limb Monocompartmental Lymphoscintigraphy in Patient with Secondary Bilateral Non-pitting Edema of the Lower Extremities, More Evident on the Left, and Left Ureteral Obstruction Due to Lymphocele

Luciano Feggi, Chiara Peterle, Corrado Cittanti, Valentina de Cristofaro, Stefano Panareo, Ilaria Rambaldi, Virginia Rossetti, Ivan Santi, and Paolo Carcoforo

Background Clinical Case

A 47-year-old woman with melanoma of the left leg and metastasis of the inguinal homolateral lymph nodes underwent surgery (removal of melanoma and left inguinal and iliac lymphadenectomy). After 7 years, during follow-up, CT detected a large pelvic mass, which remained undiagnosed (lymphocele? ovarian cyst?). Two years later, the patient suffered from left ureteral obstruction by compression of a pelvic mass on the third tract of the ureter. Patient reported bilateral swelling in the lower limbs, more evident on the left. Therefore her clinical presentation includes bilateral non-pitting edema of the lower extremities, more evident on the left, and left ureteral obstruction, which needs nephrostomy.

Anatomic location of edema: Lower limbs (more evident in left one).

Lymphoscintigraphy

Lymphoscintigraphy was performed following administration of two aliquots of 2 mL containing 111 MBq ^{99m}Tc-albumin nanocolloid. Radiopharmaceutical injections were performed superficially and bilaterally (injection in first, second, and fourth interdigital spaces and in the outer retromalleolar space in each foot). A dual-detector SPECT gamma camera (E-cam Siemens Medical Solutions, Hoffman Estates, IL) equipped with low-energy high-resolution (LEHR) collimators was used to obtain planar images. Planar images were acquired 5 min, 1 h, 4 h, and 24 h, respectively, after injection in an anterior view (256 × 256 matrix, zoom factor 1.00, acquisition time 200 s for each view). SPECT/CT was acquired 24 h after radiopharmaceutical administration (60 s for each frame, CT slice thickness: 1 mm, tube current of 30 mA, tube voltage of 13 kV).

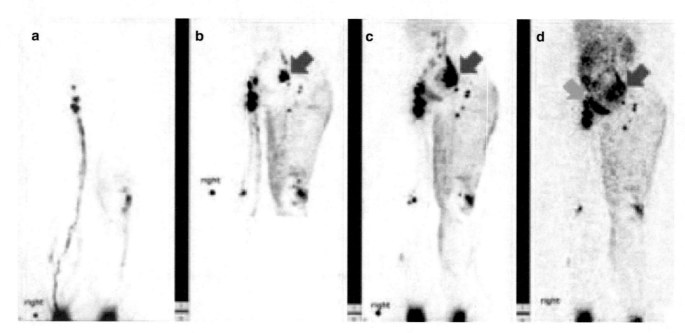

Fig. 5.39 "Whole-body" images extending from the feet to the lower abdomen. From left to right: (**a**) 5 min after radiocolloid injection, normal drainage is noted in the right limb (visualization of a main lymphatic channel and inguinal lymph nodes), whereas in the left limb lymphatic drainage is delayed (the radiocolloid almost stops at the knee). (**b**) 1 h after injection, acquisition from knees to abdomen: normal drainage in right limb with "dermal flow/backflow" in the left thigh, without visualization of the inferior inguinal lymph nodes (prior lymphadenectomy). Bilateral iliac nodes and an area of tracer uptake only on the left (*red arrow*) are visualized. (**c**) Planar scan (feet to abdomen) at 4 h: normal lymphatic drainage on the right limb; popliteal lymph nodes are visualized bilaterally (mostly on the left side), with "dermal flow/backflow" in the thigh; faint radiocolloid uptake in the left inguinal region; in this scan, the pelvic area of radiocolloid accumulation on the left (*red arrow*) appears more evident and larger; there is slight visualization of the bladder and the reticuloendothelial system. (**d**) 24-h scan: the radiocolloid has cleared almost completely from the right lower limb; radioactivity accumulation in the left pelvic area (*red arrow*) has expanded to a larger area. Radioactivity accumulation in the bladder is more evident (*green arrow*), whereas the other sites of uptake remain almost identical. SPECT/CT was performed in order to better characterize this pattern of distribution of the radiocolloid

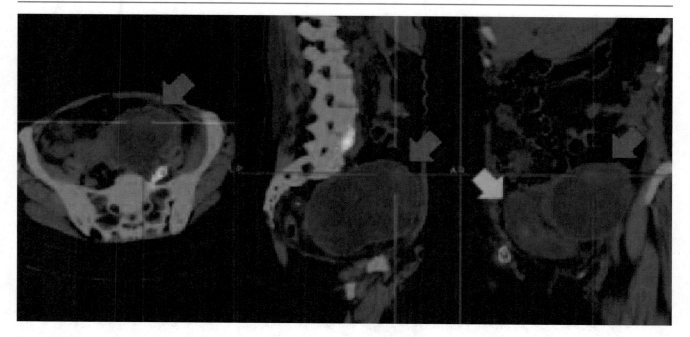

Fig. 5.40 Multiplanar reconstruction (MPR) fusion SPECT/CT (24 h after injection): a large pelvic mass is seen on the left (*red arrow*), near to the bladder (*green arrow*), with retention of a very low amount of radioactivity

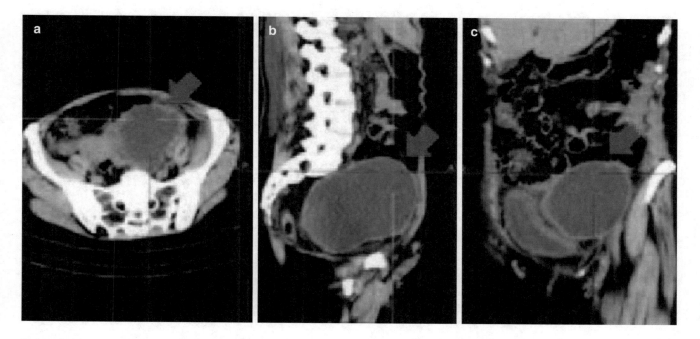

Fig. 5.41 MPR SPECT/CT acquisition (CT only). In the CT component of the acquisition, the content of the pelvic mass (*red arrow*) has radiodensity Hounsfield Unit values typical of a fluid (**a–c**). In a diagnostic CT the pelvic mass does not show contrast enhancement: **d** contrast-enhanced transaxial section; **e** corresponding noncontrast CT section

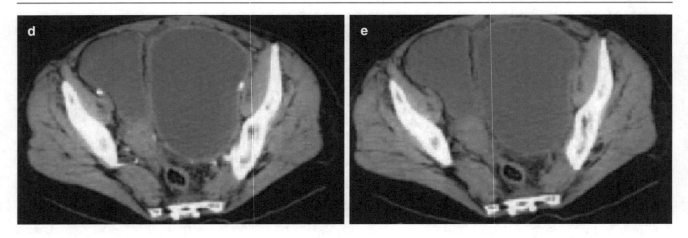

Fig. 5.41 (continued)

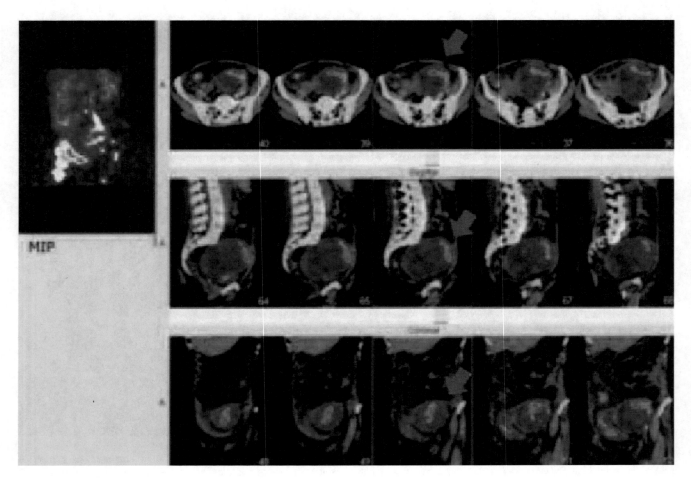

Fig. 5.42 MPR SPECT/CT fusion images. Lymphoscintigraphy confirmed the suspicion that the pelvic mass was a lymphocele. Therefore, the patient underwent surgery, which restored a normal left nephro-ureteral function

Case 5.17: Lower Limb Bicompartmental Lymphoscintigraphy in Patient with Posttraumatic Edema of the Left Leg Associated with Disability Grade 3 According to Ricci Scale, at Baseline and After 5 Years of Multiple Surgeries and Cycles of Therapy

Paola Anna Erba and Luisa Locantore

Background Clinical Case

A 36-year-old man with posttraumatic edema of the left leg. After crush injury, the patient had multiple surgical procedures for the presence of tissue necrosis and cheloids, with cutaneous graft. Before the accident, the patient had had a left leg saphenectomy performed. There is stage V lymphedema of the lower left limb with cutaneous retraction of the proximal and medial portion of the leg, hyperkeratosis, lymphatic vesicles, eczema, and ulcerations. A disability grade 3 according to Ricci scale was present.

Anatomic location of edema: Lower left limb.

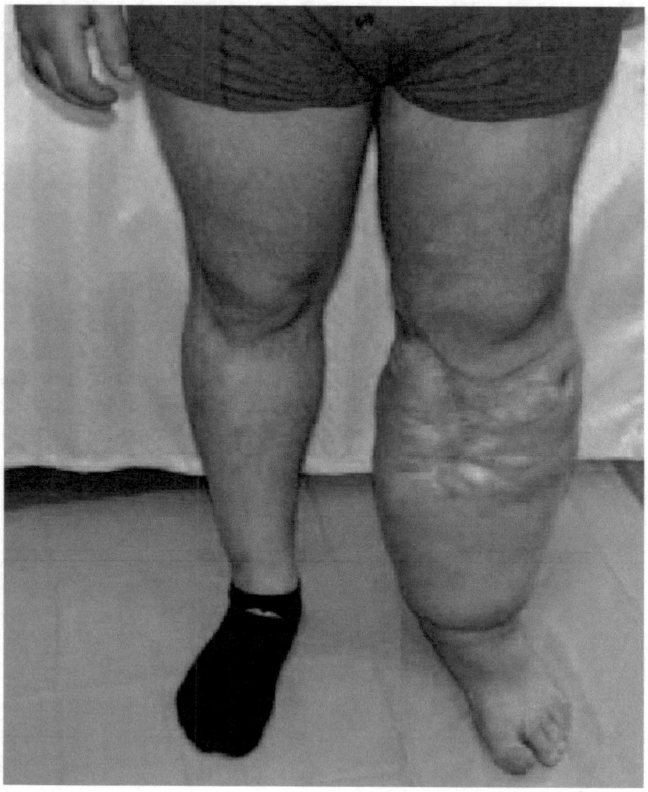

Lymphoscintigraphy
Lower Limbs

For the deep lymphatic circulation (DLC): two aliquots of ^{99m}Tc-nanocolloid, 7 MBq each of injection in 0.1 mL in the first and second intermetatarsal spaces, identified by palpating the soles of both feet immediately proximal to the distal heads of the metatarsal bones on each side, inserting the needle by about 12–13 mm to reach the intermetatarsal muscles below the deep fascia plantaris.

For the superficial lymphatic circulation (SLC): three aliquots of about 10 MBq in 0.1 mL on the dorsum of each foot, inserting the needle subdermally in sites corresponding approximately to the prior palmar injections, about 1–2 cm proximally to the interdigital web. Spot and whole-body images were obtained from the distal feet up to the abdomen.

Spot images: 180 s/view, matrix 128 × 128, zoom 1.33.

Whole-body images: matrix 256 × 1024, zoom 1, speed: 12 cm/min

Fig. 5.43 The patient's legs at baseline scan

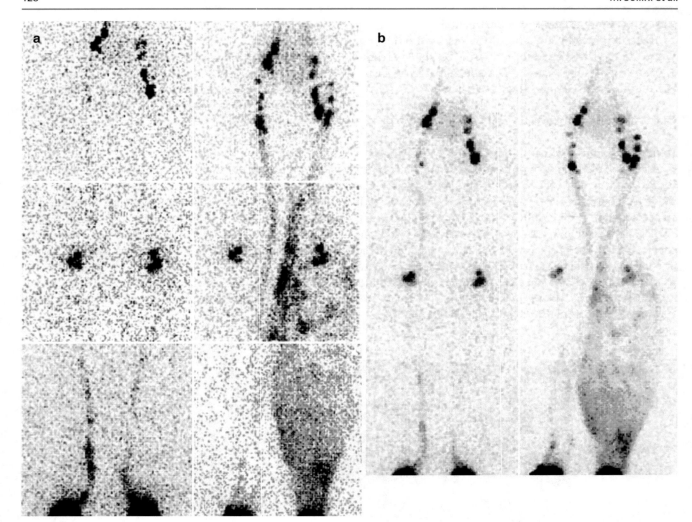

Fig. 5.44 Baseline lymphoscintigraphy. The spot images (**a**, *right*) and the whole-body image (**b**, *right*) show a normal deep lymphatic circulation with a relatively delayed right distal flow; normal popliteal and inguinal lymph nodes are detected with only faint visualization of the inferior right inguinal lymph nodes. After radiocolloid injection for assessing the superficial lymphatic circulation, a normal right lymph flow was depicted. Conversely, "dermal flow" and "dermal backflow" up to mid-thigh are present at the left limb, with preservation of the main lymphatic vessel. New lymph nodes appear in the inguinal region. No radiocolloid progression through the lumbo-aortic lymph nodes is detected and liver uptake of the radiocolloid is not observed

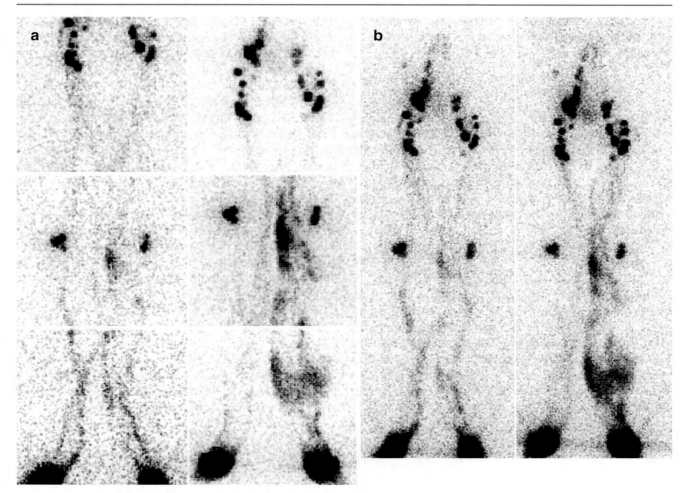

Fig. 5.45 Follow-up lymphoscintigraphy performed after 5 years of subsequent surgical procedures and multiple cycles of therapy. Spot images (anterior view, **a** *left column* DLC, *right column* DLC and SLC) and whole-body images (**b**, *left column* DLC, *right column* DLC and SLC) demonstrated a significant reduction of the left limb "dermal flow" and "dermal backflow" with enhanced lymphatic flow through both the deep and the superficial lymphatic circulation. However, col-lateral lymphatic channels are still visualized after injection for evaluation of the SLC, with enhanced uptake at the site of popliteal lymph nodes; furthermore, increased radiocolloid accumulation along the soft tissue of the lower part of the leg is still present. The pattern of lymphatic drainage for the right leg remains normal. Based on these findings, a new, less aggressive treatment plan was designed, to maintain these favorable results

Case 5.18: Upper and Lower Limb Bicompartmental Lymphoscintigraphy in Patient with Bilateral Feet and Ankle Edema, More Prevalent on Left Side

Paola Anna Erba and Luisa Locantore

Background Clinical Case

A 62-year-old woman with bilateral edema mainly at the distal part of the leg and the feet, worsening in the last 10 months. Doppler ultrasound negative. Ultrasound of the soft tissue showing an increased thickening of the derma, which is hypoechogenic, representing an interstitial edema.

Anatomic location of edema: Bilateral feet and ankles, major at the left side.

Lymphoscintigraphy

Upper Limbs

For the deep lymphatic circulation (DLC): two aliquots of 99mTc-nanocolloid, 7 MBq each of injection in 0.1 mL in the first and second intermetacarpal spaces, identified by palpating the palms of both hands immediately proximal to the distal heads of the metacarpal bones on each side, inserting the needle by about 12–13 mm to reach the intermetacarpal muscles below the deep fascia. *For the superficial lymphatic circulation (SLC)*: three aliquots of about 10 MBq in 0.1 mL on the dorsum of each hand, inserting the needle subder-

mally in sites corresponding approximately to the prior palmar injections, about 1–2 cm proximally to the interdigital web. Spot and whole-body images of both arms, thorax, and upper abdomen.

Lower Limbs

For the DLC: two aliquots of 99mTc-nanocolloid, 7 MBq each of injection in 0.1 mL in the first and second intermetatarsal spaces, identified by palpating the soles of both feet immediately proximal to the distal heads of the metatarsal bones on each side, inserting the needle by about 12–13 mm to reach the intermetatarsal muscles below the deep fascia plantaris.

For the SLC: three aliquots of about 10 MBq in 0.1 mL on the dorsum of each foot, inserting the needle subdermally in sites corresponding approximately to the prior palmar injections, about 1–2 cm proximally to the interdigital web. Spot and whole-body images were obtained from the distal feet up to the abdomen.

Spot images: 180 s/view, matrix 128 × 128, zoom 1.33

Whole-body images: matrix 256 × 1024, zoom 1, speed: 12 cm/min

This is a typical example of lower limb lymphedema due to an impairment of the DLC with conserved function of the SLC; however, signs of overload of the SLC are also present at the left lower limb. Arm circulation is normal.

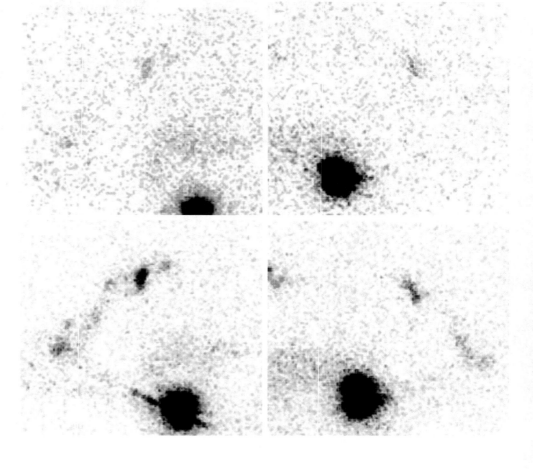

Fig. 5.46 Lymphoscintigraphy of upper limbs, spot images (*upper panel*: DLC; *lower panel*: SLC). A normal deep and superficial lymphatic circulation of the left upper limb is present with mild delay of the superficial circulation. Faint uptake is present at epitrochlear lymph nodes, while axillary lymph nodes are bilaterally visualized, despite being low in number

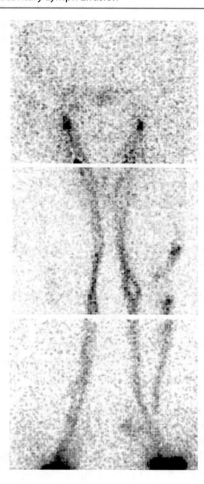

Fig. 5.47 Spot images of lymphoscintigraphy of the lower limbs of the DLC from the distal feet to the inguinal region of the lower limbs. No radiocolloid migration from the injection sites

Fig. 5.48 Spot images of lymphoscintigraphy of the lower limbs of the DLC and SLC from the distal feet to the inguinal region. Images show a normal SLC at the right lower limb, while at the left limb collateral channels are visualized, with sites of uptake representing lymphatic collection along the external margin thigh. No popliteal lymph nodes can be detected, while only few lymph nodes are detected at the inguinal region

Case 5.19: Upper and Lower Limb Bicompartmental Lymphoscintigraphy in Patient with Right Pelvic Paravesical and Inguinal Swelling

Paola Anna Erba and Luisa Locantore

Background Clinical Case

A 33-year-old man with right pelvic (alongside the bladder) and right inguinal swelling. CT finding of multiple cystic lesions suspected for cystic lymphangiomatosis, localized in the retroperitoneal space, at the splenic lodge, in the bone (ribs, vertebral bodies, and pelvic bones of maximum 23 mm) and in the pelvis (about 10 cm). Negative [18F] FDGPET/CT findings.

Anatomic location of edema: Right inguinal.

Lymphoscintigraphy

Upper Limbs

For the deep lymphatic circulation (DLC): two aliquots of 99mTc-nanocolloid, 7 MBq each of injection in 0.1 mL in the first and second intermetacarpal spaces, identified by palpating the palms of both hands immediately proximal to the distal heads of the metacarpal bones on each side, inserting the needle by about 12–13 mm to reach the intermetacarpal muscles below the deep fascia.

For the superficial lymphatic circulation (SLC): three aliquots of about 10 MBq in 0.1 mL on the dorsum of each hand, inserting the needle subdermally in sites corresponding approximately to the prior palmar injections, about 1–2 cm proximally to the interdigital web. Spot and whole-body images of both arms, thorax, and upper abdomen.

Lower Limbs

For the DLC: two aliquots of 99mTc-nanocolloid, 7 MBq each of injection in 0.1 mL in the first and second intermetatarsal spaces, identified by palpating the soles of both feet immediately proximal to the distal heads of the metatarsal bones on each side, inserting the needle by about 12–13 mm to reach the intermetatarsal muscles below the deep fascia plantaris.

For the SLC: three aliquots of about 10 MBq in 0.1 mL on the dorsum of each foot, inserting the needle subdermally in sites corresponding approximately to the prior palmar injections, about 1–2 cm proximally to the interdigital web. Spot and whole-body images were obtained from the distal feet up to the abdomen.

Spot images: 180 s/view, matrix 128 × 128, zoom 1.33

Whole-body images: matrix 256 × 1024, zoom 1, speed: 12 cm/min

Normal bilateral lymph flow was depicted, with only mild delay for the right SLC in the medial and distal part of the leg. Interestingly, two sites of radiopharmaceutical accumulation are evident. The first is at the pelvis localized near the bladder, at the right side, and which is receiving the lymph from the deep lymphatic system. The second is in the upper abdominal area, at the level of the upper right kidney portion which is supplied by the SLC. Normal lymph node images were seen for the popliteal lymph nodes bilaterally and for the left inguinal node. Progression through the lumbo-aortic lymph nodes is present, as well as faint liver uptake of the radiocolloids.

The exam demonstrated the lymphatic nature of both the pelvic and the abdominal collections, therefore confirming the clinical diagnosis of cystic lymphangiomatosis.

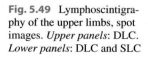

Fig. 5.49 Lymphoscintigraphy of the upper limbs, spot images. *Upper panels*: DLC. *Lower panels*: DLC and SLC

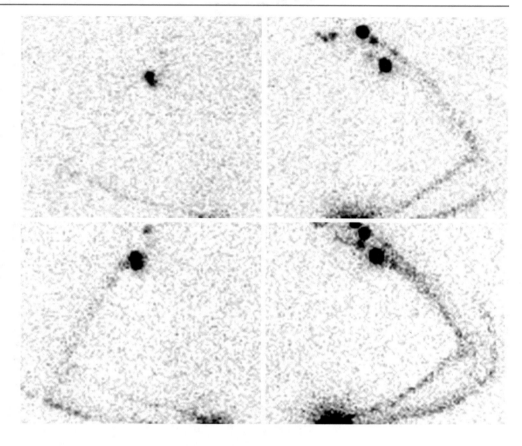

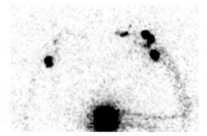

Fig. 5.50 Anterior view of the thoracic and upper abdominal regions, showing a normal deep and superficial lymphatic circulation of the right upper limb; for the left upper limb simultaneous visualization of DLC and SCL was observed immediately after the first injection (for DLC). No epitrochlear lymph nodes were detected and also the right axillary lymph nodes were faintly visualized (mainly first-level nodes). The left axillary nodes were normal. At the end of this phase of the scan radiocolloids had not yet localized in the liver

Fig. 5.51 Spot images of lower limbs during lymphoscintigraphy from the distal feet to the inguinal region. *Left column*: DLC. *Right column*: SLC

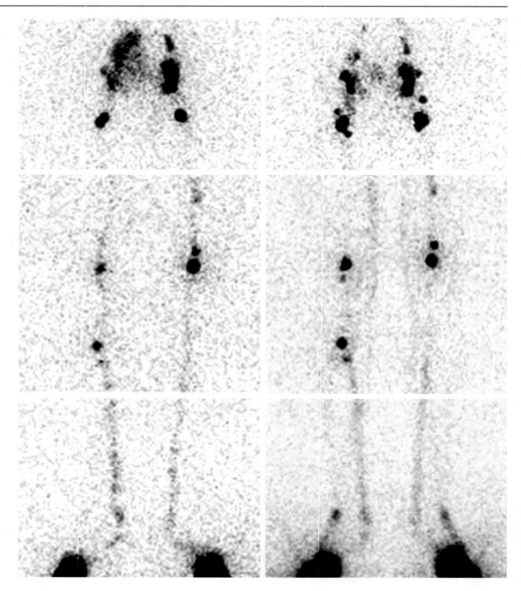

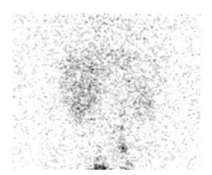

Fig. 5.52 Spot images of the abdomen, anterior view

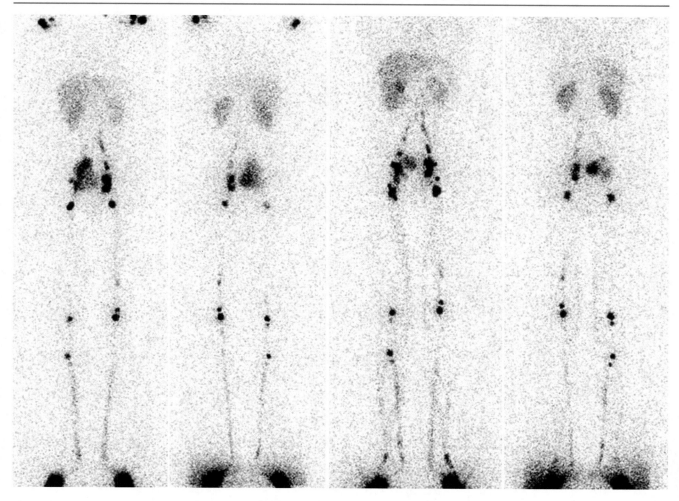

Fig. 5.53 Whole-body images (*left column*, anterior view; *right column*, posterior view) after radiocolloid injection for the assessment of DLC

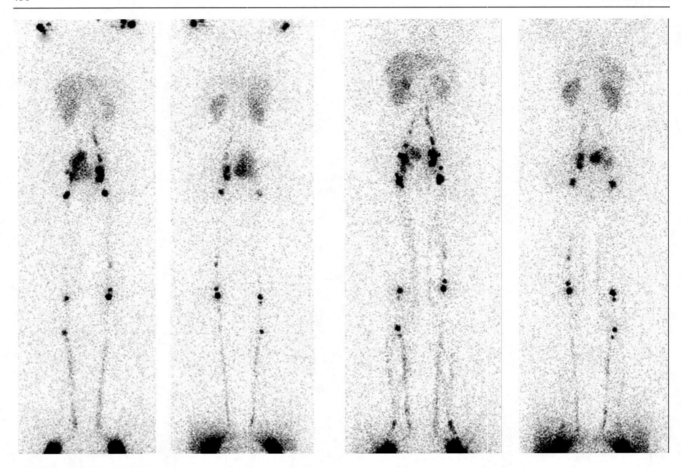

Fig. 5.54 With both DLC and SLC

Case 5.20: Lower Limb Bicompartmental Lymphoscintigraphy in Patient with Edema of the Scrotum

Paola Anna Erba and Luisa Locantore

Background Clinical Case

A 72-year-old man with edema of the scrotum but no edema of upper or lower extremities. Previous surgery for left inguinal hernia.

Anatomic location of edema: Scrotum.

Lymphoscintigraphy

For the deep lymphatic circulation (DLC): two aliquots of 99mTc-nanocolloid, 7 MBq each of injection in 0.1 mL into the first and second intermetatarsal spaces, identified by palpating the soles of both feet immediately proximal to the distal heads of the metatarsal bones on each side, inserting the needle by about 12–13 mm to reach the intermetatarsal muscles below the deep fascia plantaris.

For the superficial lymphatic circulation (SLC): three aliquots of about 10 MBq in 0.1 mL on the dorsum of each foot, inserting the needle subdermally in sites corresponding approximately to the prior palmar injections, about 1–2 cm proximally to the interdigital web. Spot and whole-body images were obtained from the distal feet up to the abdomen.

Spot images: 180 s/view, matrix 128 × 128, zoom 1.33

Whole-body images: matrix 256 × 1024, zoom 1, speed: 12 cm/min

After injections for assessment of the SLC, a normal right lymph flow was depicted, with only mild delay in the medial and distal part of the leg. Conversely, at the left limb, multiple collateral vessels are evident with lymph collection at the proximal left leg; preservation of the main lymphatic vessel is present. New images of the lymph nodes appear at the inguinal region. The lymph collection at the left scrotum persists, without increasing significantly the uptake of the radiocolloid. Progression through the lumbo-aortic lymph nodes is present, as well as faint liver uptake of the radiocolloids.

The exam demonstrated the lymphatic origin of the edema of the scrotum, which is alimented by both the deep and the superficial lymphatic circulation and is evident after injection at the intermetatarsal space. Therefore, the same technique of injection was used for the subsequent injection of the blue dye during surgery performed to detect the site of lymphatic leakage. After the injection, which was performed after the preparation of the main operative field, a passive movement of the patient's leg was performed to allow the blue dye to reach the site of leak. As soon as the operative field became blue, indicating blue dye extravasation, the surgeon searched for the site of leakage, and then performed the suture.

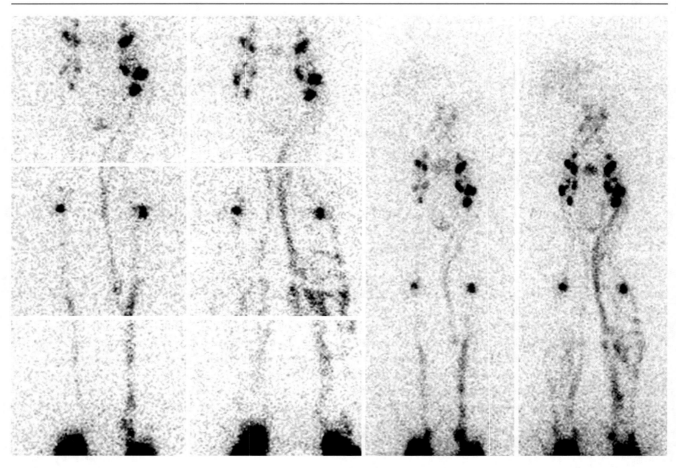

Figs. 5.55 and 5.56 Lymphoscintigraphy, spot images (Fig. 5.55), and whole-body images (Fig. 5.56) of the lower limbs (*left column*, DLC; *right column* DLC and SLC). Normal deep lymphatic circulation of the right lower limbs with a relatively slow right distal flow; normal popliteal and inguinal nodes are detected, with only faint visualization of the inferior right inguinal lymph nodes. At the left lower limb, con- comitant DLC and SLC are visible, both delayed as compared to the right DLC and SLC. In addition, radiocolloid accumulation is also clearly depicted, localized medially at the left proximal thigh, which is consistent with the edema of the scrotum. Normal popliteal and ingui- nal nodes are detected also on the left side

Case 5.21: Lower Limb Monocompartmental Lymphoscintigraphy in Patient with Postsurgical Chylopericardium (Ductus Arteriosus), Treated with Thoracentesis

Paola Anna Erba and Luisa Locantore

Background Clinical Case

Girl, aged 1 year, with postsurgical chylopericardium (ductus arteriosus), treated with thoracentesis.

Anatomic location of edema: Pericardium.

Lymphoscintigraphy
Lower Limbs

For the superficial lymphatic circulation (SLC): three aliquots of about 10 MBq in 0.1 mL on the dorsum of each foot, inserting the needle subdermally, about 1–2 cm proximally to the interdigital web. Spot and whole-body images were obtained from the distal feet up to the abdomen.

Spot images: 180 s/view, matrix 128 × 128, zoom 1.33

Whole-body images: matrix 256 × 1024, zoom 1, speed: 12 cm/min

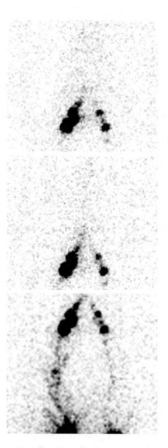

Fig. 5.57 Early spot lymphoscintigraphic acquisitions (SLC) of the lower limbs from the distal feet to the liver, acquired immediately after subdermal radiocolloid administration. A normal lymphatic drainage pattern is present at the left side. At the right side, there are indirect signs of overloaded drainage with delayed radiocolloid migration along dilated lymphatic vessels and delayed appearance of dermal backflow at the leg. Popliteal and inguinal lymph nodes are detected (mainly at right side). At this time, no radiocolloid accumulation is detectable in the thorax

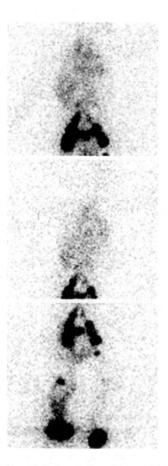

Fig. 5.58 Delayed spot lymphoscintigraphic acquisitions (SLC) of the lower limbs from the distal feet to the liver acquired 2 h after radiocolloid injection. A clear pattern of dermal backflow at the leg is observed, with persisting uptake in lymph nodes. Physiological visualization of the liver. In these images, faint radiocolloid accumulation can be detected in the thorax, localized in the mediastinal space and cardiac region, demonstrating the persistence of chylopericardium. A sample of pleuropericardial fluid was withdrawn from a mediastinal catheter; gamma counting of this sample confirmed radiocolloid localization, further confirming the lymphatic origin of the effusion

References

1. Mortimer PS. Managing lymphedema. Clin Dermatol. 1995;13:499–505.
2. Ely JW, Osheroff JA, Chambliss ML, et al. Approach to leg edema of unclear etiology. J Am Board Fam Med. 2006;19:148–60.
3. Tiwari A, Cheng KS, Button M, et al. Differential diagnosis, investigation, and current treatment of lower limb lymphedema. Arch Surg. 2003;138:152–61.
4. Nakazono T, Kudo S, Matsuo Y, et al. Angiosarcoma associated with chronic lymphedema (Stewart-Treves syndrome) of the leg: MR imaging. Skelet Radiol. 2000;29:413–6.
5. Executive Committee. The diagnosis and treatment of peripheral lymphedema: 2016 consensus document of the International Society of Lymphology. Lymphology. 2016;49:170–84.
6. Gasbarro V, Michelini S, Antignani PL, et al. The CEAP-L classification for lymphedemas of the limbs: the Italian experience. Int Angiol. 2009;28:315–24.
7. Mortimer PS. Swollen lower limb-2: lymphoedema. BMJ. 2000;320:1527–9.
8. Stemmer R. A clinical symptom for the early and differential diagnosis of lymphedema. Vasa. 1976;5:261–2.
9. Fries R. Differential diagnosis of leg edema. MMW Fortschr Med. 2004;146:39–41.
10. Brorson H, Ohlin K, Olsson G, et al. Adipose tissue dominates chronic arm lymphedema following breast cancer: an analysis using volume rendered CT images. Lymphat Res Biol. 2006;4:199–210.
11. Ghanta S, Cuzzone DA, Torrisi JS, et al. Regulation of inflammation and fibrosis by macrophages in lymphedema. Am J Physiol Heart Circ Physiol. 2015;308:H1065–77.
12. Ly CL, Kataru RP, Mehrara BJ. Inflammatory manifestations of lymphedema. Int J Mol Sci. 2017;18.
13. Savetsky IL, Torrisi JS, Cuzzone DA, et al. Obesity increases inflammation and impairs lymphatic function in a mouse model of lymphedema. Am J Physiol Heart Circ Physiol. 2014;307:H165–72.
14. Weitman ES, Aschen SZ, Farias-Eisner G, et al. Obesity impairs lymphatic fluid transport and dendritic cell migration to lymph nodes. PLoS One. 2013;8:e70703.
15. Greene AK, Grant FD, Slavin SA. Lower-extremity lymphedema and elevated body-mass index. N Engl J Med. 2012;366:2136–7.
16. Goss JA, Greene AK. Sensitivity and specificity of the Stemmer sign for lymphedema: a clinical lymphoscintigraphic study. Plast Reconstr Surg Glob Open. 2019;7:e2295. https://doi.org/10.1097/GOX.0000000000002295.
17. Kaulesar Sukul DM, den Hoed PT, Johannes EJ, et al. Direct and indirect methods for the quantification of leg volume: comparison between water displacement volumetry, the disk model method and the frustum sign model method, using the correlation coefficient and the limits of agreement. J Biomed Eng. 1993;15:477–80.
18. Mikes DM, Cha BA, Dym CL, et al. Bioelectrical impedance analysis revisited. Lymphology. 1999;32:157–65.
19. Cornish BH, Bunce IH, Ward LC, et al. Bioelectrical impedance for monitoring the efficacy of lymphoedema treatment programmes. Breast Cancer Res Treat. 1996;38:169–76.
20. Cornish BH, Chapman M, Thomas BJ, et al. Early diagnosis of lymphedema in postsurgery breast cancer patients. Ann N Y Acad Sci. 2000;904:571–5.
21. Cha K, Chertow GM, Gonzalez J, et al. Multifrequency bioelectrical impedance estimates the distribution of body water. J Appl Physiol (1985). 1995;79:1316–9.
22. Cavezzi A, Schingale F, Elio C. Limb volume measurement: from the past methods to optoelectronic technologies, bioimpedance analysis and laser based devices. Int Angiol. 2010;29:392–4.

23. Mayrovitz HN, Sims N, Macdonald J. Assessment of limb volume by manual and automated methods in patients with limb edema or lymphedema. Adv Skin Wound Care. 2000;13:272–6.
24. Mellor RH, Bush NL, Stanton AW, et al. Dual-frequency ultrasound examination of skin and subcutis thickness in breast cancer-related lymphedema. Breast J. 2004;10:496–503.
25. Gniadecka M. Localization of dermal edema in lipodermatosclerosis, lymphedema, and cardiac insufficiency. High-frequency ultrasound examination of intradermal echogenicity. J Am Acad Dermatol. 1996;35:37–41.
26. Hu D, Phan TT, Cherry GW, et al. Dermal oedema assessed by high frequency ultrasound in venous leg ulcers. Br J Dermatol. 1998;138:815–20.
27. Naouri M, Samimi M, Atlan M, et al. High-resolution cutaneous ultrasonography to differentiate lipoedema from lymphoedema. Br J Dermatol. 2010;163:296–301.
28. Cambria RA, Gloviczki P, Naessens JM, et al. Noninvasive evaluation of the lymphatic system with lymphoscintigraphy: a prospective, semiquantitative analysis in 386 extremities. J Vasc Surg. 1993;18:773–82.
29. Hreshchyshn MM, Sheehan FR. Lymphangiography in advanced gynecologic cancer. Obstet Gynecol. 1964;24:525–9.
30. Guermazi A, Brice P, Hennequin C, et al. Lymphography: an old technique retains its usefulness. Radiographics. 2003;23:1541–58; discussion 59–60.
31. Jackson RJ. Complications of lymphography. Br Med J. 1966;1:1203–5.
32. Weil GJ, Ramzy RM. Diagnostic tools for filariasis elimination programs. Trends Parasitol. 2007;23:78–82.
33. Rockson SG, Miller LT, Senie R, et al. American Cancer Society Lymphedema Workshop. Workgroup III: diagnosis and management of lymphedema. Cancer. 1998;83:2882–5.
34. Vignes S, Trévidic P. Role of surgery in the treatment of lymphedema. Rev Med Interne. 2002;23 Suppl 3:426s–30s.
35. Andréjak M, Gersberg M, Sgro C, et al. French pharmacovigilance survey evaluating the hepatic toxicity of coumarin. Pharmacoepidemiol Drug Saf. 1998;7:S45–50.
36. Campisi C. Lymphoedema: modern diagnostic and therapeutic aspects. Int Angiol. 1999;18:14–24.
37. Hwang JH, Choi JY, Lee JY, et al. Lymphoscintigraphy predicts response to complex physical therapy in patients with early stage extremity lymphedema. Lymphology. 2007;40:172–6.
38. Lee BB, Laredo J, Neville R. Current status of lymphatic reconstructive surgery for chronic lymphedema: it is still an uphill battle! Int J Angiol. 2011;20:73–80.
39. Lee BB, Laredo J, Neville R. Reconstructive surgery for chronic lymphedema: a viable option, but. Vascular. 2011;19:195–205.
40. Pecking AP, Albérini JL, Wartski M, et al. Relationship between lymphoscintigraphy and clinical findings in lower limb lymphedema (LO): toward a comprehensive staging. Lymphology. 2008;41:1–10.
41. Watt H, Singh-Grewal D, Wargon O, et al. Paediatric lymphoedema: a retrospective chart review of 86 cases. J Paediatr Child Health. 2017;53:38–42.
42. Ter SE, Alavi A, Kim CK, et al. Lymphoscintigraphy. A reliable test for the diagnosis of lymphedema. Clin Nucl Med. 1993;18:646–54.
43. Williams WH, Witte CL, Witte MH, et al. Radionuclide lymphangioscintigraphy in the evaluation of peripheral lymphedema. Clin Nucl Med. 2000;25:451–64.
44. Weissleder H, Weissleder R. Lymphedema: evaluation of qualitative and quantitative lymphoscintigraphy in 238 patients. Radiology. 1988;167:729–35.
45. Kandeel AA, Ahmed Younes J, Mohamed ZA. Significance of popliteal lymph nodes visualization during radionuclide lymphoscintigraphy for lower limb lymphedema. Indian J Nucl Med. 2013;28:134–7.

46. Karaçavuş S, Yılmaz YK, Ekim H. Clinical significance of lymphoscintigraphy findings in the evaluation of lower extremity lymphedema. Mol Imaging Radionucl Ther. 2015;24:80–4.

47. Maclellan RA, Zurakowski D, Voss S, et al. Correlation between lymphedema disease severity and lymphoscintigraphic findings: a clinical-radiologic study. J Am Coll Surg. 2017;225:366–70.

48. Hassanein AH, Maclellan RA, Grant FD, et al. Diagnostic accuracy of Lymphoscintigraphy for lymphedema and analysis of false-negative tests. Plast Reconstr Surg Glob Open. 2017;5:e1396.

49. Forner-Cordero I, Oliván-Sasot P, Ruiz-Llorca C, et al. Lymphoscintigraphic findings in patients with lipedema. Rev Esp Med Nucl Imagen Mol. 2018;37:341–8.

50. Gould DJ, El-Sabawi B, Goel P, et al. Uncovering lymphatic transport abnormalities in patients with primary lipedema. J Reconstr Microsurg. 2020;36:136–41.

51. Frühling JG, Bourgeois P. Axillary lymphoscintigraphy: current status in the treatment of breast cancer. Crit Rev Oncol Hematol. 1983;1:1–20.

52. Das IJ, Cheville AL, Scheuermann J, et al. Use of lymphoscintigraphy in radiation treatment of primary breast cancer in the context of lymphedema risk reduction. Radiother Oncol. 2011;100:293–8.

53. Yoo JN, Cheong YS, Min YS, et al. Validity of quantitative lymphoscintigraphy as a lymphedema assessment tool for patients with breast cancer. Ann Rehabil Med. 2015;39:931–40.

54. Szuba A, Chacaj A, Koba-Wszedybyl M, et al. Upper extremity lymphedema after axillary lymph node dissection: prospective lymphoscintigraphic evaluation. Lymphology. 2016;49:44–56.

55. de Oliveira MM, Sarian LO, Gurgel MS, et al. Lymphatic function in the early postoperative period of breast cancer has no short-term clinical impact. Lymphat Res Biol. 2016;14:220–5.

56. Cintolesi V, Stanton AW, Bains SK, et al. Constitutively enhanced lymphatic pumping in the upper limbs of women who later develop breast cancer-related lymphedema. Lymphat Res Biol. 2016;14:50–61.

57. Kim P, Lee JK, Lim OK, et al. Quantitative lymphoscintigraphy to predict the possibility of lymphedema development after breast cancer surgery: retrospective clinical study. Ann Rehabil Med. 2017;41:1065–75.

58. Yoo J, Choi JY, Hwang JH, et al. Prognostic value of lymphoscintigraphy in patients with gynecological cancer-related lymphedema. J Surg Oncol. 2014;109:760–3.

59. Boccardo F, De Cian F, Campisi CC, et al. Surgical prevention and treatment of lymphedema after lymph node dissection in patients with cutaneous melanoma. Lymphology. 2013;46:20–6.

60. Feldman S, Bansil H, Ascherman J, et al. Single institution experience with lymphatic microsurgical preventive healing approach (LYMPHA) for the primary prevention of lymphedema. Ann Surg Oncol. 2015;22:3296–301.

61. Boccardo F, Casabona F, De Cian F, et al. Lymphatic microsurgical preventing healing approach (LYMPHA) for primary surgical prevention of breast cancer-related lymphedema: over 4 years follow-up. Microsurgery. 2014;34:421–4.

62. Roman MM, Barbieux R, Nogaret JM, et al. Use of lymphoscintigraphy to differentiate primary versus secondary lower extremity lymphedema after surgical lymphadenectomy: a retrospective analysis. World J Surg Oncol. 2018;16:75. https://doi.org/10.1186/s12957-018-1379-5.

63. Notohamiprodjo M, Weiss M, Baumeister RG, et al. MR lymphangiography at 3.0 T: correlation with lymphoscintigraphy. Radiology. 2012;264:78–87.

64. Proby CM, Gane JN, Joseph AE, et al. Investigation of the swollen limb with isotope lymphography. Br J Dermatol. 1990;123:29–37.

65. Hwang JH, Kwon JY, Lee KW, et al. Changes in lymphatic function after complex physical therapy for lymphedema. Lymphology. 1999;32:15–21.

66. Kim DI, Huh S, Hwang JH, et al. Venous dynamics in leg lymphedema. Lymphology. 1999;32:11–4.

67. Kafejian-Haddad AP, Perez JM, Castiglioni ML, et al. Lymphoscintigraphic evaluation of manual lymphatic drainage for lower extremity lymphedema. Lymphology. 2006;39:41–8.

68. Chang L, Cheng MF, Chang HH, et al. The role of lymphoscintigraphy in diagnosis and monitor the response of physiotherapeutic technique in congenital lymphedema. Clin Nucl Med. 2011;36:e11–2.

69. Partsch H, Stöberl C, Wruhs M, et al. Indirect lymphography with iotrolan. Fortschr Geb Rontgenstrahlen Nuklearmed Erganzungsbd. 1989;128:178–81.

70. Baulieu F, Baulieu JL, Vaillant L, et al. Factorial analysis in radionuclide lymphography: assessment of the effects of sequential pneumatic compression. Lymphology. 1989;22:178–85.

71. Olszewski WL, Cwikla J, Zaleska M, et al. Pathways of lymph and tissue fluid flow during intermittent pneumatic massage of lower limbs with obstructive lymphedema. Lymphology. 2011;44:54–64.

72. Liu NF, Olszewski W. The influence of local hyperthermia on lymphedema and lymphedematous skin of the human leg. Lymphology. 1993;26:28–37.

73. Pecking AP, Février B, Wargon C, et al. Efficacy of Daflon 500 mg in the treatment of lymphedema (secondary to conventional therapy of breast cancer). Angiology. 1997;48:93–8.

74. Moore TA, Reynolds JC, Kenney RT, et al. Diethylcarbamazine-induced reversal of early lymphatic dysfunction in a patient with bancroftian filariasis: assessment with use of lymphoscintigraphy. Clin Infect Dis. 1996;23:1007–11.

75. Szuba A, Cooke JP, Yousuf S, et al. Decongestive lymphatic therapy for patients with cancer-related or primary lymphedema. Am J Med. 2000;109:296–300.

76. Ho LC, Lai MF, Yeates M, et al. Microlymphatic bypass in obstructive lymphoedema. Br J Plast Surg. 1988;41:475–84.

77. Campisi C, Davini D, Bellini C, et al. Lymphatic microsurgery for the treatment of lymphedema. Microsurgery. 2006;26:65–9.

78. Gloviczki P, Fisher J, Hollier LH, et al. Microsurgical lymphovenous anastomosis for treatment of lymphedema: a critical review. J Vasc Surg. 1988;7:647–52.

79. François A, Richaud C, Bouchet JY, et al. Does medical treatment of lymphedema act by increasing lymph flow? Vasa. 1989;18:281–6.

80. Ciudad P, Manrique OJ, Adabi K, et al. Combined double vascularized lymph node transfers and modified radical reduction with preservation of perforators for advanced stages of lymphedema. J Surg Oncol. 2019;119:439–48.

81. Gironet N, Baulieu F, Giraudeau B, et al. Lymphedema of the limb: predictors of efficacy of combined physical therapy. Ann Dermatol Venereol. 2004;131:775–9.

82. Slavin SA, Upton J, Kaplan WD, et al. An investigation of lymphatic function following free-tissue transfer. Plast Reconstr Surg. 1997;99:730–41; discussion 42–3.

83. Seo KS, Suh M, Hong S, et al. The new possibility of lymphoscintigraphy to guide a clinical treatment for lymphedema in patient with breast cancer. Clin Nucl Med. 2019;44:179–85.

84. Weiss M, Baumeister RG, Hahn K. Planning and monitoring of autologous lymph vessel transplantation by means of nuclear medicine lymphoscintigraphy. Handchir Mikrochir Plast Chir. 2003;35:210–5.

85. Mikami T, Hosono M, Yabuki Y, et al. Classification of lymphoscintigraphy and relevance to surgical indication for lymphaticovenous anastomosis in upper limb lymphedema. Lymphology. 2011;44:155–67.

86. Burnand KM, Glass DM, Mortimer PS, et al. Lymphatic dysfunction in the apparently clinically normal contralateral limbs of patients with unilateral lower limb swelling. Clin Nucl Med. 2012;37:9–13.

87. Bourgeois P, Frühling J, Henry J. Postoperative axillary lympho-scintigraphy in the management of breast cancer. Int J Radiat Oncol Biol Phys. 1983;9:29–32.

88. Hara H, Mihara M. Postoperative changes in lymphoscintigraphic findings after lymphaticovenous anastomosis. Ann Plast Surg. 2019;83:548–52.

89. Weiss M, Baumeister RG, Frick A, et al. Lymphedema of the upper limb: evaluation of the functional outcome by dynamic imaging of lymph kinetics after autologous lymph vessel transplantation. Clin Nucl Med. 2015;40:e117–23.

90. Baumeister RG, Mayo W, Notohamiprodjo M, et al. Microsurgical lymphatic vessel transplantation. J Reconstr Microsurg. 2016;32: 34–41.

91. Ciudad P, Agko M, Perez Coca JJ, et al. Comparison of long-term clinical outcomes among different vascularized lymph node trans-fers: 6-year experience of a single center's approach to the treat-ment of lymphedema. J Surg Oncol. 2017;116:671–82.

92. Zhang W, Wu P, Li F, et al. Potential applications of using ^{68}Ga-Evans blue PET/CT in the evaluation of lymphatic disorder: preliminary observations. Clin Nucl Med. 2016;41:302–8.

93. Aström KG, Abdsaleh S, Brenning GC, et al. MR imaging of pri-mary, secondary, and mixed forms of lymphedema. Acta Radiol. 2001;42:409–16.

94. Hadjis NS, Carr DH, Banks L, et al. The role of CT in the diagnosis of primary lymphedema of the lower limb. AJR Am J Roentgenol. 1985;144:361–4.

95. Monnin-Delhom ED, Gallix BP, Achard C, et al. High resolution unenhanced computed tomography in patients with swollen legs. Lymphology. 2002;35:121–8.

96. Lohrmann C, Földi E, Bartholomä JP, et al. MR imaging of the lymphatic system: distribution and contrast enhancement of gado-diamide after intradermal injection. Lymphology. 2006;39:156–63.

97. Suga K, Yuan Y, Okada M, et al. Breast sentinel lymph node map-ping at CT lymphography with iopamidol: preliminary experi-ence. Radiology. 2004;230:543–52.

98. Yamada K, Shinaoka A, Kimata Y. Three-dimensional imaging of lymphatic system in lymphedema legs using interstitial computed tomography-lymphography. Acta Med Okayama. 2017;71:171–7.

99. Lohrmann C, Foeldi E, Speck O, et al. High-resolution MR lym-phangiography in patients with primary and secondary lymph-edema. AJR Am J Roentgenol. 2006;187:556–61.

100. Lohrmann C, Kautz O, Speck O, et al. Chronic lymphedema: detected with high-resolution magnetic resonance lymphangiog-raphy. J Comput Assist Tomogr. 2006;30:688.

101. Lohrmann C, Foeldi E, Langer M. MR imaging of the lym-phatic system in patients with lipedema and lipo-lymphedema. Microvasc Res. 2009;77:335–9.

102. Liu NF, Lu Q, Jiang ZH, et al. Anatomic and functional evalua-tion of the lymphatics and lymph nodes in diagnosis of lymphatic circulation disorders with contrast magnetic resonance lymphan-giography. J Vasc Surg. 2009;49:980–7.

103. Bull RH, Gane JN, Evans JE, et al. Abnormal lymph drainage in patients with chronic venous leg ulcers. J Am Acad Dermatol. 1993;28:585–90.

104. Bae JS, Yoo RE, Choi SH, et al. Evaluation of lymphedema in upper extremities by MR lymphangiography: comparison with lymphoscintigraphy. Magn Reson Imaging. 2018;49:63–70.

105. White RD, Weir-McCall JR, Budak MJ, et al. Contrast-enhanced magnetic resonance lymphography in the assessment of lower limb lymphoedema. Clin Radiol. 2014;69:e435–44.

106. Kiang SC, Ahmed KA, Barnes S, et al. Direct contrast-enhanced magnetic resonance lymphangiography in the diagnosis of persis-tent occult chylous effusion leak after thoracic duct embolization. J Vasc Surg Venous Lymphat Disord. 2019;7:251–7.

107. Long X, Zhang J, Zhang D, et al. Microsurgery guided by sequen-tial preoperative lymphography using ^{68}Ga-NEB PET and MRI in patients with lower-limb lymphedema. Eur J Nucl Med Mol Imaging. 2017;44:1501–10.

108. Hou G, Hou B, Jiang Y, et al. ^{68}Ga-NOTA-Evans Blue TOF PET/MR lymphoscintigraphy evaluation of the severity of lower limb lymphedema. Clin Nucl Med. 2019;44:439–45.

109. Giacalone G, Yamamoto T, Belva F, et al. The application of vir-tual reality for preoperative planning of lymphovenous anastomo-sis in a patient with a complex lymphatic malformation. J Clin Med. 2019;8.

The Sentinel Lymph Node Concept

6

Omgo E. Nieweg

Contents

6.1 **History** 143

6.2 **Concept** 145

6.3 **Definition of a SLN** 145

6.4 **Other Definitions** 145

6.5 **Concluding Remarks** 148

References 148

Learning Objectives
- To become familiar with how lymphatic mapping evolved into current practice
- To comprehend the physiologic principle on which lymphatic mapping is based
- To become familiar with the concept of lymphatic mapping
- To appreciate the technical challenges of the sentinel lymph node biopsy (SLNB)
- To learn and understand the definition of a sentinel lymph node (SLN)
- To realize that there is no consensus on the definition of a SLN
- To beware of other definitions

- To appreciate why some alternative definitions are associated with an increased risk of false-negative SLNB
- To understand how some definitions are associated with unnecessary removal of innocent lymph nodes

6.1 History

For many years, regional lymph node dissection was a routine component of the surgical treatment of various solid cancers, even if the nodes appeared clinically normal. Common examples include head and neck cancer, breast cancer, melanoma, and tumors of the gastrointestinal tract. This practice was rooted in the observations by the German pathologist Rudolf L. K. Virchow (1821–1902) that lymph nodes filter particulate matter from lymph fluid and that cancer metastasizes via lymph ducts to such nodes [1]. These fundamental findings inspired the American surgeon William S. Halsted to develop the mastectomy with *en bloc* axillary lymph node dissection for breast cancer at the end of the nineteenth century [2]. Halsted's concept was based on the notion that cancer generally metastasizes first to regional lymph nodes. These nodes act as filters that temporarily prevent further spread of cancer cells. This barrier

O. E. Nieweg (✉)
Department of Surgery, Melanoma Institute of Australia, Sydney, NSW, Australia

Faculty of Medicine and Health, The University of Sydney, Sydney, NSW, Australia

Department of Melanoma and Surgical Oncology, Royal Prince Alfred Hospital, Sydney, NSW, Australia
e-mail: omgo.nieweg@melanoma.org.au

© Springer Nature Switzerland AG 2020
G. Mariani et al. (eds.), *Atlas of Lymphoscintigraphy and Sentinel Node Mapping*,
https://doi.org/10.1007/978-3-030-45296-4_6

creates a window of opportunity for radical local-regional surgery to cure the patient.

These general concepts eventually led to the current concept of SLNB. The term "sentinel" lymph node was first mentioned in 1923 by the British surgeon Braithwaite, who studied lymph drainage. He dripped a blue dye onto the omentum and removed the lymph node to which the blue-stained lymphatic drained and called this the "gland sentinel" [3]. In 1960, Gould et al. used the term SLN to describe a lymph node at the junction of the anterior and posterior facial veins [4]. In a study of parotid cancer, they found that this node was the first one to be involved when a parotid tumor spread, and they designated this node the SLN [1]. A radical lymph node neck dissection was performed if frozen section examination revealed metastatic disease in this node.

In the 1980s, work of Dr. Bernard Fisher and others appeared to refute Halsted's postulation [5, 6]. They advocated that cancer does not spread in an orderly fashion. The Fisher hypothesis indicates rather that lymph nodes and distant sites tend to become involved simultaneously and that lymph nodes are ineffective as barriers to further dissemination. As a result, lymph node metastasis was presumed to indicate that the disease had spread to various sites and that curative surgery was no longer an option.

Against the common opinion at that time, some surgeons held on to the Halstedian view. A few developed his concept further in attempts to avoid the—in hindsight—often unnecessary, elective regional lymph node dissections that were routinely performed for various cancer types. The purpose was to identify and remove the lymph nodes that were the first to be involved, so that regional node dissection could be reserved for patients who really had metastases. This way, patients without lymph node metastases could be spared a full dissection. One of these surgeons was Ramon Cabañas from Paraguay, who had a special interest in penile cancer, a common tumor in his country. Squamous cell carcinoma of the penis tends to metastasize to lymph nodes but not to distant sites until at a late stage. In 1977, Cabañas found that penile cancer initially drains to a particular lymph node that is always at the same location in the groin and termed this node the SLN [7]. So, the node was defined by its constant anatomic position, which appears plausible for penile cancer, because the primary cancer is always situated in the exact same location, on the glans. However, the hypothesis that lymph drainage rigorously follows a pattern to a lymph node that is always in the exact same location did not hold. False-negative procedures occurred and urologists found that results with biopsy of this SLN were not reliable enough to make the technique routine clinical practice [8, 9].

In the late 1980s, the surgeon Donald L. Morton at the John Wayne Cancer Center in Santa Monica and his pathologist Alistair J. Cochran from the University of California,

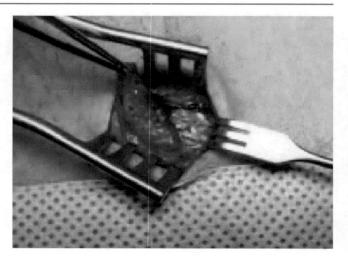

Fig. 6.1 Blue afferent lymph channel with SLN

Los Angeles, took the SLN procedure a major step forward when they proposed the innovative concept of "lymphatic mapping with SLNB" for melanoma [10]. They suggested that a melanoma could drain to any lymph node in a particular lymph node field or even outside a nodal field, depending on the location of the primary lesion and with a certain individual variability. They developed a technique to identify and remove this lymph node after administration of patent blue dye at the tumor site. The dye is taken up by the lymphatic system. Delicate dissection of the afferent blue lymph duct guided Morton to the SLN (Fig. 6.1). Subsequently, lymphoscintigraphy was added to reliably identify the field to which the tumor drained and to indicate the number of SLNs actually present. The radiopharmaceutical enabled an alternative technique to retrieve the SLN. Intraoperatively, the radioactivity was gauged with a gamma ray detection probe and guided the surgeon to it. The pathologist obtained multiple sections from the lymph node and used sensitive immunohistochemistry staining techniques to detect even minute deposits of malignant cells.

It has been demonstrated that the hypothesis of Morton and Cochran is correct and that lymphatic dissemination generally occurs in a sequential fashion [11, 12]. The SLN is indeed the first node to be involved and its tumor status reflects the status of the entire lymph node field.

Key Learning Points
- Lymphatic mapping is based on the Halstedian principle, which entails that cancer generally metastasizes first to regional lymph nodes. In the absence of metastases elsewhere, removal of affected lymph nodes cures the patient.
- Modern-day SLNB is based on the physiology of lymphatic drainage.

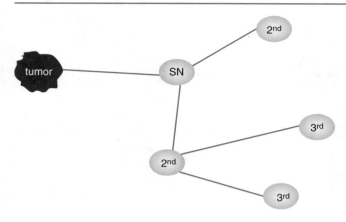

Fig. 6.2 The concept of lymphatic mapping is based on the notion that lymph fluid from a primary cancer drains to a particular regional lymph node. *SN* SLN, *2nd* second-tier lymph node, *3rd* third-tier lymph node

6.2 Concept

Cancer cells that are shed from the primary tumor enter the lymphatic system with the excess of interstitial fluid. The fluid in the lymph vessels passes through a number of lymph nodes on the way to the upper chest, where the fluid is returned to the bloodstream. Lymph nodes act as filters that temporarily prevent further spread of cancer cells. As lymph node metastases commonly precede blood-borne metastases, this barrier creates a window of opportunity for radical local-regional surgery to cure the patient. In order to fully utilize this opportunity, lymph node involvement must be detected at the earliest possible stage.

The concept of lymphatic mapping is based on the notion that lymph fluid from a primary cancer drains through an afferent lymph vessel to at least one particular regional lymph node (Fig. 6.2). This is the SLN, also known as first-tier node or first-echelon node. From this lymph node, lymph fluid passes through efferent lymph vessels to other lymph nodes in the nodal field. When tumor cells spread, they will first lodge in the SLN. So, this is the node at greatest risk of harboring tumor cells. Other nodes downstream may subsequently become involved in a stepwise fashion.

Lymphatic mapping identifies and removes this SLN, and determines whether it contains metastatic disease. Knowledge of the tumor status of the lymph nodes facilitates informed decisions on completion of regional lymph node dissection to remove other potentially involved lymph nodes and on adjuvant systemic therapy.

> **Key Learning Points**
> - Many cancers spread in a stepwise fashion through the lymphatic system.
> - The SLN is the first lymph node to be involved with metastasis.

> - The purpose of SLNB is to detect lymph node metastases at an early stage.
> - SLNB is used to select patients who may benefit from completion lymph node dissection.
> - SLNB is used to select patients who may benefit from adjuvant systemic therapy.

6.3 Definition of a SLN

Morton et al. used the definition "a SLN is the initial lymph node upon which the primary tumor drains" [10]. The word "initial" was prone to misinterpretation. For instance, multiple lymph vessels may link the tumor to multiple nodes that may not necessarily light up simultaneously on the lymphoscintigrams, yet they all are directly at risk of receiving tumor cells. To avoid confusion, the definition was slightly modified to the following: "a SLN is any lymph node on the direct drainage pathway from the primary tumor." This definition reflects the physiology of lymphatic drainage and the stepwise dissemination of cancer through the lymphatic system. This is the definition most experts adhere to.

6.4 Other Definitions

Later, the definition of a SLN being any lymph node on the direct drainage pathway was challenged [13–17]. Some investigators have come up with their own definitions (see Table 6.1) [18–21]. This development is understandable, since specialists from different fields are involved and each is addressing the concept from their own background and perspective. Also, lymphoscintigrams may be difficult to interpret, as they tend to depict multiple lymph nodes and do not always clearly indicate the order of lymph drainage. Moreover, the surgical procedure can be challenging. SLNB requires a considerable ability to think in a three-dimensional fashion. The surgeon needs to translate the one-dimensional probe readings and the two-dimensional scintigrams into a three-dimensional image in his/her mind. Furthermore, when using the blue dye the stained lymphatic vessel that visually

Table 6.1 Less appropriate definitions of a SLN

Lymph node closest to the primary lesion
First lymph node depicted on the lymphoscintigrams
Lymph node with the highest count rate
Any radioactive lymph node
Lymph node with a count rate that is a certain factor higher than the background or compared to non-SLNs
Lymph node with a count rate that exceeds a certain fraction of the hottest node
Any blue-stained lymph node

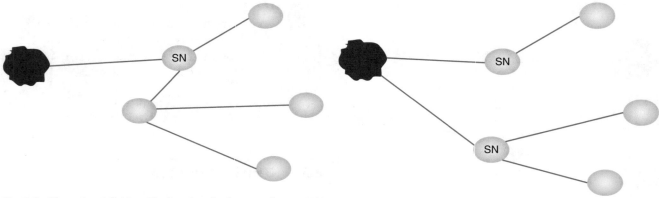

Fig. 6.3 Alternative definition. The lymph node closest to the cancer is not necessarily directly at risk of receiving tumor cells

Fig. 6.4 Two lymph vessels originating in the tumor draining upon separate lymph nodes

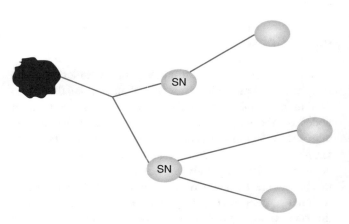

Fig. 6.5 Lymph duct dividing into two channels leading to separate lymph nodes

guides the surgeon to the SLN is very fragile. It requires considerable experience and finesse to dissect this delicate structure in a small, confined space, through a small incision, in a sometimes-deep lymph node field. For these reasons, some surgeons sought easier criteria to determine which lymph node(s) to remove in the situation that lymphoscintigraphy depicts multiple nodes.

Developing a more practical procedure using the definition that is based on the concept was problematic. Instead, the color of the node and its radioactivity were used as criteria. In the process, some investigators changed the definition. Some defined the SLN as the lymph node closest to the primary lesion [22]. Oftentimes, the node closest to the tumor is indeed (the) one into which the lymph vessel from the tumor drains, but this is not always the case (Fig. 6.3). So, this anatomy-based definition does not take into account the physiology of lymph drainage and the wrong lymph node could be removed.

Other investigators defined the SLN as the first lymph node that becomes visible on the lymphoscintigraphic images. It is inevitable that the first node that is depicted lies on a direct drainage pathway from the cancer and must be classified as SLN. However, this definition does not acknowledge the facts that more lymph nodes than a single one can be on a direct drainage pathway and that there may be reasons that prevent them from becoming visible simultaneously. For instance, there may be two lymph vessels originating in the tumor that drain upon different lymph nodes (Fig. 6.4). Sometimes, a single lymph duct divides into two channels going to separate lymph nodes (Fig. 6.5). Tumor cells may follow either route and both lymph nodes are at direct risk of being involved. Because the lymph flow speed may be quite different in the two channels, lymphoscintigraphy may visualize one lymph node before the other, but this does not imply that the other node need not be removed. All lymph nodes in direct drainage contact with the primary tumor are directly at risk of harboring tumor cells. All these first-tier lymph nodes should be harvested and

examined by the pathologist. Therefore, the definition of the SLN being the first node to be visualized is too narrow; too few nodes are designated as SLN and metastases may be left unnoticed.

When lymphoscintigraphy shows multiple lymph nodes, some people considered only the brightest on the scintigrams or the one that yields the highest probe reading as SLN [21]. This definition of the "hottest" lymph node being the SLN has several drawbacks. Again, lymph can drain directly to multiple lymph nodes and one can collect more of the radiopharmaceutical than another (Fig. 6.6). The size of the lymph node is one parameter that determines the amount of radioactivity that can be accumulated. Its location is also relevant; a superficial lymph node has a short distance to the gamma camera or the gamma ray detection probe. Such a lymph node yields more counts than a node that contains three times as much of the tracer but lies at twice the distance. Some of the radiopharmaceutical may pass through the first lymph node and move on to subsequent nodes. A large second-echelon lymph node—or one with more active macrophages—

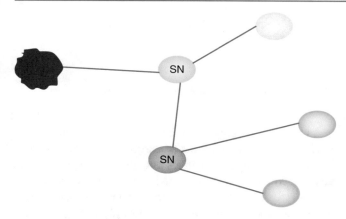

Fig. 6.6 Lymph fluid can drain directly to multiple lymph nodes and one may accumulate more of the radiopharmaceutical than another

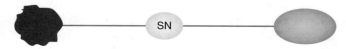

Fig. 6.7 A large second-echelon lymph node—or one with more active macrophages—may accumulate more of the radiopharmaceutical than a small first-echelon lymph node

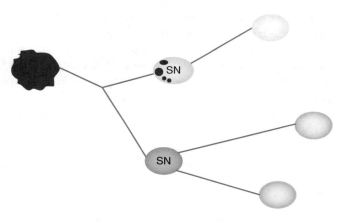

Fig. 6.8 Lymph flow to SLN hampered by metastatic disease

may accumulate more of the tracer than a small first-echelon lymph node (Fig. 6.7).

The amount of radiopharmaceutical that is accumulated by a lymph node depends on not only its position in the drainage order, but also the number of lymphatic channels that enter the node and parameters such as lymph flow speed. Another reason for a node to receive a sparse lymph supply is that the flow to that particular lymph node is hampered by metastatic disease obstructing its ingress (Fig. 6.8) [23]. So, there are a number of reasons not to classify a lymph node as a SLN based on its superior brightness on the scintigram or on the highest probe reading.

Certain surgeons relied on their gamma probe to find the SLN without preoperative imaging or use of a blue dye. They assumed that any radioactive node identified with the gamma ray detection probe is a SLN, and they defined a SLN as such. This point of view does not acknowledge the notion that some of the tracer fluid may pass through the first-tier lymph node and lodge in secondary nodes downstream that are not directly at risk of harboring metastatic disease. This definition is too liberal and too many lymph nodes may be removed as a result. One report indicated that up to 37 SLNs were to be removed from a single basin [24].

Another definition was based on the SLN-to-background count ratio. This definition also has shortcomings. Various factors determine the accumulation of the radiopharmaceutical in a lymph node, like type of tracer, size of the colloid particles if a radiocolloid is used and their surface features, size of the lymph node, metabolic activity of its macrophages, and lymph flow speed. The lymph flow speed fluctuates and depends on factors like physical exercise, time of day, medication, massaging of the injection site, and hydration state of the patient. As a result, radioactivity uptake in a lymph node to which the cancer drains is variable. In breast cancer patients, 95% of the SLNs are within an uptake range that varies from 0.001 to 2.5% of the injected radioactivity, and in melanoma patients this range is 0.06–3.6% [25]. Different surgeons used different sites for their background count reading to calculate the node-to-background ratio. Some surgeons obtained the background reading in the lymph node basin, and others used a location elsewhere in the body or even outside the body.

The SLN-to-non-SLN ratio was another parameter used to determine whether a lymph node is a SLN. This approach implies that one has to find a non-SLN first and then examine the other nodes with the probe to determine whether the designated count rate is reached. The node-to-hottest node ratio was yet another criterion. The approaches exploiting aspects of the radiopharmaceutical accumulation cannot be used in the 15–30% of the lymph nodes on a direct drainage pathway from a primary breast cancer that are not radioactive at all [26, 27]. One is left with the conclusion that the definition of a SLN cannot reliably be based on factors measurable with the gamma ray detection probe alone.

Some surgeons considered every lymph node that is stained blue to be a SLN. However, unlike the radioactive tracer, the blue dye is not retained by the macrophages in a lymph node. It just flows through and moves on to the next lymph node downstream. Rapidly, there will be a string of blue lymph nodes of which only the first one is directly at risk of containing tumor cells (Fig. 6.9).

In summary, all these alternative definitions may be correct most of the time, but they are not based on the physiol-

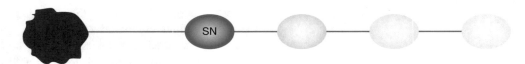

Fig. 6.9 Blue dye is not retained in the SLN. It flows through downstream and stains a string of subsequent-tier lymph nodes

ogy of lymph drainage, nor on the biology of the disease and they all have their flaws [16]. The SLN is not always the node closest to the tumor. The SLN is not just the node that is depicted first on the images, neither is it necessarily the most radioactive node, nor a radioactive node per se, nor is it always a node that is a certain number of times more radioactive or less radioactive than another node or compared to some other tissue. Not every SLN is blue, and not every blue node is a SLN.

In conclusion, the definition that a SLN is any lymph node that receives afferent lymphatic drainage directly from a primary tumor best reflects the route that the tumor cells travel and the concept of stepwise spread of cancer through the lymphatic system. However, this definition requires a meticulous technique of lymphoscintigraphy, a conscientious interpretation of the images, and a precise dissection of the afferent lymphatic ducts [28, 29]. In the occasional situation in which it is unclear whether a certain lymph node is a SLN or not, one should proceed and remove such a node.

> **Key Learning Points**
> - A SLN is best defined as any lymph node on the direct lymphatic drainage pathway from the primary tumor.
> - SLNB calls for detailed lymphoscintigraphy to visualize the afferent lymphatics that identify SLNs and requires specific surgical expertise.
> - A multitude of other definitions are used to simplify the procedure, but these are less accurate.

6.5   Concluding Remarks

Lymphatic mapping exploits the notion that cancer generally metastasizes first to lymph nodes and later on to distant sites. A lymph node that receives lymphatic drainage directly from the primary tumor is a SLN. SLNB was devised to identify the lymph nodes that are directly at risk and to assess whether these are involved in an early phase. A multitude of other definitions is used to simplify the procedure, but these are less accurate.

Lymphatic mapping requires a concerted effort from nuclear medicine physician, surgeon, and pathologist. Lymphoscintigraphy visualizes the afferent lymph vessel(s) and the lymph node(s) receiving lymph fluid from the lesion site and tells the surgeon where to look and how many nodes to expect. The surgeon visualizes the physiology of lymphatic drainage using a dye and exploits the radioactivity trapped in the node. The pathologist examines the node in detail.

The procedure provides prognostic information and enables more accurate staging, which guides further management. This improves the chance of survival in patients with nodal involvement from penile cancer or melanoma [30, 31]. The morbidity of the procedure is limited. Many patients with breast cancer or vulvar cancer are spared an unnecessary lymph node dissection and more patients are identified who may benefit from adjuvant systemic therapy. After description of its success in patients with these diseases, lymphatic mapping was quickly explored in other cancer types, as described in the subsequent chapters. One can conclude that lymphatic mapping with SLNB is one of the most interesting and important developments in clinical oncology in recent years and it fits in perfectly with the current trend for more individualized and conservative surgery in patients with cancer.

References

1. Tanis PJ, Nieweg OE, Valdés Olmos RA, et al. History of sentinel node and validation of the technique. Breast Cancer Res. 2001;3:109–12.
2. Halsted WS. The results of operations for the cure of cancer of the breast performed at the Johns Hopkins Hospital from June 1889 to January 1894. Johns Hopkins Hosp Bull. 1894;4:297–323.
3. Braithwaite LR. The flow of lymph from the ileocaecal angle, and its possible bearing on the cause of duodenal and gastric ulcer. Br J Surg. 1923;11:7–26.
4. Gould EA, Winship T, Philbin PH, et al. Observations on a 'sentinel node' in cancer of the parotid. Cancer. 1960;20:77–8.
5. Cancer Research Campaign Working Party. Cancer research campaign (King's/Cambridge) trial for early breast cancer. A detailed update at the tenth year. Lancet. 1980;ii:55–60.
6. Fisher B, Redmond C, Fisher ER, et al. Ten-year results of a randomized clinical trial comparing radical mastectomy and total mastectomy with or without radiation. N Engl J Med. 1985;312:674–81.
7. Cabañas RM. An approach for the treatment of penile cancer. Cancer. 1977;39:456–66.

8. Bouchot O, Bouvier S, Bochereau G, et al. Cancer of the penis: the value of systematic biopsy of the superficial inguinal lymph nodes in clinical N0 stage patients. Prog Urol. 1993;3:228–33.

9. Pettaway CA, Pisters LL, Dinney CPN, et al. Sentinel lymph node dissection for penile carcinoma: M.D. Anderson Cancer Center experience. J Urol. 1995;154:1999–2003.

10. Morton DL, Wen D-R, Wong JH, et al. Technical details of intra-operative lymphatic mapping for early stage melanoma. Arch Surg. 1992;127:392–9.

11. Reintgen D, Cruse CW, Wells K, et al. The orderly progression of melanoma nodal metastases. Ann Surg. 1994;220:759–67.

12. Kapteijn BA, Nieweg OE, Peterse JL, et al. Identification and biopsy of the sentinel lymph node in breast cancer. Eur J Surg Oncol. 1998;24:427–30.

13. Morton DL, Bostick PJ. Will the true sentinel node please stand? Ann Surg Oncol. 1999;6:12–4.

14. Balch CM, Ross MI. Sentinel lymphadenectomy for melanoma—is it a substitute for elective lymphadenectomy? Ann Surg Oncol. 1999;6:416–7.

15. Thompson JF, Uren RF. What is a 'sentinel' lymph node? Eur J Surg Oncol. 2000;26:103–4.

16. Nieweg OE, Tanis PJ, Kroon BBR. The definition of a sentinel node. Ann Surg Oncol. 2001;9:538–41.

17. Coit DG. The "true" sentinel lymph node: in search of an operational definition of a biological phenomenon. Ann Surg Oncol. 2001;8:187–9.

18. Veronesi U, Paganelli G, Galimberti V, et al. Sentinel-node biopsy to avoid axillary dissection in breast cancer with clinically negative lymph-nodes. Lancet. 1997;349:1864–7.

19. De Cicco C, Sideri M, Bartolomei M, et al. Sentinel node detection by lymphoscintigraphy and gamma detecting probe in patients with vulvar cancer. J Nucl Med. 1997;38:33p.

20. Gershenwald JE, Tseng CH, Thompson W, et al. Improved sentinel lymph node localization in patients with primary melanoma with the use of radiolabeled colloid. Surgery. 1998;124:203–10.

21. Boxen I, McCready D, Ballinger JR. Sentinel node detection and definition may depend on the imaging agent and timing. Clin Nucl Med. 1999;24:390–4.

22. Taylor AT, Murray D, Herda S, et al. Dynamic lymphoscintigraphy to identify the sentinel and satellite nodes. Clin Nucl Med. 1996;21:755–8.

23. Leijte JAP, Van der Ploeg IMC, Valdés Olmos RA, et al. Visualization of tumor-blockage and rerouting of lymphatic drainage in penile cancer patients using SPECT/CT. J Nucl Med. 2009;50:364–7.

24. Liu LC, Parrett BM, Jenkins T, et al. Selective sentinel lymph node dissection for melanoma: importance of harvesting nodes with lower radioactive counts without the need for blue dye. Ann Surg Oncol. 2011;18:2919–24.

25. Jansen L. Sentinel node biopsy: evolving from melanoma to breast cancer. Thesis, University of Amsterdam; 2000.

26. Cox CE, Pendas S, Cox JM, et al. Guidelines for sentinel node biopsy and lymphatic mapping of patients with breast cancer. Ann Surg. 1998;227:645–61.

27. De Vries J, Doting MHE, Jansen L, et al. Sentinel node localisation in breast cancer in two institutions. Eur J Nucl Med. 1999;26 Suppl:S67.

28. Rutgers EJT, Jansen L, Nieweg OE, et al. Technique of sentinel node biopsy in breast cancer. Eur J Surg Oncol. 1998;24:316–9.

29. Nieweg OE, Jansen L, Kroon BBR. Technique of lymphatic mapping and sentinel node biopsy for melanoma. Eur J Surg Oncol. 1998;24:520–4.

30. Kroon BK, Horenblas S, Lont AP, et al. Patients with penile carcinoma benefit from immediate resection of clinically occult lymph node metastases. J Urol. 2005;173:816–9.

31. Morton DL, Thompson JF, Essner R, et al. Immediate versus delayed lymphadenectomy in the management of primary melanoma. N Engl J Med. 2006;355:1307–17.

General Concepts on Radioguided Sentinel Lymph Node Biopsy: Preoperative Imaging, Intraoperative Gamma Probe Guidance, Intraoperative Imaging, Multimodality Imaging

Federica Orsini, Federica Guidoccio, Sergi Vidal-Sicart, Renato A. Valdés Olmos, and Giuliano Mariani

Contents

7.1   **Introduction** 151

7.2   **Preoperative Imaging** 153

7.3   **Intraoperative Gamma Probe Guidance** 157

7.4   **Intraoperative and Multimodality Imaging** 159

References 167

Learning Objectives
- To acquire basic knowledge about the role of nuclear medicine imaging in the sentinel lymph node (SLN)
- To understand the SLN concept
- To learn the different steps of sentinel lymph node biopsy (SLNB) consisting of preoperative and intraoperative imaging
- To become familiar with the practical aspects of SLN mapping
- To understand the nuclear medicine issues involved in the mini-invasive surgical approach
- To become familiar with the main steps of intraoperative gamma camera imaging with real-time scintigraphic imaging of the surgical field

F. Orsini (✉)
Nuclear Medicine Unit, "Maggiore della Carità" University Hospital, Novara, Italy
e-mail: federica.orsini@maggioreosp.novara.it

F. Guidoccio · G. Mariani
Regional Center of Nuclear Medicine, Department of Translational Research and Advanced Technologies in Medicine and Surgery, University of Pisa, Pisa, Italy

S. Vidal-Sicart
Nuclear Medicine Department, Hospital Clinic Barcelona, Barcelona, Catalonia, Spain

Institut d'Investigacions Biomèdiques August Pi Sunyer (IDIBAPS), Barcelona, Catalonia, Spain

R. A. Valdés Olmos
Department of Radiology, Section of Nuclear Medicine and Interventional Molecular Imaging Laboratory, Leiden University Medical Center, Leiden, The Netherlands

7.1 Introduction

SLNB is a diagnostic staging procedure which is routinely employed in the current clinical practice for decision-making in a variety of solid tumor types, above all breast cancer [1] and melanoma [2], in order to assess the tumoral involvement of lymph nodes not only for staging (parameter N of the TNM system) and prognostic stratification, but also for therapeutic purposes [3]. This procedure is part of the so-called radioguided surgery, a whole spectrum of nuclear medicine applications based on the combination of preoperative imaging, intraoperative detection, and postoperative techniques, involving close collaboration between at least three different specialties (nuclear medicine, surgery, pathology, and sometimes radiology and health physics as well) that have rapidly expanded over the last decades [4].

Originally introduced in the early 1990s, the SLN procedure optimizes the detection of occult lymph node metastases in patients without clinical evidence of locoregional involvement. Histopathology of the SLNs so identified and

© Springer Nature Switzerland AG 2020
G. Mariani et al. (eds.), *Atlas of Lymphoscintigraphy and Sentinel Node Mapping*,
https://doi.org/10.1007/978-3-030-45296-4_7

resected can distinguish macrometastases (>2 mm in size), micrometastases (between 0.2 and 2 mm), isolated tumor cells (malignant cell clusters <0.2 mm), or positive molecular analysis findings as specified in the eighth edition of the AJCC cancer staging manual [5]. This is possible because attention of the pathologist can now focus on much fewer lymph nodes than those normally retrieved during complete lymph node dissection of a given lymphatic station as customarily done with conventional surgery, so that a more detailed histopathologic examination of the SLNs can be carried out, using more histologic sections (to encompass virtually the entire lymph node) and more sensitive techniques (immunohistochemistry in addition to hematoxylin and eosin staining, and even molecular analysis) [5].

Radioguided surgical procedures are generally less invasive and/or less aggressive than traditional surgical approaches. In the case of radioguided SLNB, instead of a total lymphadenectomy de novo (for example of the homolateral axilla in breast cancer), patients undergo surgical removal of only one (or a few) lymph node(s), thus reducing both immediate and long-term postsurgical complications, such as lymphedema, motor/sensory nerve damage, and functional impairment of the shoulder/arm. This novel surgical strategy is based on the hypothesis that lymphatic drainage to a regional lymph node basin follows an orderly, predictable pattern, and on the function of lymph nodes on a direct drainage pathway as effective filters for tumor cells. This leads us to consider as SLNs all lymph nodes with direct drainage from the primary tumor.

The presence or absence of metastasis in the SLNs has a significant impact on therapeutic strategy. In fact, in patients with early cancer, if the SLN does not contain metastasis, the surgical approach should aim at removing the primary tumor avoiding unnecessary regional node dissection. The likelihood that non-SLNs contain metastasis when the SLN is free from tumor cells is extremely low, thus making extensive lymph node dissection unnecessary in this circumstance. Instead, patients whose SLN contains metastasis usually require dissection of regional lymph nodes. However there is increasing evidence that lymph node dissection can be avoided when the tumor burden in the SLNs is minimal or moderate, such as in particular conditions of early breast cancer [3]. These patients can be managed with different therapeutic strategies, without differences in terms of prognosis than patients treated with axillary dissection. In any case, the SLN status remains a crucial step for the choice of the most appropriate therapeutic strategy [6].

Imaging is made possible by tumoral or peritumoral interstitial administration of a radiopharmaceutical that drains from the injection site through the lymphatic system, and then selectively accumulates by phagocytosis into the macrophages of the SLNs, with consequent prolonged retention.

Colloid particles labeled with ^{99m}Tc are currently used for this purpose. The general term "colloid" indicates a class of macromolecules of micellar size varying in size between about 5 and 1000 nm (0.005–1 μm), with similar physicochemical and biological patterns. The speed of lymphatic drainage from the site of interstitial injection and the amount retained in the SLN depend mainly on the size of the radiocolloids, which may be either an inorganic substance (^{198}Au-colloid, ^{99m}Tc-antimony sulfur, ^{99m}Tc-sulfur colloid, ^{99m}Tc-stannous fluoride, ^{99m}Tc-rhenium sulfur) or derived from biological substances (^{99m}Tc-labeled nano- or micro-colloidal human serum albumin). Small-size radiocolloids (smaller than about 100 nm) migrate quite fast from the injection site through the lymphatic system, but they are not efficiently retained in the SLN. On the other hand, larger size radiocolloids are retained more efficiently in the SLN, but their migration from the interstitial administration site is slower.

^{99m}Tc-albumin nanocolloid (that has a quite narrow range of particle size, with over 90% of the particles being smaller than 80 nm) is commercially available and most widely employed in Europe, while ^{99m}Tc-sulfur colloid (with a wide range of particle size between about 20 and 400 nm) is widely employed in the USA.

A novel non-colloidal tracer has recently been introduced in the clinical practice, ^{99m}Tc-tilmanocept. This receptor-targeted radiopharmaceutical consists of a small-sized macromolecule (average diameter 7 nm) of a dextran backbone with multiple units of DTPA (for labeling with ^{99m}Tc) and mannose residues, each covalently attached to the dextran backbone. The uptake mechanism of this radiopharmaceutical in lymph nodes does not depend on the particle size but on avid binding to the CD206 receptors for mannose expressed on the surface of macrophages and dendritic cells in lymph nodes [7].

The advantages of this novel radiopharmaceutical include rapid clearance from the injection site, high SLN extraction, and high SLN retention, with consequent low migration to second-echelon lymph nodes [7, 8].

More recently the hybrid radioactive and fluorescent tracer ICG-^{99m}Tc-nanocolloid has been extensively validated in various malignancies [9]. This bimodal tracer enables preoperative lymphatic mapping thanks to its radioactive component adding intraoperative high resolution based on its fluorescence component. Due to a similar distribution in comparison with ^{99m}Tc-nanocolloid both time schedule and imaging protocol with the hybrid tracer remain unchanged [10].

Lymphoscintigraphy, a mandatory preoperative step of the entire SLNB procedure [11], is normally performed with conventional gamma cameras. When the gamma camera is combined with a CT component to constitute a hybrid SPECT/CT tomograph, the fused images so obtained are highly useful [12], especially in case of complex anatomical

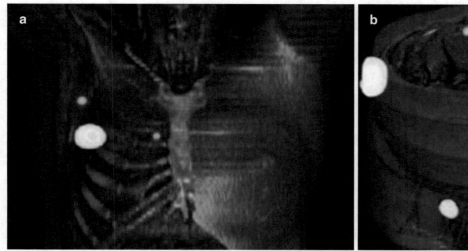
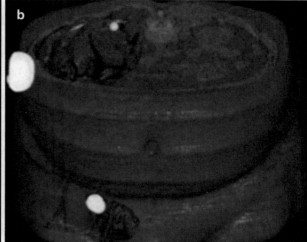

Fig. 7.1 Example of post-processing elaboration of SPECT/CT images. In both cases layers of the tegument have been focally "removed/canceled" asymmetrically between the two sides of the body so as to show the underlying anatomy. (**a**) Lymphoscintigraphy for SLN mapping in a patient with breast cancer, clearly showing migration of ^{99m}Tc-nanocolloid both to an axillary SLNs and to an internal mammary chain SLN. (**b**) Lymphoscintigraphy for SLN mapping in a patient with melanoma at the right flank, clearly showing migration of ^{99m}Tc-nanocolloid both to SLN in the right groin and to a SLN in the retroperitoneal area of the abdomen

regions and/or in case of unusual lymphatic drainage patterns (Fig. 7.1). In fact, hybrid images provide to the surgeon a morphologic and functional roadmap (CT component and SPECT component, respectively) for planning the SLNB procedure with minimal surgical access and operating time.

For immediate decision-making during surgery, intraoperative exploration of the surgical field is performed with the widely validated procedure based on the so-called handheld gamma probe. While this instrumentation produces a numerical readout and an acoustic signal proportional to radioactivity accumulation as a guide in the surgical field, the recently developed portable gamma cameras enable real-time scintigraphic imaging of the surgical field. All these instrumentations allow selective identification of the SLNs to be removed by the surgeon and analyzed by the pathologist. This interaction between technologies and medical disciplines permits to continuously refine the methodology and to improve the outcomes of radioguided surgery.

isolated tumor cells (malignant cell clusters <0.2 mm), or positive molecular analysis findings.
- The interactions between different medical disciplines permit to improve the outcomes of radioguided surgery during SLNB.
- Radioguided surgical procedures are generally less invasive and/or less aggressive than traditional surgical approaches.
- The presence or absence of metastasis in the SLN has a significant impact on therapeutic strategy.
- Imaging is made possible by tumoral or peritumoral interstitial administration of a radiopharmaceutical that drains from the injection site through the lymphatic system, and then selectively accumulates by phagocytosis into the macrophages of the SLNs.
- The radiopharmaceuticals most frequently employed for SLNB are ^{99m}Tc-sulfur colloid, ^{99m}Tc-albumin nanocolloid, and ^{99m}Tc-tilmanocept.

Key Learning Points
- SLNB is a diagnostic staging procedure that is applied in a variety of tumor types with the aim to determine the tumor status of the SLNs.
- Histopathology of the SLNs so identified and resected can distinguish macrometastases (>2 mm in size), micrometastases (between 0.2 and 2 mm),

7.2 Preoperative Imaging

Lymphoscintigraphy is generally performed in the afternoon of the day preceding surgery if the operation is scheduled in the early morning, or on the same day 4–6 h prior to surgery, depending on logistics of the institution. For same-day procedures, a smaller activity of radiocolloid is generally administered (at least 15–20 MBq) compared to the two-day procedure (at least 37–74 MBq).

The gamma camera energy selection peak is centered on the 140 keV of ^{99m}Tc (with ±10% window), and the use of high-resolution collimator(s) and of a 256 × 256 acquisition matrix is preferred; a pinhole collimator may occasionally be used to improve spatial resolution.

While dynamic acquisition is needed especially when a fast lymphatic drainage is expected (head and neck, melanoma, penile, testis, or vulvar cancers), it can nevertheless provide relevant information for identifying the actual SLNs (versus higher echelon nodes) also in the case of other malignancies, particularly breast cancer. Concerning in particular breast cancer, the patient is positioned supine with her arms raised above the head, and the collimator is placed as close as possible to the axillary region. Anterior, anterior-oblique, and lateral images are acquired. A ^{57}Co flood source can be positioned beneath the patient's body in order to obtain some reference anatomic landmarks in the scintigraphic image (Figs. 7.2 and 7.3). Alternatively, the body contour can be identified by moving a ^{57}Co or ^{99m}Tc point

source along the patient's body during scintigraphic acquisition (Fig. 7.4).

Besides SLN identification, lymphoscintigraphy is also useful to identify other possible unusual paths of lymphatic draining, such as the internal mammary chain or even intra-mammary, interpectoral, or infraclavicular lymph nodes in case of breast cancer [11] (Fig. 7.5), or in case of additional SLNs in areas of deep lymphatic drainage such as the pelvis, abdomen, or mediastinum. Especially in these cases, SPECT/CT imaging is important since it directly demonstrates anatomical localization of SLNs and obviates the problem of identifying anatomic landmarks as a reference for topographic intraoperative location of the SLNs [12–14]. Moreover, SPECT/CT imaging is highly recommended to localize SLNs in areas with complex anatomy and a high number of lymph nodes (such as the head and neck) and/or in case of absent visualization of SLN at planar imaging. In this occurrence, it is only SPECT/CT imaging that can allow SLN identification; in fact, due to the correction for tissue attenuation SPECT/CT imaging is more sensitive than planar imaging and is generally particularly useful in obese patients (Fig. 7.6).

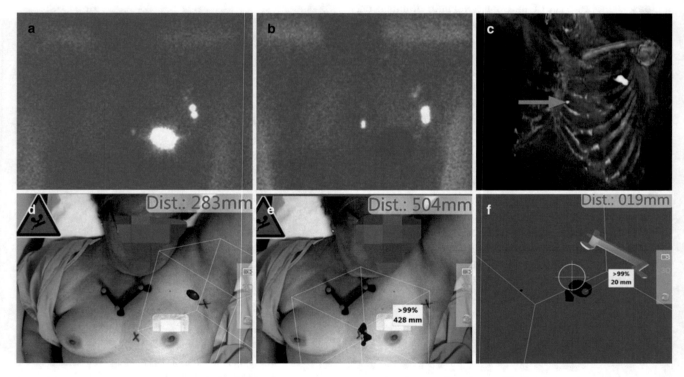

Fig. 7.2 Upper panels: planar scintigraphy (with flood phantom for body contour, see further below) obtained in a breast cancer patient about 30 min after injecting ^{99m}Tc-nanocolloidal albumin intratumorally (a). Besides intense radioactivity remaining at the injection site, left image shows migration of the radiocolloid to axillary SLNs and to the internal mammary chain area. Central image (b) was taken 2 h later, using a lead plate to cover the injection site. Axillary hot spots are clearly depicted, as well as the hot spot in left parasternal area. Right

image (c) shows a 3D volume rendering displaying the SLNs: two in left axilla and one (arrow) in the third left intercostal space. Lower panels show overlay of the freehand SPECT 3D image on the intraoperative video image of the same patient, for easier anatomical correlation. Panel (d) shows the axilla with visualization of lymph nodes. Panel (e) shows the display of internal mammary node. Panel (f) shows intraoperative visualization of the SLN in the left axilla when gamma probe is 19 mm away

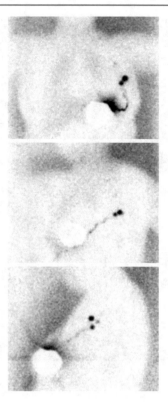

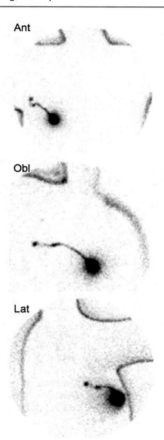

Fig. 7.3 Planar lymphoscintigraphy of breast cancer patient obtained between 20 and 30 min after injecting about 111 MBq of ^{99m}Tc-nanocolloidal albumin peri-areolarly in a patient with cancer of left breast. Upper row shows anterior projection, central row depicts oblique view, and lower row shows lateral projection. Images were taken using a lead circle to cover the injection site. All images were acquired using a single-head gamma camera and a high-resolution, low-energy collimator (acquisition time 2 min). The ^{99m}Tc flood phantom placed opposite to the gamma camera head produces the body contour delineation. While two axillary SLNs are visualized in the anterior and oblique projection, three nodes are visualized in the lateral projection

Fig. 7.4 Body contour delineation obtained by moving a ^{57}Co point source along the body of the patient during acquisition of the planar scintigraphic images. In this patient with cancer of the right breast, ^{99m}Tc-nanocolloidal albumin was injected peri-areolarly. Images acquired in the anterior projection (upper panel), right anterior oblique projection (central panel), and right lateral view (lower panel) visualize migration of the radiocolloid through a lymphatic channel to a single SLN in the axilla

However, SPECT/CT imaging does not replace planar lymphoscintigraphy, but it must rather be considered as a complementary imaging modality. In fact, contrary to SPECT/CT, planar lymphoscintigraphy allows to mark the cutaneous projection of the SLN with a dermographic pen, in order to help the surgeon to localize the site for the best surgical access. In current protocols SPECT/CT imaging is performed following delayed planar imaging (mostly 2–4 h after radiocolloid administration). This sequence of acquisitions is helpful to clarify the role of both modalities. Sequential planar acquisitions allow better visualization of the routes of lymphatic drainage. Dynamic planar acquisition usually consists of sets of serial frames (generally 1–5 min each) or sequential sets of static images in the preset count mode (generally 300,000–500,000 counts) acquired starting immediately after radiocolloid injection and up to clear scintigraphic visualization of the lymphatic routes and SLNs.

Multiplanar reconstruction enables two-dimensional display of fusion images in relation to CT and SPECT, and the use of cross-reference lines allowing the navigation between axial, coronal, and sagittal views. At the same time this tool leads to correlate radioactive SLNs seen on fused SPECT/CT with lymph nodes seen on CT (Fig. 7.7a, b). This information is helpful during the intraoperative procedure, as well as to assess completeness of excision—using portable gamma cameras or probes.

Fused SPECT/CT images can also be displayed using maximum intensity projection reconstruction. This tool enables three-dimensional display, and improves anatomical localization of SLNs (Fig. 7.7c).

When using volume rendering for three-dimensional display, different colors are assigned to anatomical structures such as muscle, bone, and skin. This leads to identifying of better anatomical reference points and incorporating of an additional dimension in the recognition of SLNs (Fig. 7.7d).

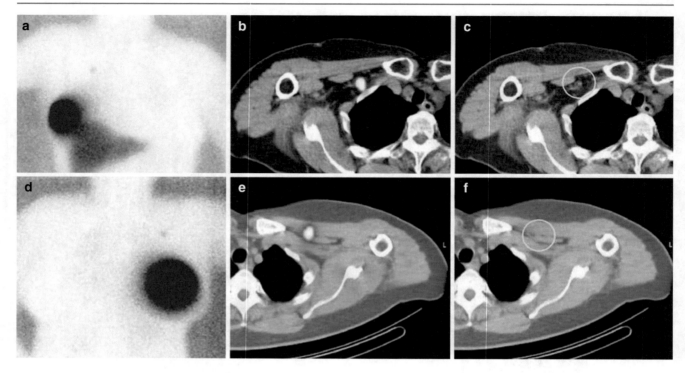

Fig. 7.5 Added value of SPECT/CT imaging in two different patients in whom planar scintigraphy shows focal uptake in the retroclavicular area; the patients had cancer located in the right breast (**a**) and in the left breast (**d**), respectively. Fused axial SPECT/CT sections (**b** and **e**), showing the location of the two SLNs between the pectoral muscles. These SLNs correspond to two single lymph nodes in the CT images (**c** and **f**, yellow circle), respectively

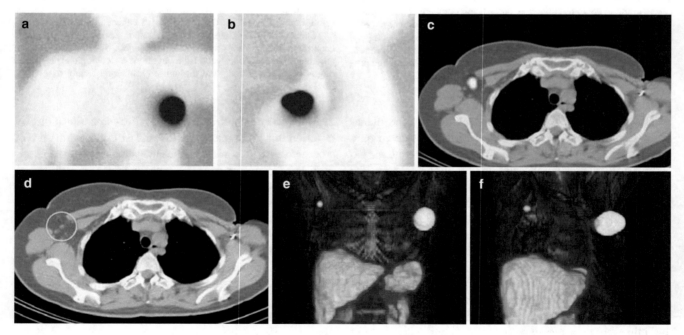

Fig. 7.6 Example of lymphatic drainage to the contralateral axilla in a patient with breast cancer. Anterior (**a**) and left lateral (**b**) planar images showing no drainage from the site of intratumoral radiocolloid injection in the left breast (body contour obtained with a flood source placed beneath the patient's body). By contrast, on the fused axial SPECT/CT image a SLN is clearly visualized at the border of the right pectoral muscle (**c**), corresponding to a single lymph node on the CT image (**d**, yellow circle). This SLN is displayed using 3D volume rendering for a better anatomical recognition in the anterior (**e**) and in the right anterior-oblique views (**f**)

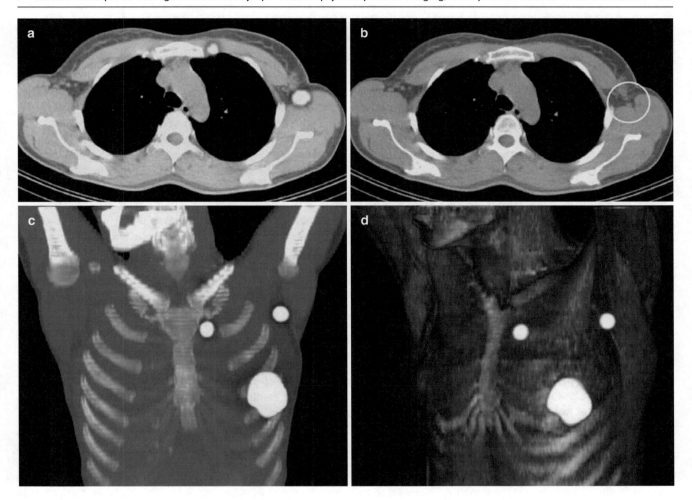

Fig. 7.7 (**a**) Fused axial SPECT/CT section obtained during lymphoscintigraphy in a patient with breast cancer, showing two SLNs, respectively, in the left internal mammary chain and in the left axilla; the yellow circle in (**b**) corresponds to a small lymph node seen on axial CT. (**c**) Fused coronal SPECT/CT displayed as maximum intensity projection (MIP), showing a SLN in the left axilla and an internal mammary chain SLN in the second left intercostal space. (**d**) SPECT/CT with volume rendering for 3D display, showing the two SLNs, respectively, in the left internal mammary chain and in the left axilla with their anatomic localizations with reference to muscles and bones

---

Key Learning Points
- Lymphoscintigraphy is a mandatory preoperative step of the SLNB procedure and it is normally performed with conventional gamma cameras.
- Added SPECT/CT images improve SLN detection by providing anatomical landmarks, especially regions with complex and/or unusual lymphatic drainage patterns.

7.3   Intraoperative Gamma Probe Guidance

The gamma probe is used to count radioactivity in the surgical field intraoperatively, without producing any scintigraphic image but yielding both a numerical readout and an audible signal, which is proportional to the counting rate.

The detector is usually of limited size, basically a long narrow cylinder with diameter of 10–18 mm, sometimes slightly angled in order to allow easier handling within the surgical field. The gamma probe can be utilized in the surgical field because it is made of a material that can be sterilized (usually metal), or it can simply be covered with a sterilized wrapping (such as those used for intraoperative ultrasound probes). Through the digital readout and acoustic signal, the gamma probe enables the surgeon to precisely localize areas of maximum radioactivity accumulation, thus guiding identification and removal of the target tissue [15, 16].

The commercially available gamma probes can be divided into crystal scintillation and semiconductor probes. Further technical features of the probe vary depending upon whether the radiopharmaceuticals are labeled with ^{99m}Tc or other radionuclides, including positron-emitting radiopharmaceuticals [17–19].

The probe is connected to a small control unit, equipped with a portable laptop or tablet, usually with a flexible cable that may also be covered with sterilized wrapping; Bluetooth-based connections have now become available, permitting easier use of the entire instrument in the operating room. Energy window for detection/counting is usually around 140 Kev (for ^{99m}Tc-labeled radiopharmaceuticals), but can vary depending on the radionuclide employed. At the same time the unit usually emits an audible signal, the pitch/tone of which varies proportionally to the counting rates. The acoustic signal helps the surgeon to explore the surgical field without looking at the control unit display.

Sensitivity (counting rate per unit of radioactivity), energy resolution (ability to detect "true" counts arising in the target versus secondary scattered radiation), spatial resolution (ability to identify very close radioactive sources as distinct from each other), and linearity of counting (it relates to the dead time) are the most important parameters of the probe in detecting radiation. Therefore, the main important tasks of a probe include sufficient sensitivity (to identify a weakly active SLN when attenuated by, typically, up to 5 cm of soft tissue), and energy and spatial resolution (to discriminate activity of a certain energy within the SLN from that originating from other sites).

More recently, with the development of PET techniques, intraoperative probes specifically designed to detect the high-energy photons originated by the annihilation process have become commercially available, thus making it possible to use radioguidance also with PET radiopharmaceuticals [20–22].

Nevertheless, major advantages of the whole process of SLN mapping in both the preoperative and the intraoperative phases have been made possible by the use of SPECT/CT and/or intraoperative imaging probes, providing a set of anatomo-topographic information that guides resection through the optimal surgical access according to the principle of least invasive surgery [23, 24]. As exemplified in Fig. 7.8, this approach is especially useful when planning surgery in complex anatomical regions such as the head and neck or the pelvis [25–31].

Just before starting surgery and with the patient already positioned on the operating table, the gamma probe is initially utilized to scan the SLN basin(s) and/or any other region where radiocolloid accumulation has been visualized, in order to confirm correct identification of the SLNs. Using the images and skin markings as guides, the probe (placed over the regions of highest counts) can be used to select the optimum location for incision. After incision, the probe is then introduced through the surgical field to explore the

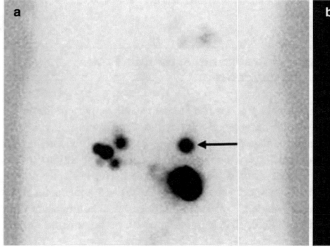 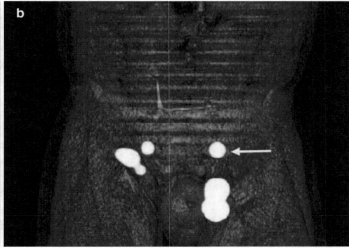

Fig. 7.8 (**a**) Planar anterior image showing lymphatic drainage to both sides, seemingly to groin lymph nodes (single SLN indicated by arrow on the left side) in a patient with penile cancer. (**b, c**) SPECT/CT with volume rendering for 3D display, respectively, in the anterior view and in a cranial view (in the latter, the bottom side corresponds to the anterior side of the body). (**d**) Fused axial SPECT/CT section showing anatomic localization of three of the lymph nodes (two on the right and one on the left) at different depths in the pelvis

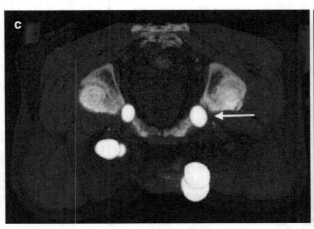
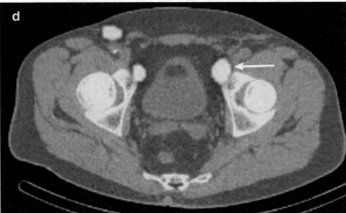

Fig. 7.8 (continued)

expected localization of the SLNs, which are usually easily identified by acoustic signal thanks to high target/background count rates. After removing the radioactive lymph nodes, the operative field is explored again with the gamma probe, assessing any residual radioactivity to confirm removal of the hot node(s). If necessary, the search must continue for possible further radioactive lymph nodes. The SLN and any other nodes so identified are then sent for complete histopathologic analysis.

Counts are recorded per unit time with the probe in the operative field, over the node before excision (in vivo) and after excision (ex vivo). A background tissue count is also recorded with the probe pointing away from the injection site, nodal activity, or other physiologic accumulations (i.e., liver) [32].

In breast cancer, once the learning phase of SLNB has been completed, the success rate of lymphoscintigraphy and intraoperative gamma probe counting in identifying SLNs is higher than 96–97% in experienced centers. This value is greater than that commonly experienced using blue dye alone (75–80%), while combining radioguidance with the blue dye leads to a 98–99% success rate in SLN identification [33]. The blue dye can be injected around the primary tumor or scar (in a similar way as the radiocolloid was injected) 10–20 min prior to the operation. Administration should be performed after the patient is anesthetized, to avoid a painful injection. Within 5–15 min the SLN is colored. Currently, the most commonly used dyes are patent blue V, isosulfan blue, and methylene blue. The additional value of dyes may be observed in cases with macrometastasis in the SLN. In fact, such SLN involvement may inhibit radiocolloid accumulation, if tumor cells have replaced most of the normal lymph node tissue [34]. In these cases a new first draining node is seen (Fig. 7.9) that can result in a false-negative finding [26]. To decrease false-negative results, the open axilla should be palpated and suspicious lymph nodes

harvested, even if they are neither hot nor blue. In cases of non-visualization or if the SLN is located outside the lower medial part of the axilla, palpation of the typical SLN area is particularly important [32, 35].

A notable disadvantage of using blue dyes instead of radiotracers is that blue dyes are not helpful when extra-axillary nodes (internal mammary or supraclavicular) are to be evaluated [36, 37].

> **Key Learning Points**
> - Intraoperative exploration of the surgical field is performed with the widely validated procedure based on the so-called handheld gamma probe.
> - This instrumentation produces a numerical readout and an acoustic signal proportional to radioactivity accumulation, as a guide in the surgical field for SLN detection and localization.

7.4 Intraoperative and Multimodality Imaging

Currently, the trend of surgery is towards adopting minimally invasive approaches for a growing spectrum of procedures. This includes oncological surgery, as it implies much faster postsurgical recovery of patients. For optimally planning and performing these approaches, the most crucial issue is accurate preoperative characterization of the surgical strategy, which is achieved through diagnostic imaging. In this regard, maximum benefit for the success of minimally invasive surgery derives from integration of anatomical (e.g., CT) and metabolic/functional imaging, the latter being typically provided by nuclear medicine procedures. These features contribute to a better characterization of the lesion to be

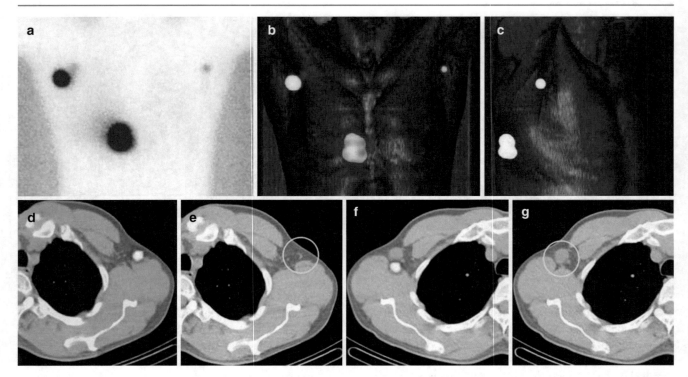

Fig. 7.9 Upper panels: (**a**) planar anterior view acquired in a patient with melanoma located in the back of the right torso, showing lymphatic drainage to both axillae, as better demonstrated by SPECT/CT with volume rendering for 3D display, respectively, in the anterior and in the right oblique view (**b** and **c**). Lower panels: fused axial SPECT/CT section at two different levels, showing the location of radioactive lymph nodes, respectively, in the left axilla (**d**) and in the right axilla (**f**).

The corresponding CT sections show that the hot lymph node in the left axilla corresponds to a normal-sized node (yellow circle in panel **e**), while in the right axilla the hot lymph node (of approximately normal size) is located posterior to a grossly enlarged, most likely metastatic lymph node not visualized by lymphoscintigraphy (yellow circle in panel **g**)

removed, and in many cases enable subsequent intraoperative guidance through the use of devices especially designed for this use [38, 39].

Over the last decade, intraoperative imaging probes have become commercially available for clinical practice, and the use of such handheld portable gamma cameras is increasing. By providing real-time imaging with a global overview of all radioactive hot spots in the whole surgical field [40], intraoperative imaging with portable gamma cameras can be used either during open surgery or during laparoscopic procedures; the information so gained can be combined with data obtained with conventional or laparoscopic gamma probe counting [41, 42].

Information provided by these devices can be combined with those ones obtained preoperatively by lymphoscintigraphy or SPECT/CT. Using the anatomic landmarks provided by SPECT/CT images, the portable device can be oriented to surgical targets in the operating room [43]. No delay has to elapse between image acquisition and display (real-time imaging), with the possibility of continuous monitoring and spatial orientation on the screen. Real-time quantification of the count rates recorded should also be displayed.

The development of such cameras is shown in Fig. 7.10. While the earliest devices were heavy handheld devices, the new generation of such equipment includes portable gamma cameras that are lighter, or equipped with stable support systems.

Among the products commercially available, one of the most used devices is equipped with a CsI(Na) scintillation crystal and different collimators (pinhole collimators, 2.5 and 4 mm in diameters, and divergent). The pinhole collimator enables to visualize the whole surgical field (depending on the distance between the camera and the source). The field of view varies between 4 cm × 4 cm at 3 cm from the source and 20 cm × 20 cm at 15 cm from the source. This device has been integrated in a mobile and an ergonomic support that is easily adjustable. The imaging head is located on one arm that allows optimal positioning on the specific area to be explored.

Another approach is based on the use of CdZnTe detectors. For instance, the detector is made of a single tile of CdZnTe, patterned in an array of 16 × 16 pixels at a pitch of 2 mm. The head is equipped with a series of interchangeable parallel-hole collimators to achieve different performances

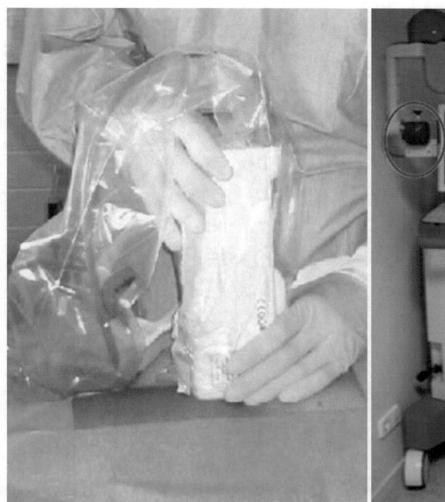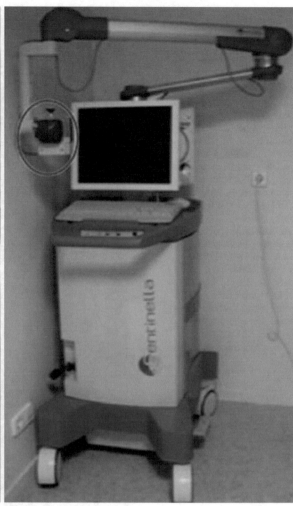

Fig. 7.10 Example of portable gamma cameras. Left panel: light-weight portable gamma camera (less than 1 kg), without support system. Right panel: recent-generation portable gamma camera with improved ergonometry and adequate and stable support system for intraoperative use; this unit incorporates a laser pointer to center the image and adjust the scanning procedure

in terms of spatial resolution and/or sensitivity. The field of view is 3.2 cm × 3.2 cm and the weight is 800 g [44].

A further development is represented by an intraoperative gamma camera that is still based on the CdZnTe pixel technology, and has originally been developed for breast imaging. The field of view is 13 cm × 13 cm and the intrinsic spatial resolution is 2 mm. This camera is also equipped with interchangeable parallel-hole collimators and is integrated in a workstand articulated arm.

However, since non-imaging probes are still the standard equipment for detection of radiolabeled tissue in the operating room, the role of intraoperative imaging is generally limited, at least so far, to constitute an additional aid to the surgeon to identify the SLN. Some authors have assessed the added value of portable gamma camera in clinical practice. The usefulness of the portable gamma cameras in breast can-

cer patients is being established in the following conditions: (a) when no conventional gamma camera is available, (b) in particular cases with difficult drainage or extra-axillary drainage (intramammary and internal mammary chain nodes) [45], (c) in case of only faint lymph nodal radiocolloid uptake, (d) when the SLN is located very close to the injection site, or (e) in case of significant photon emission and scatter from the injection site. In fact, the position of the portable gamma camera can be moved and adjusted in such a manner so as to acquire special-angle views in order to also show SLNs near the injection area.

The use of an intraoperative imaging device implies the possibility to monitor the lymphatic basin before and after removal of the hot nodes, to verify completeness of lymph node excision [46] (Fig. 7.11). After excision of each lymph node, a new image is acquired and compared

Fig. 7.11 Preoperative images in a 42-year-old patient with a T1 cancer in her left breast. (**a**) 3D reconstruction image after processing SPECT/CT data. (**b**) A scintigraphic anterior view is acquired by placing the portable gamma camera in previously marked points on the skin (inner mammary chain, see laser cross pointers). (**c**) The portable gamma camera can be placed in different positions to better depict the lymph nodes; in this picture it is tilted in an oblique view. (**d**) Visualization of an inner mammary chain lymph node, with partial vision of the injection site (image corresponding to the position of the gamma camera as in panel **b**). (**e**) Visualization of an axillary lymph node depicted with the gamma camera positioned as in panel **c**

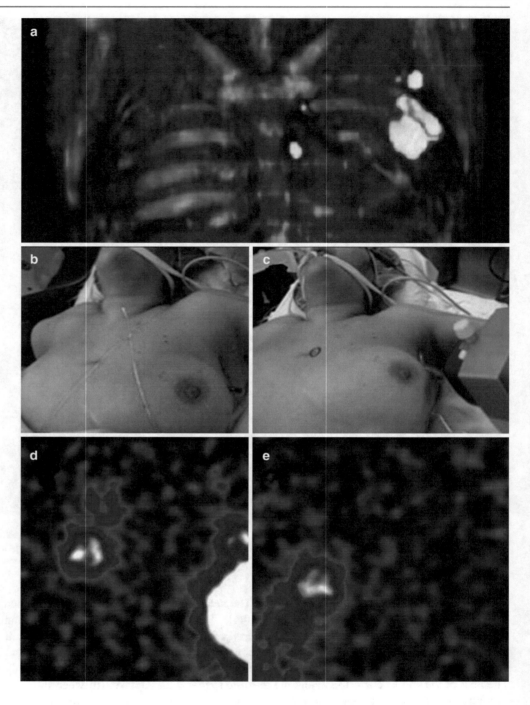

with the image acquired before excision (Fig. 7.12). If focal radioactivity remains at the same location, it is concluded that another possible SLN is still in place. Thus, the use of a portable gamma camera in addition to the gamma probe is important to provide certainty on whether all SLNs have been adequately removed (Fig. 7.13) [47].

In the operation room, the gamma camera can be placed above the previously marked SLN locations using some external point sources (like ^{133}Ba, ^{153}Gd, or ^{125}I); alternatively, in some gamma cameras a laser pointer is fitted to the device. In those devices where a laser pointer is included, it is displayed as a red cross over the patient's skin. The position of this red cross is visible on the computer screen of the equipment.

During surgery, an initial 30–60-s image is acquired with the gamma camera to assess the surgical field and validate SLN uptake. This time can be longer when the lymph nodes are depicted as areas with faint focal uptake. After incision, if there is any difficulty in finding the precise location of the

Fig. 7.12 (**a**) Lymphoscintigraphic image acquired with a conventional, large-field-of-view gamma camera 2 h after intratumoral injection of 111 MBq of ^{99m}Tc-nanocoll in a 57-year-old patient with breast cancer in her left upper outer quadrant; at least one axillary SLN is clearly depicted (yellow circle). (**b**) The same image without lead shielding of the injection site shows similar radiocolloid distribution. (**c**) Operating room image obtained with a portable gamma camera prior to starting the SLN procedure, confirming similar findings (yellow arrow). (**d**) Image obtained with the portable gamma camera after completing radioguided SLN excision, showing no residual activity except the intratumoral injection site. The use of the portable gamma camera, in addition to the handheld, non-imaging gamma probe, was especially useful to confirm the completeness of SLN removal

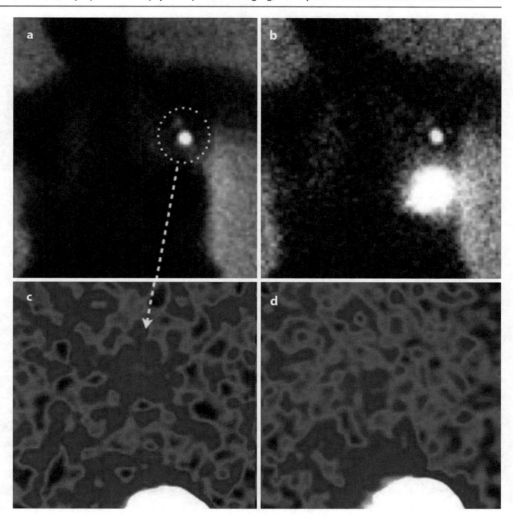

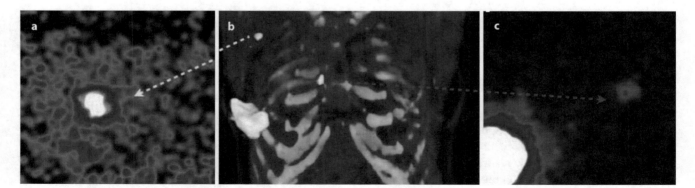

Fig. 7.13 Utility of the portable gamma camera during surgery for the certainty of SLN resection. Radiotracer uptake displayed on gamma camera (**a**), corresponding to the node depicted in the axillary area (yellow arrow) on the 3D volume-rendering reconstruction of a breast cancer patient with lymphatic drainage to axilla and inner mammary chain (**b**). Parasternal SLN (red arrow) is depicted with the gamma camera as well (**c**). Preoperative image of the axilla shows a highly active SLN (**d**). Image after axillary node retrieval informs about the absence of other significant tracer uptake (**e**). Similar approach in the internal mammary chain SLN (**f, g**)

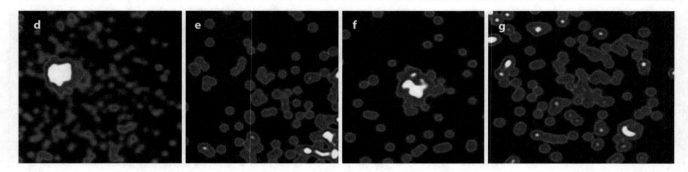

Fig. 7.13 (continued)

SLN using the gamma probe, another 30–120-s image, depending on the level of lymph node uptake, is acquired using the portable gamma camera.

The use of the external point sources facilitates SLN localization, as these sources can be depicted separately on the screen of the portable gamma camera, thus functioning as a pointer in the search for the nodes. The matching of two signals ([99mTc] signal and [153Gd], [133Ba], or [125I] pointer signals) indicates the correct location of the SLNs. This location is then checked using the gamma probe. After SLN retrieval, another set of images is acquired to ascertain the absence of the previously visualized SLNs, or to ascertain the presence of remaining radioactive nodes (additional SLNs or second-tier nodes, see Fig. 7.14).

Thanks to novel technological possibilities, combining a spatial localization system and two tracking targets to be fixed on a conventional, handheld gamma probe results in new 3D visualization of the traditional acoustic signal of the gamma probe. This feature, together with the real-time information on depth that the system may provide, would expand the applications of radioguided SLNB in oncology, particularly for malignancies with deep lymphatic drainage [48, 49]. In this regard, the most interesting development in radioguided surgery is the so-called system free-hand SPECT, in which a continuous positioning system installed in the operating room is based on a fix pointing device, on the patient's body, and, respectively, on the handheld gamma counting probe, thus permitting a virtual reconstruction in a 3D environment. Position of the gamma probe relative to the fix device is tracked by infrared positioning technology, and the output of the intraoperative gamma probe is spatially co-registered in the surgical field (depicted by a video camera) and displayed on a monitor in which the surgeon can easily check location and depth of the foci of radioactivity accumulation to be resected. This 3D information may be further used for precise localization and targeting of the radioactive SLNs and of tumor tissue, thus implementing a radioguided navigation system. The device can ensure permanent assistance and transparent documentation of soft-tissue removal during the intervention (Figs. 7.15 and 7.16).

On the other hand, the possibility of combining the current radiopharmaceuticals with other agents opens new fields to explore. In this regard, a radiolabeled nanocolloid agent has been combined with ICG, a fluorescent agent, for SLN detection in robot-assisted lymphadenectomy [50].

In contrast to the use of a single-fluorescent agent [51, 52], this bimodal tracer may allow the surgeons to integrate the standard approach based on radioguided detection with a portable gamma camera with a new optical modality based on fluorescent signal detection. This approach is being successfully applied in various malignancies (Fig. 7.17) [53], since the hybrid approach (ICG-[99mTc]-nanocolloid) provides the ability to perform radioguidance and enhance it by fluorescence imaging of the exact same features. This results in a further refinement of the surgical SLN identification, e.g., the ability to surgically identify SLNs in close proximity to the injection site. The synergistic approach also yields enhanced intraoperative SLN identification/retrieval rates.

Key Learning Points

- Portable gamma cameras enable real-time scintigraphic imaging of the surgical field and helps in SLN identification and verification of completeness of SLN excision.
- Products commercially available support different technologies such as CsI(Na) scintillating crystal, CdZnTe detectors, and combinations of spatial localization system and tracking targets fixed on a conventional handheld gamma probe, the latter resulting in new 3D visualization of the surgical field.
- During surgery, an initial fast image is acquired with the portable gamma camera to assess the surgical field and validate SLN uptake; after the incision, a second image is acquired to confirm complete resection of radioactive lymph nodes.
- Combining current radiopharmaceuticals with other agents, such as fluorescent agents, opens new fields to explore different compounds for SLN identification and removal.

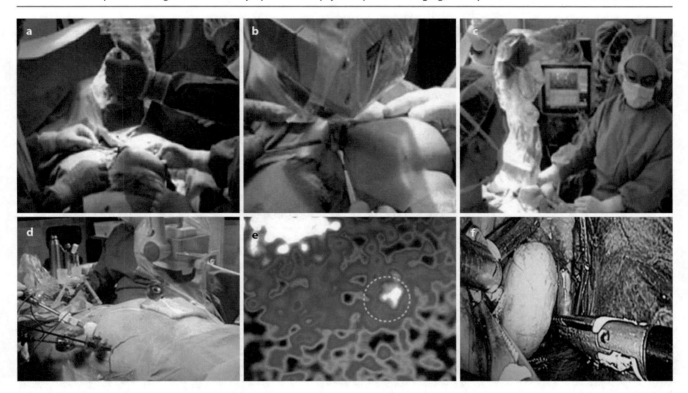

Fig. 7.14 Portable gamma camera intraoperative approach. The device is placed over the interest area in the most convenient way (**a**). A red cross shows the central position of image on the gamma camera's screen (**b**). This feature allows a better comprehension and awareness about the potential SLNs on the surgical field (**c**). Lower row: Laparoscopic approach. The portable gamma camera is positioned over abdominal wall to continuously assess the tracer uptake (**d**). Usual uptake in a SLN close to the common iliac vein (green circle; **e**). This node was clearly located in that area and subsequently removed (**f**)

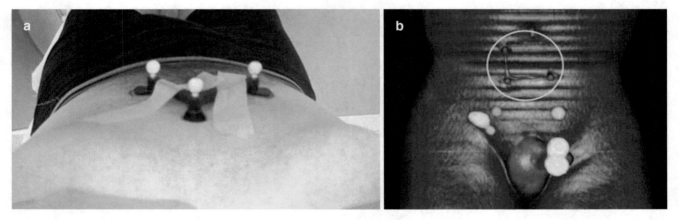

Fig. 7.15 (**a**) Positioning of the tracking device positioned on the patient's body for radioguided SLNB in a patient with penile cancer (same patient as in Fig. 7.8). (**b**) 3D volume-rendering SPECT/CT, showing the pattern of lymphatic drainage in a patient with penile cancer (approximate position of the tracking device on the patient's body is also indicated in the yellow circle). (**c**) Tracking device attached to a gamma probe in order to generate freehand SPECT data. (**d**) By integrating preoperative SPECT/CT data it is possible to overlay the generated 3D image to the patient's body with simultaneous display of the SLNs on the right side of the pelvis

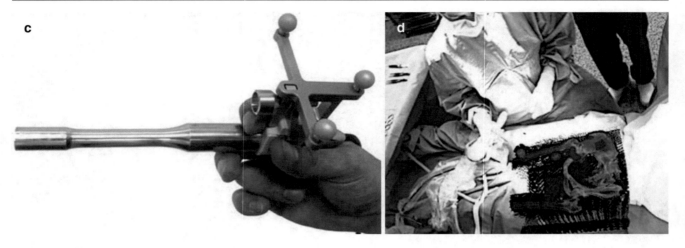

Fig. 7.15 (continued)

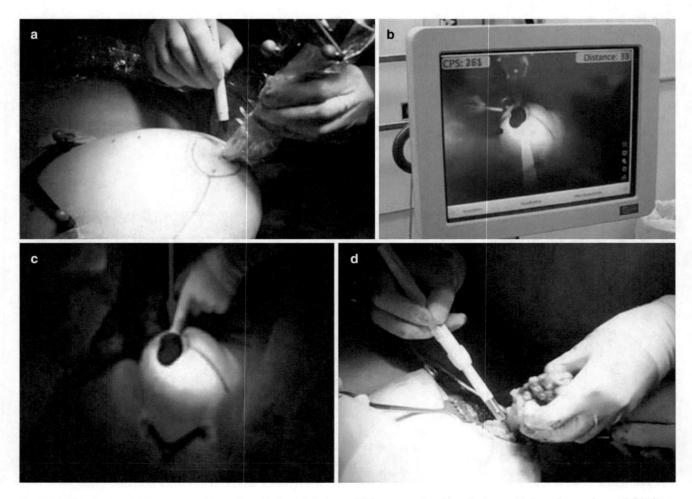

Fig. 7.16 Free-hand SPECT system used for radioguided occult lesion localization (ROLL) in a patient with non-palpable breast cancer. (**a**) Surgical approach for ROLL; the tracking device positioned on the patient's body is visible on the left. (**b, c**) Overlay of freehand SPECT 3D images on the video displays, with the red arrow in panel C indicating the site of the tumor. (**d**) Completion of lumpectomy guided by the freehand SPECT-based system

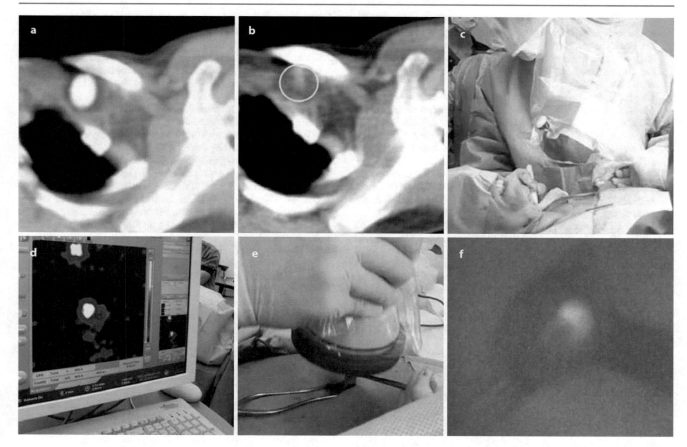

Fig. 7.17 (**a**) Fused axial SPECT/CT section showing a radioactive SLN in the left cervical area. (**b**) This focus of radioactive accumulation corresponds to a solitary lymph node seen in the CT section (circle). (**c**) The use of a portable gamma camera permits the surgeon to select the site for incision, and (**d**) also to monitor the procedure with intraopera- tive imaging guidance. The recent introduction of bimodal tracers for simultaneous radioguided (**e**) and fluorescent (**f**) detection is leading to the additional use of a fluorescence camera to better distinguish the SLN in anatomically complex areas

References

1. NCCN clinical practice guidelines in oncology (NCCN guide-lines®) breast cancer, version 3.2019. https://www.nccn.org/profes-sionals/physician_gls/pdf/breast.pdf.
2. NCCN clinical practice guidelines in oncology (NCCN guide-lines®) cutaneous melanoma, version 2.2019. https://www.nccn.org/professionals/physician_gls/pdf/cutaneous_melanoma.pdf.
3. Giuliano AE, Hunt KK, Ballman KV, et al. Axillary dissection vs no axillary dissection in women with invasive breast cancer and sentinel node metastasis: a randomized clinical trial. JAMA. 2011;305:569–75.
4. Giammarile F, Vidal-Sicart S, Orsini F, et al. In: Volterrani D, Erba PA, Carrió I, Strauss HW, Mariani G, editors. Nuclear medicine textbook—methodology and clinical applications. Basel: Springer Nature; 2019. p. 351–90.
5. Galimberti V, Cole BF, Viale G, et al. Axillary dissection versus no axillary dissection in patients with breast cancer and sentinel-node micrometastases (IBCSG 23-01): 10-year follow-up of a ran-domised, controlled phase 3 trial. Lancet Oncol. 2018;19:1385–93.
6. Giuliano AE, Han SH. Local and regional control in breast cancer: role of sentinel node biopsy. Adv Surg. 2011;45:101–16.
7. Orsini F, Puta E, Mariani G. Single-photon emitting radiopharma-ceuticals. In: Volterrani D, Erba PA, Carrió I, Strauss HW, Mariani G, editors. Nuclear medicine texbook—methodology and clinical applications. Basel: Springer Nature; 2019. p. 21–56.
8. Vidal-Sicart S, Vera D, Valdés Olmos RA. Next generation of radio-tracers for sentinel lymph node biopsy: what is still necessary to establish new imaging paradigms? Rev Esp Med Nucl Imagen Mol. 2018;37:373–9.
9. KleinJan GH, van Werkhoven E, van den Berg NS, et al. The best of both worlds: a hybrid approach for optimal pre- and intraopera-tive identification of sentinel lymph nodes. Eur J Nucl Med Mol Imaging. 2018;45:1915–25.
10. Brouwer OR, Buckle T, Vermeeren L, et al. Comparing the hybrid fluorescent-radioactive tracer indocyanine green-99mTc-nanocolloid with 99mTc-nanocolloid for sentinel node identification: a validation study using lymphoscintigraphy and SPECT/CT. J Nucl Med. 2012;53:1034–40.

11. Goyal A, Newcombe RG, Mansel RE, et al. Role of routine preoperative lymphoscintigraphy in sentinel node biopsy for breast cancer. Eur J Cancer. 2005;41:238–43.

12. Even-Sapir E, Lerman H, Lievshitz G, et al. Lymphoscintigraphy for sentinel node mapping using a hybrid SPECT/CT system. J Nucl Med. 2003;44:1413–20.

13. Lerman H, Metser U, Lievshitz G, et al. Lymphoscintigraphic sentinel node identification in patients with breast cancer: the role of SPECT/CT. Eur J Nucl Med Mol Imaging. 2006;33:329–37.

14. Lerman H, Lievshitz G, Zak O, et al. Improved sentinel node identification by SPECT/CT in overweight patients with breast cancer. J Nucl Med. 2007;48:201–6.

15. Zanzonico P, Heller S. The intraoperative gamma probe: basic principles and choices available. Semin Nucl Med. 2000;30:33–48.

16. Mathelin CE, Guyonnet JL. Scintillation crystal or semiconductor gamma-probes: an open debate. J Nucl Med. 2006;47:373.

17. Meller B, Sommer K, Gerl J, et al. High energy probe for detecting lymph node metastases with ^{18}F-FDG in patients with head and neck cancer. Nuklearmedizin. 2006;45:153–9.

18. Curtet C, Carlier T, Mirallié E, et al. Prospective comparison of two gamma probes for intraoperative detection of ^{18}F-FDG: in vitro assessment and clinical evaluation in differentiated thyroid cancer patients with iodine-negative recurrence. Eur J Nucl Med Mol Imaging. 2007;34:1556–62.

19. Schneebaum S, Essner R, Even-Sapir E. Positron-sensitive probes. In: Mariani G, Giuliano AE, Strauss HW, editors. Radioguided surgery—a comprehensive team approach. New York: Springer; 2008. p. 23–8.

20. Valdés Olmos RA, Vidal-Sicart S, Manca G, et al. Advances in radioguided surgery. Q J Nucl Med Mol Imaging. 2017;61:247–70.

21. Rauscher I, Horn T, Gschwend JE, et al. Novel technology of molecular radio-guidance for lymph node dissection in recurrent prostate cancer by PSMA-ligands. World J Urol. 2018;36:603–8.

22. Van Oosterom MN, Rietbergen DDD, Welling MM, et al. Recent advances in nuclear and hybrid detection modalities for image-guided surgery. Expert Rev Med Devices. 2019;16:711–34.

23. Vermeeren L, van der Ploeg IM, Valdés Olmos RA, et al. SPECT/CT for preoperative sentinel node localization. J Surg Oncol. 2010;101:184–90.

24. Israel O, Pellet O, Biassoni L, et al. Two decades of SPECT/CT—the coming of age of a technology. An updated review of the literature evidence. Eur J Nucl Med Mol Imaging. 2019;46:1990–2012.

25. Kobayashi K, Ramirez PT, Kim EE, et al. Sentinel node mapping in vulvovaginal melanoma using SPECT/CT lymphoscintigraphy. Clin Nucl Med. 2009;34:859–61.

26. Leijte JA, van der Ploeg IM, Valdés Olmos RA, et al. Visualization of tumor blockage and rerouting of lymphatic drainage in penile cancer patients by use of SPECT/CT. J Nucl Med. 2009;50:364–7.

27. van der Ploeg IM, Valdés Olmos RA, Kroon BB, et al. The yield of SPECT/CT for anatomical lymphatic mapping in patients with melanoma. Ann Surg Oncol. 2009;16:1537–42.

28. Vermeeren L, Valdés Olmos RA, Meinhardt W, et al. Value of SPECT/CT for detection and anatomic localization of sentinel lymph nodes before laparoscopic sentinel node lymphadenectomy in prostate carcinoma. J Nucl Med. 2009;50:865–70.

29. Pandit-Taskar N, Gemignani ML, Lyall A, et al. Single photon emission computed tomography SPECT-CT improves sentinel node detection and localization in cervical and uterine malignancy. Gynecol Oncol. 2010;117:59–64.

30. Vermeeren L, Meinhardt W, Valdés Olmos RA. Prostatic lymphatic drainage with sentinel nodes at the ventral abdominal wall visualized with SPECT/CT: a case series. Clin Nucl Med. 2010;35:71–3.

31. Vermeeren L, Valdés Olmos RA, Klop WM, et al. SPECT/CT for sentinel lymph node mapping in head and neck melanoma. Head Neck. 2011;33:1–6.

32. Giammarile F, Alazraki N, Aarsvold JN, et al. The EANM and SNMMI practice guideline for lymphoscintigraphy and sentinel node localization in breast cancer. Eur J Nucl Med Mol Imaging. 2013;40:1932–47.

33. Cox CE, Cox JM, Mariani G, et al. Sentinel lymph node biopsy in patients with breast cancer. In: Mariani G, Giuliano AE, Strauss HW, editors. Radioguided surgery—a comprehensive team approach. New York: Springer; 2008. p. 87–97.

34. Estourgie SH, Nieweg OE, Valdés Olmos RA, et al. Eight false negative sentinel lymph node procedures in breast cancer: what went wrong? Eur J Surg Oncol. 2003;29:336–40.

35. Serrano Vicente J, Infante de la Torre JR, Domínguez Grande ML, et al. Optimization of sentinel lymph node biopsy in breast cancer by intraoperative axillary palpation. Rev Esp Med Nucl. 2010;29:8–11.

36. Varghese P, Abdel-Rahman AT, Akberali S, et al. Methylene blue dye—a safe and effective alternative for sentinel lymph node localization. Breast J. 2008;14:61–7.

37. Rodier JF, Velten M, Wilt M, et al. Prospective multicentric randomized study comparing periareolar and peritumoral injection of radiotracer and blue dye for the detection of sentinel lymph node in breast sparing procedures: FRANSENODE trial. J Clin Oncol. 2007;25:3664–9.

38. Valdés Olmos RA, Vidal-Sicart S, Nieweg OE. SPECT-CT and real-time intraoperative imaging: new tools for sentinel node localization and radioguided surgery? Eur J Nucl Med Mol Imaging. 2009;36:1–5.

39. Vermeeren L, Valdés Olmos RA, Meinhardt W, et al. Intraoperative radioguidance with a portable gamma camera: a novel technique for laparoscopic sentinel node localisation in urological malignancies. Eur J Nucl Med Mol Imaging. 2009;36:1029–36.

40. Hoffman EJ, Tornai MP, Janecek M, et al. Intra-operative probes and imaging probes. Eur J Nucl Med. 1999;26:913–35.

41. Mathelin C, Salvador S, Huss D, et al. Precise localization of sentinel lymph nodes and estimation of their depth using a prototype intraoperative mini gamma-camera in patients with breast cancer. J Nucl Med. 2007;48:623–9.

42. Scopinaro F, Tofani A, di Santo G, et al. High-resolution, hand-held camera for sentinel-node detection. Cancer Biother Radiopharm. 2008;23:43–52.

43. Zaknun JJ, Giammarile F, Valdés Olmos RA, et al. Changing paradigms in radioguided surgery and intraoperative imaging: the GOSTT concept. Eur J Nucl Med Mol Imaging. 2012;39:1–3.

44. Vermeeren L, Klop WM, van den Brekel MW, et al. Sentinel node detection in head and neck malignancies: innovations in radioguided surgery. J Oncol. 2009;2009:681746.

45. Duch J. Portable gamma cameras: the real value of an additional view in the operating theatre. Eur J Nucl Med Mol Imaging. 2011;38:633–5.

46. Vidal-Sicart S, Paredes P, Zanón G, et al. Added value of intraoperative real-time imaging in searches for difficult-to-locate sentinel nodes. J Nucl Med. 2010;51:1219–25.

47. Leong SP, Wu M, Lu Y, et al. Intraoperative imaging with a portable gamma camera may reduce the false-negative rate for melanoma sentinel lymph node surgery. Ann Surg Oncol. 2018;25:3326–33.

48. Wendler T, Herrmann K, Schnelzer A, et al. First demonstration of 3-D lymphatic mapping in breast cancer using freehand SPECT. Eur J Nucl Med Mol Imaging. 2010;37:1452–61.

49. Rieger A, Saeckl J, Belloni B, et al. First experiences with navigated radio-guided surgery using freehand SPECT. Case Rep Oncol. 2011;4:420–5.

50. van der Poel HG, Buckle T, Brouwer OR, et al. Intraoperative laparoscopic fluorescence guidance to the sentinel lymph node in prostate cancer patients: clinical proof of concept of an integrated functional imaging approach using a multimodal tracer. Eur Urol. 2011;60:826–33.

51. Keereweer S, Kerrebijn JD, van Driel PB, et al. Optical image-guided surgery—where do we stand? Mol Imaging Biol. 2011;13:199–207.

52. Polom K, Murawa D, Rho YS, et al. Current trends and emerging future of indocyanine green usage in surgery and oncology: a literature review. Cancer. 2011;117:4812–22.

53. Namazov A, Volchok V, Liboff A, et al. Sentinel nodes detection with near-infrared imaging in gynecological cancer patients: ushering in an era of precision medicine. Isr Med Assoc J. 2019;21:390–3.

SPECT/CT Image Generation and Criteria for Sentinel Lymph Node Mapping

8

Renato A. Valdés Olmos and Sergi Vidal-Sicart

Contents

8.1	**Introduction**	171
8.2	**The Clinical Problem**	172
8.3	**Image Generation with SPECT/CT**	172
8.4	**General Indications for SPECT/CT Imaging**	173
8.5	**Comprehensive Interpretation of Preoperative SLN Imaging**	174
8.6	**SPECT/CT as a Roadmap for Intraoperative SLN Detection**	179
8.7	**Imaging Report Combining Planar Lymphoscintigraphy and SPECT/CT**	179
	References	183

Learning Objectives
- To acquire basic knowledge about the role of nuclear medicine imaging in the sentinel lymph node (SLN) procedure
- To understand the role of lymphoscintigraphy in incorporating time sequential aspects to differentiate SLNs from higher echelon nodes
- To learn when it is necessary to acquire SPECT/CT imaging and how these images can be used to localize SLNs in an anatomical environment
- To preoperatively identify SLNs and to learn how this information can be transferred to surgeons for the intraoperative procedure
- To learn basic knowledge about imaging report generation combining lymphoscintigraphy and SPECT/CT imaging
- To become familiar with the role of SPECT/CT imaging and of its CT component in the SLN procedure

R. A. Valdés Olmos (✉)
Department of Radiology, Section of Nuclear Medicine and Interventional Molecular Imaging Laboratory, Leiden University Medical Center, Leiden, The Netherlands
e-mail: R.A.Valdes_Olmos@lumc.nl

S. Vidal-Sicart
Nuclear Medicine Department, Hospital Clinic Barcelona, Barcelona, Catalonia, Spain

Institut d'Investigacions Biomèdiques August Pi Sunyer (IDIBAPS), Barcelona, Catalonia, Spain

8.1 Introduction

Since the introduction of the SLN procedure, lymphoscintigraphy has constituted an essential component for the preoperative SLN identification in melanoma and breast cancer patients.

With the integration of spiral CT scanners with the modern large-field-of-view gamma cameras, SPECT/CT became possible in the first decennium of this century with increasing popularity in clinical practice and in the medical literature. In the same period SPECT/CT was incorporated in the SLN procedure combining the functional information from SPECT with the morphological CT imaging by applying both techniques simultaneously in one session. The resulting SPECT/CT fused images can depict SLNs in

© Springer Nature Switzerland AG 2020
G. Mariani et al. (eds.), *Atlas of Lymphoscintigraphy and Sentinel Node Mapping*,
https://doi.org/10.1007/978-3-030-45296-4_8

their anatomical environment, thus generating a helpful roadmap to be used by surgeons in the operating room. In the early years of validation of SPECT/CT imaging in the SLN procedure, its use was limited to melanoma and breast cancer patients with unusual or complex drainage. This is the case in melanomas of the neck or the upper part of the trunk, and in breast cancer patients with drainage outside the axilla. SPECT/CT has also been found to be useful in visualizing SLNs in the axilla when lymph nodes are not depicted on planar images [1]. In areas such as the pelvis, retroperitoneum and upper abdomen for gynaecological, urological and gastrointestinal malignancies, SPECT/CT is becoming essential to localize SLNs.

Due to the increasing role of SPECT/CT imaging, the evaluation of this modality in relation to planar lymphoscintigraphy for SLN detection and localization is necessary. On the other hand, the preoperative anatomical information obtained by SPECT/CT is currently essential for generating roadmaps for SLN procedures in the operation room, leading at the same time to a more effective use of portable devices for SLN localization [2].

8.2　The Clinical Problem

The SLN procedure is based on the hypothesis of an orderly and predictable pattern of lymphatic drainage to a regional lymph node basin, and on the functioning of lymph nodes on a direct drainage pathway as effective filters for tumour cells [3]. This leads to considering as SLNs all lymph nodes with direct drainage from the primary tumour. In this respect, the most important contribution of nuclear medicine is to identify SLNs based on the mapping of lymphatic drainage. This is accomplished by sequential lymphoscintigraphy including images acquired immediately after tracer injection as well as delayed images in order to distinguish between SLNs receiving lymph directly from the primary lesion from second-tier lymph nodes—receiving the tracer in a later phase. A subsequent SPECT/CT acquisition helps to confirm the identification of SLNs and also provides anatomical landmarks for surgeons to plan skin incision and to recognize SLN location during the surgical act. This approach of "see and open" can be considered a logical complement of the above-mentioned modern SLN concept initially developed by Morton [4].

Another important notion is that the SLN procedure is a multidisciplinary modality based on the combination of preoperative imaging, intraoperative detection and refined histopathological analysis. For preoperative imaging, colloid particles labelled with ^{99m}Tc are currently used. Radioactive colloid particles are incorporated into the macrophages by phagocytosis, thus enabling prolonged lymph node retention. This leads to an adequate detection window enabling not only delayed planar images and SPECT/CT, but also

intraoperative SLN localization using portable devices based on gamma ray detection.

Furthermore, the SLN procedure aims at detecting lymph node metastases in patients without clinical evidence of regional metastasis [5]. An adequate preoperative selection can currently identify patients with palpable lymph nodes at clinical examination, suspected lymph nodes at ultrasound or CT or tumour-positive lymph nodes at cytological aspiration. In clinical practice this leads to considering the SLN biopsy as a procedure principally oriented to the detection of subclinical metastasis. For practical reasons, this category mainly includes small macrometastases (>2 mm and <5 mm), micrometastases (>0.2 mm and <2 mm) and submicrometastases (<0.2 mm). This approach originally designed for breast cancer has gradually been incorporated in other malignancies [6].

> **Key Learning Points**
> - Based on the hypothesis of an orderly and predictable pattern of lymphatic drainage to a regional lymph node basin, and on the functioning of lymph nodes on a direct drainage pathway as effective filters for tumour cells, all lymph nodes receiving direct radiocolloid drainage from the primary tumour-related injection are considered SLNs.
> - The SLN procedure is a multidisciplinary modality based on the combination of preoperative imaging, intraoperative detection and refined histopathological analysis.
> - Radioactive colloid particles reaching the SLNs are incorporated into the macrophages by phagocytosis, thus enabling prolonged lymph node retention and imaging with lymphoscintigraphy and SPECT/CT.
> - The SLN procedure is oriented to the detection of subclinical lymph node metastases which include small macrometastases (>2 mm and <5 mm), micrometastases (>0.2 mm and <2 mm) and submicrometastases (<0.2 mm).

8.3　Image Generation with SPECT/CT

Use of SPECT/CT in this scenario is principally oriented to the anatomical localization of SLNs. This is the principal reason why SPECT/CT is acquired using a low-dose CT. The use of a diagnostic high-dose CT, with or without intravenous contrast, is not necessary because the SLN procedure primarily aims to detect subclinical metastasis in non-enlarged lymph nodes.

However, for SLN localization the CT component of SPECT/CT must be able to provide optimal anatomical information. SPECT/CT has evolved from the original devices based on a low-end slow CT scanner to a second generation of SPECT/CT gamma cameras that include an improved fast high-end CT component. This modern equipment enables the simultaneous evaluation of the lymph nodes corresponding to the radioactive nodes on fused SPECT/CT images with a low-dose CT (40 mAs). For superficial areas such as the groin and the axilla, slices of at least 5 mm are recommended. For more complex anatomical areas (head and neck, pelvis, abdomen), 2 mm slices may be necessary. With this approach, SPECT/CT imaging can accurately localize SLNs in relation to the vascular and muscular structures in deep anatomical areas.

The CT component is also used to correct the SPECT signal for tissue attenuation and scattering. After these corrections, SPECT is fused with CT [7]. A grey scale is used to display the morphology (anatomy) in the background image (CT), whereas a colour scale is used to display the SLN in the foreground anatomic image (SPECT).

The display of SPECT/CT is similar to that of conventional tomography. Multiplanar reconstruction (MPR) enables two-dimensional display of fusion images in relation to CT and SPECT. The use of cross-reference lines allows the navigation between axial, coronal and sagittal views. At the same time, this tool facilitates the correlation of radioactive SLNs seen on fused SPECT/CT with lymph nodes identified on CT. This information may be helpful for the intraoperative procedure and the post-excision control using portable gamma cameras or handheld gamma probes.

Fused SPECT/CT images may also be displayed using maximum intensity projection (MIP). MIP is a specific type of rendering in which the brightest voxels are projected into a three-dimensional image, thus allowing improved anatomical SLN localization and recognition by the surgeon. One limitation of MIP is that the presence of other high-attenuation voxels on CT may obscure the recognition of the vasculature and of other anatomical structures. Another limitation is that the MIP display is a two-dimensional representation that cannot accurately depict the actual anatomical correlates with the vessels and other structures [8].

When using volume rendering for three-dimensional display, different colours are assigned to anatomical structures such as vessels, muscle, bone and skin. This leads to obtaining of better anatomical reference points and to incorporating of an additional dimension in the recognition of SLNs. By incorporating a colour display, volume rendering improves visualization of complex anatomy and of 3D relationships (Fig. 8.1).

Key Learning Points

- Since SPECT/CT imaging is principally oriented to the localization of SLNs, its CT component must be able to provide optimal anatomical information.
- After correction for tissue attenuation and scattering, SPECT is fused with CT using a grey scale to display the morphology in the background image (CT) and with a colour scale for SLNs in the foreground image (SPECT).
- Multiplanar reconstruction (MPR) enables two-dimensional display of SPECT/CT fusion images in relation to separate CT and SPECT. The use of cross-reference lines allows the navigation between axial, coronal and sagittal views, thus facilitating the correlation of radioactive SLNs seen on fused images with lymph nodes identified on CT.
- When using volume rendering for 3D SPECT/CT display, the different colours assigned to anatomical structures such as vessels, muscle, bone and skin enable an adequate recognition of the vasculature and of other anatomical structures.

8.4 General Indications for SPECT/CT Imaging

Indications for SPECT/CT imaging in the SLN procedure depend on the type of malignancy and on the complexity of lymphatic drainage. They will also depend on the criteria adopted by surgeons and nuclear physicians in different hospitals. In general, indications for SPECT/CT in the SLN procedure are as follows:

1. Detection of SLNs in cases without visualization or with poor visualization on planar imaging [9] (Fig. 8.2): Due to the correction for tissue attenuation, SPECT/CT is usually more sensitive than planar imaging and may be particularly useful in obese patients.
2. Localization of SLNs in areas with complex anatomy and a high number of lymph nodes, such as the head and neck or in cases with unexpected lymphatic drainage (e.g. between the pectoral muscles, internal mammary chain, level II or III of the axilla, in the vicinity of the scapula) at planar imaging: Examples of unexpected patterns of lymphatic drainage in patients with various cancers are shown in Figs. 8.3, 8.4 and 8.5.
3. Anatomical localization and detection of additional SLNs in areas of deep lymphatic drainage, such as the pelvis (Fig. 8.6), abdomen or mediastinum [10].

Fig. 8.1 A 51-year-old woman with a non-palpable T1 carcinoma in the medial lower quadrant of the left breast. SPECT/CT performed 3 h after ultrasound-guided intratumoural injection of 121 MBq ^{99m}Tc-nanocolloid. The use of maximum intensity projection (MIP) generated for the area between the green lines (**a**) enables a better anatomical recognition of an internal mammary SLN at the first intercostal space (**b**). Volume rendering (**c**) allows a 3D display of the SLN and the tumour site in relation to the anatomical structures

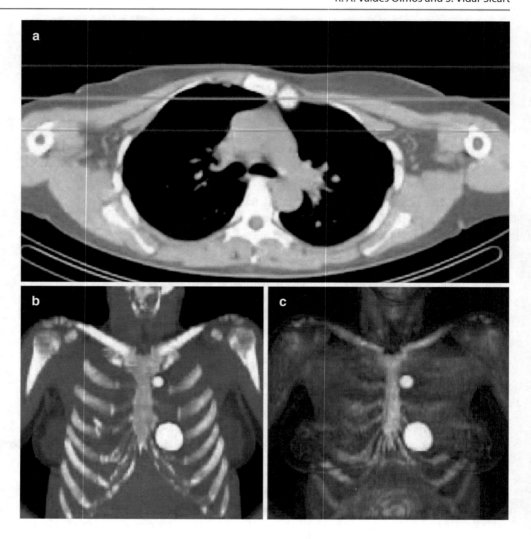

8.5   Comprehensive Interpretation of Preoperative SLN Imaging

SPECT/CT imaging does not replace planar lymphoscintigraphy, but should rather be considered as a complementary modality. In fact, SPECT/CT is intended to anatomically localize SLNs already visualized on planar imaging, although in some cases SPECT/CT can detect additional SLNs. In order to better understand the combined use of planar lymphoscintigraphy and SPECT/CT imaging, it is necessary to elucidate some issues [11]. First of all, by acquiring early and delayed planar images lymphoscintigraphy can identify SLNs in most cases. In current protocols, SPECT/CT is acquired following delayed planar imaging (mostly 2–3 h after radiocolloid administration). This sequential acquisition helps to clarify the role of both modalities. However, it

is necessary to specify the criteria for SLN identification on preoperative images. Major criteria to identify lymph nodes as SLNs are (1) the visualization of lymphatic ducts, (2) the time of appearance, (3) the lymph node basin and (4) the intensity of lymph node uptake [12]. Following these criteria, visualized radioactive lymph nodes may be classified as follows:

1. Definitely SLNs: This category includes all lymph nodes draining from the site of the primary tumour through their own lymphatic vessel, or a single radioactive lymph node in a lymph node basin [4, 11, 13].
2. Highly probable SLNs: This category includes lymph nodes appearing between the injection site and a first draining node, or nodes with increasing uptake appearing in other lymph node stations.

Fig. 8.2 A 79-year-old man with a 1.6 Breslow melanoma on the left in the back. The lateral planar image (**c**), performed after injection of 80 MBq ^{99m}Tc-nanocolloid, shows drainage to the left axilla, with visualization of various lymphatic ducts and nodes. Volume rendering (**a**) also depicts additional lymph nodes in the vicinity of the injection site. These additional SLNs are localized in subcutaneous fat and in the muscle, as seen on axial SPECT/CT and CT (**b**, **d**, **e**, **f**). All SLNs were tumour free at histopathology

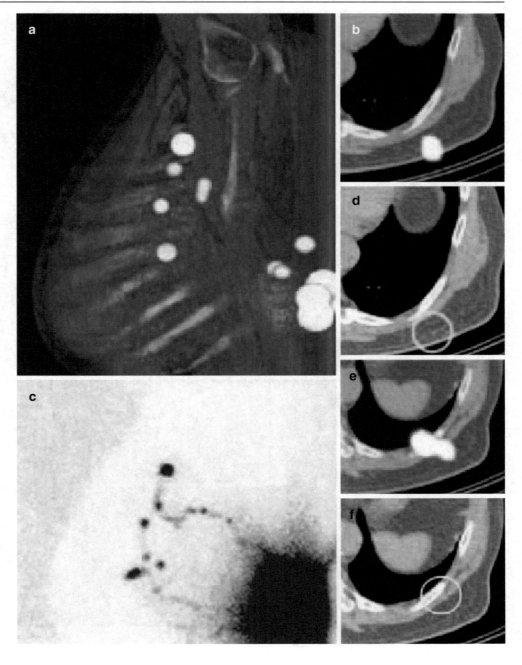

3. Less probable SLNs: All higher echelon nodes (in trunk and extremities) or lower echelon nodes (head and neck) may be included in this category.

An example of lymph nodes visualized at lymphoscintigraphy with different degrees of probability to actually be SLNs is shown in Fig. 8.7.

Early planar images are essential to identify the first draining lymph nodes as SLNs by visualization of lymphatic ducts. These nodes (category 1) can be distinguished from secondary lymph nodes (category 3), mostly appearing on delayed planar images.

In other cases a single lymph node is seen in early and/or delayed images. This lymph node is also considered as a definite SLN (category 1). However, in some cases SPECT/CT can detect additional lymph nodes in other basins. These nodes can be considered as definitely (category 1) or highly probable SLNs (category 2). Less frequently, a radioactive

Fig. 8.3 A 42-year-old woman with recurring breast cancer in the upper inner quadrant of the left breast. Eight years earlier the patient had been treated with mastectomy and left axillary dissection due to a T1N1 breast carcinoma. SPECT/CT was performed 3 h after intratumoural injection of 114 MBq ^{99m}Tc-nanocolloid. Orthogonal multiplanar reconstruction (MPR) and use of cross-reference lines, as shown in SPECT/CT and CT axial images, facilitate the localization of an internal mammary SLN on the right (**a**, **b**). Volume rendering (**c**) allows a 3D display of the contralateral drainage, with the SLN at the first intercostal space on the right. Radiocolloid accumulation into the tumour recurrence is seen in the vicinity of the prosthesis in the left breast on axial SPECT/CT (**d**) and CT (**e**)

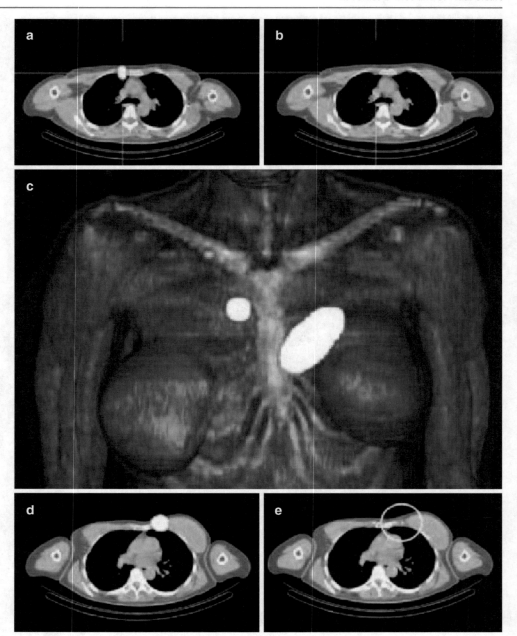

Fig. 8.4 A 60-year-old man with a T1 carcinoma of the right border of the tongue. Lymphoscintigraphy and SPECT/CT performed after injection of 84 MBq ^{99m}Tc-nanocolloid divided into four aliquots injected around the tumour. Early planar anterior image (**a**) shows bilateral drainage to both sides of the neck, with visualization of two lymph nodes with an own lymphatic duct. These two nodes are considered as definitively SLNs. A third lymph node seen in the vicinity of the injection on the left is also considered as a SLN, due to its location in a different basin. Delayed planar imaging (**b**) shows no other additional nodes. On volume rendering (**c**) and axial SPECT/CT fusion images (**d**, **e**), these SLNs, free of tumour at histopathology, are localized in levels II and III on the left and level III on the right

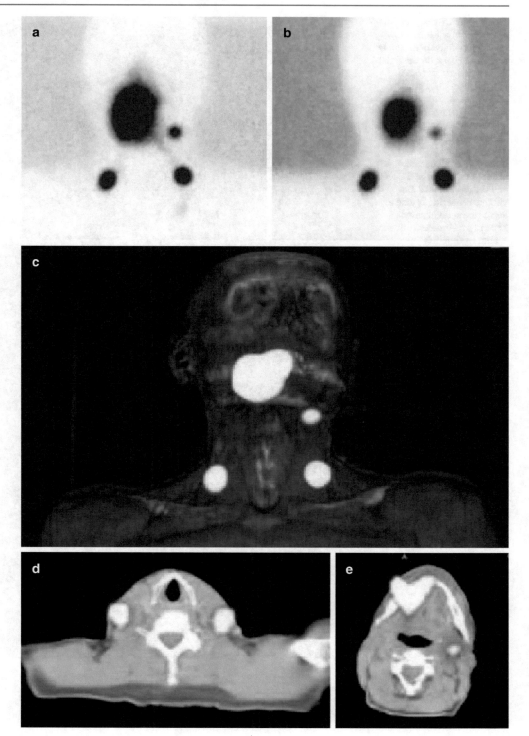

Fig. 8.5 A 15-year-old woman with a 1.9 Breslow melanoma in the periscapular area of the back on the right. A total activity of 67 MBq ^{99m}Tc-nanocolloid was administered. Volume rendering (**a**) and planar anterior image (**b**) depict drainage to both axillae and to the left supraclavicular area. The supraclavicular SLN is also seen on axial SPECT/CT and CT (**c**, **d**). Note that volume rendering is able to depict the supraclavicular node in a 3D context allowing spatial recognition

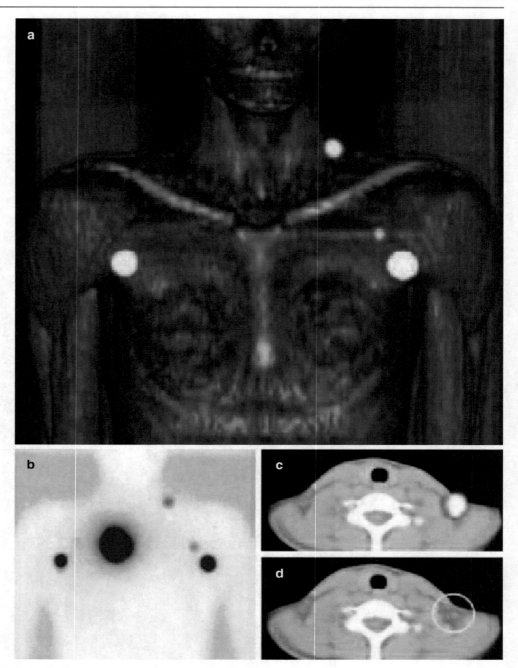

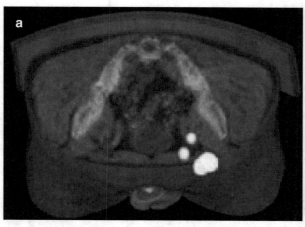
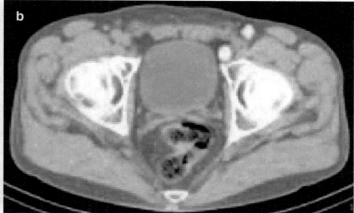

Fig. 8.6 A 59-year-old man with a 1.4 mm Breslow melanoma in the left lower area of the back. SPECT/CT performed 2 h after injection of 79 MBq ^{99m}Tc-nanocolloid. Volume rendering displayed with cranial tilt (**a**) is able to differentiate inguinal SLNs from iliac second-echelon lymph nodes in a 3D context. On the axial SPECT/CT fusion image (**b**) two of the lymph nodes are also displayed. SLNs of the groin were tumour free at histopathology

lymph node may appear between the injection site and a first draining node; its increasing uptake can confirm this node as a highly probable SLN (category 2) and it helps to differentiate this lymph node from prolonged valve activity in a lymphatic duct.

> **Key Learning Points**
> - Preoperative lymphoscintigraphy provides time sequential aspects to differentiate SLNs from higher echelon nodes.
> - SPECT/CT imaging is essential to localize SLNs in relation to anatomical landmarks (blood vessels, muscles, surgical levels).
> - SPECT/CT has an added value particularly when planar scintigraphy fails to adequately visualize the lymphatic drainage pathways.
> - Different visual criteria categorizing radioactive lymph nodes as definitely, high-probable and less probable SLNs must be considered in order to identify which lymph nodes should be removed to maximize the likelihood of harvesting the "true" SLN for pathology analysis.

8.6 SPECT/CT as a Roadmap for Intraoperative SLN Detection

The use of the scintigraphic categories defined above to characterize radioactive lymph nodes also contributes to surgical decision-making. Lymph nodes of the first two categories (definitely SLN or highly probable SLN) are the nodes recognized by the nuclear physician and subsequently marked on skin, or indicated in SPECT/CT key images. These SLNs must be removed in the operation room by the surgeon. Less probable SLNs may sometimes be removed, depending on the degree of remaining radioactivity measured by the gamma probe or the portable gamma camera during the control of the excision fossa [14].

Another important issue is the need to correlate findings of fused SPECT/CT with those of CT. In many cases radioactive SLNs correspond to single lymph nodes. However, in some cases a single radioactive focus on SPECT/CT corresponds to a cluster of lymph nodes on CT (Fig. 8.8). This preoperative information may lead to a careful post-excision control after removal of the first radioactive nodes by the surgeon, particularly for areas such as the pelvis and head and neck [14].

The continuous display of SPECT/CT images on screen in the operation room can help the surgeons in their intraoperative search, by identifying anatomical structures adjacent to the SLN. In the future, the incorporation of co-registered SPEC/CT to 3D navigation devices will probably improve these features even more.

The use of volume rendering for 3D display enables to assign different colours to different anatomical structures such as muscle, bone and skin. This configuration offers a multidimensional roadmap to the surgeon and facilitates interpretation of the SPECT/CT images.

8.7 Imaging Report Combining Planar Lymphoscintigraphy and SPECT/CT

Specific practical guidelines to generate imaging report in the SLN procedure have been recently described for oral cavity cancer [15]. This approach is applicable to all SLN

Fig. 8.7 A 64-year-old patient with a T2 carcinoma in the central area of the right breast. After intratumoural injection of 120 MBq ^{99m}Tc-nanocolloid, early drainage to the internal mammary chain is observed on planar imaging (**a**); the most caudal lymph node is considered as definitively a SLN. However, on delayed planar imaging (**b**) another lymph node in the internal mammary shows increasing uptake; this lymph node is considered as high-probable SLN. In volume-rendering (**c**) and axial SPECT/CT fusion images (**d–f**) the most cranial node of the internal mammary chain is identified as a mediastinal lymph node (**e**). This leads to considering the lymph node of the infraclavicular basin, seen in delayed planar image and SPECT/CT, also as a SLN

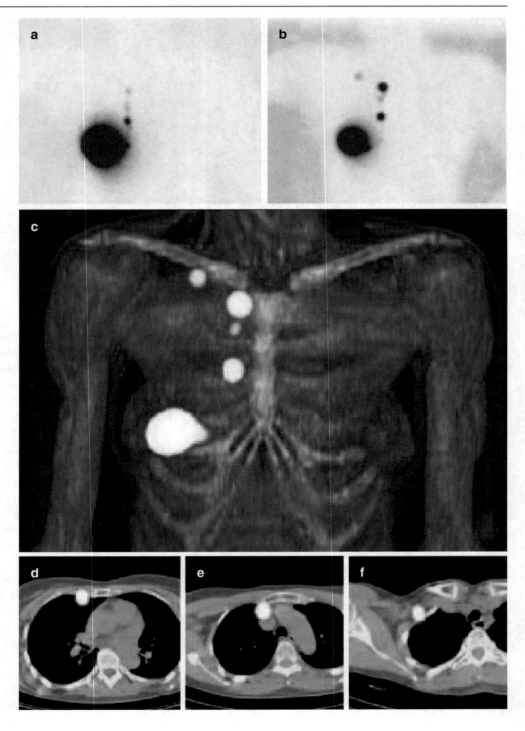

procedures and includes the description of each component of the lymphatic mapping procedure incorporating the above-mentioned criteria (Fig. 8.9).

For dynamic studies it is necessary to define and describe:

(a) Lymphatic ducts directly draining from the injection site to lymph nodes
(b) Bilateral or unilateral drainage

For early and delayed static images:

(a) Number and intensity uptake of first-echelon lymph nodes
(b) Number of second-echelon lymph nodes
(c) Additional lymph nodes appearing on delayed images in other basins

Fig. 8.8 An 84-year-old man with a 3 mm Breslow melanoma of the right cheek. SPECT/CT performed 2 h after injection of 77 MBq ^{99m}Tc-nanocolloid. Volume rendering (**a**) shows a radioactive node in level II of the neck, with drainage from the injection site through an own lymphatic vessel. In axial SPECT/CT fusion images (**b**) the radioactive node corresponds to a cluster of small lymph nodes on CT (**c**)

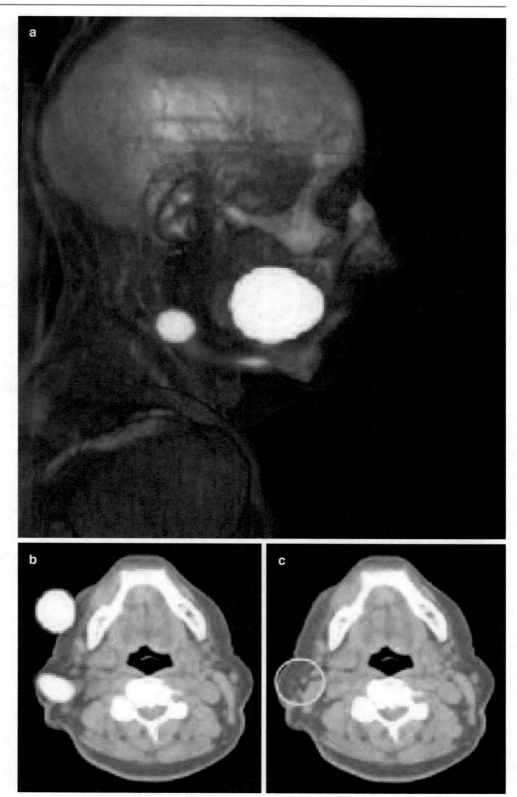

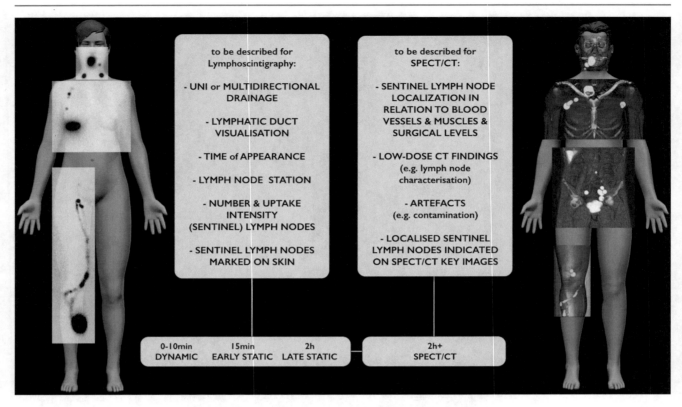

Fig. 8.9 Schematic generation of the report including a summary of key aspects for SLN mapping. For planar lymphoscintigraphy (*on the left*) examples of drainage patterns to both sides of the neck for oral cavity cancer (top), right axilla for melanoma of the flank (middle) and groin for right leg (bottom) are shown. On SPECT/CT displayed with volume rendering (*on the right*) anatomical SLN localization in neck for oral cavity cancer (top), both axillae for melanoma of the upper part of the back (middle), bilateral in pelvis for prostate cancer (middle) and right popliteal area for leg melanoma (bottom) is illustrated

For SPECT/CT imaging:

(a) Identification of additional SLNs
(b) Localization of SLNs with description of lymph node stations and reference to anatomical landmarks (vessels and muscles): Correlating fused SPECT/CT with CT images, the likelihood of a nodal cluster behind a single hot spot must be indicated
(c) Localization in reference to surgical levels (e.g. head and neck, axilla, groin) or lymph node groups (e.g. pelvis, abdomen, mediastinum)
(d) Secondary findings on low-dose non-enhanced CT including enlarged lymph nodes, cluster of lymph nodes, incidental findings and other abnormalities

The conclusion of the report must include:

- Number, uptake intensity and anatomical localization of SLNs in relation to lymph nodal groups and surgical level
- Order of appearance of lymph nodes
- Cutaneous marking with description of the localization of the SLNs

- SPECT/CT labelling based on anatomical landmarks including SLN location in reference to vessels and muscles
- Volume-rendered SPECT/CT images
- Second-echelon lymph nodes considered as low-probability SLNs

Selected key images to be uploaded to the PACS (or printed if PACS is not readily available to the multidisciplinary team) include dynamic, static and 3D SPECT/CT images, in which the SLNs are indicated.

Key Learning Points
- For the dynamic part of lymphoscintigraphy, describe if drainage is unilateral or bilateral and whether lymphatic ducts directly drain from the injection site to lymph nodes.
- For the static images of lymphoscintigraphy, indicate both the number and intensity uptake of first-echelon lymph nodes as well as the number of

second-echelon nodes and the possible appearance of additional SLNs on delayed images in other basins.

- For SPECT/CT indicate (additional) SLNs in relation to anatomical landmarks (vessels and muscles).
- Localize SLNs on SPECT/CT in relation to surgical levels (e.g. head/neck, axilla, groin) or lymph node groups (e.g. pelvis, abdomen, mediastinum).
- Correlate SPECT/CT with low-dose CT images to characterize (sentinel) lymph nodes and to estimate the likelihood of a nodal cluster behind a single hot spot.
- Select key images indicating the SLNs to upload in PACS (or printed if PACS is not readily available to the multidisciplinary team) including dynamic, static and 3D SPECT/CT images.
- Cutaneous marking with description of the localization of the SLNs will maximize the likelihood of harvesting the "true" SLN for pathology analysis.

References

1. Valdés Olmos RA, Rietbergen DDD, Vidal-Sicart S. SPECT/CT and sentinel node lymphoscintigraphy. Clin Transl Imaging. 2014;2:491–504.
2. Vidal-Sicart S, Valdés Olmos RA. Synergism of SPECT/CT and portable gamma cameras for intraoperative sentinel lymph node biopsy in melanoma, breast cancer and other malignancies. Clin Transl Imaging. 2016;5:313–27.
3. Morton DL, Wen DR, Wong JH, et al. Technical details of intraoperative lymphatic mapping for early stage melanoma. Arch Surg. 1992;127:392–9.
4. Valdés Olmos RA, Rietbergen DD, Vidal-Sicart S, et al. Contribution of SPECT/CT imaging to radioguided sentinel lymph node biopsy in breast cancer, melanoma, and other solid cancers: from "open and see" to "see and open". Q J Nucl Med Mol Imaging. 2014;58:127–39.
5. Giuliano AE, Connolly JL, Edge SB, et al. Breast cancer—Major changes in the American Joint Committee on Cancer eighth edition cancer staging manual. CA Cancer J Clin. 2017;67:290–303.
6. Brierley JD, Gospodarowicz MK, Wittekind C, editors. TNM classification of malignant tumours. 8th ed. Hoboken: Wiley-Blackwell; 2017.
7. Israel O, Pellet O, Biassoni L, et al. Two decades of SPECT/CT—the coming of age of a technology: an updated review of literature evidence. Eur J Nucl Med Mol Imaging. 2019;46:1990–2012.
8. Fishman EK, Ney DR, Heath DG, et al. Volume rendering versus maximum intensity projection in CT angiography: what works best, when, and why. Radiographics. 2006;26:905–22.
9. Jimenez-Heffernan A, Ellmann A, Sado H, et al. Results of a prospective multicenter International Atomic Energy Agency sentinel node trial on the value of SPECT/CT over planar imaging in various malignancies. J Nucl Med. 2015;56:1338–44.
10. Vermeeren L, van der Ploeg IM, Valdés Olmos RA, et al. SPECT/CT for preoperative sentinel node localization. J Surg Oncol. 2010;101:184–90.
11. Vidal-Sicart S, Valdés Olmos RA. Evaluation of the sentinel lymph node combining SPECT/CT with the planar images and its importance for the surgical act. Rev Esp Med Nucl. 2011;30:331–7.
12. Valdés Olmos RA, Vidal-Sicart S, Manca G, et al. Advances in radioguided surgery in oncology. Q J Nucl Med Mol Imaging. 2017;61:247–70.
13. Alazraki N, Glass EC, Castronovo F, et al. Procedure guideline for lymphoscintigraphy and the use of intraoperative gamma probe for sentinel lymph node localization in melanoma of intermediate thickness 1.0. J Nucl Med. 2002;43:1414–8.
14. Hellingman D, de Wit-van der Veen LJ, Klop WM, et al. Detecting near-the-injection-site sentinel nodes in head and neck melanomas with a high-resolution portable gamma camera. Clin Nucl Med. 2015;40:e11–6.
15. Giammarile F, Schilling C, Gnanasegaran G, et al. The EANM practical guidelines for sentinel lymph node localization in oral cavity squamous cell carcinoma. Eur J Nucl Med Mol Imaging. 2019;46:623–37.

Preoperative and Intraoperative Lymphatic Mapping for Radioguided Sentinel Lymph Node Biopsy in Breast Cancer

9

Lenka M. Pereira Arias-Bouda, Sergi Vidal-Sicart, and Renato A. Valdés Olmos

Contents

9.1   **Introduction** 186

9.2   **The Clinical Problem** 186

9.3   **Lymphatic Drainage of the Breast** 187

9.4   **Lymphoscintigraphy: Technical Controversies** ... 189

9.5   **Intraoperative SLN Detection in Patients with Breast Cancer** 195

9.6   **Indications and Controversies for SLN Mapping in Patients with Breast Cancer** 196

9.7   **Clinical Impact of SLNB in Breast Cancer** 200

Clinical Cases 203

References 215

Learning Objectives
- To understand the pathophysiologic basis of the sentinel lymph node (SLN) concept in breast cancer
- To acquire basic knowledge on the lymphatic drainage routes in the breast and draining lymph node stations
- To become familiar with the lymphoscintigraphy procedure in breast cancer patients concerning radiotracer type, injection procedure, and lymphatic mapping acquisition, including the indications and advantages of SPECT/CT
- To understand the differences between superficial and deep tumor-related injections including advantages, limitations, and consequences
- To become familiar with the intraoperative aspects of radioguided SLN localization procedure inside and outside the axilla aided by the use of the hand-held gamma-detecting probe
- To gain knowledge on the advantages of intraoperative usage of portable gamma cameras
- To become familiar with the clinical indications for sentinel lymph node biopsy (SLNB) in breast cancer patients
- To become aware of the benefits and risks of the SLNB procedure in other, controversial clinical situations
- To understand the pros and cons concerning the treatment of the internal mammary chain if involved, related to clinical outcome

L. M. Pereira Arias-Bouda (✉)
Department of Radiology, Section of Nuclear Medicine, Leiden University Medical Centre, Leiden, Netherlands

Department of Nuclear Medicine, Alrijne hospital, Leiderdorp, Netherlands
e-mail: L.M.Pereira_Arias-Bouda@lumc.nl

S. Vidal-Sicart
Nuclear Medicine Department, Hospital Clinic Barcelona, Barcelona, Catalonia, Spain

Institut d'Investigacions Biomèdiques August Pi Sunyer (IDIBAPS), Barcelona, Catalonia, Spain

R. A. Valdés Olmos
Department of Radiology, Section of Nuclear Medicine and Interventional Molecular Imaging Laboratory, Leiden University Medical Center, Leiden, The Netherlands

© Springer Nature Switzerland AG 2020
G. Mariani et al. (eds.), *Atlas of Lymphoscintigraphy and Sentinel Node Mapping*,
https://doi.org/10.1007/978-3-030-45296-4_9

- To understand the advantages and limitations of the SLNB procedure when applied before or after treatment in patients pretreated with chemotherapy and to gain knowledge on how to improve the accuracy of the procedure in these situations
- To become familiar with the management strategies of the axilla, related to the result of the SLN procedure

9.1 Introduction

Axillary lymph node status still is a major prognostic factor in early-stage breast cancer, providing information that is important for tailoring postsurgical treatment [1, 2].

Since imaging techniques have limited sensitivity for detecting metastases in axillary lymph nodes, the axilla must be explored surgically. Histology of all resected nodes at the time of axillary lymph node dissection (ALND) has traditionally been thought to be the most accurate method for assessing metastatic spread of disease to the locoregional lymph nodes. However, the anatomic disruption caused by ALND may result in lymphedema, nerve injury, shoulder dysfunction, and other short-term and long-term complications that may compromise function and quality of life.

SLNB is a less invasive method of assessing nodal involvement [3]. The concept of the SLN is intimately embedded in the notion that, as a consequence of the orderly pattern of lymph flow, metastatic spread of solid tumors through the lymphatic route follows a predictable pattern [4]. According to this concept, early systematic studies in breast cancer patients [5, 6] have suggested that the use of SLNB can be reliably performed in selected patients with early-stage breast cancer by a carefully trained multidisciplinary team (surgeon, pathologist, nuclear physician), thus reducing the need for ALND and avoiding the associated morbidity [6]. While nowadays the SLNB procedure is considered "standard of care" in patients with early-stage breast cancer without cytologically or histologically proven axillary lymph node metastases, controversy remains concerning its use in patients with ductal carcinoma in situ (DCIS), in patients with large or multifocal/multicentric tumors, in recurrent disease, and in the neoadjuvant setting.

With the implementation of SLNB, not only the technique itself but also the histologic processing and SLNB-based management of the axilla have evolved over time, resulting in a paradigm shift in patient management [7, 8]. In contrast to the axilla, the importance of treatment of the internal mammary nodes (IMNs) is still a highly debated issue [9].

Recent guidelines and reviews have updated the field, which encompasses a growing body of literature dealing with several aspects of the procedure, from technical modalities to immediate and long-term clinical implications [9–13].

9.2 The Clinical Problem

ALND has been an integral part of the management of breast cancer since Halsted described the radical mastectomy in the 1890s [14]. This operation was designed to achieve locoregional control in women with large locally advanced tumors metastatic to the axillary lymph nodes. Since then, breast cancer is detected earlier, with smaller tumors and less nodal involvement [15]. Since Halsted's time, operations on the breast itself have become less radical. Radical mastectomy was replaced by modified radical mastectomy, which in turn has been largely replaced by lumpectomy in patients with early breast cancer. Despite the revolution in surgery on the breast itself, ALND continued largely unchanged until the 1990s, when SLNB was first introduced [16].

Accurate lymph node staging is essential for both prognosis and treatment in patients with breast cancer. Axillary nodal status is the most important predictor of overall survival, and control of the axilla remains essential to patient well-being. Axillary dissection, however, is associated with a number of significant morbidities and complications such as seroma, infection, decreased range of motion, axillary web syndrome, shoulder pain, paresthesias, and lymphedema [17].

The SLNB procedure was introduced as a means of accurately identifying axillary metastases by removing only a few lymph nodes, usually one or two, and avoiding the complications and morbidity of ALND. The rate and severity of complications such as lymphedema and sensory loss are markedly less after SLNB compared to ALND (2% versus 13% and 12% versus 44%, respectively), while patients are dealing with less adverse effects in terms of range of motion, quality of life, and resumption of normal activities of daily life after surgery [8, 18].

Numerous prospective single-institutional and multicenter randomized controlled studies have shown the accuracy and safety of SLNB in early breast cancer [6, 19, 20]. With the increasing use of neoadjuvant chemotherapeutic agents in order to preserve the breast in patients with locally advanced cancer, a new, highly debated issue is the appropriate timing of the SLNB, pre- or post-neoadjuvant chemotherapy [21].

SLNB has radically changed the management of the axilla for patients with early breast cancer. After more than a century, axillary management has finally changed to a less morbid and less radical approach. Patients have far fewer complications after SLNB alone than they do after ALND, and quality of life and time missed from the activities of daily living are markedly improved with this less radical operation.

Key Learning Points
- Axillary nodal status is the most important predictor of overall survival.
- Accurate lymph node staging is essential for both prognosis and treatment in patients with breast cancer.
- Axillary lymph node dissection is associated with significant morbidity and complications.
- The SLNB procedure can accurately identify axillary metastases while avoiding the complications and morbidity of axillary dissection.
- SLNB has radically altered the management of the axilla for patients with early breast cancer with fewer complications and better quality of life than ALND.

9.3 Lymphatic Drainage of the Breast

9.3.1 Lymphatic System of the Breast

Anatomical knowledge of the breast lymphatics is primarily derived from the work of Sappey in the 1850s. Sappey identified two groups of lymphatic vessels with extensive interconnections: one group draining the superficial aspect of the breast, primarily the skin and subcutaneous tissue, while a deep lymphatic vessel group draining the gland itself to a subareolar

plexus, which in turn drains to the axilla [22]. Subsequent and more contemporary studies of breast lymphatics involved not only postmortem injections, but also metastatic routes and, more recently, lymphangiography and lymphoscintigraphy. Suami and coworkers investigated the lymph drainage of the breast in cadavers and found no evidence of a centripetal lymphatic pathway to a subareolar plexus; instead, their study showed that different areas of the breast frequently drained to different lymph nodes [23]. This finding has been supported by clinical studies involving lymphoscintigraphy using tumor-related injections (see below) [24–26].

9.3.2 Draining Lymph Node Stations

The breast drains to lymph nodes at different sites. Most of the breast lymph drains to the axilla. A subareolar plexus-related injection will not identify sites of metastases outside the axilla. In fact, a subareolar plexus-related injection rarely identifies lymphatic drainage to the internal mammary, parasternal, or intramammary lymph nodes. Posterior to the breast parenchyma itself is a second plexus in the retromammary space, which drains not only to the axilla, but also to the internal mammary chain as well as to the intercostal and diaphragmatic lymph nodes. Drainage to the internal mammary basin occurs in 20% of patients after intratumoral or peritumoral radiocolloid injection. Other unusually located SLNs are also seen in a non-negligible fraction of patients: intramammary (pre-pectoral) in 6%, inter-pectoral in 2%, and infraclavicular (axilla level III) in 3% [27]. There is overlap of drainage areas and extensive anastomoses of the lymphatics of the breast [28]. In each quadrant, a breast cancer may drain to SLNs in various locations [24] (Fig. 9.1). When drainage to the internal mammary chain occurs, most

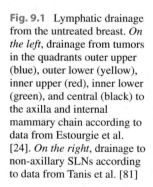

Fig. 9.1 Lymphatic drainage from the untreated breast. *On the left*, drainage from tumors in the quadrants outer upper (blue), outer lower (yellow), inner upper (red), inner lower (green), and central (black) to the axilla and internal mammary chain according to data from Estourgie et al. [24]. *On the right*, drainage to non-axillary SLNs according to data from Tanis et al. [81]

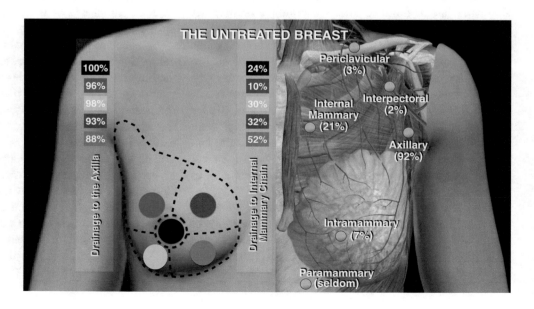

Fig. 9.2 Lymphatic drainage from malignant tumors in the untreated breast. *On the right*, drainage to the internal mammary chain according to data from Estourgie et al. [24] showing most frequent drainage to SLNs in the second, third, and fourth intercostal spaces. *On the left*, drainage to the axilla according to data from Uren et al. [29] with level I (89%) and II as the most frequent SLN sites

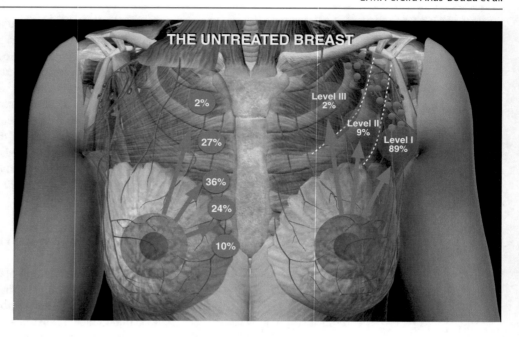

SLNs are found in the second, third, and fourth intercostal spaces (Fig. 9.2).

There are three groups of axillary nodes, arbitrarily defined by their anatomic relationship to the pectoralis major and minor muscles. These nodes are caudal to the axillary vein. Level I lymph nodes extend from the lateral edge of the pectoralis major muscle to the lateral edge of the pectoralis minor muscle. Level II lymph nodes are those directly posterior to the pectoralis minor muscle, and level III are the lymph nodes medial to the medial border of the pectoralis minor muscle and extending to the Halsted's ligament at the chest wall. There are very few lymph nodes in level III.

Within level I, there are a number of nodal groups. The external mammary lymph node group runs parallel and along the lateral thoracic artery, draining primarily the lateral breast. The lateral axillary vein group is located posteriorly along the anterior border of the latissimus dorsi and contains the largest amount of nodal tissue. The subscapular nodal group runs parallel to the scapular vessels and drains the lower posterior neck, posterior trunk, and posterior shoulder as well as the breast. The axillary vein group medial and posterior to the axillary vein receives drainage primarily from the upper extremity and not the breast. Axillary dissections for breast cancer should not routinely remove tissue posterior or superior to the axillary vein.

Level II nodes may receive lymphatic drainage directly from the breast, but also drainage from afferent vessels of level I nodes. Level III lymph nodes are the most medial nodal group in the axilla, which not only drain the other axillary nodal groups, but also merge with lymphatic vessels

from the subclavicular group and form the subclavian trunk. Rotter's lymph nodes are located between the pectoralis major and minor muscles. Some lymphatics from the retro-mammary plexus penetrate the pectoralis major muscle and travel along the thoracoacromial vessel, terminating directly in level III. Superior and medial aspects of the breast may also drain directly to level III. However, isolated nodal metastases are rarely seen in level III nodes without extensive involvement of the level I and level II lymph nodes. For this reason, most surgeons perform a level I and level II axillary dissection without removing level III, unless palpable lymph nodes are encountered or there is extensive nodal disease in the first two levels. SLNs are encountered primarily in level I, less so in level II, and rarely in level III [29] (Fig. 9.2). Good exposure of level III lymph nodes often requires partial or full transection of the pectoralis minor muscle.

Lymph nodes of the internal mammary chain (IMNs) primarily drain the posterocentral and posteromedial aspects of the breast. Usually nodal metastases are seen in the internal mammary chain only when there are concomitant axillary metastases. Only about 3–5% of the patients have nodal metastases identified in the internal mammary SLN without axillary involvement.

The ipsilateral supraclavicular nodal metastases are no longer considered stage IV disease in the American Joint Commission on Cancer (AJCC) Staging System, because of the direct drainage of the upper inner portion of the breast to the supraclavicular nodes. Involvement of these lymph nodes results in classification of these patients as AJCC nodal stage N3. IMN metastases result in classification as N1, N2, or N3 [30].

Key Learning Points

- There is no evidence of a centripetal lymphatic pathway to a subareolar plexus as proposed by Sappey; instead, most of the lymph from the breast flows toward the nodal basins with a direct course.
- There are three groups of axillary lymph nodes, defined by their anatomic relationship to the pectoralis major and minor muscles: levels I, II, and III.
- SLNs are encountered primarily in level I, less so in level II, and rarely in level III.
- Drainage to the internal mammary basin occurs in 20% of patients after intratumoral or peritumoral radiocolloid injection with 3–5% of the patients having nodal metastases identified in the internal mammary SLN without axillary involvement.
- Ipsilateral supraclavicular nodal metastases are no longer considered stage IV disease in the AJCC Staging System, because of the direct drainage of the upper inner portion of the breast to the supraclavicular nodes.

9.4 Lymphoscintigraphy: Technical Controversies

Although SLNB is widely employed in patients with breast cancer, several technical issues remain unresolved. The main areas of controversy concern the radiopharmaceuticals to be used, the site and mode of radiocolloid injection, and the use of preoperative imaging with or without SPECT/CT imaging.

9.4.1 Radiopharmaceuticals

Three types of radiocolloid preparations are commonly used for lymphoscintigraphy and intraoperative identification of the SLN with a handheld γ-probe. ^{99m}Tc-sulfur colloid is the most commonly used agent in the United States, either unfiltered (particle size about 15–5000 nm) or filtered (particle size depending on the filter employed, usually 220 nm). Most European investigators use a ^{99m}Tc-nanocolloidal preparation of human serum albumin with particles ranging in size between 4 and about 100 nm (95% of the particles being <80 nm). At present, this radiopharmaceutical offers the best range of particle size, approaching the ideal range, and offers the additional benefits of instant labeling at room temperature and stability both in vitro and in vivo. ^{99m}Tc-antimony trisulfide (3–30 nm) is commercially available in Australia

and Canada, where it is widely used for SLN procedures [31].

It is generally considered that a radiocolloid with most of the particles ranging in size between 100 and 200 nm represents a practical compromise between fast and efficient lymphatic drainage from the site of interstitial injection and satisfactory retention in the SLN. The activity of the radiotracer depends on the timing of surgery relative to lymphoscintigraphy, with an approximate amount of 37–111 MBq (1–3 mCi).

A novel radiopharmaceutical has been approved in 2013 for lymphatic mapping, ^{99m}Tc-tilmanocept (Lymphoseek®) [32]; Lymphoseek® accumulates in lymphatic tissue by binding to a receptor on the surface of macrophage cells within LNs. Due to its properties, Lymphoseek® has faster clearance from the injection site, prolonged retention in SLNs, and a smaller amount of excised lymphatic nodes than ^{99m}Tc-sulfur colloid [32–34]. Although Lymphoseek® appears to have all the desired properties for SLN mapping, the low yield of excised lymph nodes could become an unfavorable factor in this new era in which the approach toward management of limited metastatic SLN disease in the axilla has changed (see below).

9.4.2 Radiocolloid Injection for SLN Mapping in Patients with Breast Cancer

No consensus exists on the optimal injection approach. Widely applied techniques include tumor-related injections (intratumoral or peritumoral) and superficial injections (intradermal, subdermal, subareolar, and periareolar) (Fig. 9.3).

Direct intratumoral injection has originally represented a natural extension of the technique developed earlier with vital blue dye [35]. For intratumoral and peritumoral administration, the radiocolloid is injected into the tumor or in a site immediately adjacent to the tumor, in the space with a supposedly normal lymphatic system that is the only possible drainage pathway for fluids, particles, and cells leaving the tumor through the extravascular route. Although in most centers such intra- or peritumoral injections are directed simply by palpation, it is advisable to inject the tracer under sonographic guidance (or stereotactic devices).

The likelihood of visualizing a lymphatic duct and a draining lymph node increases when the radiocolloid is injected in the skin overlying the mammary gland (subdermal/intradermal injection) [36]. Therefore, axillary SLNs can be efficiently visualized as early as 20–30 min after intradermal injection of radiocolloid (versus 30–40 min for the peritumoral and 40–60 min for the intratumoral routes of

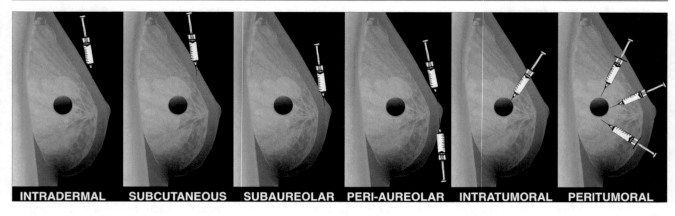

| INTRADERMAL | SUBCUTANEOUS | SUBAUREOLAR | PERI-AUREOLAR | INTRATUMORAL | PERITUMORAL |

Fig. 9.3 Radiotracer administration modalities for SLN mapping illustrating superficial (first four images) and deep (last two images) injection options

administration), thus making the entire lymphoscintigraphic procedure highly practicable.

Finally, periareolar/subareolar radiocolloid injection [37] is based on the presence of a lymphatic plexus around each lobule of the mammary gland that follows the path of the galactophore ducts, converging to the areola to form the Sappey subareolar plexus, which is part of the general subcutaneous plexus.

As mentioned above, any drainage pattern from any quadrant of the breast can occur, and most of the lymph from the breast flows toward the nodal basins with a direct course, not necessarily passing through the subareolar plexus [23, 24, 28]. These variations in lymphatic drainage of the breast have important implications for the performance of lymphoscintigraphy (Fig. 9.4). Superficial injections will result in primarily axillary nodal drainage. Injection at the level of the tumor in the breast or more posteriorly can identify internal mammary, supraclavicular, or even intramammary SLNs.

Although some have suggested that the site of injection does not necessarily affect the accuracy of axillary SLN detection [38], conflicting results have been published. Noushi and coworkers found a high level of discordance in the localization of SLNs after performing both lymphoscintigraphy using a superficial injection and repeated lymphatic mapping after a tumor-related injection in the same patient. The discordance rate in the axilla and internal mammary chain was 21% and 39%, respectively; the overall discordance rate in this study of 39 patients was quite high, 59% [26]. A second clinical study investigated whether lymphoscintigraphy after intralesional injection in two separate tumors in the same breast of patients with multifocal/multicentric disease yielded additional SLNs compared to intralesional injection of only the largest tumor; they found a high incidence of additional SLNs draining from tumors other than the largest one, mainly in

the axilla [25], which is in line with the investigations by Noushi and coworkers. However, in only 2 out of 50 patients studied, metastatic disease was found in the additional SLNs only, so the clinical implication of these discrepancies is not yet clear.

As mentioned before, the peritumoral, intraparenchymal route of radiocolloid injection results in a high rate of visualization of SLNs in the internal mammary chain, an occurrence reported in an average 20% of the patients, with a maximum of about 30% [39]. Although the long-term clinical impact of identifying pathways of lymphatic drainage to the internal mammary chain in patients with early breast cancer is still unclear (see further below), this finding is a definite plus of the peritumoral administration route when one compares its merits with those of the superficial injection technique. On the contrary, advantages of the superficial injection technique are represented by its high practicability with minimum training, small volume administered as a single injection, fast visualization of lymphatic drainage pathways, and a high SLN detection rate.

Choosing the optimal approach depends on the aim of the lymphatic mapping in the individual patient [28]; in patients at low risk for lymph node metastases, especially with small and/or superficially located tumors in the upper lateral quadrant of the breast in whom the purpose is to spare an unnecessary ALND, a superficial injection technique may be adequate. On the contrary, in high-risk patients with large or multifocal tumors or tumors located deep or medio-caudally in the mammary gland, in whom the purpose of lymphatic mapping is to determine the stage as accurately as possible and to identify also SLNs outside the axilla, a tumor-related injection technique may be more appropriate. Another reasonable approach is to combine both injection techniques (deep and superficial), which may improve SLN detection and decrease false-negative findings.

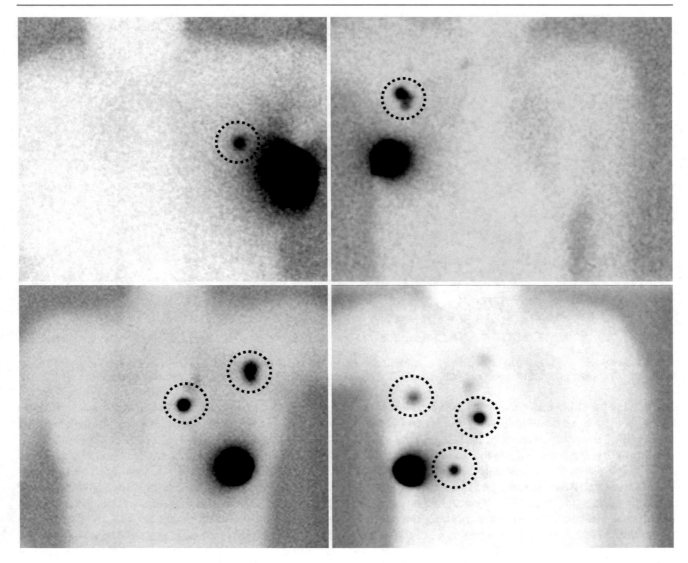

Fig. 9.4 Patterns of radiocolloid migration from untreated breast cancer to SLNs (circles) with a single axillary lymph node (*left above*), two axillary nodes (*right above*), single nodes in axilla and internal mammary chain (*left bottom*), and single axillary, internal mammary, and intramammary SLNs (*right bottom*)

9.4.3 Preoperative Imaging for SLN Mapping in Patients with Breast Cancer

The addition of a radiotracer to the lymphatic mapping procedure with blue dye has transformed lymphoscintigraphy into a visual roadmap for surgeons. This preoperative imaging is essential to determine which lymph nodes should be considered as a SLN and to identify unpredictable lymph drainage patterns leading to SLNs in unusual drainage areas, improving the accuracy and reducing morbidity relative to γ-probing alone [40].

There is general consensus on how to perform lymphoscintigraphic acquisitions for SLN identification. The energy setting of the gamma camera should be centered on the 140 keV emission peak of ^{99m}Tc, with a ±5% window. The use of a low-energy (ultra-)high-resolution collimator and an acquisition matrix of 256 × 256 pixels is highly recommended. Large-field-of-view gamma cameras are useful to depict the lymphoscintigraphic pattern of the entire lymphatic basin in a single image.

Planar static images are acquired 15–30 min and 2–4 h after injection, and if necessary in case of non-visualization after 18–24 h as well. At each acquisition time point at least two or three images are acquired: anterior, lateral, and 45° anterior oblique. The use of radioactive flood sources (^{57}Co or ^{99m}Tc) helps to provide a basic anatomical reference, especially when SPECT/CT is not performed or available (Fig. 9.5). A final, integral phase of lymphoscintigraphy is to mark the exact position of the

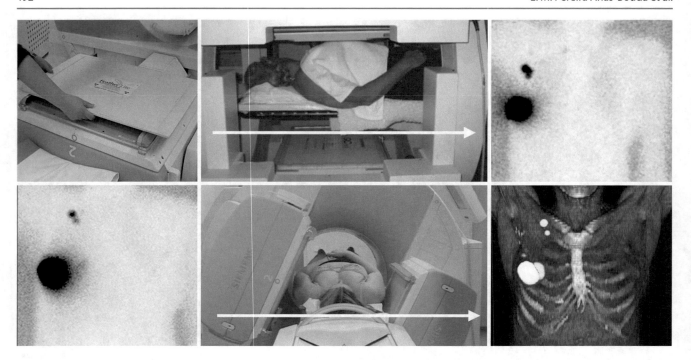

Fig. 9.5 Incorporation of anatomical aspects to preoperative SLN mapping in breast cancer. A ^{57}Co flat source, placed under the patient's trunk, provides body contour information (upper row) whereas SPECT/CT incorporates more specific anatomical landmarks (lower row)

SLNs using indelible ink, either with the aid of a radioactive point source or preferably using the probe (or both) for counting the axilla externally, focusing on the spot(s) visualized by lymphoscintigraphy. In this topographic localization phase, the arm should be abducted at about 90°, approximately in the same position as on the operating table during surgery, to identify accurate topographic coordinates that the surgeon can use during the surgical procedure. Marking the skin projection of the SLN and having the images available may assist the surgeon in reducing the operating time to locate the SLN, thus keeping the surgical incision to a minimum (Fig. 9.6).

9.4.4 Contribution of SPECT/CT Imaging for SLN Mapping in Patients with Breast Cancer

With the new generation of large-field gamma cameras, hybrid SPECT/CT has been incorporated in the SLN procedure. The functional information provided by SPECT can be combined with the morphological information provided by CT by employing such hybrid imaging in a single session. The fused SPECT/CT images depict the SLNs (visualized by lymphoscintigraphy) in an anatomical landscape, thus providing additional helpful roadmaps for surgeons. In recent years, SPECT/CT has been used in breast cancer patients with unusual or complex drainage, for example in patients with lymphatic drainage outside the axilla [41]. SPECT/CT

imaging can also visualize SLNs within the axilla when no nodes are visualized by planar imaging (including lateral images after breast displacement or with hanging breast) or if high activity at the injection site masks adjacent lymph nodes (Fig. 9.7). SPECT/CT also helps to identify SLNs in case of inconclusive planar images and especially when SLNs appear to be located in uncommon sites (Fig. 9.8). Table 9.1 gives an overview of the overall advantages of SPECT/CT versus planar imaging during lymphoscintigraphy in breast cancer [41–43]. SPECT/CT is principally oriented to the anatomical localization of SLNs, by acquiring a low-dose CT. For SLN localization, the CT component of SPECT/CT must provide optimal anatomical information. For superficial areas such as the axilla, 5 mm slices are recommended. The CT component is also used to correct the SPECT signal for tissue attenuation and scattering. After these corrections, SPECT is fused with CT [41].

A gray scale is used to display the anatomic information in the background image (CT), whereas a color scale is used to depict lymphoscintigraphic mapping in the foreground image (SPECT). Multiplanar reconstruction (MPR) enables two-dimensional display of fusion images in relation to CT and SPECT. The use of cross-reference lines allows the navigation between axial, coronal, and sagittal views. At the same time, this procedure enables to correlate radioactive SLNs seen on fused SPECT/CT images with lymph nodes seen on the CT portion. This information may be helpful for the intraoperative procedure, as well as for post-excision control using portable gamma cameras or

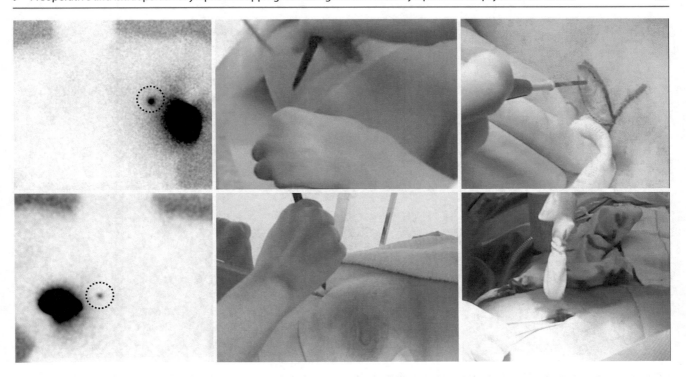

Fig. 9.6 Importance of cutaneous marking during preoperative imaging to guide skin incision in the operating room for SLNs (circles) in the left axilla (upper row) and right internal mammary chain (lower row)

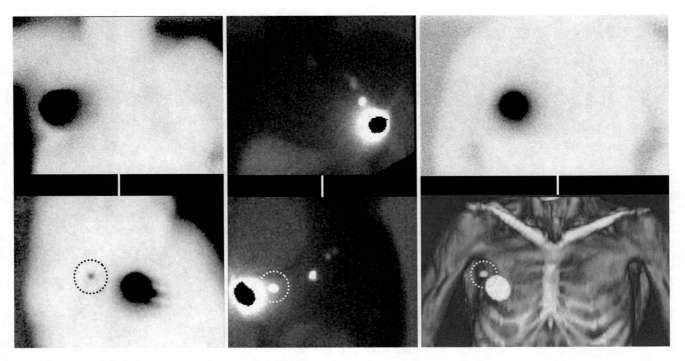

Fig. 9.7 Intervention possibilities (lower row) to depict no visualized SLNs (circles) during standard lymphoscintigraphy (upper row): in the right axilla by means of displacement of the breast with the opposite hand of the patient (left column), left intramammary by means of additional hanging breast patient position (middle column) and right axillary by means of SPECT/CT (right column)

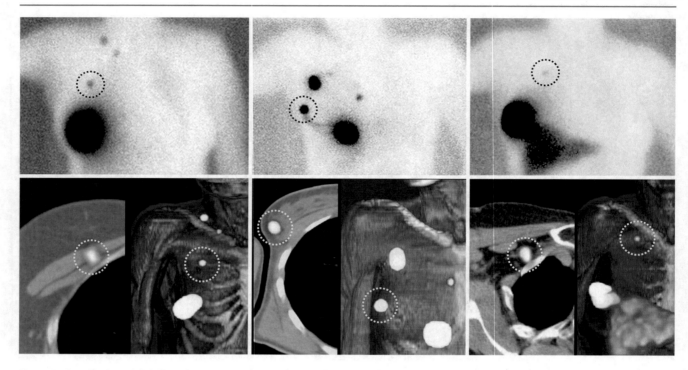

Fig. 9.8 Contribution of SPECT/CT to anatomically localize SLNs (circles) in cases with interpectoral (left column), intramammary (middle column), and axillary level III (right column) lymphatic drainage

Table 9.1 Advantages of SPECT/CT imaging versus planar imaging in breast cancer

1. Improved anatomical localization of SLNs, especially outside the axilla
2. Improved recognition of non-lymph node radiocolloid accumulation
3. Improved characterization of equivocal findings
4. Greater sensitivity, resulting in detection of additional SLNs
5. Greater specificity, resulting in fewer false-positive findings

Adapted from Ref [42]

probes. The use of 3D volume rendering enables identification of better anatomical reference points and incorporates an additional dimension in the recognition of SLNs (Fig. 9.8).

Key Learning Points

- A radiocolloid with particles ranging in size between 100 and 200 nm represents a practical compromise between fast and efficient lymphatic drainage and satisfactory retention in the SLN.
- ^{99m}Tc-tilmanocept (Lymphoseek®) is a new radio-tracer for lymphatic mapping with faster clearance from the injection site and prolonged retention in SLNs compared to conventional radiocolloid tracers.
- Variations in lymphatic drainage of the breast have important implications for the performance of lymphoscintigraphy: a subareolar plexus-related injection rarely identifies SLNs outside the axilla.
- In patients at low risk for lymph node metastases a superficial injection technique may be adequate, while in high-risk patients in whom the purpose of lymphatic mapping is to determine the stage as accurately as possible, a tumor-related injection technique may be more appropriate.
- Preoperative imaging is essential to determine which lymph nodes should be considered as a SLN and to identify unpredictable lymph drainage patterns.
- The addition of SPECT/CT to standard lymphoscintigraphy is indicated in specific situations, such as in cases of unusual or complex drainage or non-visualization of SLNs at planar imaging or when the injection site masks adjacent lymph nodes.

9.5 Intraoperative SLN Detection in Patients with Breast Cancer

After positioning the patient on the operating table before starting the surgical procedure, location of the SLNs should be confirmed further by external counting with the γ-probe. Minor variations in the sequence of operating procedures exist: some surgeons remove the primary tumor first and then proceed to perform SLNB, whereas other surgeons perform SLNB first and then proceed to remove the tumor while waiting for the results of intraoperative frozen section histopathology, although routine intraoperative pathologic assessment has become unnecessary and less indicated after the appearance of large trial results showing that ALND is not indicated in all patients with positive SLNs (see below).

In most recent reports, the overall success rate of lymphoscintigraphy for SLN identification is very high, around 95%. Usually the radioguided procedure is combined with blue dye, using the blue dye in the lymphatics as a roadmap helping to find the radioactive SLN, especially when a non-involved lymph node is only few millimeters in diameter and very soft to palpation. A γ-probe-guided search of the SLN is based on detecting a focal spot of radioactivity accumulation in the area of interest (open surgical field). The probe is now in direct contact with the hot spot and is adequately shielded from radiation scattered from the injection site.

Thus, counting rates change almost instantly from tens or hundreds of counts per second to nearly zero (as the patient's background virtually corresponds to room background) when moving the detector—for instance, simply changing the angle—from the hot spot (lymph node) to nearby tissues. Therefore, the concept of target-to-background ratio as commonly used for in vivo nuclear medicine procedures takes on a new meaning; typically, the ratio of counts in the hot spot relative to background is in the 10–100 range, though with wide variations depending on the activity injected, type of radiocolloid injected, time elapsed between radiocolloid injection and surgery, and type of γ-probe used.

Reexamination of the operative site should then be performed to ensure that the area of focal radioactivity accumulation has been removed and that a second lymph node is not also active; if this is the case, such lymph node should also be removed and the axilla reexamined. Complete removal of the SLNs is confirmed by reduction of the counting rate in the axilla to background levels. Reduction of the activity to 10–20% of the counting rate in the most active SLN is commonly accepted as background level [44, 45].

9.5.1 Combining Existent Technologies with New Modalities for SLN Mapping in Patients with Breast Cancer

Although high identification rates are achieved using the combination of dye and γ-probe, together with optimal preoperative imaging including SPECT/CT when indicated, intraoperative detection can be further improved using portable imaging devices, such as portable gamma cameras, freehand SPECT, and hybrid approaches (Fig. 9.9). This is especially helpful in case of complex drainage, deep-seated lymph nodes or when lymph nodes are located close to the injection site [46, 47].

Appropriate perioperative use of a portable gamma camera enhances the reliability of the SLNB, by providing high-resolution imaging of the surgical field. The use of these techniques implies the possibility to better plan the surgical approach, to localize surgical targets just before making the surgical incision, to monitor the lymphatic basin before and after removal of the SLNs, and, above all, to verify completeness of SLNB.

The freehand SPECT-based device integrates a positioning system attached to the conventional gamma probe and permits a virtual reconstruction in a 3D environment [47]. This 3D information may be further used for precise localization and targeting of radioactive SLNs. The device can ensure permanent assistance and transparent documentation of soft-tissue removal during surgery. Although the contribution of these new portable devices in breast cancer surgery is still unclear, they definitely will play an increasing role in the future within the evolving GOSTT (guided intraoperative scintigraphic tumor targeting) concept.

The use of hybrid tracers has been shown to improve further the accuracy of lymphatic mapping and SLN localization. A hybrid compound has been developed combining ^{99m}Tc-albumin nanocolloid with indocyanine green (ICG) [48]. In contrast to single-fluorescent agents [49], this bimodal tracer procedure may allow the surgeons to integrate the standard approach based on radioguided detection with a portable gamma camera with a new optical modality based on fluorescent signal detection. This approach is being successfully applied in various malignancies with promising results; it makes the SLNB procedure more accurate and independent of the use of blue dye [50], although its role in breast cancer still needs to be elucidated.

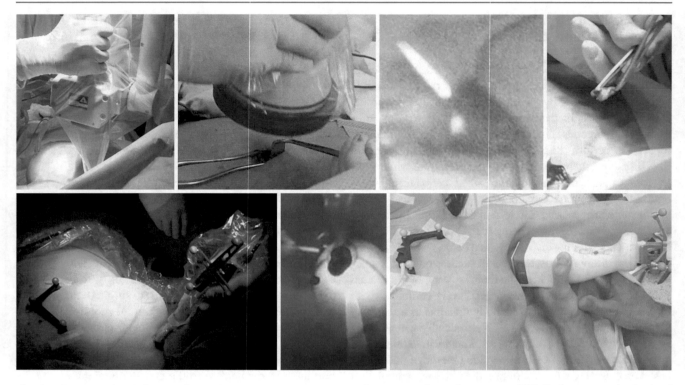

Fig. 9.9 Intraoperative SLN procedure using new modalities. The images of the *upper row* illustrate the hybrid approach following administration of ICG-^{99m}Tc-nanocolloid, which enables the combination of a portable gamma camera with a fluorescence camera to localize and remove an internal mammary SLN. In *lower row*, the freehand SPECT technology using a tracked gamma probe (left image) or hand-held gamma camera (right image) to generate an augmented reality navigation protocol for breast radioguided surgery

Key Learning Points
- The overall success rate of lymphoscintigraphy in SLN identification is very high, around 95%.
- The radioguided procedure is frequently combined with blue dye, using the blue dye in the lymphatics as a roadmap helping to find the radioactive SLN.
- Complete removal of the SLNs is confirmed by reduction of the counting rate in the axilla to background levels.
- Reduction of the activity to 10–20% of the counting rate in the most active SLN is commonly accepted as background level.
- Intraoperative detection of SLNs may be further improved using portable gamma cameras and freehand SPECT cameras and/or hybrid radiofluorescent tracers, although their role in breast cancer patients needs to be elucidated.

9.6   Indications and Controversies for SLN Mapping in Patients with Breast Cancer

There is general consensus that the SLNB procedure is indicated in patients with early-stage breast cancer (cT1-2 tumors) without cytological or histological evidence of axillary lymph node metastases; SLNB is contraindicated in patients with inflammatory breast cancer.

9.6.1   Pregnancy

The international guidelines concerning the use of lymphatic mapping in pregnant and/or lactating women are inconsistent; while the ASCO guidelines do not recommend SLNB in pregnant women, the EANM and SNMMI guidelines state that SLNB is justified in these women by the low risks of the procedure relative to the risks of axillary dissection. However, vital blue dye should only be included if there is a clear medical need to do so.

9.6.2   Internal Mammary Chain

Although, like the axilla, the IMN are a first-echelon nodal drainage site, the importance of its treatment has long been debated in breast cancer. Parasternal recurrences are uncommon and studies in the past have failed to demonstrate a survival benefit from IMN treatment. However, more recent studies provided evidence that lymphatic drainage toward the internal mammary chain is associated with a worse disease-free survival (DFS) [51]. The results of the Early Breast Cancer Trialists' Collaborative Group (EBCTCG) established the importance of locoregional control (including the internal mammary chain) on long-term survival even when systemic therapy is given [52]. Large randomized trials have demonstrated a limited but significant improvement in DFS, metastatic-free survival (MFS), and to a smaller extent overall survival (OS), when additional regional radiotherapy was applied on the IMNs and medial supraclavicular nodes in patients with increased risk for IMN metastases [53].

Hence, this suggests that besides patients with macroscopic disease in these lymph nodes, a selective group of breast cancer patients at high risk for subclinical involvement of the internal mammary chain might also benefit from parasternal irradiation, for example in patients with proven metastatic axillary SLNs in combination with parasternal lymphatic drainage identified on lymphoscintigraphy. Other recent studies have also led to renewed interest in IMN staging, regarding particularly its implications for systemic therapy. Madsen and coworkers found that patients with metastatic IMNs without axillary involvement tended to have a significantly worse outcome than patients with no regional lymph node metastases at all [54]. Therefore, the development of the SLNB aided by lymphoscintigraphy, providing a less invasive method of assessing the IMNs than surgical dissection, may affect decisions regarding not only locoregional treatment, but also systemic therapy. In this regard, one could plead for performing lymphoscintigraphy with tumor-related injections only, since the rate of parasternal drainage reflects the method of tracer injection used.

9.6.3   Large and Multifocal/Multicentric Breast Cancers

The application of SLNB in T3–T4 tumors and multifocal disease is controversial. The debate is related to the lack of consensus on the drainage routes in the breast. If drainage from any site of the breast would pass the sub-areolar plexus, the presence of more than one tumor or a large tumor would not affect the accuracy of the SLN procedure when a single (superficial) injection is performed. However, if multiple drainage routes exist, this actually would theoretically affect the accuracy and could lead to a higher false-negative rate, which is undesirable considering that multifocality and multicentricity are associated with a higher rate of lymph node metastases, as is the case in large tumors. Studies addressing this issue show heterogenic results, with false-negative rates ranging from 4 to 14% [55–57]. Moreover, application of multiple tumor-related injections in patients with multiple tumors in the breast leads to a significant amount of additional SLNs after the second injection: 64% in the study of Brouwer and coworkers [25]. However, in only 4% of these patients, metastatic disease was found in the additional SLNs only, so the clinical implication of these discrepancies is not yet clear. In summary, one should be aware of the fact that the accuracy of the SLN procedure in multifocal disease is probably lower, while these patients have a higher risk of lymph node metastases, which has to be weighed up against the benefits of SLNB in the individual patient.

9.6.4   Ductal Carcinoma In Situ

Ductal carcinoma in situ (DCIS) is an intraductal proliferation of malignant cells, without invasion of the stroma, and is considered as a precursor of invasive ductal carcinoma. Still, in one out of four patients upstaging to micro-invasion or invasion cancer occurs after surgery [58], leading to unexpected lymph node metastases in 10% of patients with pure DCIS in the biopsy specimen (macro-metastases in 2.4%). The strongest predictor for lymph node metastases is occult invasion; other risk factors include a lesion >2–2.5 cm, palpable DCIS lesion, high-grade DCIS, contrast enhancement on MRI, and age >55 years [58, 59].

Although SLNB should not be considered a standard procedure in the treatment of all patients with DCIS, it should be considered if risk factors for lymph node metastases are present, independent of the type of surgery (breast conserving or mastectomy).

Fig. 9.10 Lymphatic drainage from the treated breast according to data from van der Ploeg et al. [62] showing increased SLN visualization outside the ipsilateral axilla

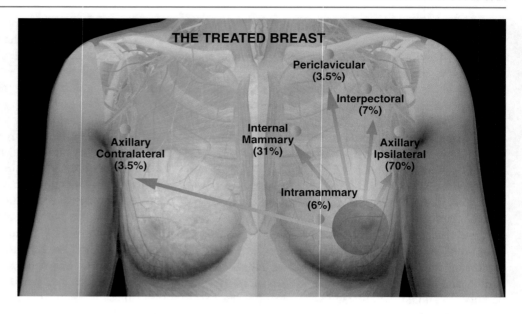

9.6.5 Recurrent Disease and SLN Mapping in Patients with Breast Cancer

Use of SLNB in patients with recurrent disease has been a debated issue, related to the consideration that the lymph drainage pathways may be disrupted by previous SLNB and therapy, presumably leading to a less reliable SLN procedure. However, based on the data of a recent meta-analysis in 1053 patients, it may be concluded that SLNB in these patients, on the contrary, is feasible. The investigators reported a SLN identification rate of 63% on lymphoscintigraphy and 60% at surgery; since metastatic disease in SLNs was found in 10% of patients, ALND could be avoided in approximately 500 of the patients studied (50%) [60]. The SLN identification rate was significantly higher in patients who underwent SLNB at primary surgery compared to ALND.

Perhaps even more important than the impact on the axilla is the identification of aberrant lymphatic drainage, providing options for targeted surgical excision of SLNs outside the ipsilateral axilla, using lymphoscintigraphy and SPECT/CT as a surgical roadmap [61]. This is relevant in light of the changes in lymphatic drainage due to previous surgery and radiotherapy with significant increase of SLN visualization outside the ipsilateral axilla [62] (Fig. 9.10). Ahmed and coworkers reported an aberrant lymphatic drainage identification rate of 26% of patients on lymphoscintigraphy, being highest in patients who had undergone ALND at primary surgery. It allows alteration of the treatment plan in patients with metastatic disease in lymph nodes outside the ipsilateral axilla, either by targeted surgery, adjuvant systemic treatment, or radiotherapy. Examples of modified radiocolloid migration on lymphoscintigraphy and SPECT/CT are shown in Fig. 9.11.

9.6.6 SLNB in the Neoadjuvant Setting

Neoadjuvant chemotherapy (NAC) is being increasingly used not only in patients with locally advanced breast cancer, but also in patients with early-stage breast cancer, raising a new dilemma: when to perform SLNB. The timing of SLNB in patients receiving NAC is under debate. SLNB before NAC is most accurate, but leads to overtreatment of the axilla, since 20–50% of patients with metastatic disease in the axilla achieve complete pathological response after NAC, with a remission rate being highest in patients with triple-negative tumors and tumors with HER2 overexpression.

Recent studies have shown that in patients without clinical evidence of axillary lymph node involvement at diagnosis (cN0), SLNB after NAC is approaching the globally accepted false-negative rate threshold of 5% without a decrease in efficacy [63]; this is generally considered as acceptable, conferring the benefit of sparing these patients from an extra surgical intervention and more important unnecessary treatment of the axilla and associated morbidity. To achieve a high accuracy, thorough examination of the axilla at diagnosis is necessary, using physical examination and ultrasound. One should take into account the fact that in cN0 patients, persistence of tumor in the breast and the luminal subtype are factors that determine lymph node involvement after NAC.

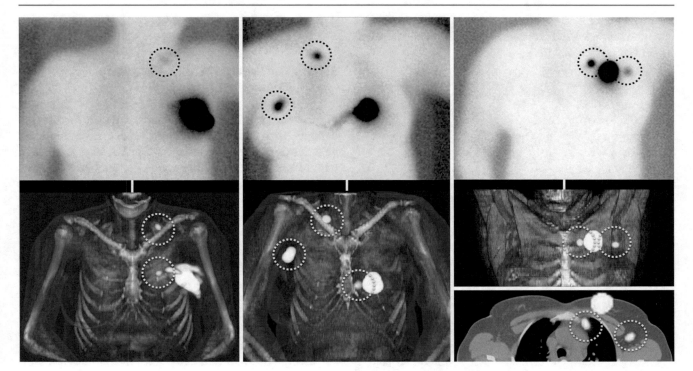

Fig. 9.11 Patterns of radiocolloid migration from the treated breast. Visualized drainage on lymphoscintigraphy (upper row) is anatomically localized using SPECT/CT (lower row) with SLNs (circles) in the ipsilateral internal mammary and supraclavicular regions (left column), ipsilateral mammary chain as well as contralateral axilla and supraclavicular (middle row), and ipsilateral in axilla as well as retrosternal (right column)

More complex is the situation in patients with lymph node involvement at diagnosis (cN+). Noninvasive staging, in the form of physical examination, ultrasound, MRI, or PET-CT, is not reliable for detection of complete pathological nodal response after NAC. In addition, the reliability of SLNB after NAC is questionable; with increasing tumor load in the first-echelon nodes, the risk of aberrant drainage increases, leading to a lower efficacy and higher FNR. This negative effect is enlarged by the chemotherapeutic treatment related to disruption of the lymph drainage. In recent years, many studies addressing this issue have been published. Two large prospective cohort studies, the SENTINA trial and ACOSOG Z1071 trial, investigated the accuracy of the SLNB procedure after NAC in patients with cT0-4N1-2 breast cancer. They reported false-negative rates of 14% and 13%, respectively, with SLN detection rates of 80% and 93%. Subgroup analyses in both trials showed that the false-negative rate could be significantly limited to <10% if (a) the radiocolloid is combined with blue dye, (b) more than two SLNs are removed, and (c) accurate clinical axillary lymph node evaluation is performed before and after chemotherapy [64, 65]. Thus, accurate evaluation of the axilla is essential after NAC and should consist of at least a thorough physical examination and ultrasound examination. With magnetic resonance imaging (MRI) and [18F]FDG PET/CT the accuracy may be increased.

A different approach is to evaluate the response to NAC by marking the involved lymph node prior to treatment. Marking methods include tattooing the node with a carbon particle suspension or placing a metallic clip or a magnetic or radioactive iodine-125 (^{125}I) seed in the involved lymph node. Marking the node with a ^{125}I seed was first described in 2010, better known as the MARI procedure [66]. Initial evaluation of this method reported a detection rate of 97% and false-negative rate of 7%, including lymph nodes with isolated tumor cells [67]. To improve the accuracy of post-NAC axillary staging, nodal clipping may be combined with the post-NAC SLNB procedure, further decreasing the false-negative rate (only 2% in the study of Caudle and coworkers) [68].

Thus, combining the MARI procedure (or other lymph node marking method) with SLNB post-NAC in patients with cN+ breast cancer at diagnosis is feasible and seems to be the most effective way to restage the axilla post-NAC, providing an approach to preserve the axilla. Other proposed axillary treatment algorithms include information regarding the nodal tumor load at diagnosis (using [^{18}F]FDG PET/CT) and result of the MARI procedure post-NAC, without including SLNB (see below) [69].

Key Learning Points

- The SLNB procedure is indicated in patients with early-stage breast cancer (cT1-2 tumors) without cytological or histological evidence of axillary lymph node metastases.
- SLNB is justified in pregnant women due to the low risks of the procedure relative to the risks of axillary dissection.
- Lymphatic drainage toward the internal mammary chain is associated with a worse disease-free survival and a selective group of breast cancer patients at high risk for subclinical involvement of the internal mammary chain might benefit from parasternal irradiation.
- The accuracy of SLNB in large and multifocal/multicentric tumors is decreased, which has to be weighed up against the benefits of SLNB in the individual patient.
- In DCIS, SLNB should be considered if risk factors for lymph node metastases are present.
- SLNB in patients with recurrent disease is feasible and may avoid ALND in a significant proportion of patients and identify aberrant lymphatic drainage in these patients, providing options for targeted therapy.
- SLNB before NAC is most accurate, but leads to overtreatment of the axilla, since 20–50% of patients with metastatic disease in the axilla achieve complete pathological response.
- In clinically negative axillary disease at diagnosis, SLNB after NAC is accurate, approaching the globally accepted false-negative threshold of 5%.
- In clinically positive axillary disease at diagnosis SLN post-NAC is less accurate, although false-negative rate may be limited to <10% when dual mapping is applied, more than two SNs are removed. and accurate clinical axillary lymph node evaluation is performed before and after chemotherapy.
- Combining the SLNB procedure post-NAC with a lymph node marking method such as the MARI procedure seems to be the most accurate way to restage the axilla post-NAC.

9.7   Clinical Impact of SLNB in Breast Cancer

9.7.1   The Paradigm Shift in Axillary Management

SLNB has become the "standard of care" for staging patients with early-stage breast cancer with clinically negative nodes. As mentioned earlier, SLNB is associated with reduced arm morbidity and better quality of life and has replaced the ALND for staging the axilla. Extensive evaluations have proven the safety of this technique showing high detection rate and acceptable false-negative rate, especially when preoperative lymphoscintigraphy and dual mapping are applied [70–72].

In the latest years an increasing tendency has emerged to preserve the axilla, based on the ALND-related arm morbidity and reduced quality of life, together with the fact that clinical presentation of the disease and (systemic) treatment have changed over time. Furthermore, there are reasons to believe that axillary metastases do not always become clinically relevant, as may be concluded from earlier studies in the 1970–1980s. For example, in the NSABP B-04 trial, a trial that did not include systemic therapy, the axillary recurrence rate in patients with no axillary treatment was approximately half of the expected rate from the prevalence of metastases found in patients in whom axillary contents were removed and examined [73]. These results are supported by more recent studies such as the ACOSOG Z0011 trial (see below), showing a non-inferior outcome in a group of patients in whom 27% had lymph node metastatic disease left in place. Besides the fact that these metastases were probably treated either by the adjuvant systemic treatment or by the whole-breast irradiation, this may also (at least partly) be related to the existence of biologic factors that determine the clinical growth of axillary metastases.

This gain in knowledge over time has resulted in the emergence of a treatment paradigm shift: not all SLN-positive patients need to receive local axillary treatment in terms of ALND or axillary radiotherapy. In addition, in the near future, SLNB will probably increasingly be omitted in specific low-risk or comorbidity situations (such as T1 luminal A, age >70 years). However, whether and how this will happen depend on the results of current ongoing studies.

9.7.2 SLN-Negative Breast Cancer

There is general consensus that patients with negative axillary SLNB by routine histopathological evaluation do not require ALND. A randomized controlled study in 516 histopathologically node-negative patients treated with either SLNB alone or SLNB plus ALND reported overt axillary metastases in only two cases in the SLNB-alone arm during 8-year follow-up and a slightly greater overall survival in the SLNB-alone arm [74]. Another large study in patients with hematoxylin-eosin (H&E)-negative, tumor-free SLNs, who did not undergo completion ALND, revealed a remarkably low axillary recurrence of 0.2% and high disease-free survival [75]. Similar long-term results were reported by the American College of Surgeons Oncology Group. This ACOSOG Z0010 trial included 3904 patients with H&E-negative SLNs and reported only 0.5% regional recurrences, 3.3% local recurrences, and 3.4% distant recurrences at a median follow-up of 8.4 years [76]. The NSABP B-32 trial showed similar results [18].

Factors associated with local-regional recurrence were younger age and hormone receptor-negative disease. Locoregional recurrence is less often seen in patients with hormone receptor-positive tumors and those who receive chemotherapy.

9.7.3 SLN-Positive Breast Cancer

The addition of immunohistochemistry (IHC) analysis to the standard H&E examination has led to increased detection of metastases (isolated tumor cells or micrometastases) in SLNs. Isolated tumor cells are defined as "small clusters of cells not greater than 0.2 mm, or single tumor cells, or a cluster of fewer than 200 cells in a single histologic cross-section" and micrometastases as "tumor deposits greater than 0.2 mm but not greater than 2.0 mm in largest dimension" [30]. These occult metastases may be found in up to 16% of H&E-negative SLNs [77]. However, large trials as the ACOSOG Z0010 and NSABP B-32 revealed that IHC detection of these H&E-occult SLN metastases does not contribute to survival [7, 77]. Ram and coworkers performed a meta-analysis pooling results of three randomized trials. They concluded that for patients with a clinically negative axilla and micrometastases in the SLN, SLNB alone was non-inferior to completion ALND [19].

While safety and efficacy of SLNB alone, with no reduction in survival, have been proven for patients with tumor-free or SLN micrometastatic disease, no consensus exists on the management of patients with "limited SLN macrometastatic" disease ("limited" commonly defined as one or two positive SLNs). As mentioned earlier, the tendency to preserve the axilla, together with the fact that clinical presentation and management of breast cancer have changed over time, has raised questions concerning the necessity of ALND in these patients. In the AMAROS trial, 1425 patients with T1 or T2 invasive primary breast cancer and positive SLNs were randomized between completion ALND and locoregional (axillar and periclavicular) radiotherapy only; they concluded that excellent and comparable axillary control was achieved with locoregional radiotherapy in this patient population [78]. The ACOSOG Z0011 trial randomized 891 patients with T1 or T2 invasive breast cancer, clinically negative axillary disease, and one or two H&E-positive SLNs between completion ALND and SLNB alone; this trial revealed that 10-year overall survival for patients treated with SLNB alone was non-inferior to overall survival for those treated with completion ALND [79]. It is important to note that most of the patients in both treatment arms received adjuvant systemic therapy. The results of both trials have changed the management of breast cancer at major centers throughout the United States and Europe. Early metastatic breast cancer patients with SLN metastases who have limited axillary disease found at operation may be spared the morbidity of ALND, further increasing the role of SLNB in the management of early breast cancer.

Based on these recent reports, neither the St. Gallen nor the American Society of Clinical Oncology (ASCO) guidelines recommend ALND in patients with isolated tumor cells in their SLNs. In addition, ASCO also recommends to omit ALND in most patients with 1–2 metastatic SLNs who are planning to undergo breast-conserving surgery with whole-breast radiotherapy, albeit controversy persists around the question whether axillary radiotherapy should be added in these cases, as appeared from a recent St. Gallen Consensus Conference in 2019 [80].

9.7.4 SLN-Positive Breast Cancer, Downstaged After Neoadjuvant Therapy

As mentioned earlier, axillary staging after NAC in patients with cN+ breast cancer at diagnosis may prevent overtreatment of the axilla in a significant number of patients. Because of the reduced accuracy of SLNB when performed after NAC, combination of SLNB with a lymph node marking method such as the MARI procedure should be considered to restage the axilla.

A different approach to spare the axilla in these patients is to implement a tailored axillary treatment algorithm based on the lymph node marking procedure together with the known axillary tumor load at diagnosis, omitting the (less accurate) SLNB in these patients. Koolen and coworkers constructed and tested a treatment algorithm for tailored axillary treatment after NAC in a cohort of axillary node-positive patients, based on the results of [^{18}F]FDG PET/CT pre-NAC and the MARI procedure in 93 patients [69]. Based on this algorithm, axillary treatment would be omitted in patients with 1–3 [^{18}F]FDG-avid axillary lymph nodes on PET/CT and a tumor-negative MARI node; those with a positive MARI node would receive axillary radiotherapy, as would patients with four or more [^{18}F]FDG-avid axillary lymph nodes and a negative MARI node. An ALND would be performed only in patients with four or more [^{18}F]FDG-avid axillary lymph nodes and a positive MARI node after NAC. In their hands, treatment according to this algorithm would have resulted in 74% of patients avoiding an ALND, with potential undertreatment in 3% and overtreatment in 17% of patients. Although promising, long-term results are lacking at the moment for both mentioned strategies.

Key Learning Points
- Occult metastases may be found in up to 16% of H&E-negative SLNs after immunohistochemistry analysis; however detection of ITCs and micrometastases in SLNs does not contribute to survival.

- An increasing tendency has emerged to preserve the axilla, based on the ALND-related morbidity on one side and the changed clinical presentation of the disease and improved (systemic) treatment on the other side.
- Treatment of the axilla has changed from a dichotomized treatment plan based on negative or positive SLNs toward a more tailored axillary treatment based on the axillary tumor load.
- Comparable axillary control seems to be achieved with locoregional radiotherapy compared to ALND in patients with SLN-positive disease.
- In patients with cT1 or T2 disease and 1–2 positive SLNs who are planned to undergo breast-conserving surgery with whole-breast radiotherapy, ALND may be omitted since ALND in these patients does not lead to improved survival.
- In patients with clinically positive axillary disease at diagnosis receiving NAC, a tailored axillary treatment algorithm based on a lymph node marking procedure pre-NAC and axillary tumor load at diagnosis ([^{18}F]FDG PET/CT) may lead to a significant reduction of ALND procedures while omitting the SLNB in these patients.

Acknowledgements The current chapter is a revision of the original chapter written by G. Manca, M. Tredici, V. Duce, S. Mazzarri, F. Orsini, S. Chiacchio, A. E. Giuliano, G. Mariani in the previous edition of the book.

Clinical Cases

Case 9.1: SLN Mapping in Breast Cancer with Ipsilateral Drainage to the Axilla

Daphne D. D. Rietbergen, Lenka M. Pereira Arias-Bouda, and Renato A. Valdés Olmos

Background Clinical Case

A 75-year-old woman with invasive ductal breast carcinoma was referred for SLNB. During staging of the left axilla no lymph node abnormalities had been detected on physical examination and ultrasonography (clinical stage T1N0).

Planar Lymphoscintigraphy and SPECT/CT Imaging

In the afternoon before surgery a subareolar injection with 78 MBq ^{99m}Tc-tilmanocept was administered in the left breast. After tracer administration, 5-min planar anterior and lateral static images were acquired at 15 min and 3 h using a dual-head gamma camera (Symbia T6, Siemens, Erlangen, Germany) equipped with low-energy high-resolution collimators. In addition, SPECT/CT imaging was acquired after acquiring the delayed planar images using the same gamma camera.

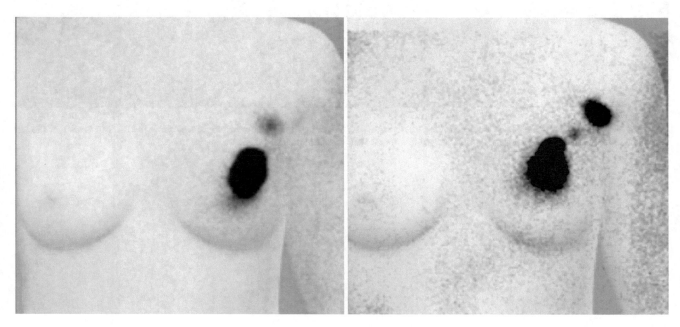

Fig. 9.12 Anterior early (on the left) and delayed (on the right) planar images, displayed in superposition to anatomical models, showing unilateral drainage to the left axilla with visualization of a single lymphatic duct and increasing uptake in a lymph node

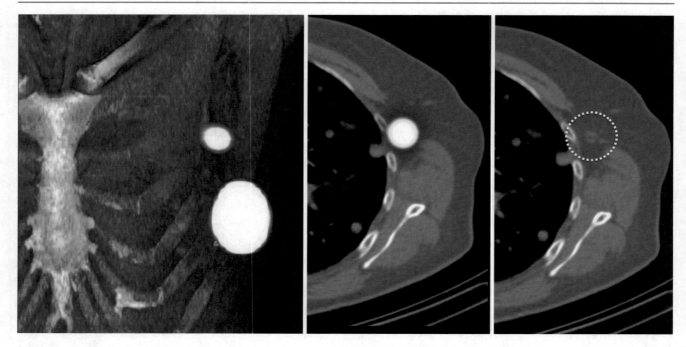

Fig. 9.13 SPECT/CT images displayed with volume rendering (first image) and transaxial (second image) show the SLN in level 1 of the left axilla and corresponding on low-dose CT (third image) to a round lymph node (circle)

Case 9.2: SLN Mapping in Breast Cancer with Ipsilateral Drainage to the Axilla

Daphne D. D. Rietbergen, Lenka M. Pereira Arias-Bouda, and Renato A. Valdés Olmos

Background Clinical Case

A 74-year-old woman with invasive ductal carcinoma of the left breast was referred for the SLN procedure. During staging no lymph node abnormalities had been detected on physical examination and ultrasonography of the ipsilateral axilla (clinical stage T2N0).

Planar Lymphoscintigraphy and SPECT/CT Imaging

In the afternoon before surgery 75 MBq ^{99m}Tc-tilmanocept was administered by means of a single subareolar injection in the left breast. After tracer administration, 5-min planar anterior and lateral static images were acquired at 15 min and 3 h using a dual-head gamma camera (Symbia T6, Siemens, Erlangen, Germany) equipped with low-energy high-resolution collimators. In addition, SPECT/CT imaging was acquired after acquiring the delayed planar images using the same gamma camera.

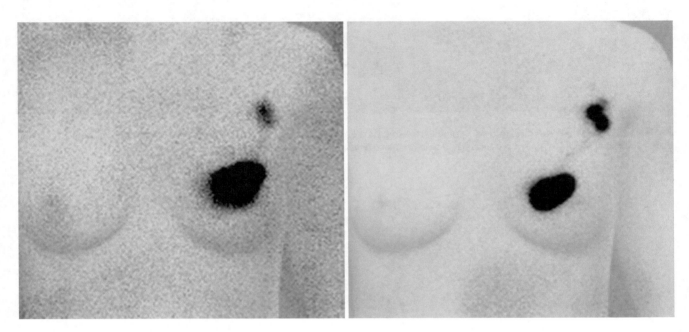

Fig. 9.14 Anterior early (on the left) and delayed (on the right) planar images, displayed in superposition to anatomical models, showing unilateral drainage to the left axilla with visualization of a single lymphatic duct and increasing uptake in two lymph nodes

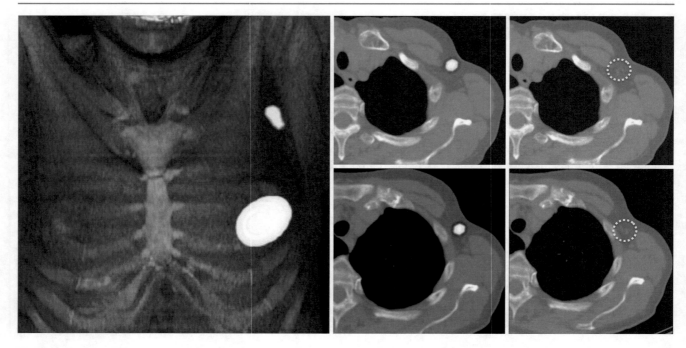

Fig. 9.15 SPECT/CT images displayed with volume rendering (first image) and transaxial (second image) show both SLNs in level 1 of the left axilla corresponding on low-dose CT (third image) to normal-size lymph nodes (circles)

Case 9.3: SLN Mapping in Breast Cancer with Ipsilateral Drainage to Interpectoral and Axillary Lymph Nodes

Lenka M. Pereira Arias-Bouda, Daphne D. D. Rietbergen, and Renato A. Valdés Olmos

Background Clinical Case

A 56-year-old woman with invasive ductal carcinoma of the right breast was referred for SLNB. During staging no lymph node abnormalities had been detected on physical examination and ultrasonography of the right axilla (clinical stage T1N0).

Planar Lymphoscintigraphy and SPECT/CT Imaging

In the afternoon of the day before surgery 112 MBq ^{99m}Tc-nanocolloid was administered by means of a single intratumoral injection in the right breast. After tracer administration, 5-min planar anterior and lateral static images were acquired at 15 min and 3 h using a dual-head gamma camera (Symbia T, Siemens, Erlangen, Germany) equipped with low-energy high-resolution collimators. In addition, SPECT/CT imaging was acquired after acquiring the delayed planar images using the same gamma camera.

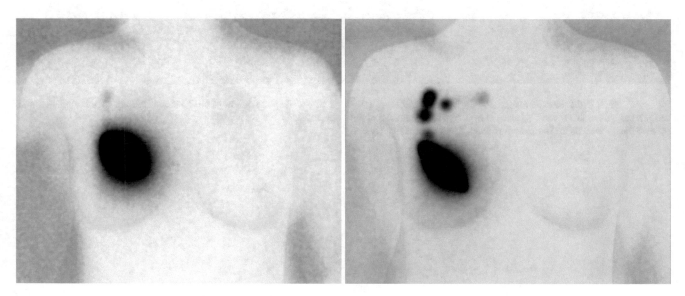

Fig. 9.16 Anterior early planar image (on the left) showing ipsilateral drainage to the right axilla with visualization of a single lymphatic duct and initial uptake in a lymph node. In the delayed planar image (on the right) multiple radioactive lymph nodes are visualized

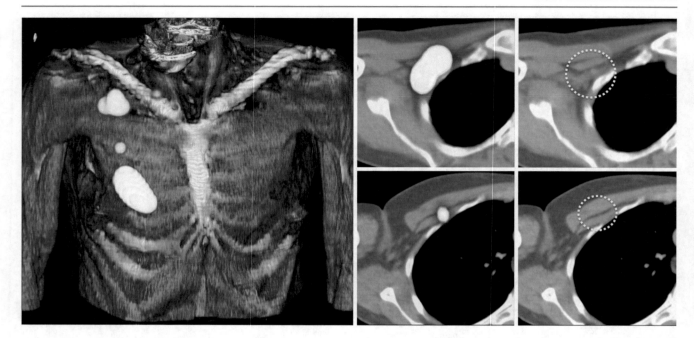

Fig. 9.17 SPECT/CT images displayed with volume rendering (first image) and transaxial (second column) show two SLNs in level 2 of the right axilla as well as an interpectoral SLN. These radioactive lymph nodes correspond on low-dose CT (third column) to normal-size lymph node (circles)

Case 9.4: SLN Mapping in Breast Cancer with Drainage to the Ipsilateral Internal Mammary Chain and Axilla

Lenka M. Pereira Arias-Bouda, Daphne D. D. Rietbergen, and Renato A. Valdés Olmos

Background Clinical Case

A 55-year-old woman with invasive ductal carcinoma of the left breast was submitted for SLNB. During staging no lymph node abnormalities had been detected on physical examination and ultrasonography of the left axilla (clinical stage T2N0).

Planar Lymphoscintigraphy and SPECT/CT Imaging

In the afternoon of the day before surgery 108 MBq ^{99m}Tc-nanocolloid was administered by means of a single intratumoral injection in the left breast. After tracer administration, 5-min planar anterior and lateral static images were acquired at 15 min and 3 h using a dual-head gamma camera (Symbia T, Siemens, Erlangen, Germany) equipped with low-energy high-resolution collimators. In addition, SPECT/CT imaging was acquired after acquiring the delayed planar images using the same gamma camera.

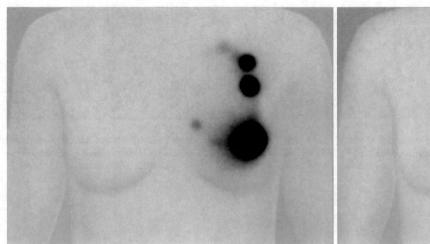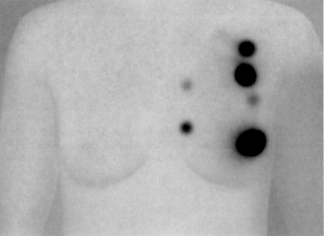

Fig. 9.18 Anterior early planar image (on the left) showing ipsilateral drainage to the left axilla and internal mammary chain with visualization of lymphatic ducts. On delayed planar imaging (on the right) mul- tiple radioactive axillary lymph nodes are visualized as well as increasing uptake in the first draining internal mammary lymph node

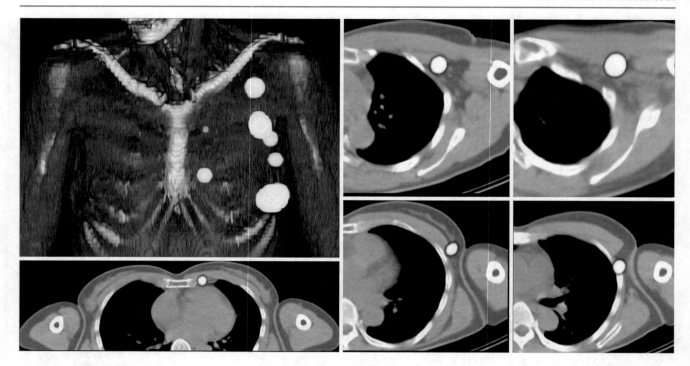

Fig. 9.19 In the SPECT/CT image displayed with volume rendering (first image left above) four radioactive lymph nodes are visualized in the area of the left axilla as well as an internal mammary lymph node with intense uptake at the left third intercostal space. On cross-sectional SPECT/CT slices the intercostal SLN is depicted (bottom on the left) as well as SLNs behind the breast, lower part of the axilla, and in level 2

Case 9.5: SLN Mapping in Relapsed Breast Cancer with Tracer Migration to the Ipsilateral Internal Mammary Chain and No Axillary Drainage

Renato A. Valdés Olmos, Lenka M. Pereira Arias-Bouda, and Daphne D. D. Rietbergen

Background Clinical Case

A 51-year-old woman with relapsed invasive ductal carcinoma of the left breast was referred for SLNB. In the past the patient had been treated with lumpectomy and SLN surgery due to a T1N0 tumor in the same breast. During current staging no lymph node abnormalities had been detected on physical examination and ultrasonography of the left axilla (clinical stage T2N0).

Planar Lymphoscintigraphy and SPECT/CT Imaging

In the afternoon of the day before surgery 110 MBq ^{99m}Tc-nanocolloid was administered by means of a single intratumoral injection in the left breast. After tracer administration, 5-min planar anterior and lateral static images were acquired at 15 min and 3 h using a dual-head gamma camera (Symbia T, Siemens, Erlangen, Germany) equipped with low-energy high-resolution collimators. In addition, SPECT/CT imaging was acquired after acquiring the delayed planar images using the same gamma camera.

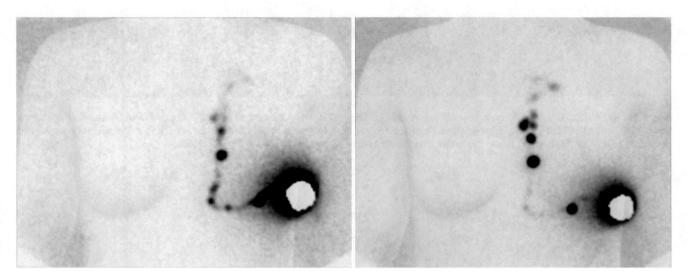

Fig. 9.20 Anterior early planar image (on the left) showing ipsilateral drainage to the internal mammary chain with visualization of a lymphatic duct. On delayed planar imaging (on the right) multiple radioactive internal mammary lymph nodes are visualized. There is no drainage to the left axilla

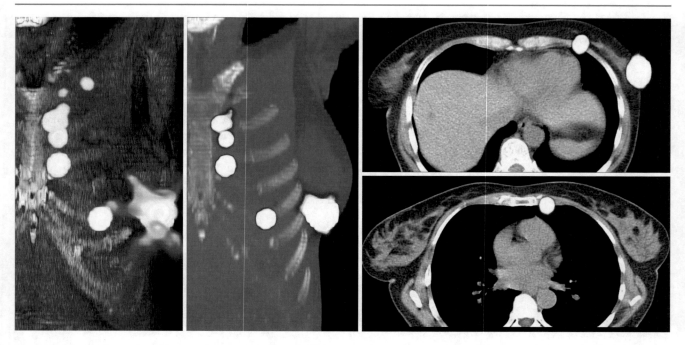

Fig. 9.21 SPECT/CT images displayed with volume rendering (first image) and coronal SPECT/CT with multiple intensity projection (second image) show drainage solely to the ipsilateral internal mammary chain. The radioactive lymph nodes at the first rib and third intercostal space were identified as SLNs, as were further displayed on cross-sectional SPECT/CT slices (third image)

Case 9.6: SLN Mapping in Relapsed Breast Cancer with Drainage to the Contralateral Axilla

Renato A. Valdés Olmos, Lenka M. Pereira Arias-Bouda, and Daphne D. D. Rietbergen

Background Clinical Case

A 56-year-old woman with relapsed invasive ductal carcinoma of the left breast was referred for SLNB. In the past the patient had been treated with lumpectomy, axillary lymph node dissection, and radiotherapy due to a T2N1 tumor in the same breast. During current staging no lymph node abnormalities had been detected on physical examination and ultrasonography of the axilla (clinical stage T1N0).

Planar Lymphoscintigraphy and SPECT/CT Imaging

In the afternoon of the day before surgery 105 MBq ^{99m}Tc-nanocolloid was administered by means of a single ultrasound-guided intratumoral injection in the left breast. After tracer administration, 5-min planar anterior and lateral static images were acquired at 15 min and 3 h using a dual-head gamma camera (Symbia T, Siemens, Erlangen, Germany) equipped with low-energy high-resolution collimators. In addition, SPECT/CT imaging was acquired after acquiring the delayed planar images using the same gamma camera.

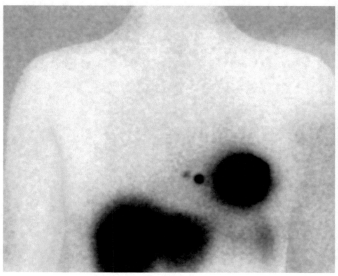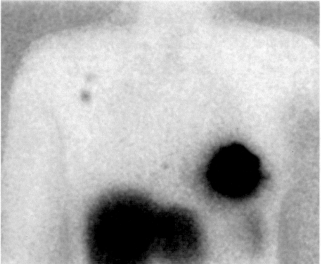

Fig. 9.22 Anterior early planar image (on the left) showing initial tracer migration close to the injection site. On delayed planar image (on the right) two radioactive lymph nodes are visualized in the contralateral axilla. Note that the radioactivity in the vicinity of the injection site has disappeared

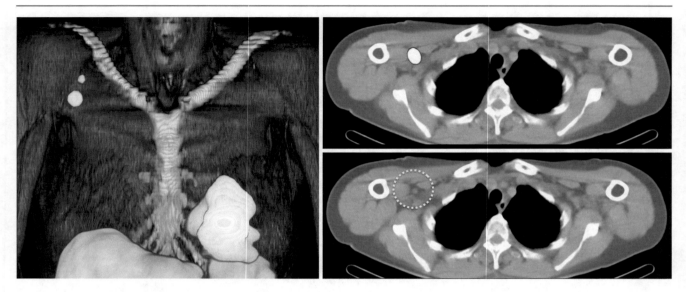

Fig. 9.23 SPECT/CT image displayed with volume rendering (first image) showing a SLN and a second-echelon lymph node in the right axilla. Cross-sectional SPECT/CT section (above on the right) shows the SLN in level 1 of the axilla. This corresponds to a normal-size lymph node (circle) on low-dose CT (bottom on the right)

References

1. Carter CL, Allen C, Henson DE, et al. Relation of tumor size, lymph node status, and survival in 24,740 breast cancer cases. Cancer. 1989;63:181–7.
2. Carlson RW, Allred DC, Anderson BO, et al. Breast cancer: clinical practice guidelines in oncology. J Natl Compr Cancer Netw. 2009;7:122–92.
3. Krag DN, Weaver DL, Alex JC, et al. Surgical resection and radiolocalization of the sentinel lymph node in breast cancer using a gamma probe. Surg Oncol. 1993;2:335–9.
4. Nathanson SD, Shah R, Rosso K. Sentinel lymph node metastases in cancer: causes, detection and their role in disease progression. Semin Cell Dev Biol. 2015;38:106–16.
5. Veronesi U, Paganelli G, Viale G, et al. A randomized comparison of sentinel-node biopsy with routine axillary dissection in breast cancer. N Engl J Med. 2003;349:546–53.
6. Morton DL, Thompson JF, Essner R, et al. Validation of the accuracy of intraoperative lymphatic mapping and sentinel lymphadenectomy for early-stage melanoma: a multicenter trial—multicenter selective lymphadenectomy trial group. Ann Surg. 1999;230:453–65.
7. Giuliano AE, Hawes D, Ballman KV, et al. Association of occult metastases in sentinel lymph nodes and bone marrow with survival among women with early-stage invasive breast cancer. JAMA. 2011;306:385–93.
8. Lucci A, McCall LM, Beitsch PD, et al. Surgical complications associated with sentinel lymph node dissection (SLND) plus axillary lymph node dissection compared with SLND alone in the American College of Surgeons Oncology Group Trial Z0011. J Clin Oncol. 2007;5:3657–63.
9. Manca G, Rubello D, Tardelli E, et al. Sentinel lymph node biopsy in breast cancer: indications, contraindications, and controversies. Clin Nucl Med. 2016;41:126–33.
10. Lyman GH, Giuliano AE, Somerfield MR, et al. American Society of Clinical Oncology guideline recommendations for sentinel lymph node biopsy in early-stage breast cancer. J Clin Oncol. 2005;23:7703–20.
11. Giammarile F, Alazraki N, Aarsvold JN, et al. The EANM and SNMMI practice guideline for lymphoscintigraphy and sentinel node localization in breast cancer. Eur J Nucl Med Mol Imaging. 2013;40:1932–47.
12. Lyman GH, Temin S, Edge SB, et al. Sentinel lymph node biopsy for patients with early-stage breast cancer: American Society of Clinical Oncology clinical practice guideline update. J Clin Oncol. 2014;32:1365–83.
13. Lyman GH, Somerfield MR, Bosserman LD, et al. Sentinel lymph node biopsy for patients with early-stage breast cancer: American Society of Clinical Oncology clinical practice guideline update. J Clin Oncol. 2017;35:561–4.
14. Halsted WS. The results of operations for the cure of carcinoma of the breast. Ann Surg. 1907;46:1–19.
15. Cady B, Michaelson JS, Chung MA. The "tipping point" for breast cancer mortality decline has resulted from size reductions due to mammographic screening. Ann Surg Oncol. 2011;18:903–6.
16. Giuliano AE, Kirgan DM, Guenther JM, et al. Lymphatic mapping and sentinel lymphadenectomy for breast cancer. Ann Surg. 1994;220:391–8.
17. Yeoh EK, Denham JW, Davies SA, et al. Primary breast cancer: complications of axillary management. Acta Radiol Oncol. 1986;25:105–8.
18. Krag DN, Anderson SJ, Julian TB, et al. Sentinel-lymph-node resection compared with conventional axillary-lymph-node dissection in clinically node-negative patients with breast cancer: overall survival findings from the NSABP B-32 randomized phase 3 trial. Lancet Oncol. 2010;11:927–33.
19. Ram R, Singh J, McCaig E. Sentinel node biopsy versus completion axillary node dissection in node positive breast cancer: systematic review and meta-analysis. Int J Breast Cancer. 2014;2014:513780. https://doi.org/10.1155/2014/513780.
20. Mansel RE, Fallowfield L, Kissin M, et al. Randomized multicenter trial of sentinel node biopsy versus standard axillary treatment in operable breast cancer: the ALMANAC trial. J Natl Cancer Inst. 2006;98:599–609.
21. Ruano Pérez R, Rebollo Aguirre AC, García-Talavera P, et al. Review of the role of the sentinel node biopsy in neoadjuvant chemotherapy in women with breast cancer and negative or positive axillary node at diagnosis. Rev Esp Med Nucl Imagen Mol. 2018;37:63–70.
22. Sappey MPC. Anatomie, physiologie, pathologie des vaisseaux lymphatiques considérés chez l'homme et les vertebrés. Paris: A. Delahaye and E. Lecrosnier; 1874.
23. Suami H, Pan WR, Mann GB, et al. The lymphatic anatomy of the breast and its implications for sentinel lymph node biopsy: a human cadaver study. Ann Surg Oncol. 2008;15:863–71.
24. Estourgie SH, Nieweg OE, Valdés Olmos RA, et al. Lymphatic drainage patterns from the breast. Ann Surg. 2004;239:232–7.
25. Brouwer OR, Vermeeren L, van der Ploeg IM, et al. Lymphoscintigraphy and SPECT/CT in multicentric and multifocal breast cancer: does each tumour have a separate drainage pattern? Results of a Dutch multicentre study (MULTISENT). Eur J Nucl Med Mol Imaging. 2012;39:1137–43.
26. Noushi F, Spillane AJ, Uren RF, et al. High discordance rates between sub-areolar and peri-tumoural breast lymphoscintigraphy. Eur J Surg Oncol. 2013;39:1053–60.
27. Van Rijk MC, Tanis PJ, Nieweg OE, et al. Clinical implications of sentinel nodes outside the axilla and internal mammary chain in patients with breast cancer. J Surg Oncol. 2006;94:281–6.
28. Tanis PJ, Nieweg OE, Valdés Olmos RA, et al. Anatomy and physiology of lymphatic drainage of the breast from the perspective of sentinel node biopsy. J Am Coll Surg. 2001;192:399–409.
29. Uren RF, Howman-Giles R, Chung DK, et al. SPECT/CT scans allow precise anatomical location of sentinel lymph nodes in breast cancer and redefine lymphatic drainage from the breast to the axilla. Breast. 2012;21:480–6.
30. Giuliano AE, Connolly JL, Edge SB, et al. Breast cancer—major changes in the American Joint Committee on Cancer eighth edition cancer staging manual. CA Cancer J Clin. 2017;67:290–303.
31. Tsopelas C. Particles size analysis of ^{99m}Tc-labeled and unlabeled antimony trisulfide and rhenium sulfide colloids intended for lymphoscintigraphic application. J Nucl Med. 2001;42:460–6.
32. Wallace AM, Hoh CK, Vera DR, et al. Lymphoseek: a molecular radiopharmaceutical for sentinel node detection. Ann Surg Oncol. 2003;10:531–8.
33. Wallace AM, Hoh CK, Limmer KK, et al. Sentinel lymph node accumulation of Lymphoseek and Tc-99m–sulfur colloid using a "2-day" protocol. Nucl Med Biol. 2009;36:687–92.
34. Kim CK, Zukotynski KA. Desirable properties of radiopharmaceuticals for sentinel node mapping in patients with breast cancer given the paradigm shift in patient management. Clin Nucl Med. 2017;42:275–9.
35. Tanis Valdés Olmos RA, Muller SH, Nieweg OE. Lymphatic mapping in patients with breast carcinoma: reproducibility of lymphoscintigraphic results. Radiology. 2003;228:546–51.

36. Borgstein PJ, Pijpers R, Comans EF, et al. Sentinel lymph node biopsy in breast cancer: guidelines and pitfalls of lymphoscintigraphy and gamma probe detection. J Am Coll Surg. 1998;186:275–83.

37. Smith LF, Cross MJ, Klimberg VS. Subareolar injection is a better technique for sentinel lymph node biopsy. Am J Surg. 2000;180:434–7; discussion 437–438.

38. Nieweg OE, Estourgie SH, van Rijk MC, et al. Rationale for superficial injection techniques in lymphatic mapping in breast cancer patients. J Surg Oncol. 2004;87:153–6.

39. Alazraki NP, Styblo T, Grant SF, et al. Sentinel node staging of early breast cancer using lymphoscintigraphy and the intraoperative gamma-detecting probe. Semin Nucl Med. 2000;30:56–64.

40. Kim SC, Kim DW, Moadel RM, et al. Using the intraoperative hand held probe without lymphoscintigraphy or using only dye correlates with higher sensory morbidity following sentinel lymph node biopsy in breast cancer: a review of the literature. World J Surg Oncol. 2005;3:64.

41. Vermeeren L, van der Ploeg IM, Valdés Olmos RA, et al. SPECT/CT for preoperative sentinel node localization. J Surg Oncol. 2010;101:184–90.

42. Valdés Olmos RA, Vidal-Sicart S, et al. Advances in radioguided surgery in oncology. Q J Nucl Med Mol Imaging. 2017;61:247–70.

43. Van der Ploeg IM, Nieweg OE, Kroon BB, et al. The yield of SPECT/CT for anatomical lymphatic mapping in patients with breast cancer. Eur J Nucl Med Mol Imaging. 2009;36:903–9.

44. Martin RC 2nd, Edwards MJ, Wong SL, et al. Practical guidelines for optimal gamma probe detection of sentinel lymph nodes in breast cancer: results of a multi-institutional study. For the University of Louisville Breast Cancer Study Group. Surgery. 2000;128:139–44.

45. Manca G, Romanini A, Pellegrino D, et al. Optimal detection of sentinel lymph node metastases by intraoperative radioactive threshold and molecular analysis in patients with melanoma. J Nucl Med. 2008;49:1769–75.

46. Vidal-Sicart S, Paredes P, Zanón G, et al. Added value of intraoperative real-time imaging in searches for difficult-tolocate sentinel nodes. J Nucl Med. 2010;51:1219–25.

47. Wendler T, Herrmann K, Schnelzer A, et al. First demonstration of 3-D lymphatic mapping in breast cancer using freehand SPECT. Eur J Nucl Med Mol Imaging. 2010;37:1452–61.

48. Van Den Berg NS, Buckle T, Kleinjan GI, et al. Hybrid tracers for sentinel node biopsy. Q J Nucl Med Mol Imaging. 2014;58:193–206.

49. Keereweer S, Kerrebijn JD, van Driel PB, et al. Optical image-guided surgery—where do we stand? Mol Imaging Biol. 2011;13:199–207.

50. KleinJan GH, Van Werkhoven E, Van den Berg NS, et al. The best of both worlds: a hybrid approach for optimal pre- and intraoperative identification of sentinel lymph nodes. Eur J Nucl Med Mol Imaging. 2018;45:1915–25.

51. Kong AL, Tereffe W, Hunt KK, et al. Impact of internal mammary lymph node drainage identified by preoperative lymphoscintigraphy on outcomes in patients with stage I to III breast cancer. Cancer. 2012;118:6287–96.

52. McGale P, Taylor C, Correa C, et al. Effect of radiotherapy after mastectomy and axillary surgery on 10-year recurrence and 20-year breast cancer mortality: meta-analysis of individual patient data for 8135 women in 22 randomised trials. Lancet. 2014;383:2127–35.

53. Budach W, Kammers K, Boelke E, et al. Adjuvant radiotherapy of regional lymph nodes in breast cancer—a meta-analysis of randomized trials. Radiat Oncol. 2013;8:267–73.

54. Madsen EVE, Aalders KC, Van der Heiden-van der Loo M, et al. Prognostic significance of tumor-positive internal mammary sentinel lymph nodes in breast cancer: a multicenter cohort study. Ann Surg Oncol. 2015;22:4254–62.

55. Ozmen V, Muslumanoglu M, Cabioglu N, et al. Increased false negative rates in sentinel lymph node biopsies in patients with multifocal breast cancer. Breast Cancer Res Treat. 2002;76:237–44.

56. Knauer M, Konstantiniuk P, Haid A, et al. Multicentric breast cancer: a new indication for sentinel node biopsy—a multi-institutional validation study. J Clin Oncol. 2006;24:3374–80.

57. Giard S, Chauvet MP, Penel N. Feasibility of sentinel lymph node biopsy in multiple unilateral synchronous breast cancer: results of a French prospective multi-institutional study (IGASSU 0502). Ann Oncol. 2010;21:1630–5.

58. Francis AM, Haugen CE, Grimes LM, et al. Is sentinel lymph node dissection warranted for patients with a diagnosis of ductal carcinoma in situ? Ann Surg Oncol. 2015;22:4270–9.

59. Groen EJ, Elshof LE, Visser LL, et al. Finding the balance between over- and under-treatment of ductal carcinoma in situ (DCIS). Breast. 2017;31:274–83.

60. Ahmed M, Baker R, Rubio IT. Meta-analysis of aberrant lymphatic drainage in recurrent breast cancer. Br J Surg. 2016;103:1579–88.

61. Borrelli P, Donswijk M, Stokkel M, et al. Contribution of SPECT/CT for sentinel node localization in patients with ipsilateral breast cancer relapse. Eur J Nucl Med Mol Imaging. 2017;44:630–7.

62. Van der Ploeg IM, Oldenburg HS, Rutgers EJ, et al. Lymphatic drainage patterns from the treated breast. Ann Surg Oncol. 2010;17:1069–75.

63. Ruano Pérez R, Rebollo Aguirre AC, García-Talavera San Miguel P, et al. Review of the role of the sentinel node biopsy in neoadjuvant chemotherapy in women with breast cancer and negative or positive axillary node at diagnosis. Rev Esp Med Nucl Imagen Mol. 2018;37:63–70.

64. Kuehn T, Bauerfeind I, Fehm T, et al. Sentinel-lymph-node biopsy in patients with breast cancer before and after neoadjuvant chemotherapy (SENTINA): a prospective, multicentre cohort study. Lancet Oncol. 2013;14:609–18.

65. Boughey JC, Suman VJ, Mittendorf EA, et al. Alliance for clinical trials in oncology. Factors affecting sentinel lymph n patients enrolled in ACOSOG Z1071 (Alliance). Ann Surg. 2015;261:547–52.

66. Straver ME, Loo CE, Alderliesten T, et al. Marking the axilla with radioactive iodine seeds (MARI procedure) may reduce the need for axillary dissection after neoadjuvant chemotherapy for breast cancer. Br J Surg. 2010;97:1226–31.

67. Donker M, Straver ME, Wesseling J, et al. Marking axillary lymph nodes with radioactive iodine seeds for axillary staging after neoadjuvant systemic treatment in breast cancer patients: the MARI procedure. Ann Surg. 2015;261:378–82.

68. Caudle AS, Yang WT, Krishnamurthy S, et al. Improved axillary evaluation following neoadjuvant therapy for patients with node-positive breast cancer using selective evaluation of clipped nodes: implementation of targeted axillary dissection. J Clin Oncol. 2016;34:1072–8.

69. Koolen BB, Donker M, Straver ME, et al. Combined PET–CT and axillary lymph node marking with radioactive iodine seeds (MARI procedure) for tailored axillary treatment in node-positive breast cancer after neoadjuvant therapy. Br J Surg. 2017;104:1188–96.

70. Goyal A, Newcombe RG, Chhabra A, ALMANAC Trialists Group, et al. Factors affecting failed localisation and false-negative rates of sentinel node biopsy in breast cancer: results of the ALMANAC validation phase. Breast Cancer Res Treat. 2006;99:203–208.

71. Pesek S, Ashikaga T, Krag LE, et al. The false negative rate of sentinel node biopsy in patients with breast cancer: a meta-analysis. World J Surg. 2012;36:2239–51.

72. Ahmed M, Purushotham AD, Horgan K, et al. Meta-analysis of superficial versus deep injection of radioactive tracer and blue dye for lymphatic mapping and detection of sentinel lymph nodes in breast cancer. Br J Surg. 2015;102:169–81.

73. Fisher B, Redmond C, Fisher ER, et al. Ten-year results of a randomized clinical trial comparing radical mastectomy and total mastectomy with or without radiation. N Engl J Med. 1985;312:674–81.

74. Veronesi U, Viale G, Paganelli G, et al. Sentinel lymph node biopsy in breast cancer: ten-year results of a randomized controlled study. Ann Surg. 2010;251:595–600.

75. Kapoor NS, Sim MS, Lin J, et al. Long-term outcome of patients managed with sentinel lymph node biopsy alone for node-negative invasive breast cancer. Arch Surg. 2015;147:1047–52.

76. Hunt KK, Ballman KV, McCall LM. Factors associated with local-regional recurrence after a negative sentinel node dissection: results of the ACOSOG Z0010 trial. Ann Surg. 2012;256:428–36.

77. Weaver DL, Ashikaga T, Krag DN, et al. Effect of occult metastases on survival in node-negative breast cancer. N Engl J Med. 2011;364:412–21.

78. Donker M, van Tienhoven G, Straver ME, et al. Radiotherapy or surgery of the axilla after a positive sentinel node in breast cancer (EORTC 10981-22023 AMAROS): a randomised, multicentre, open-label, phase 3 non-inferiority trial. Lancet Oncol. 2014;15:1303–10.

79. Giuliano AE, Ballman KV, McCall L, et al. Effect of axillary dissection vs no axillary dissection on 10-year overall survival among women with invasive breast cancer and sentinel node metastasis: the ACOSOG Z0011 (Alliance) randomized clinical trial. JAMA. 2017;318:918–26.

80. Morigi C. Highlights of the 16th St. Gallen International Breast Cancer Conference, Vienna, Austria, 20–23 March 2019: personalised treatments for patients with early breast cancer. Ecancermedicalscience. 2019;13:924.

81. Tanis PJ, Nieweg OE, Valdés Olmos RA, et al. Impact of non-axillary sentinel node biopsy on staging and treatment of breast cancer patients. Br J Cancer (2002) 87:705-710.

Preoperative and Intraoperative Lymphatic Mapping for Radioguided Sentinel Lymph Node Biopsy in Cutaneous Melanoma

10

Sergi Vidal-Sicart, Andrés Perissinotti, Daphne D. D. Rietbergen, and Renato A. Valdés Olmos

Contents

10.1   **Introduction** 220

10.2   **The Clinical Problem** 220

10.3   **Lymphatic Drainage of Skin and Lymph Nodal Groups** 222

10.4   **Indications and Contraindications for SLNB in Melanoma** 223

10.5   **Technical Issues** 224

10.6   **Preoperative Imaging of SLNs** 227

10.7   **Contribution of SPECT/CT Imaging** 231

10.8   **Intraoperative Approach** 233

10.9   **Practical Considerations for SLN Mapping in Melanoma** 243

10.10   **Technical Pitfalls in Lymphatic Mapping for Melanoma Patients** 245

10.11   **The Dawn of a New Era?** 245

Clinical Cases 246

References 256

S. Vidal-Sicart (✉)
Nuclear Medicine Department, Hospital Clinic Barcelona, Barcelona, Catalonia, Spain

Institut d'Investigacions Biomèdiques August Pi Sunyer (IDIBAPS), Barcelona, Catalonia, Spain
e-mail: svidal@clinic.cat

A. Perissinotti
Nuclear Medicine Department, Hospital Clinic Barcelona, Barcelona, Catalonia, Spain

Biomedical Research Networking Center in Bioengineering, Biomaterials and Nanomedicine (CIBER-BBN), Barcelona, Catalonia, Spain

D. D. D. Rietbergen
Department of Radiology, Section of Nuclear Medicine, Leiden University Medical Centre, Leiden, Netherlands

R. A. Valdés Olmos
Department of Radiology, Section of Nuclear Medicine and Interventional Molecular Imaging Laboratory, Leiden University Medical Center, Leiden, The Netherlands

Learning Objectives
- To acquire basic knowledge about the role of nuclear medicine imaging in the sentinel lymph node (SLN) procedure in cutaneous melanoma
- To learn the clinical indications and contraindications of sentinel lymph node biopsy (SLNB) in patients with melanoma
- To understand the variability in lymphatic drainage of the skin and the need to use preoperative lymphatic mapping to assess the different individual patterns
- To know the role of lymphoscintigraphy including SPECT/CT imaging to identify and localize SLNs

© Springer Nature Switzerland AG 2020
G. Mariani et al. (eds.), *Atlas of Lymphoscintigraphy and Sentinel Node Mapping*,
https://doi.org/10.1007/978-3-030-45296-4_10

- To understand the importance of SPECT/CT to localize SLNs in different anatomical scenarios for cutaneous melanoma
- To understand the possible use of different "signatures" for SLN mapping based on the combination of intraoperative radioguidance and visual guidance with fluorescent tracers
- To preoperatively identify SLNs and to learn how this information can be transferred to surgeons for the intraoperative procedure

10.1   Introduction

Melanoma is one of the most aggressive and treatment-resistant cancers, and its incidence is growing throughout the world [1].

In recent years the melanoma incidence stands for 10–14 new cases/100,000 inhabitants per year in Central Europe and 6–10/100,000 inhabitants in Southern Europe. In the USA the incidence has risen to 10–25/10,000 inhabitants, and Australia and New Zealand show the highest incidence with 60 new cases/100,000 inhabitants per year [2].

According to the American Cancer Society, more than 71,000 new cases of melanoma are currently diagnosed each year in the USA, and about 9500 deaths occur due to metastatic disease.

Regional lymph nodes are frequently the first site of metastasis before systemic spreading of the disease. Metastatic involvement of lymph nodes is of paramount importance for prognosis in patients with intermediate-thickness (0.8–4 mm) melanomas. Other factors that worsen the prognosis include higher tumour thickness, presence of ulceration, and increasing mitotic rate [3].

Radioguided surgery plays an important role in melanoma, as SLNB is currently the procedure of choice for assessing regional lymphatic staging of these patients. This procedure includes lymphatic mapping by means of presurgical lymphoscintigraphy, which allows a precise SLN anatomical localization [4].

The first descriptions of the lymphatic drainage of the skin were based on the work of the French anatomist Sappey, who injected mercury into cadavers to visualize the lymphatic channels. He reported drainage to the axilla and groin from the skin of the trunk, and identified a vertical midline zone anteriorly and posteriorly where drainage to lymphatic basins in both sides of the body tended to overlap. A similar zone was observed horizontally around the waist from the umbilicus to the area of the second lumbar vertebra. In these zones, called "Sappey's lines", drainage

was said to be possible to either side in the case of the vertical zone, or to either the groin or the axilla in the case of the horizontal zone [5].

Sappey's concept of the predictability of lymphatic drainage of the trunk was accepted as correct for more than a century, until it was modified by Haagensen et al. who enlarged the ambiguous zone to a 5 cm band down the midline and around the waist. The later addition of lymphoscintigraphy enabled to identify the great variability of lymphatic drainage throughout individuals not only for the different areas of the trunk, but also for areas with minor (e.g. extremities) or major (e.g., head and neck, scapular) unpredictability of drainage [6]. This superiority of lymphoscintigraphy in the delineation of the ambiguous zones of lymphatic drainage is illustrated in Fig. 10.1.

Presurgical lymphoscintigraphy currently constitutes the "roadmap" for guiding surgeons toward draining lymph nodes potentially harbouring metastasis and is extremely useful for identifying unpredictable drainage patterns that otherwise would not be considered.

New refinements have recently been added to this approach in order to improve the clinical results. In particular, the incorporation of SPECT/CT imaging to preoperative mapping has resulted in improved detection of additional SLNs not visualized in planar images, as well as in an accurate anatomical localization providing to the surgeon specific landmarks for SLN excision. This advance has been accompanied by the development of novel tracers, such as ^{99m}Tc-tilmanocept (Lymphoseek®) or ICG-^{99m}Tc-nanocoll (bimodal or hybrid tracer), aimed at increasing the intraoperative SLN identification rate.

10.2   The Clinical Problem

The clinical outcome for patients with intermediate-thickness melanoma relies on adequate surgical control of the primary melanoma site and on the accuracy of regional and systemic staging at diagnosis. SLNB was initially indicated for patients with intermediate Breslow thickness (>1–4 mm). However, more recently, the biopsy may also be considered for thin melanomas that are T1b (0.8–1 mm or <0.8 mm thickness with ulceration) after a thorough discussion with the patient of the potential benefits and risks of harm associated with the procedure [7]. Due to the low risk of finding lymph nodal metastasis in melanoma lesions that are T1a (non-ulcerated lesions <0.8 mm thickness), SLN staging can be omitted in these patients. In lesions >4 mm SLNB is currently also offered, because it yields valuable prognostic information with positive SLN rates ranging from 30 to 40% in spite of the risk of synchronous distant metastases reported for this patients' category [8].

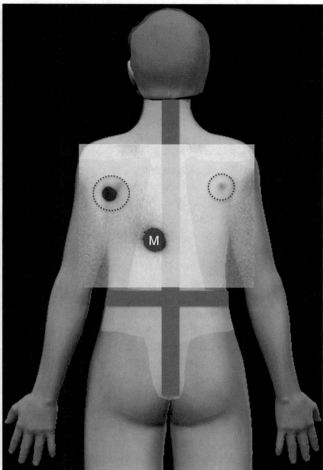

Fig. 10.1 Superiority of mapping with lymphoscintigraphy (slightly brown) in comparison to classical skin watershed Sappey's areas (pink) to define ambiguous drainage in the trunk. On the *left*, bilateral periclavicular drainage (circles) is seen on superimposed lymphoscintigraphy for a parasternal primary melanoma (M), located definitely outside the Sappey's area. On the *right*, bilateral axillary drainage (circles) is observed for a dorsal melanoma (M), located just outside of the Sappey's line

Regional lymph nodes are the most common site of metastatic dissemination from melanoma, and it is well known that physical examination of lymph nodes is inaccurate in up to 40% of patients. Non-invasive diagnostic imaging procedures (CT, MRI, US, PET-CT) have been employed to rule out nodal involvement (stage N0), but their findings are not accurate enough to avoid invasive techniques, because small lymph node metastases cannot be reliably detected with any imaging modalities [9].

Nearly 20% of patients who present with a melanoma with Breslow thickness >1 mm have occult metastases in regional nodes (clinically non-palpable and difficult to be detected by ultrasound). Hence, a thorough pathological evaluation for early detection of metastasis is crucial. In the past, regional lymphadenectomy was routinely performed to stage clinically node-negative melanoma patients. However,

a remarkable percentage (>75%) of patients with <4 mm Breslow thickness melanomas did not present lymph node metastases.

Therefore, lymphadenectomy exposed many patients to unnecessary surgical complications such as lymphedema, hematoma, seroma, wound infection and pain. Moreover, several randomized studies revealed no clear advantages of performing prophylactic regional lymph node dissection in terms of survival. The therapeutic value of immediate lymphadenectomy in the clinically node-negative patient has been one of the longest standing and most controversial issues in the clinical management of cutaneous melanoma [10, 11].

In the last 20 years, lymphadenectomy has progressively been replaced by the SLNB procedure, a minimally invasive method based on the hypothesis of stepwise spreading of melanoma through the lymphatic system, and on the definition of the SLN as the node with a direct lymphatic drainage pathway from the primary tumour [12]. The classical SLNB concept implies that, in case of no SLN metastatic involvement, the rest of the lymph nodes in the same regional basin could be considered as disease free, thus sparing these patients regional lymphadenectomy, which remains reserved only for those cases with SLN-containing metastases; the procedure therefore avoids unnecessary surgical complications in patients with tumour-free SLN.

In the past presurgical lymphoscintigraphy was used as a guide to determine which lymph node basins were to be subjected to elective lymphadenectomy. Preoperative lymphoscintigraphy depicts all lymph node stations that might be at risk for metastases, thus providing a roadmap to guide the intervention. The continuous use of this technique disclosed lymphatic drainage to some basins not often considered as potential metastatic sites based on clinical judgement. Several studies have widened the zone of ambiguity around Sappey's lines, and also demonstrated that drainage in the head and neck was quite unpredictable [13].

SLNB was introduced in 1992 by Morton and co-workers who used intradermal injection of vital blue dye intraoperatively to identify SLNs at the lymph node stations previously mapped with lymphoscintigraphy. In 1993, the use of the handheld gamma probe for intraoperative SLN detection was reported. Ever since, radioguided detection has been incorporated into SLNB in combination with intraoperative blue dyes. More recently gamma probe detection has overshadowed the use of vital blue dye, which is currently omitted by some groups [6, 14].

The SLN procedure is currently widely adopted by surgical oncologists as an alternative to elective lymphadenectomy and to observation of patients with clinically negative regional lymph nodes, but at high risk of nodal metastasis.

One of the goals of SLNB is to identify those 20–25% of patients with clinically negative nodes who present with occult lymphatic regional disease at diagnosis. This minimally invasive procedure can also identify those patients that are most likely to benefit from lymphadenectomy, thus minimizing the morbidity associated with elective lymphadenectomy, such as lymphedema and other complications. The technique also increases the identification rate of occult lymph node metastases, by guiding the pathologist to the lymph node (or nodes) most likely to contain metastatic disease, although there is a non-negligible false-negative rate [15, 16].

Regarding the therapeutic implications of this procedure, the Multicenter Selective Lymphadenectomy Trial-1 (MSLT-1) compared the outcome of patients with melanoma ≥1.20 mm thick, who were randomly assigned to a SLNB arm (with complete lymph node dissection if the SLN harboured metastasis) or an observation arm (elective lymph node dissection in case of clinical nodal relapse).

At the 10-year follow-up, the rate of nodal relapse in cases with a negative SLNB was much lower than the nodal relapse rate in the observation arm (4% versus 17.4%). These results confirm that the SLN procedure is an effective and accurate staging tool capable of identifying patients with clinically occult metastases and selecting them for lymphadenectomy and locoregional disease control. As a consequence, the SLN status was shown to be the single most important prognostic factor in patients with clinically node-negative disease [17].

On the other hand, indication for complete regional lymphadenectomy is currently limited taking into account the recent results from MSLT-II and DeCOG-SLT trials, which showed no melanoma-specific survival benefits between immediate lymphadenectomy and active ultrasound surveillance in patients with metastatic SLN melanoma.

The MSLT-II trial compared complete lymph node dissection versus ultrasound-based observation in 1755 SLN-positive melanoma patients. Even though the lymphadenectomy group after 3 years showed a slightly higher disease-free survival than the observation group (68% vs. 63%) due to a higher rate of disease control in the regional nodes (92% vs. 77%), no statistically significant 3-year melanoma-specific survival between the two groups was observed [18, 19].

The data of these two studies indicate that the decision to perform regional lymphadenectomy should not be made when a positive SLN is detected, but rather at the time when recurrence is discovered. These results have shown that active surveillance of the nodal basin is a safe and efficient way to identify patients who have more probability to benefit from delayed lymph node-directed treatment [7].

Anyway, SLNB clearly remains a cornerstone in the current staging system with, either for SLN excision or for surveillance, lymphoscintigraphy as an essential part of the approach in order to offer the best lymphatic mapping in every patient, particularly for avoiding potential misleading results.

10.3 Lymphatic Drainage of Skin and Lymph Nodal Groups

The skin has a very dense network of lymphatic capillaries and vessels. The paths followed by the collecting vessels on their way to the lymph basins vary from patient to patient and for every cutaneous location. These ducts can sometimes be very complex and unexpected. Lymphatic vessels join to form larger vessels or multiple vessels. These collecting ducts pass through the subcutaneous fat layer and penetrate into the deep fascia after reaching the lymph node basin.

On the other hand, the velocity of lymphatic flow is not the same in all regions of the body. Thus, the average lymph flow velocity in the head and neck region is 1.5 cm/min; it increases in the posterior trunk to 3.9 cm/min, and is even higher in the forearm and hand (5.5 cm/min). The highest velocity of lymph flow is seen in the lower limb (10.2 cm/min) [20].

Lymphatic drainage from the primary tumour is quite predictable when this malignancy is located in the extremities. Hence, a melanoma located in the lower limb usually drains to the ipsilateral groin, while a melanoma of the upper limb will drain to the ipsilateral axilla. However, drainage to alternative lymph node stations (such as the popliteal or the epitrochlear groups) may be observed and the drainage patterns from lesions in the head and neck area or in the trunk are less predictable. The concept developed by Sappey in the nineteenth century has remained unaltered until the last years of twentieth century, when new information became available from lymphatic mapping studies using lymphoscintigraphy.

In fact, the more recent data from lymphoscintigraphy have modified the concept of Sappey's lines, markedly widening the area of ambiguous drainage up to 20 cm or more instead of the original 5 cm (Fig. 10.1). In fact, lymphoscintigraphy better reflects the high variability among different patients and more accurately depicts lymphatic drainage than the Sappey's approach, which would predict drainage to the wrong node basin in 30% of patients [21, 22].

As lymphatic cutaneous drainage is highly variable, lymphoscintigraphy is currently mandatory. The reproducibility of this technique is very high, ranging from 84 to 96% in several studies [23].

The predictability of lymphatic drainage in cutaneous melanoma depends on the location of the primary lesions, being approximately 98% in the lower limbs, 88% in the upper extremities, 56% in the anterior thorax and 39% in the posterior trunk. Lymphatic drainage is almost completely unpredictable in the head and neck region. However, when a strict injection protocol is followed and the time interval for tracer administration is limited to just a few days, reproducibility can reach 100% as demonstrated in a head-to-head comparison in melanomas with different anatomical locations [13, 24, 25].

Nevertheless, learning the physiologic and "lymphoscintigraphic" drainage patterns of the primary tumour's location is crucial to estimate the draining basins most likely to be investigated preoperatively with lymphoscintigraphy (Table 10.1).

With increasing experience, interpretation of lymphoscintigrams becomes more and more reliable. This means that fewer SLNs will go unnoticed by the nuclear medicine physician and by the surgeon. Since spatial resolution of gamma cameras is not expected to dramatically improve in the near future, advances in lymphoscintigraphy will most likely derive from the use of better radiopharmaceuticals (used

Table 10.1 Possible lymphatic drainage and potential SLN location depending on the site of cutaneous melanoma

Melanoma location	Expected drainage	Unexpected
Foot, leg	Femoral, inguinal	Popliteal, external iliac
Hand, arm	Axillary	Epitroclear, arm, supraclavicular
Mammary	Axillary	Supraclavicular, parasternal
Thorax (anterior-posterior)	Axillary	Subcutaneous, supraclavicular, parasternal, diaphragmatic, mediastinal
Head	Pre- and post-auricular, submandibular	Cervical
Neck	Cervical, supraclavicular	Axillary
Abdomen	Axillary, inguinal	Subcutaneous, paravertebral, para-aortic, parasternal

either alone or in combination with non-radioactive compounds) and from the improvement in SPECT/CT acquisition and reconstruction [26].

Key Learning Points
- In patients with cutaneous melanoma, SLNB has replaced regional lymphadenectomy, which exposes patients to unnecessary immediate and long-term surgical complications in >75% of patients with <4 mm Breslow thickness melanomas and a clinically negative lymph node basin.
- The extensive use of presurgical lymphoscintigraphy has demonstrated failure in the Sappey's concept to accurately predict the pathway of lymphatic drainage for melanomas located in ambiguous areas around Sappey's lines.
- High inter-patient variability in the patterns of lymphatic cutaneous drainage makes the use of preoperative lymphoscintigraphy a mandatory component of radioguided SLNB in patients with cutaneous melanoma.

10.4 Indications and Contraindications for SLNB in Melanoma

The indication for SLNB in melanoma should be offered to and discussed with all patients with melanomas >1.0 mm in thickness and clinically negative regional lymph nodes on physical examination, and in whom the morbidity and risk are considered to be acceptable. However, SLNB can also be offered to patients with melanomas <1.0 mm and high risk of micrometastasis in the regional node basin (presence of ulceration, high mitotic index and/or Clark IV/V invasion). Even though the indication for SLNB may be questioned in cases of very thick melanomas (>4 mm) due to a higher risk of systemic spread of the disease (via haematogenous dissemination) and concurrent lymphatic spread, SLNB can be performed as a strong predictive factor also in this subgroup of patients [27, 28].

The seventh edition of the AJCC/UICC Cancer Staging Manual published in 2010 has been widely adopted, although the eighth edition published in 2018 has introduced some changes in the classification system, concerning especially stages I–III [29]. The basic changes introduced can be summarized as follows:

- Category T thickness is now rounded to the 10th decimal instead of the 100th decimal.
- The T1a and 1b stage border is at 0.8 mm.
- The mitotic rate (MR) is removed as a T1 staging criterion.
- The pT1b tumours now belong to stage IA disease.

The other T stages are subcategorized by tumour thickness and presence of ulceration (a and b), as follows:

- T0: No evidence of primary melanoma.
- Tx: Breslow thickness cannot be determined.
- T1a: Non-ulcerated melanomas <0.8 mm Breslow thickness.
- T1b: Ulcerated melanomas of any Breslow thickness and non-ulcerated 0.8–1 mm Breslow thickness melanomas.
- T2a: Non-ulcerated melanomas >1 mm and <2 mm Breslow thickness.
- T2b: Ulcerated melanomas >1 mm and <2 mm Breslow thickness.
- T3a: Non-ulcerated melanomas >2 mm and ≤4 mm Breslow thickness.
- T3b: Ulcerated melanomas >2 mm and ≤4 mm Breslow thickness.
- T4a: Non-ulcerated melanomas >4 mm Breslow thickness.
- T4b: Ulcerated melanomas >4 mm Breslow thickness.

Regarding lymph node status (category N), the following changes in definitions have been adopted:

- The "microscopic" and "macroscopic" descriptors are redefined as clinically hidden (occult) and clinically detected (evident) metastases, respectively.
- Tumour burden is not used to determine groups in category N.
- The presence of microsatellitosis, satellitosis or metastasis in transit is now classified as Nc (N1c, N2c or N3c depending on the number of regional lymph nodes affected).

- Extranodal extension is not included in category N (Fig. 10.2).

Finally, regarding the metastatic status (category M), the following changes in definitions have been adopted:

- M1 is now defined by the anatomical site of metastatic disease and the serum lactate dehydrogenase (LDH) value for all subcategories of the anatomical site.
- A new designation of M is added (d) to include metastases in the CNS.

Among the main changes proposed in the eighth edition of the AJCC/UICC, mitosis is excluded as a prognostic factor; tumours with 0.8 mm Breslow thickness and ulceration have an indication to perform the SLNB, as do all those with Breslow thickness ≥1 mm. Thickness and ulceration remain the factors with the most predictive value. Any positive nodal state, including in-transit metastases, is considered stage III [30]. Table 10.2 summarizes the current indications and contraindication of SLNB for cutaneous melanoma patients.

10.5 Technical Issues

10.5.1 Radiotracers

After initial studies using blue dyes, lymphoscintigraphy was incorporated in the SLN procedure in melanoma using radiocolloids varying between 5 and 1000 nm in particle size. In general, radiocolloids used for preoperative lymphoscintigraphy are mostly trapped in the SLN by the phagocytic activity of the macrophages and tissue histiocytes that line the subcapsular sinus of lymph nodes. Therefore, retention of radiocolloids in the lymph node is a physiological process, and it does not indicate the presence or absence of metastatic involvement in the node [22].

The speed of radiotracer migration from the injection site and the amount retained in the SLN depend on the size of the radiocolloids. Choice of the radiotracer for performing preoperative lymphoscintigraphy and SLNB has been a controversial issue. The ideal radiotracer would be the one with the highest uptake in the SLN, low retention at the injection site and minimal distribution to the upper tier lymph nodes. Optimally, small-sized radiocolloids (less than about 100 nm) migrate quite fast from the injection site through the lymphatic system visualizing lymphatic vessels with the ability to cover more lymph node stations, which may be important in anatomical areas of expected multidirectional drainage. Intermediate-sized particles (50–200 nm) migrate more slowly from the primary lesion, but exhibit a more prolonged retention in the SLN. Larger sized radiocolloids are retained longer in the SLN, and

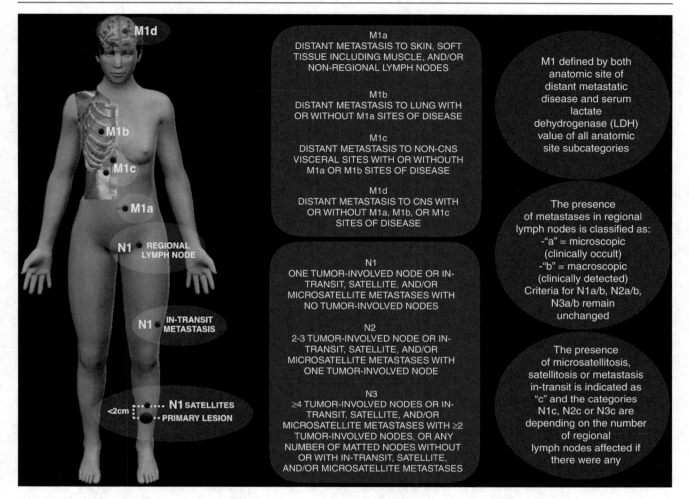

Fig. 10.2 Schematic illustration of metastatic dissemination of cutaneous melanoma according to the eighth edition of TNM AJCC/UICC classification. Criteria for regional disease have been specified (framework and circles) for N1, N2 and N3. Concerning distant metastases, the M1d category, concerning central nervous system (CNS), has been added to the M1a, M1b and M1c categories

Table 10.2 Indications and contraindications for SLNB in cutaneous melanoma

Indications

1. Breslow thickness 0.8–1 mm with presence of ulceration. The risk of lymph node metastasis is approximately 5%
2. Breslow thickness 1–4 mm. The risk of lymph node metastases increases from 8 to 30% and there is a consensus on the need to offer the option of radioguided biopsy for correct staging of these patients
3. Breslow thickness >4 mm. Thicker melanomas have a high risk of distant metastases (about 40%), although lymph nodes are usually not clinically palpable. For this reason, the status of the SLN still offers valuable prognostic information and can be considered

Contraindications

1. Extensive previous surgery in the region of the primary lesion or in the selected lymphatic region
2. Patients with known metastases
3. Breslow thickness <0.8 mm. It is usually not recommended to perform the SLN procedure in these patients because the risk of metastasis in the draining lymph nodes is 1%
4. Poor general condition and serious concurrent diseases
5. Known allergy to dyes or radiotracers
6. Radiation therapy on the lesion or the lymph node area

lymphoscintigraphy usually visualizes only 1–2 nodes; in principle, this aspect can lead to an underestimation in the mapping of lymph node stations considered at risk of metastases. On the other hand, migration of larger particles from the interstitial administration site is very slow and therefore a longer acquisition time will be necessary to complete lymphoscintigraphy. Nevertheless, the choice of radiopharmaceutical varies according to geographic region and is usually guided by local legislation and commercial availability [31].

In Europe, the most commonly used radiotracer is the ^{99m}Tc-labelled albumin nanocolloid, while in the USA ^{99m}Tc-sulphur colloid is used and in Australia ^{99m}Tc-antimony sulphide. Available radiotracers for SLN mapping in Europe include Nanocoll® (particle size range 5–80 nm), Nanoscan® (≤80 nm), Nanocis® (100 nm) and Sentiscint® (100–600 nm range, with average 200 nm).

There is no specific consensus regarding the activity to be injected, which should be adapted to the local logistics and to the time lapse between the injection and surgery. Activities

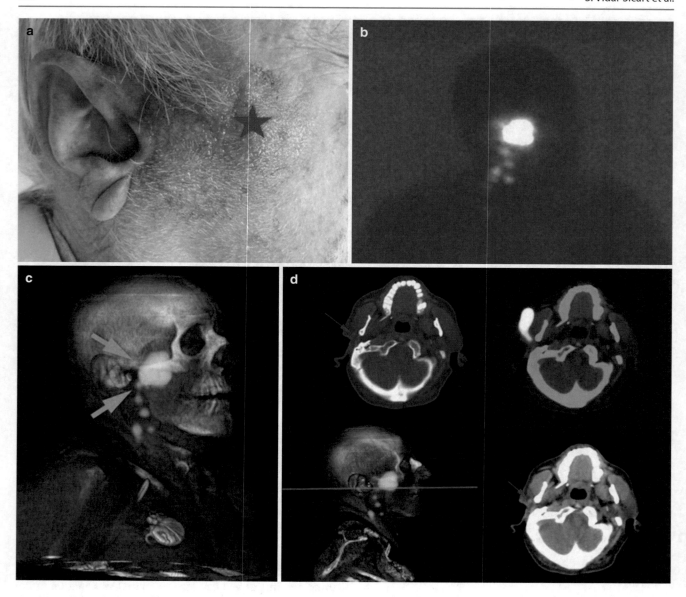

Fig. 10.3 Four intradermal ^{99m}Tc-tilmanocept injections (74 MBq) were performed around the excision scar of a melanoma of the right cheek (**a**). Right lateral view on planar image showing injection site and several faint uptakes caudally (**b**). Volume-rendering reconstruction of SPECT/CT images shows focal uptake in right preauricular and level IIa cervical regions considered as SLNs (green arrows) and radiotracer progression to secondary cervical lymph echelons (not considered SLNs) (**c**). Due to the rapid washout from the injection site of ^{99m}Tc-tilmanocept, activity from injection site did not interfere with the intraoperative identification of the right preauricular SLNs (red arrows) (**d**)

usually range from 60 to 120 MBq, depending on the specific 1-day or 2-day protocol employed. It has been demonstrated that both procedures are equally effective for SLN detection [32, 33].

Use of ^{99m}Tc-tilmanocept (Lymphoseek®), a new radiotracer designed specifically for SLN identification, has recently been approved by the Food and Drug Administration (FDA) in the USA (since 2013) and by the European Medicines Agency (EMA) in Europe (since 2017). This tracer has unique properties for the identification of SLN and lymphatic mapping, with the potential to overcome the difficulties observed with conventional radiotracers used until now [34] (Fig. 10.3). In particular, ^{99m}Tc-tilmanocept is a mannosyl diethylene triamine penta-acetate (DTPA) dextran small 18 kDa molecule with a 3.5 nm hydrodynamic radius designed for selective molecular imaging of CD206 mannose receptor carrier tissues. It has an average molecule size of 7 nm, which allows rapid entry into the lymphatic channels as well as into the blood capillaries, resulting in rapid clearance from the site of injection allowing the detection of SLNs located near the injection site.

Concerning melanoma, ^{99m}Tc-tilmanocept has been prospectively evaluated in two non-randomized phase III trials in comparison with vital blue dye. These trials showed that ^{99m}Tc-tilmanocept has a very high rate of SLN identification. Besides its rapid clearance from the injection site and SLN uptake, there is also low further migration to second-echelon lymph nodes [35–37].

> **Key Learning Points**
> - Suitable candidates for SLNB are those patients with melanomas with a Breslow thickness ≥0.8 mm with the presence of ulceration and with negative lymph nodes (clinically or by imaging methods).
> - While there is an accepted consensus on the indication in patients with melanomas of intermediate Breslow thickness (0.8–4 mm), its indication in thinner (<0.8 mm) or thicker melanomas (>4 mm) is still a matter under investigation.
> - In Europe the standard radiotracer for lymphoscintigraphy is ^{99m}Tc-nanocolloid, in Australia ^{99m}Tc-antimony trisulphide and in the USA ^{99m}Tc-sulphur colloid.

10.5.2 Radiotracer Injection

Usually the radiotracer is intradermally administered with 4 or more (in some cases 2–4) injections (depending on the anatomic site) around the primary melanoma or around the excisional biopsy site. According to the EANM guidelines, radiotracer injection into the dermis raising a bleb within 1 cm from the melanoma or the excisional biopsy scar is the most appropriate technique [38] (Fig. 10.4).

Subcutaneous injection is also feasible and probably easier to accomplish, but its application is not recommended because it is not able to delineate the route of lymphatic drainage from the overlying cutaneous site.

Use of Luer-Lock tuberculin syringes is recommended. The intradermal injection should be performed using a 25- or 27-gauge needle. The needle is inserted in a direction as tangent as possible to the skin surface at a few mm inside the skin; this technique avoids patient's skin contamination and entails small volumes of radiotracer, just enough to produce a bleb in the skin.

Injections should surround the lesion or biopsy site to best provide lymphatic drainage in all directions. Alternatively, in upper limbs mapping may be accomplished by performing two injections proximal to the biopsy scar, an approach that can be employed also for lesions located in the foot and leg. When lesions are located in the thigh, it is advisable to inject in both sides of the scar or tumour. In other sites (the trunk, head and neck), it is mandatory to inject at least four aliquots around the lesion. In these latter patients, radiocolloid injections must be applied roughly equatorially around the lesion (at 3, 6, 9, 12 h), because lymphatic drainage may occur both cranially and caudally, as well as across the midline of the body. In the case of large excision scars, more injection depots must be given (Table 10.3).

Cutaneous lymphoscintigraphy is highly reproducible when the injection distance from the border of tumour/scar does not exceed 10 mm. On the other hand, increasing such distance may lead to injecting of the radiocolloid across a lymphatic watershed, thus visualizing other lymph nodes not reflecting the dissemination route of the primary melanoma. A larger distance from the primary lesion is only recommended in patients with hypertrophic scars and inflammation after biopsy, or in patients without lymph node visualization after the first set of injections (Fig. 10.5).

Topical anaesthetic medications may be used to diminish the pain, especially when the primary melanoma is in a sensitive location (or when using a radiocolloid with low pH, such as ^{99m}Tc-sulphur colloid).

To avoid contamination, a sheet should be placed next to the injection site, and after each injection the skin should be covered with a swab before the needle is removed. In some patients lymphatic drainage is slow. If no tracer drainage is observed in dynamic or early static images, massage of the injection site or along the lymphatic vessels can be helpful.

The tracer is injected the day before surgery or, alternatively, on the same day. Although no differences in SLN detection rate or false-negative rate have been found between these two protocols, the 2-day protocol may present some advantages with flexibility in the timing of lymphoscintigraphy and surgery. The 1-day protocol requires a good cooperation between the nuclear medicine staff and surgeons with respect to the estimated speed of lymphatic drainage in the affected region and the time to surgery. Intraoperative injection is not recommended because lymphatic drainage in melanoma may be aberrant or delayed to more than one nodal basin and because it is not always possible to obtain intraoperative imaging [38, 39].

10.6   Preoperative Imaging of SLNs

Preoperative lymphoscintigraphy is the first mandatory step in the SLN mapping procedure of melanomas and is considered to be an essential part of the procedure. It displays the flow of radioactive tracers through the lymphatic channels and discloses any alternative routes to different regional lymphatic basins. Depiction of lymph nodes located along the route of lymph drainage can be displayed and other nodes or

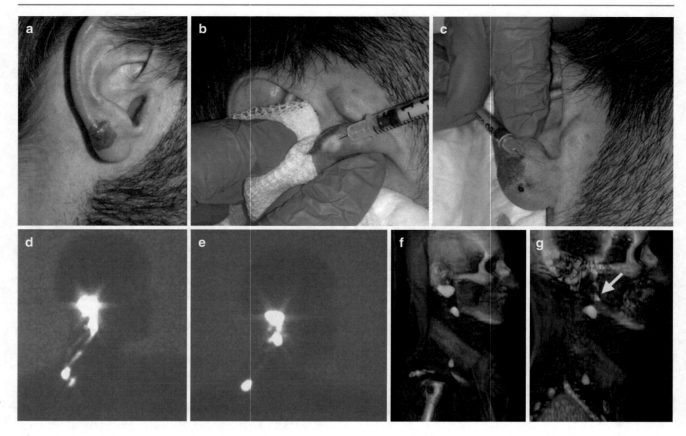

Fig. 10.4 (**a**) A superficial spread melanoma located at the bottom of the right ear. (**b**, **c**) Radiotracer injection around the margins of the lesion with a raising wheal upon injection of 0.1 mL of ^{99m}Tc-tilmanocept. Early planar images show radiotracer drainage to upper and lower ipsilateral cervical echelons (**d**). Delayed planar images reveal an additional small focus of activity located between the injection site and the upper cervical SLN (**e**). SPECT/CT (**f**, **g**) better identifies this finding as an additional SLN adjacent to the mandibular ramus (yellow arrow)

Table 10.3 Recommended modalities of tracer injection for lymphoscintigraphy according to the location of the melanoma/scar

Toes and fingers

Generally, the radiotracer is injected in 2–4 sites at the base of the nail. Local injections with lidocaine or xylocaine, surrounding the nail, are enough to provide anaesthesia in patients with subungual melanoma. After anaesthesia is obtained, the radiocolloid can be injected

Foot's sole

The sole of the foot is difficult to inject due to the characteristics of the skin. Anaesthesia involves local block of the sole of the foot, but generally a lidocaine injection suffices (though remaining painful). The area is quite bloody when the needle is inserted. Injecting radiocolloid into a callus or hyperkeratosis would show no migration

Scalp

It is useful to shave the area to be injected. The skin of the scalp is difficult to inject, but should be kept in the intradermal site as the needle tends to penetrate slightly deeper than optimal. Contamination of the injection area is a real problem and a good coverage by a sheet around the injection site is required. Care must be given to avoid any leakage from the injection, since it can be a source of significant contamination

Ear

The site of previous biopsy on the ear may be difficult to recognize. When patients are not able to precisely indicate the site of the excision scar, it is recommended to ask the surgeon or dermatologist to indicate the exact site of the biopsy. The injection is carried out at four poles surrounding the tumour, or the biopsy scar. The skin is quite loose, and thus the amount of anaesthesia and radiocolloid are generally increased in volume. Special care must be taken in the helix area, and preventing contamination of the injection site is of utmost importance

Trunk

Injection in midline melanomas is not different than in other areas but image acquisition can be problematic, because the radiocolloid can drain to almost any lymphatic basin: axillary, groin or even supraclavicular, paravertebral or intra-abdominal nodes. In-transit or aberrant lymph nodes can also be found (parascapular area, paracostal nodes, submammary)

Other areas

Injecting in areas of induration, inflammation or infection should be avoided, and these special circumstances should be discussed with the surgeon. Before injecting near the eye, it is convenient to place a gauze over the eye and to take adequate care of possible contamination

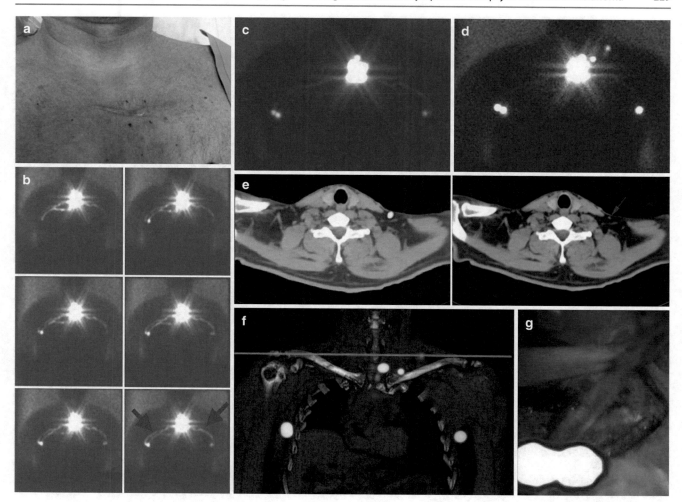

Fig. 10.5 Four intradermal injections of ^{99m}Tc-nanocolloid (111 MBq) were administered in close proximity to the excision scar in a 62-year-old man with cutaneous melanoma of the anterior trunk (**a**). Dynamic images showed direct migration of the radiotracer to the right axilla through two independent lymphatic channels and through a single channel to the left axilla (**b**). Even though early planar images showed only bilateral axillar drainage of the radiotracer (**c**), delayed planar images disclosed additional left supraclavicular drainage to lymphatic echelons also considered as SLNs (**d**). SPECT/CT images (**e**) with volumetric reconstructions (**f**) improved anatomical localization of all axillary and left supraclavicular SLNs. A portable gamma camera was used during surgery to identify and confirm SLN resection of the left supraclavicular area adjacent to the injection site (**g**)

paths could be observed if the original lymphatic flow pattern has been altered or rerouted due to massive metastatic blockage of the lymph nodes or by other causes such as fibrotic changes related to previous interventions.

Lymphoscintigraphy provides a visual roadmap of lymph node locations prior to surgery and may show the timely order in which lymphatic flow reaches those nodes, especially when a dynamic study is acquired [20, 26, 40–42]. Following injection, image acquisition is started as soon as possible covering all possible drainage routes and regions. A large field-of-view gamma camera is preferable, and dual-head cameras may be useful principally in the dynamic phase of the acquisition. The use of flood sources (^{57}Co or ^{99m}Tc) placed beneath the patient's body in order to highlight the body contours is helpful to provide some anatomical information for the surgeon. If flood sources are not available, the use of a pointer to draw the silhouette of the patient's body is recommended to give some anatomical reference. Low-energy high-resolution or ultrahigh-resolution collimators are recommended to better distinguish individual SLNs and to prevent star artefact of the injection place. The energy window in gamma camera settings should be 15% or 20% centred on the 140 keV photopeak of ^{99m}Tc.

Dynamic lymphoscintigraphy is essential to identify regional lymphatic basins and to differentiate true SLN from non-SLNs, which sequentially follow on the same lymphatic duct. A 10–20-min dynamic acquisition at the rate of 1 frame/min in a 128 × 128 matrix is suggested to determine

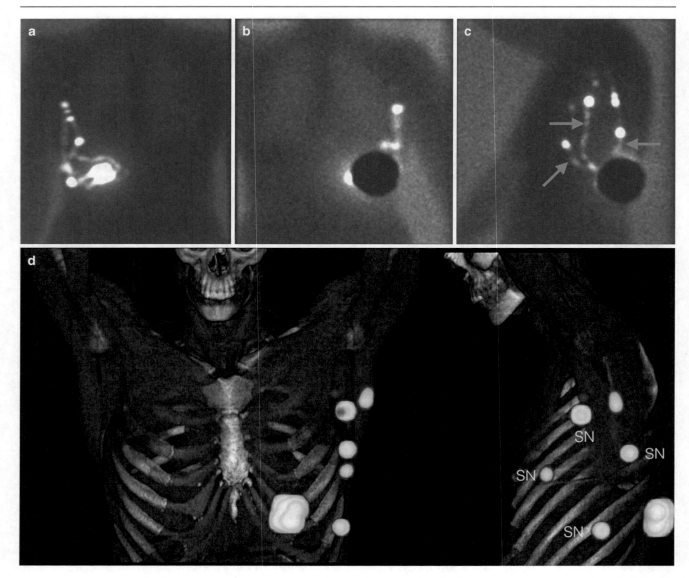

Fig. 10.6 Early dynamic planar images showing radiotracer drainage (^{99m}Tc-nanocolloid) to three SLNs through independent lymphatic channels (green arrows) in a 39-year-old man with melanoma of the right thorax (**a–c**). Delayed SPECT/CT study revealed an additional SLN closer to the injection site (**d**) that was hidden under the lead used during acquisition of planar images to mask injection activity

where the lymphatic collectors are directed. Lead shielding covering the injection site may be helpful during static image acquisition, in order to detect lymph nodes close to the injection site. However, the lead shield itself carries a risk of masking draining lymph nodes (Fig. 10.6).

Although somewhat time consuming, acquisition of dynamic images is crucial because a lymphatic channel directly draining to a lymph node may help to identify this node as a true SLN.

In melanomas of the hand/forearm or foot/leg, dynamic imaging should start over the injection site and follow the lymphatic drainage to the elbow and axilla or the knee/groin, respectively, to reveal ectopic basins and in-transit lymph nodes (popliteal, epitrochlear, etc.). For head and neck mela-

nomas, immediate imaging reduces the chance of missing a SLN because of rapid drainage from intradermal injections with uptake by superimposed lymph nodes.

After the dynamic acquisition, static early (30 min) and delayed (2–4 h) images after injection are obtained. For delayed imaging, 5-min static acquisitions in a 256 × 256 matrix size should be recorded over the potential lymph node field, in order to identify the collectors as they reach the actual SLNs (Fig. 10.7). This procedure is important since sometimes, especially in the groin for leg melanomas, some tracer will be seen passing through the SLN on to a second-tier lymph node. Usually SLNs are identified within 30 min after radiocolloid injection, but it is advisable to record 2-h images as well, due to the possibility of delayed or slow

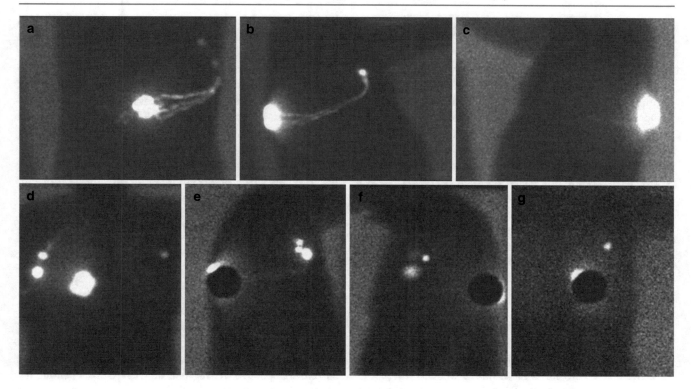

Fig. 10.7 Early dynamic planar images show exclusive radiotracer drainage to right axillary lymph nodes in a 57-year-old patient with melanoma of the right back (**a–c**). However, delayed planar images dis-played additional drainage to a contralateral axillary node, also considered SLN (**d–g**)

drainage to other SLNs in different areas/basins and to distinguish first draining from second-echelon lymph nodes.

If no radiocolloid drainage is observed from the injection site during dynamic imaging, gentle massage for 5 min can help. If lymph nodes are not seen or are weakly visualized, additional delayed imaging may be considered up to 24 h after injection. If no visualization persists, reinjection of the radiocolloid is necessary. Reinjection must be also considered when SLN uptake is faint and patient will be operated on the second day.

Finally, the site of each SLN must be marked on the skin of the patient with the help of a ^{57}Co or ^{99m}Tc point source. The study can be completed by confirming the exact location of the SLNs with the aid of a handheld gamma probe [43–45].

Lymphoscintigraphy is claimed to predict the metastatic burden in lymph nodes. Regarding this issue, a study in 509 melanoma patients scheduled for SLNB showed that clear depiction of an afferent lymph vessel may be a sign of micro-metastasis. On the other hand, the presence of macrometas-tasis was associated with prominent afferent vessels, delayed display of the first radioactive lymph node and higher number of detected hot spots. In patients with bidirectional or lymphatic drainage to three basins, the SLN metastatic involvement rates for the first, second and third basin were 25%, 12% and 0%, respectively [46].

Again, multiple lymphatic basin drainage is frequently observed in patients with trunk melanoma undergoing SLNB. Conflicting data regarding the prognostic association of this finding in SLN-negative and SLN-positive patients have been discussed. Some studies have reported that patients with negative SLNB results have better prognosis when two or more lymphatic basins are identified and analysed [47, 48].

In positive SLN patients, visualization of multiple lymphatic drainage basins is not correlated with survival, which is mainly related to AJCC prognostic factors [49].

10.7 Contribution of SPECT/CT Imaging

When the pattern of lymphatic drainage is unclear or the SLNs are deeply located or located closely next to the injection site, conventional planar lymphoscintigraphy can sometimes be challenging to interpret for SLN identification. SPECT/CT involves scatter and attenuation correction of the images, thus resulting in superior scintigraphic contrast and higher resolution than planar imaging; the end result of these features is the possibility to provide accurate anatomical localization. The SPECT/CT information is capable of modifying the evaluation of planar images in terms of number and localization of SLNs. Furthermore, SPECT/CT may discriminate more precisely the activity arising from two closely placed nodes that are usually depicted as one single hot spot on planar images [50].

SPECT/CT also provides anatomical localization of SLNs and is performed in addition to lymphoscintigraphy. A requirement for accurate SLN localization is that the CT component of SPECT/CT system must be of sufficient quality to provide adequate anatomical landmarks to be recognized by surgeons. SPECT/CT is especially useful in obese patients to demonstrate SLNs not detected on planar images, as well as to show additional SLNs in other areas. Usually, a radioactive hot spot corresponds to a single lymph node on CT, but in some cases this image corresponds to a cluster of lymph nodes adjacent one to each other [51].

SPECT/CT imaging is remarkably useful for SLNB of head and neck melanomas, because in this anatomical area lymph nodes are often small and located close to the injection site, where the bulk of the injected radioactivity is retained for a long time. The high variability of lymphatic drainage pathways is the reason why in many cases elective neck dissections and/or parotid gland excision do not detect the SLN. Knowing whether the node is located deep or superficial and whether it is within or outside the parotid gland has important surgical implications. The additional value of SPECT/CT is clear for patients with non-visualization on conventional planar scintigraphy and for patients with SLNs close to the tumour injection site. The benefit of SPECT/CT is also relevant for patients with melanoma of the trunk (Figs. 10.8, 10.9 and 10.10), while it is lower in patients with melanoma of the extremities [52].

A prospective multicentre trial of 262 patients demonstrated the added value of SPECT/CT in melanoma as well as in other solid tumours, as SPECT/CT revealed 70 additional SLNs in 53 patients (25% additional nodes in head and neck melanoma, 25.5% in patients with upper limb melanoma, 20.5% in patients with trunk melanoma and 12.9% in patients with lower limb melanoma). The surgical approach was modified in 97 patients (37%): 41%, 39%, 33% and 30% of head and neck, trunk, lower limb and upper limb lesions, respectively. Based on these results, the authors of the study recommend the use of SPECT/CT imaging in all patients with melanoma of the head and neck and trunk and in all melanoma patients with unexpected drainage on planar images [53].

Even though the addition of SPECT/CT to SLN mapping in patients with cutaneous melanoma can increase the preoperative imaging costs, its implementation was associated with a 30% reduction in overall costs achieved by decreasing operative time and duration of hospital stay [54].

The SPECT images fused with the CT images show the SLN in 2D and 3D modalities, thus facilitating the recognition of non-lymph node foci of radiotracer accumulation. Volumetric rendering techniques with 3D viewing provide high anatomical detail images that assist in the interpretation of planar lymphoscintigraphy in anatomically complex areas of the body [55, 56] (Figs. 10.11 and 10.12).

In a study based on the retrospective evaluation of two historical cohorts, Stoffels et al. showed higher frequency of metastatic involvement and higher rate of disease-free survival associated with the use of SPECT/CT-aided SLNB compared with SLN mapping without SPECT/CT imaging [57].

Following the findings described above, a new multicentre trial has been proposed in order to compare distant metastasis-free survival and metastatic lymph node detection in patients with cutaneous melanoma undergoing SLNB with preoperative SPECT/CT versus without preoperative SPECT/CT imaging [58].

Based on the advantages described above, SPECT/CT imaging is recommended in combination with planar lymphoscintigraphy. SPECT/CT acquired independently does not replace the sequential information provided by dynamic lymphoscintigraphy and subsequent planar imaging, which is the standard technique to identify the individual lymphatic collectors reaching the SLN, an essential aspect to distinguish an SLN from a secondary radioactive lymph node [59].

Key Learning Points

- The radiopharmaceuticals for lymphatic mapping (^{99m}Tc-nanocolloid, ^{99m}Tc-sulphur colloid or ^{99m}Tc-tilmanocept) are injected intradermally in several (2–4) aliquots around the primary melanoma or around the excisional biopsy scar.
- Lymphoscintigraphy usually includes an early dynamic acquisition for identifying regional lymphatic basins and to distinguish the true SLNs from second-echelon lymph nodes.
- Delayed static images acquired at 30 min and 2 h post-injection are generally sufficient for adequate preoperative imaging.
- SPECT/CT imaging provides an added value over planar imaging, to detect more SLNs and for more accurate anatomical localization of the SLNs; furthermore, it enables to distinguish focal tracer uptake in a single lymph node from clustered lymph nodes.
- SPECT/CT imaging is highly recommended in patients with melanomas of the head and neck region, of the trunk, or in areas with high probability of unexpected lymphatic drainage and non-visualization.
- SPECT/CT should always be performed in combination with planar lymphoscintigraphy.

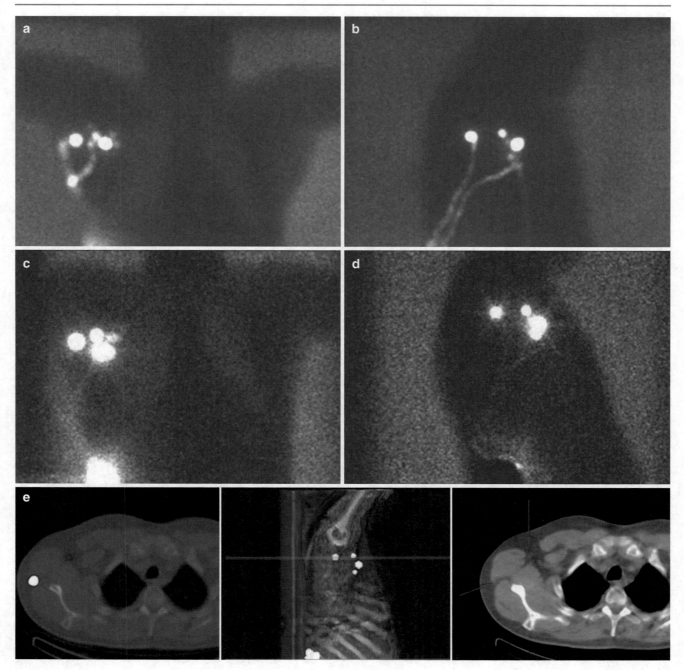

Fig. 10.8 Early (**a**, **b**) and delayed (**c**, **d**) planar images showing ipsilateral axillary drainage of the radiotracer through three independent lymphatic channels in a 48-year-old man with 1 mm Breslow thickness superficial spread melanoma of the lower right back. SPECT/CT images with 3D reconstruction depicted high radiotracer uptake in right axillary SLNs and also improved anatomical localization of a more posterior additional SLN adjacent to the anterior aspect of the right deltoid muscle (**e**)

10.8   Intraoperative Approach

10.8.1 Intraoperative Use of Handheld Gamma Probe for SLNB in Melanoma

Besides the information provided by preoperative lymphoscintigraphy, the other main cornerstone of the technique is the ability of the gamma-detecting probe to guide the dissection and to identify the SLN. It is recommended to make a preliminary search with the gamma probe on the skin surface, with the patient properly positioned on the operating table, prior to making the incision.

The scan with the gamma probe should be slow, thorough and systematic across the whole surgical field and should

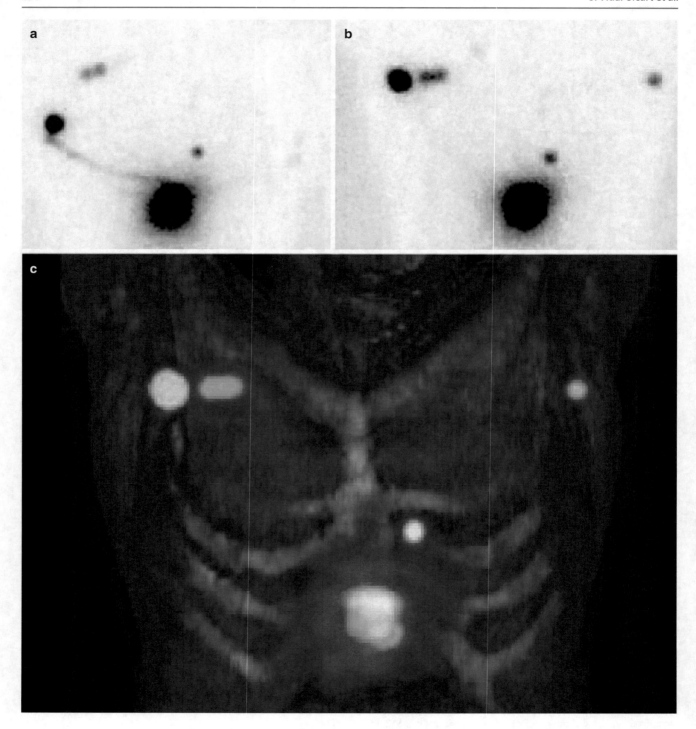

Fig. 10.9 A 42-year-old man with a 1.25 mm Breslow melanoma in the abdominal skin at the level of the xiphoid process. Planar lymphoscintigraphy and SPECT/CT performed after administration of 74 MBq ^{99m}Tc-nanocolloid in four intradermal injections around the excision scar. Anterior planar image (**a**) shows drainage to both axillae, with visualization of lymphatic ducts. In the right axilla there is initial uptake in a first draining lymph node and in 2-s echelon nodes. In the left axilla SLN uptake is only visualized on delayed planar imaging (**b**). At the third intercostal space there is a parasternal SLN, anatomically localized on volume-rendering image (**c**). The axillary SLN on the right (**d**) was found to contain metastasis at histopathology, whereas the SLNs of the internal mammary chain (**e**) and left axilla (**d**) were tumour free. Note the focal radioactivity in the liver region behind the injection site (**f**), which is probably related to drainage through the falciform ligament

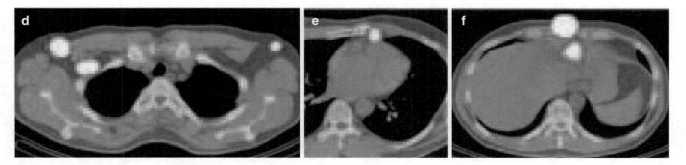

Fig. 10.9 (continued)

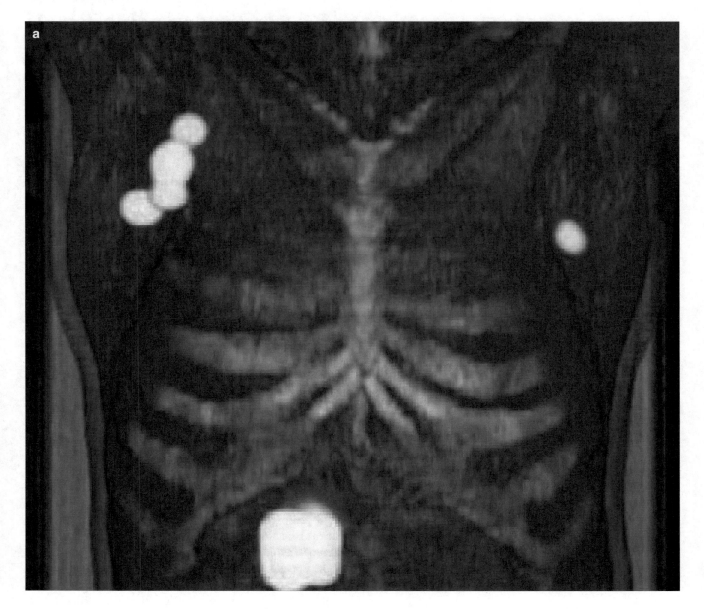

Fig. 10.10 A 66-year-old patient with a 2.1 mm Breslow melanoma of the abdominal skin. Planar lymphoscintigraphy and SPECT/CT performed after administration of 108 MBq ^{99m}Tc-nanocolloid in four intradermal injections around the excision scar. Volume rendering image (**a**) shows radioactive lymph nodes in both axillae. Early anterior planar imaging (**b**) shows three lymphatic ducts from the injection site to lymph nodes of the right axilla, and one to the left axilla. Four SLNs in the right axilla and one in the left axilla were removed, and found to be free of metastases. Note on the fused axial SPECT/CT image (**c**) a radioactive accumulation behind the injection site, which is probably related to uptake in a mesenterial lymph node

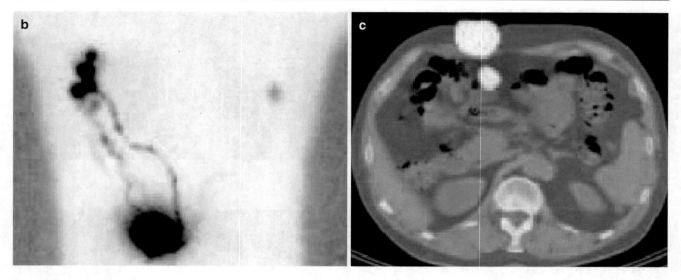

Fig. 10.10 (continued)

start between the injection site and the area of drainage visualized in the lymphoscintigraphy. Ideally, a low activity gap should be identified between the injection site and the increased activity corresponding to the SLN. This activity should be optimally matched with the skin marking(s) made by the nuclear medicine staff at the time of lymphoscintigraphic imaging.

Special precaution should be taken when the injection site overlies or is within the field of view of the detector probe; in this regard, if possible, mobilization manoeuvres or attempts to direct the gamma probe opposite to the injection site should be made. Also, removal of the primary tumour prior to the SLN can help to reduce the activity arising from the injection site.

SLN-to-background ratios are usually between 10:1 and 20:1, depending on the activity injected, time to surgery, etc. After in vivo SLN identification and excision, the ex vivo activity of the SLN should be recorded, as should also be the remaining activity in the surgical fields, to rule out the presence of other potential SLNs. Although a single SLN can be identified on planar lymphoscintigraphy, in practice there may be two adjacent lymph nodes seen as a single radioactive focus on planar imaging (especially if SPECT/CT imaging is not available); therefore, the lymphatic bed should always be reassessed. It is also mandatory to palpate the lymphatic region searching for enlarged or matted lymph nodes that could not be radioactive due to metastatic blockage, especially if an ultrasound study has not previously been performed [38, 45].

10.8.2 Vital Dyes

Vital dyes can help in the operation room to visually confirm the lymphatic vessels connecting the primary tumour to the SLN. Combining the information provided by presurgical lymphoscintigraphy with the intraoperative use of dyes and with the detector gamma probe offers the highest accuracy for SLN identification (Fig. 10.13). Their use in combination is recommended, although the additional benefit compared to the use of the radiotracer alone is less than 1% [60].

The vital dye may be especially important when the primary tumour is very close to the lymphatic basin, since the injected radioactivity (even after lesion removal) causes a high background count rate, which does not allow the detector probe to distinguish the SLN. Isosulfan blue (Lymphazurin) and Patent Blue are the dyes of choice for SLN mapping. Methylene blue is also used because of its lower cost, its lower risk of inducing anaphylaxis and its similar ability to detect the SLN compared with the other two dyes [61].

The blue dye can be injected around the primary tumour or scar (in a similar manner as the radiocolloid has been injected) 10–20 min prior to starting surgery, in a volume of 0.5–1 mL. The injection should be performed after the patient is anaesthetized (with either local or general anaesthesia) to avoid a painful injection. Five minutes of massage of the injection site enhances movement of the dye through the lymphatics to the SLNs. Blue dye is contraindicated in pregnant women and when earlier allergic reaction to blue

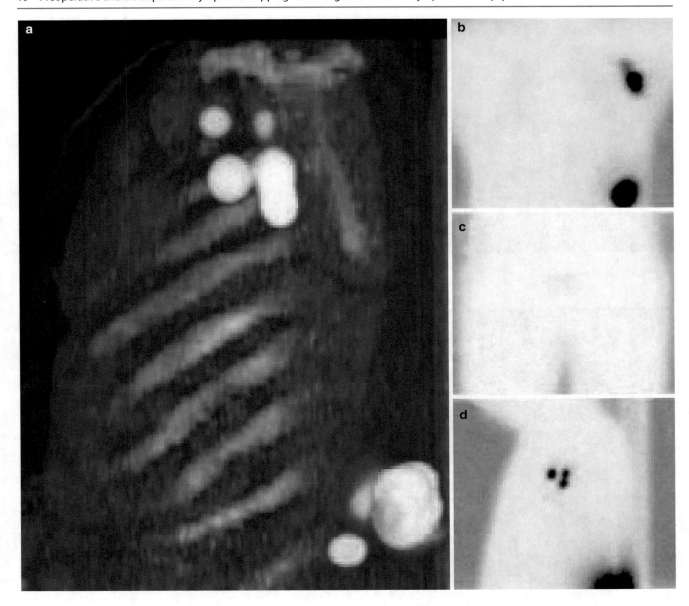

Fig. 10.11 A 36-year-old man with a 2.8 mm Breslow melanoma of the left side of the back. Planar lymphoscintigraphy and SPECT/CT performed after administration of 71 MBq ^{99m}Tc-nanocolloid in four intradermal injections around the excision scar. On volume-rendering image (**a**) not only axillary lymph nodes are seen, but also a lymph node close to the injection site. This SLN was not depicted on planar imaging (**b**–**d**) and was localized by axial SPECT/CT (**e**) and CT (**f**) between the muscles in the intercostal space. All SLNs were surgically removed and found to be tumour free at histopathology

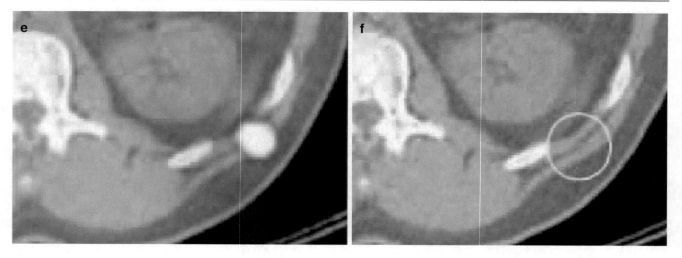

Fig. 10.11 (continued)

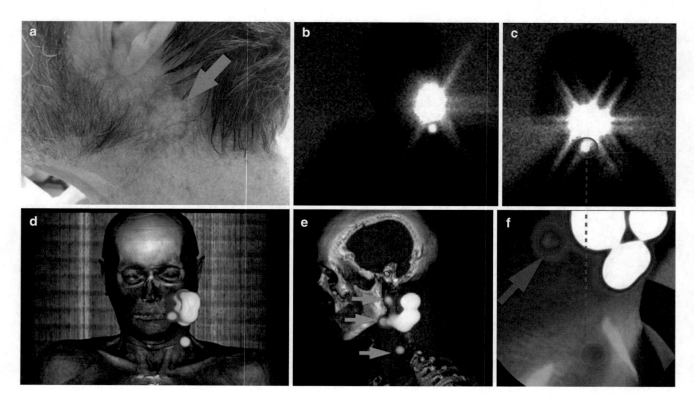

Fig. 10.12 The day before SLNB, four intradermal ^{99m}Tc-nanocolloid injections (111 MBq) were performed around the skin graft after the excision of a 2.8 mm Breslow thickness left cervical melanoma in a 41-year-old man (**a**). Planar images (**b**, **c**) showed drainage to a single left cervical lymphatic echelon (red circle) considered to be a single SLN (cervical level Vb). However, SPECT/CT images depicted three SLNs (green arrows), revealing two additional anterior SLNs (level Ib and IIa) in close proximity to the injection site (**d**, **e**). Intraoperative imaging with a portable gamma camera helped to discriminate activity arising from the injection site between the low laterocervical SLNs of the level Vb (connected with the red circle by a dotted line) and the additional anterior SLN (red arrow) (**f**)

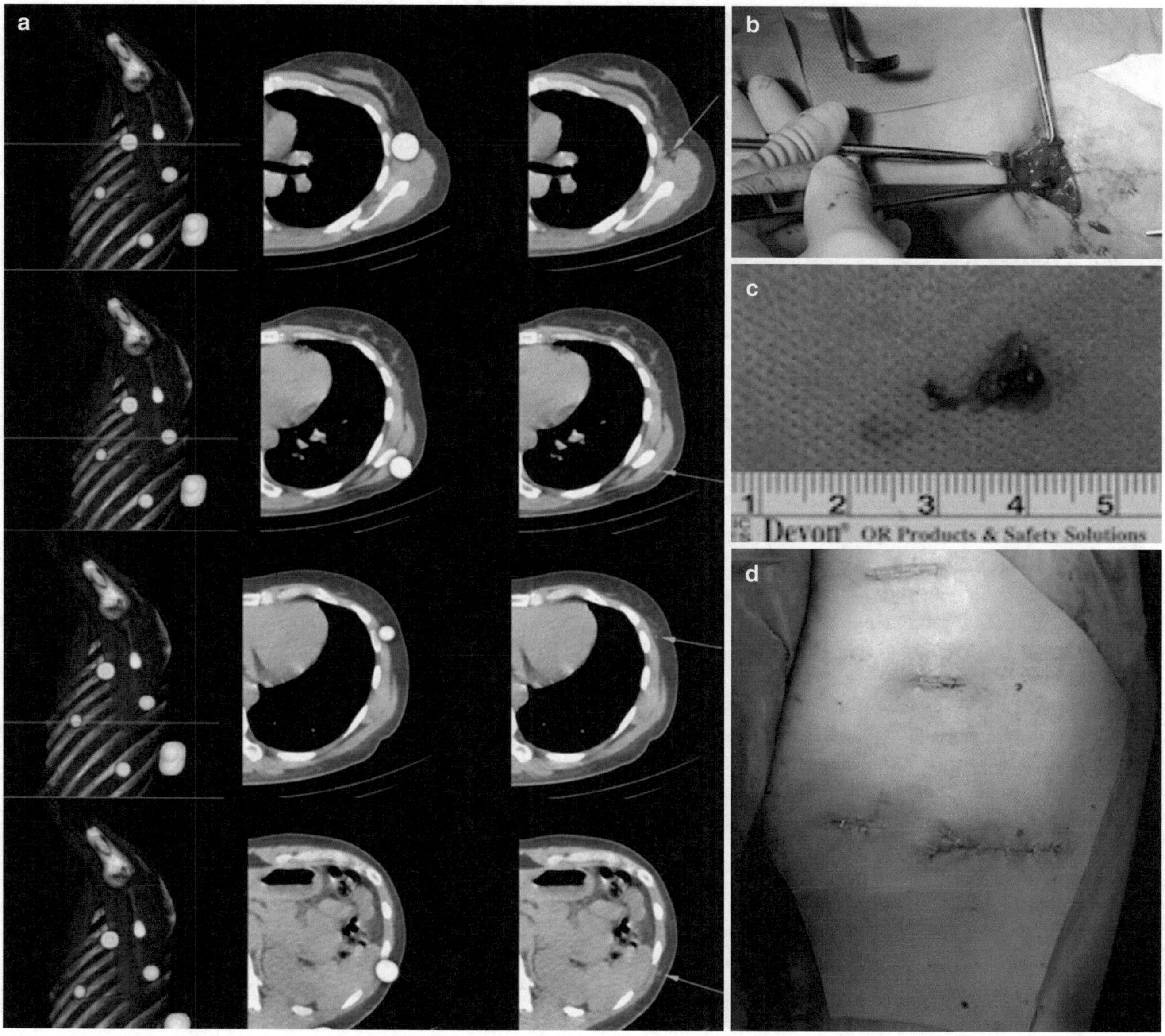

Fig. 10.13 SPECT/CT imaging of the same patient shown in Fig. 10.6 aided in the precise anatomical localization of all four SLNs, showing in the CT images three small subcutaneous lymphatic nodes and one left axillary lymph node corresponding to all four focal uptakes identified on the SPECT (**a**). Blue dye was injected in the operation room as a complementary method for visual identification of the SLNs (**b**, **c**). All in-transit nodes were found; all of them were blue-stained and were negative for metastases. (**d**) Final surgical picture of excision scars of the resected SLNs

dye has occurred. Another disadvantage is that the blue dye may cause, in some cases, a long-term tattooing of the wide excision skin limits; this is especially relevant in cases of head and neck melanoma patients.

It is important to note that vital dyes provide a small time window (approximately 45 min during surgery) before washing out from the SLNs [14].

10.8.3 Intraoperative Imaging

Although a handheld gamma probe is helpful in the majority of radioguided SLNBs, intraoperative imaging may provide a clear perspective of the location of the SLN in its anatomical surroundings, thus further facilitating the operation. The current technological advances in portable devices and the

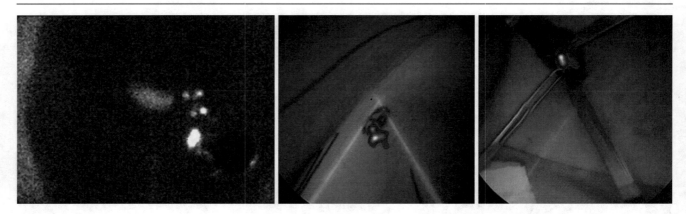

Fig. 10.14 After administration of 111 MBq of ^{99m}Tc-tilmanocept, planar images showed inguinal drainage of the radiotracer in a 74-year-old woman with melanoma of the left thigh (**a**). Portable gamma cam-era provided preoperative localization (**b**) and intraoperative confirmation of left inguinal SLN excision (**c**)

possibility of using new signatures (i.e., fluorescence) in addition to the conventional radiotracers have led to a changing paradigm: from the "see to open" approach to the "see, open and see again" approach. The combination of SPECT/CT information with new portable imaging devices enhances the reliability of the gamma probe, especially in complex drainage regions and in areas where the SLN is very close to the injection site.

However, there is further room for improvement during the intraoperative approach, because these images are "static" and, although the classical tracer + blue dye combination enables to detect the SLNs in most cases, under some circumstances SLN retrieval is complicated or even impossible.

The combination of "hot" and "blue" in the operating room has been successful in localizing the SLN in the expected lymph drainage basin. The blue dye is less effective in areas of aberrant drainage and also has a limited value in deep nodal basins. In cutaneous melanoma it is well known that the SLN identification rate in the head and neck is about 85%, which is considerably less than the almost 100% success rate commonly experienced for other locations. The head and neck as the site of a primary cutaneous melanoma has been found to be a predictive factor for a false-negative SLNB, as the false-negative procedures in this region have been reported to vary between 12 and 44% [62].

Portable small-field-of-view gamma cameras have been introduced to improve intraoperative detection of SLNs in addition to the handheld gamma probe. These devices allow real-time SLN visualization and confirmation of a complete lymph node resection. Some portable small-field-of-view gamma cameras can make a significant contribution, by indicating the SLN location in the skin by means of laser or external radioactive pointers. This issue is especially valuable when the melanoma is located in the head or neck as well as for SLNs located close to the injection site, which is difficult to locate by the gamma probe on its own.

The use of these imaging devices in the surgical theatre enables to precisely adapt in real time the surgical incision to the skin marks previously made in the nuclear medicine suite at the time of lymphoscintigraphy and confirms the exact SLN location, considering that the position of the patients on the operating table may differ from that on the imaging table [63] (Fig. 10.14).

With these devices, an overview image is recorded before the start of SLNB in the operating room. To verify the completeness of SLN removal, another image must be acquired after excision. If a residual radioactive spot is visualized at the location of a previously harvested SLN, this additional node must also be resected and be assessed as a part of a cluster of nodes to be considered as additional SLNs. Furthermore, when positioned close to the skin, a high-resolution portable gamma camera can detect SLNs at distances as small as only 3 mm from the injection site [64].

The acquisition of additional real-time scintigraphic images implies that the overall surgical time may increase depending on the level of team coordination. On the other hand, if a portable camera is not available, the surgeon may need to spend a significant amount of additional time seeking additional nodes or confirming that no more SLNs are likely to be found. Nevertheless, even when additional time is needed, this extra time could be worthwhile in this scenario of SLN procedures that are likely to be difficult, as the use of the gamma camera might reduce the possibility of missing a metastatic SLN [59].

It should be emphasized that portable gamma cameras do not serve as an intraoperative guidance in the same manner as conventional handheld gamma probes, since their size does not permit insertion in the surgical bed through the surgical incision.

The added value in the use of these devices is that they allow resection of additional SLNs, some of which result to be metastatic. Therefore, this technique may reduce the false-negative rate of SLNB, while the SLN identification rate is increased and correct application of this intraoperative imaging procedure ensures that no SLNs are left in the surgical field [65].

New multimodality system configurations have been introduced combining optical and gamma imaging. Some groups proposed different solutions for better correlation of optical imaging with gamma imaging. Haneishi et al. have proposed a parallel optical and gamma camera configuration resulting in a bimodal system that projects the scintigraphic image onto an optical image. On the other hand, Hellingman et al. evaluated a system that integrates an optical device with a portable gamma camera equipped with a pinhole collimator. Fused optical and gamma imaging makes it easier to relate in real time the position of the radioactive hot spots and the image field of view with the real-life situation [66–68].

Another device using the freehand SPECT technology has been introduced to allow for intraoperative 3D navigation by using a tracked handheld gamma probe or gamma camera with other fiducial markers in the patient. When using this device, the surgeon must scan the area of interest with the probe or gamma camera; facilitating the readings in counts per second supplied by these devices, the tracking system records these signals permitting a direct visualization of the distribution of radioactivity in the surgical field and providing exact lesion depth assessment. After all data are collected, a reconstruction algorithm generates a 3D image which is finally co-registered in real time with the image captured by a video camera focused on the surgical field. Location and depth of scanned radiolabelled tissue targets can be easily checked on the screen by the surgical team. This tool permits the generation of intraoperative 3D images of the radioactive SLN, also offering the possibility to load and fuse them in real time with tracked SPECT/CT studies previously acquired. This information can be visually superimposed on the patient's body using incorporated augmented reality devices. Specific training in the use of the technique is required for data acquisition and for making several readings during surgery, a procedure that may prolong the operation time. Nevertheless, in both cases the results might improve the conventional technique [69].

Sulzbacher et al. found that freehand SPECT was able to not only provide precise anatomical information of the SLN location, but also reveal additional SLNs compared to SPECT/CT. They studied 39 patients with the primary lesion in different sites of the body. Surgery using radioguided freehand SPECT was performed the day after acquisition of preoperative lymphoscintigraphy (planar + SPECT/CT). Most interestingly, SPECT/CT data were integrated into the 3D navigation system to enable fast and direct localization of the SLN by displaying the depth of the node from the skin surface to the gamma probe. Comparable preoperative imaging and intraoperative localization were observed in 18/39 patients. Intraoperative freehand SPECT revealed additional lymph node sites in 10 of 14 patients in whom more SLNs were resected during surgery than those visualized preoperatively. The total mean surgical time using this device was 66 min (range 36–133) [70].

Technological advances have been introduced not only in the intraoperative scenario. Different tracers and signatures are being continuously explored in order to reduce or solve the drawbacks observed with the use of radiotracers. In particular, the use of fluorescent agents for lymphatic mapping and SLN localization is expanding rapidly. Fluorescence has the advantage of providing real-time imaging, being relatively cheap and user friendly and not interfering with the surgical area. Organic fluorescent dyes such as fluorescein or indocyanine green (ICG) have been used in human studies as an alternative to nuclear imaging methods. Nevertheless, intraoperative fluorescence guidance also has several drawbacks, such as the limited penetration depth (maximum 1 cm) in tissues [71].

The radiolabelled nanocolloid has been combined with ICG (ICG-^{99m}Tc-nanocoll) to assist the intraoperative identification of SLNs located in areas of difficult surgical access. These hybrid agents for bimodal imaging combine radioactivity and fluorescence in one signature, providing the best of both worlds. In particular, preoperative lymphoscintigraphy and SPECT/CT are possible because of the radioactive "signature" of the hybrid agent, while the fluorescent "signature" allows recording high-resolution images in the operating room (Figs. 10.15 and 10.16). These hybrid tracers are capable of reproducing the exact pattern of lymphatic drainage as the parental ^{99m}Tc-colloid-radioactive tracer, thus allowing the combined use of presurgical lymphoscintigraphic planning and intraoperative near-infrared (NIR) optical detection [25, 72, 73].

A Dutch study compared this hybrid tracer with blue dye in 104 patients with melanoma. Optical SLN identification rate, made possible by the fluorescent signature of the hybrid tracer, was superior to that achieved with the blue dye, since SLNs were intraoperatively visualized in 97% of the cases with fluorescence, whereas only 62% of these nodes were stained blue. Interestingly, ex vivo examination of the excised SLNs confirmed the combined presence of a radioactive and fluorescent signature [74]. These findings are consistent with other studies showing that, although fluorescence imaging allows intraoperative identification of the SLNs, the limited tissue penetration does not allow accurate SLN mapping prior to surgery.

Nevertheless, it should be emphasized that each type of signal (radioactive or optical) must be explored with dedicated, single-modality imaging/detection devices. Ongoing efforts aim at developing multimodal devices capable of providing all the potential of intraoperative imaging, thereby achieving greater reliability in the surgical procedures [75].

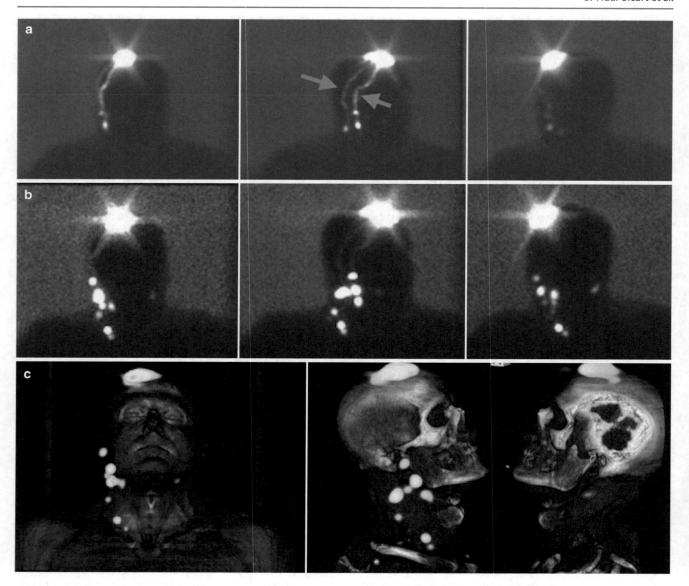

Fig. 10.15 Hybrid radiotracer (111 MBq ICG-^{99m}Tc-nanocolloid) was injected in a 54-year-old man with a 2.3 mm superficial spread melanoma located in right frontal scalp. Early dynamic planar images showed right cervical drainage of the radiotracer through two independent channels (green arrows) (**a**). Delayed planar images disclosed contralateral drainage to an additional left cervical SLN (**b**) localized in level IIa by SPECT/CT imaging (**c**)

Key Learning Points
- Handheld gamma probes are the most used devices to intraoperatively assess the SLN location.
- Blue dyes have been often used as a complementary agent for visual confirmation of SLN.
- Intraoperative imaging with portable gamma cameras or freehand SPECT helps to solve very complicate cases, although its use depends on each facility. The added value in the use of these devices is that they allow resection of additional SLNs.
- Fluorescent tracers as well as hybrid tracers are the step forward in the operating room, as the results obtained are better than those achieved with conventional dyes.
- Hybrid tracers allow the combination of preoperative lymphoscintigraphy and SPECT/CT imaging with intraoperative depiction of the SLN, thanks to their high resolution.

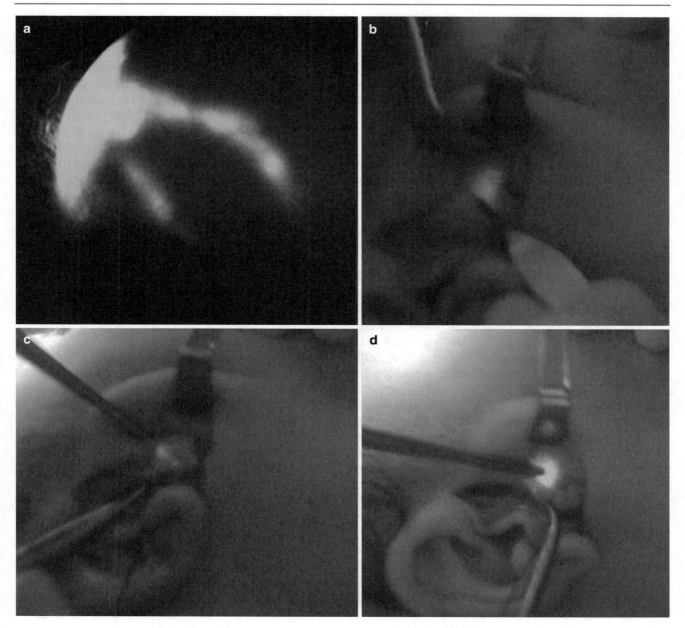

Fig. 10.16 Same patient shown in Fig. 10.8. At the time of injection, real-time images were obtained with a fluorescence camera (Hamamatsu FIS-00, Hamamatsu Photonics K.K., Shizuoka, Japan), showing drainage to the right preauricular region through two independent lymphatic vessels (**a**). Fluorescence provided visual confirmation during the intraoperative identification of a preauricular SLN (**b–d**)

10.9   Practical Considerations for SLN Mapping in Melanoma

10.9.1   In-Transit, Aberrant or Ectopic Lymph Nodes

Although the majority of cutaneous melanomas scheduled for SLNB drain to a predictable regional lymphatic basin based on localization of the primary tumour, drainage to lymph nodes outside of the expected lymphatic basins is frequently observed. The majority of SLNs are found in the major nodal basins (axilla, inguinal and cervical); in particular, predictable lymphatic drainage to the inguinal or axillary basins is observed in the majority of patients with cutaneous melanoma located in an extremity. In the groin, lymphatic drainage usually occurs to two or three superficial SLNs below the inguinal ligament. Sometimes lymph flow goes directly to Cloquet's node or to obturator or iliac nodes, bypassing the aforementioned superficial lymph nodes. In the axilla there are most often one or two SLNs located in Berg's level I.

A lymph node visualized along the lymphatic duct between the primary melanoma site and a regional lymphatic basin is called in-transit, interval, aberrant or ectopic lymph node (depending on the definitions set by different investigators) and must be considered as a SLN regardless of its location. This SLN can also be found in aberrant areas of drainage, such as the epitrochlear/epicondyleal nodal basin in the upper extremities, or the popliteal nodal basin in the lower extremities. In the thoracic-abdominal region, lymphoscintigraphy has deeply modified Sappey's concept of lymphatic watersheds and ambiguous drainage.

Likewise, preoperative lymphoscintigraphic localization of in-transit (interval, aberrant) SLNs has been demonstrated in 6–12% of these patients. Metastatic disease is found in approximately 18% of these in-transit SLNs (a rate which is similar to the rate found in conventional lymph node basins), and the status of one basin does not predict the status of the other. The highest incidence of in-transit SLNs occurs in the posterior trunk, followed by the anterior trunk, the head and neck, the upper limbs and the lower limb areas. On the other hand, the use of preoperative lymphoscintigraphy has shown discordant results with clinical predictions of nodal drainage. In fact, the SLN is not always found in the closest nodal basin. Accurate SLN mapping helps to identify all nodes receiving direct lymphatic drainage from a primary tumour site, regardless of the location.

The presence of such lymph nodes has been reported in all regions, particularly in the parascapular and supraclavicular spaces (lying between muscles or in the subcutaneous fat); para-aortic, paravertebral and retroperitoneal regions; intercostal zones; parasternal area; epitrochlear; popliteal; and even surrounding the skull (mainly in occipital area) [26, 76].

The incidence of metastasis in in-transit/aberrant SLNs appears to be quite similar in most studies, in the 14–22% range. In a review of 900 melanoma patients, it was reported that 19.5% of in-transit/aberrant lymph nodes harboured metastasis; 11 out of 15 of these patients also had metastatic involvement of at least one SLN in the expected lymphatic region, while the remaining 4 patients only had metastasis in the in-transit/aberrant SLN [77, 78].

When a cutaneous melanoma is located in the trunk region, preoperative lymphoscintigraphy drainage to multiple nodal basins has been demonstrated in 17–32% of patients undergoing radioguided SLNB. A melanoma in the flank may drain to the groin or to the axilla, or to both. Melanomas located in the scapular region often drain to the axilla, but may also drain to a supraclavicular fossa or to an interval node located in the shoulder's intermuscular space. In patients with melanoma of the lower trunk or lumbar region, there is often one SLN located cranially with respect to the inguinal ligament.

Several studies have demonstrated that the lymphatic drainage of melanomas of the head, neck and trunk cannot be reliably predicted. Multiple-basin drainage or interval lymph nodes may also be identified. This possibility highlights the importance of preoperative lymphoscintigraphy for these patients. Bilateral drainage can be seen in about 10–15% of patients, and visualization of multiple SLNs is frequent. It is also important to notice that the highly concentrated radioactivity remaining at the injection site can obscure a nearby SLN. Therefore, lateral and oblique views are mandatory (as is SPECT/CT whenever available). In this regard, the aid of precise anatomical localization (SPECT/CT) and intraoperative checking of a definite area of the body with a portable gamma camera may refine the procedure, especially in those cases where the SLNs are difficult to find [79–81].

In the current scenario, the management of in-transit/aberrant basins when a positive SLN is found is still controversial. Some authors consider that there is no need for a second procedure after obtaining a positive in-transit/aberrant SLN, while others perform a lymphadenectomy even with a low chance to find additional positive nodes. Considering this and the results of MSLT II, it seems clear that surgeons should refrain from routinely performing lymphadenectomy [82].

10.9.2 Head and Neck Location

SLNB of tumours in the head and neck region is especially challenging because of the great number of lymph nodes (>300) and because of the wide network of lymphatic vessels and vital structures that contributes to the complexity of lymphatic drainage in this area [83]. Furthermore, during lymphoscintigraphy the radioactivity remaining at the injection site can mask a SLN on planar imaging, and it is often hard to distinguish SLNs from second-echelon nodes.

A comparison between melanomas located in head or neck area and the results of presurgical lymphoscintigraphy with the expected drainage pattern derived from a predictive software showed a complete concordance in 80.4% of patients and partial in 12.2%, while discrepancy was observed in 7.4% of patients. In this regard, lymphoscintigraphy provides an added value to personalize lymphatic mapping in each individual patient and this imaging step is crucial to accurately detect the SLNs in head and neck melanomas, especially when faced with aberrant lymphatic drainage in unpredictable locations [24].

SPECT/CT imaging is currently considered to be mandatory for better assessing and depicting SLNs located in the head and neck area. SPECT/CT is able to precisely discriminate between parotid zone and cervical level II lymph nodes and visualized additional nodes not seen on planar lymphoscintigraphy, as observed in 28% of the cases [84]. A more refined technique, if available, may include preoperative SPECT/CT, intraoperative imaging using portable devices and hybrid tracer (multimodal approach). This combined approach has demonstrated to be useful especially for tumours located approximately in the expected area of lymphatic drainage and/or close to the injection site [85].

10.10   Technical Pitfalls in Lymphatic Mapping for Melanoma Patients

Although advances in the lymphoscintigraphic technique have led to a high SLN visualization in melanoma patients (virtually 100%), there remain some pitfalls when interpreting lymphoscintigraphic images. In particular, there is the need to confirm a true nodal versus non-nodal sites of uptake, such as skin folds, radiopharmaceutical contamination and lymphangiomas, which are common causes of false-positive results on conventional planar imaging. Addition of SPECT/CT to the SLN mapping has contributed to solving many of these conditions.

Contamination will occur if the needle is not tightly set, or the injection site leaks under pressure. Furthermore, leakage can result from high resistance to penetration of the injectate in the skin (typically, on the head, nose and sole skin). Injection of part of the radiocolloid into a blood vessel is another pitfall frequently observed. On the other hand, in some patients no apparent radiocolloid migration with absence of hot spot identification can occur, a situation that can be caused by several reasons: unsatisfactory radiocolloid quality, small amount of radioactivity injected, older patients, lymphatic blockade by metastatic cells, tumour involvement of the SLN, long interval between injection and lymphoscintigraphy, and also when a skin graft has been applied to cover the skin resection. Delayed images (up to 20 h after injection) can solve many of these cases, although a second set of radiocolloid administrations may be another option without postponing the operation.

Image acquisition must cover all areas draining from the injection site, since in-transit nodes can be missed if the path of radiocolloid is not followed. In areas below the knee, evaluation of the popliteal area is important. For sites below the elbow, the epitroclear and arm areas must be explored since SLNs at these locations can occur in about 10% of the patients. If a lead shield is placed over the injection site to reduce the shine-through effect, care must be taken not to mask a nearby SLN.

Dynamic and early static images are essential for identifying SLNs as the nodes that receive direct lymphatic drainage from the tumour site. SLNs are not necessarily the hottest nodes, although it may often be the case. In melanoma, lymph nodes with a lymphatic duct of their own or single nodes in a basin may frequently be visualized and identified as definitely SLNs. Lymph nodes with increasing intensity or appearing between the injection site and the first draining nodes are considered high-probable SLNs. Nodes indicated as definitively or high-probable SLNs on lymphoscintigraphy must be sampled by surgeons, regardless of count rate. Some authors maintain that the surgical bed activity after lymph node resection should be <10% of the hottest SLN. However, this practical rule can only be applied in the SLN areas indicated or marked by nuclear physicians on the basis of preoperative imaging.

Delayed images are helpful for detecting SLNs close to the primary tumour (the injection site), which may have been obscured on early imaging, as well as for detecting lymphatic drainage to multiple nodal basins. After recording an anterior view, a lateral view in the groin is often helpful to identify collectors passing to deep iliac or obturator lymph nodes. In the head and neck region other views (such as oblique or vertex views) are often necessary after acquiring the conventional orthogonal views. Nevertheless, as summarized above all these features today are more successfully solved by using SPECT/CT imaging.

10.11   The Dawn of a New Era?

The prognostic value of the SLN tumour status is no longer debated and has proven to be very useful for staging patients with melanoma [17]. In nearly all adjuvant phase III randomized controlled trials to date, completion lymphadenectomy has been mandatory; however, two recent randomized controlled trials were unable to demonstrate improved survival with regional lymphadenectomy versus nodal observation in patients with positive SLN. Patients with SLN metastases greater than 1 mm might benefit more from observation than from immediate lymph node dissection, and could potentially be considered for adjuvant systemic therapy instead of lymphadenectomy [18, 19].

These results open a new scenario for accurate patient staging. Only 5% of patients with stage III melanoma are upstaged after lymphadenectomy compared to stratification based on ulceration versus non-ulceration of the primary tumour and diameter of SLN metastasis (>1 mm versus <1 mm) [86]. Thus, lymphadenectomy does not appear to be necessary for recommending adjuvant therapy.

Adjuvant immunotherapy with ipilimumab has led to improvements in overall survival, whereas therapy with nivolumab and pembrolizumab has improved relapse-free survival. Adjuvant therapy with dabrafenib and trametinib has improved survival outcomes in BRAF V600E- and BRAF V600K-mutated melanomas. Thus, routine lymphadenectomy in case of positive SLNs should be reconsidered, because recommending adjuvant therapy for these patients without lymphadenectomy is the next logical step and can reduce the associated surgical morbidity [87]. It is envisioned that the use of SLN staging will increase because of the introduction of effective adjuvant (and promising neoadjuvant) therapies. As stated in a recent consensus melanoma meeting in this era of modern adjuvant therapy, patients with a positive SLN will be upstaged to stage 3 and will be eligible for adjuvant treatment [88].

Clinical Cases

Case 10.1: SLN Mapping in Melanoma of the Upper Back: Exclusive Drainage to SLNs in the Supraclavicular Fossa

Sergi Vidal-Sicart, Núria Sánchez, Andrés Tapias, and Antoni Bennássar

Background Clinical Case

A 67-year-old man with a black, non-ulcerated lesion on the upper back region (near the right scapula) with dermatoscopic features compatible with nodular melanoma, underwent excisional biopsy. Pathological analysis of the mole revealed nodular melanoma (7.0 mm Breslow thickness, IV Clark). Physical and preoperative examinations (ultrasonography) did not reveal suspicious regional lymph nodes.

Lymphoscintigraphy

Lymphoscintigraphy was performed 20 h before SLNB, to define the draining lymphatic basin at risk for metastatic disease and to identify the corresponding SLN. Four aliquots of 0.1 mL containing 27.5 MBq of ICG-^{99m}Tc-albumin nanocolloid were injected intradermally around the margins of the surgical scar, since the primary lesion had already been excised for biopsy. A dual-detector SPECT/CT gamma camera (Infinia Hawkeye GE Healthcare, Milwaukee, WI) equipped with low-energy general-purpose (LEGP) collimators was used to obtain planar images of the abdominal region by early dynamic imaging (2 frames/min for 10 min, 128 × 128 matrix, zoom 1.0) and 180-s delayed static imaging in anterior, and lateral views (256 × 256 matrix, zoom 1.00) at 15 min and 2 h after injection. SPECT/CT imaging was recorded after acquiring the delayed images (2 h). Image reconstruction was performed using a Xeleris (GE Healthcare) Workstation and 3D volume-rendering images were generated with a dedicated software (OsiriX MD, Pixmeo, Geneva, Switzerland).

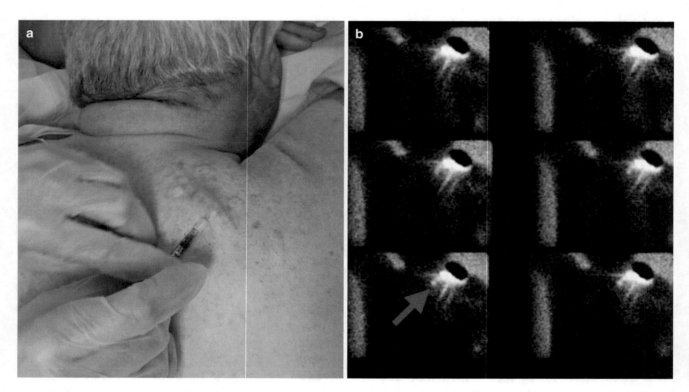

Fig. 10.17 Intradermal injection of four doses of ICG-^{99m}Tc-nanocolloid around the biopsy scar on right parascapular area. (**a**) Dynamic lymphoscintigraphy showed the progression of tracer to a "caudal" to injection site uptake (red arrow) that was considered the SLN (**b**)

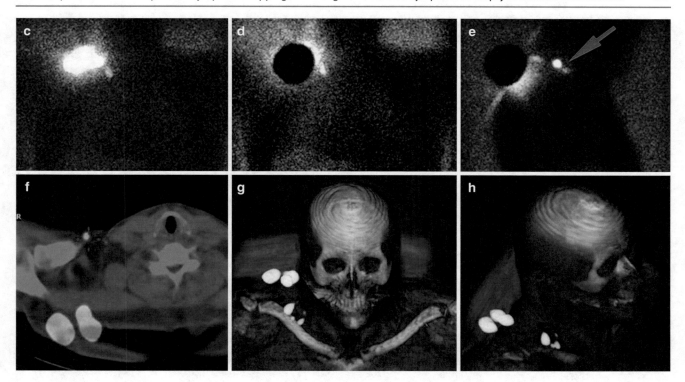

Fig. 10.18 Planar anterior view (**a–c**), with a lead covering injection site (**d**), and right lateral views (**e**) were subsequently acquired. The uptake was located anteriorly to injection site (red arrow). The fused axial SPECT/CT image (**f**) and volume-rendering images (**g** and **h**), precisely located two different foci of tracer uptake in the right supraclavicular fossa. This information was crucial to plan the optimal surgical approach

Case 10.2: SLN Mapping in Melanoma of the Perianal Area: Drainage to Inguinal and Iliac Lymph Nodes

Sergi Vidal-Sicart, Antonio Seva, and Antoni Bennássar

Background Clinical Case

A 56-year-old man with a black- and brown-pigmented area in the left gluteus underwent excisional biopsy. Histology revealed a heavily pigmented dermal, asymmetric superficial spread melanoma, involving the dermo-epidermal junction (Breslow 1.5 mm, Clark's level IV). Preoperative computed tomography (CT) of chest and abdomen was normal.

Lymphoscintigraphy

Lymphoscintigraphic delayed images were acquired 16 h before SLNB, to define the draining lymphatic basin at risk for metastatic disease and to identify the corresponding SLN. Four aliquots of 0.1 mL each, containing in total 111 MBq of ICG-^{99m}Tc-albumin nanocolloid, were injected intradermally around the margins of the surgical scar, since the primary lesion had already been excised for biopsy. A one-detector gamma camera (E-Cam, Siemens, Erlangen, Germany) equipped with low-energy high-resolution (LEHR) collimators was used to obtain planar images of the abdominal and chest regions by early dynamic imaging (1 frame/30 s for 10 min) and delayed static imaging (anterior and lateral views), with a 256 × 256 matrix and zoom factor 1.00.

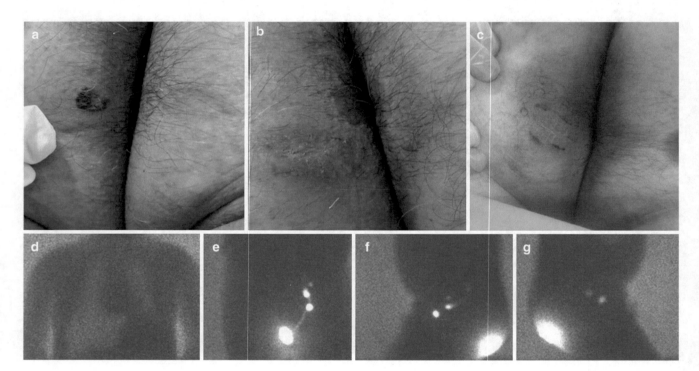

Fig. 10.19 Pigmented lesion located on the inner part of the left buttock, near the anal margin (**a**). Same location after excisional biopsy of the lesion (**b**). Schematic representation of the area of injection, around the biopsy scar (**c**). Anterior static acquisition of the thorax 30 min after radiotracer injections showing no drainage to potential in-transit or axillary nodes. Although very infrequent drainage has been observed coming from gluteal area, acquisition of one scan is recommended in order to rule out any uptake (**d**). A lymphatic duct, connecting inguinal and iliac lymph nodes, is clearly depicted in the anterior abdominal view (**e**). Left (**f**) and right (**g**) lateral views showing the different depth of these foci of uptake. Right lateral view showed the activity coming from the left nodes, but no right nodes appeared

Case 10.3: SLN Mapping in Melanoma of the Back: Drainage to In-Transit Paravertebral, Flank Lymph Nodes and Bilateral Inguinal Basins

Sergi Vidal-Sicart, Antoni Bennássar, and Antonio Seva

Background Clinical Case

A 38-year-old woman with a lesion of the central lumbar region (L3 level) underwent excisional biopsy. Histology showed that the melanoma was in vertical growth phase, with epithelioid cells, and extended to the reticular dermis (Breslow 0.8 mm; Clark's level III). No axillary or groin lymphadenopathy was detected at ultrasonography examination.

Lymphoscintigraphy

Lymphoscintigraphy was performed 17 h before SLNB, to assess the lymphatic drainage and identify the basins at risk for metastatic disease and to identify the corresponding SLN. Aliquots of 0.4 mL containing in total 111 MBq of ^{99m}Tc-albumin nanocolloid were injected intradermally around the margins of the surgical scar located in lumbar zone. Dynamic study and delayed planar images were obtained with a single-headed gamma camera (E-Cam, Siemens, Erlangen, Germany) immediately after tracer injection (dynamic study lasting for 10 min and planar static images at 15 min and 2 h after injection). After the 2-h delayed images, a dual-detector SPECT gamma camera (Infinia Hawkeye GE Healthcare, Milwaukee, WI) equipped with low-energy general-purpose (LEGP) collimators was used to acquire SPECT/CT imaging (SPECT acquisition: 120 3° frames, and 30 s/frame in a 128 × 128 matrix, zoom 1.0).

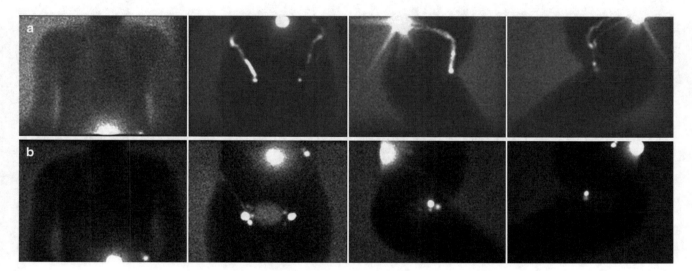

Fig. 10.20 *Upper row: Early planar images acquired 15 min after tracer injection (a).* Anterior thoracic view showing the injection site (left image, bottom) and a tiny focus of uptake left to injection site, but no axillary drainage at all. Abdominal and inguinal area scan showed bilateral inguinal drainage through two well-defined lymphatic channels. A hot spot was clearly observed in both inguinal areas (central image). Right and left lateral views nicely demonstrated the lymphatic channels to inguinal area (right images). *Lower row: Delayed planar images at 2 h after tracer injection (b).* Anterior thoracic view showing no changes to the early image (left image). Abdominal and inguinal area scan showing bilateral inguinal drainage and the appearance of second-echelon nodes in every inguinal basin. A well-defined focus of uptake is now clearly identified in left flank at the same level of injection site. It was considered an in-transit SLN (central image). Right and left lateral views nicely demonstrated the corresponding SLNs in every area and the in-transit left flank (right images)

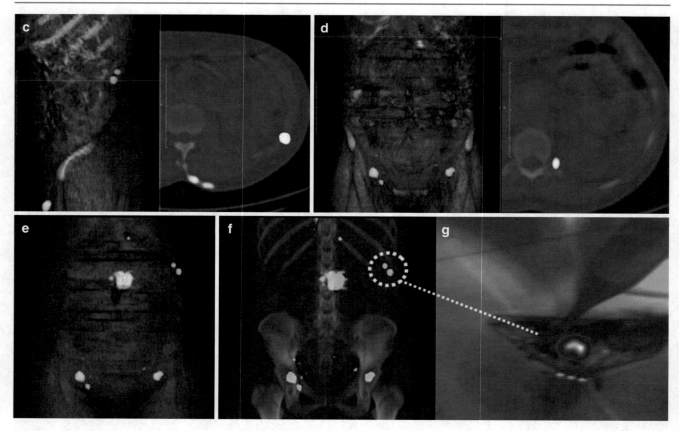

Fig. 10.21 SPECT/CT reconstruction with axial slices, 3D volume-rendering and MIP images showing the complex drainage from the injection site. The images demonstrate the importance of SPECT/CT in this case. Two subcutaneous in-transit left flank hot spots were clearly seen in the volume-rendering image and in the corresponding axial slice (**c** left and right, respectively). Two different faint hot spots were observed in dorsal paravertebral area (**d** left and right) that were unno-ticed in planar images. Volume-rendering and MIP images depicted all different tracer hot spots. A right paravertebral uptake (L3 level, near injection site) was discovered (**e** and **f**). During surgery, the in-transit left flank SLNs were intraoperatively imaged with a portable gamma camera equipped with an optical camera (**g**). Paravertebral nodes were not surgically pursued, although activity was demonstrated both with a portable gamma camera and with a handheld gamma probe

Case 10.4: SLN Mapping in Melanoma of the Neck: Bilateral Drainage to Right Submandibular and Right Axillary Lymph Nodes

Sergi Vidal-Sicart, Antoni Bennássar, Núria Sánchez, Erika Padilla-Morales, and John Orozco

Background Clinical Case

A 50-year-old woman with desmoplastic melanoma of the right-central neck, already surgically removed for biopsy. Histology showed that the melanoma was in radial growth stage and extended to the reticular dermis (Breslow 3.0 mm; Clark's level IV, no mitosis per mm^2 was present).

Lymphoscintigraphy

Lymphoscintigraphy was performed 17 h before SLNB, to define the draining lymphatic basin at risk for metastatic disease and to identify the corresponding SLN. Four aliquots of 0.1 mL each, containing a total activity of 111 MBq of ^{99m}Tc-albumin nanocolloid, were intradermally injected around the margins of the surgical scar. Dynamic study and delayed planar images were obtained with a single-headed gamma camera (E-Cam, Siemens, Erlangen, Germany) immediately after tracer administration (dynamic study lasting for 10 min and planar static images at 15 min and 2 h after injection). After acquiring the 2-h delayed images, a dual-detector SPECT gamma camera (Infinia Hawkeye GE Healthcare, Milwaukee, WI) equipped with low-energy general-purpose (LEGP) collimators was used to obtain tomographic images (SPECT/CT). SPECT acquisition: 120 3° frames, 30 s/frame in a 128 × 128 matrix and zoom 1.0.

Preoperative assessment was also performed with the Declipse freehand SPECT (SurgicEye, Munich, Germany) and a portable gamma camera (Sentinella, Oncovision, Valencia, Spain) in order to precisely mark the SLN localization on the patient's skin.

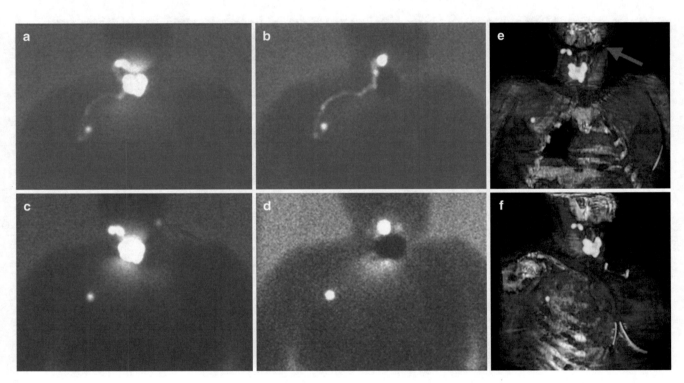

Fig. 10.22 *Upper row: Early planar images performed at 15 min after tracer injection (**a, b**).* Anterior and right lateral thoracic views showing the injection site and two lymphatic channels going cranially and caudally to different lymphatic basins (neck and axilla). *Lower row: Delayed planar images at 2 h after tracer injection (**c, d**).* Anterior and right lateral thoracic views showing two hot spots in right cervical area (cranially to injection site). A faint uptake is depicted on the left-hand side, at similar level, corresponding to a new SLN (arrow). A right hot spot, caudally to injection site, is well depicted as axillary SLN. Volume-rendering images showing the precise anatomical location of these SLNs (**e, f**)

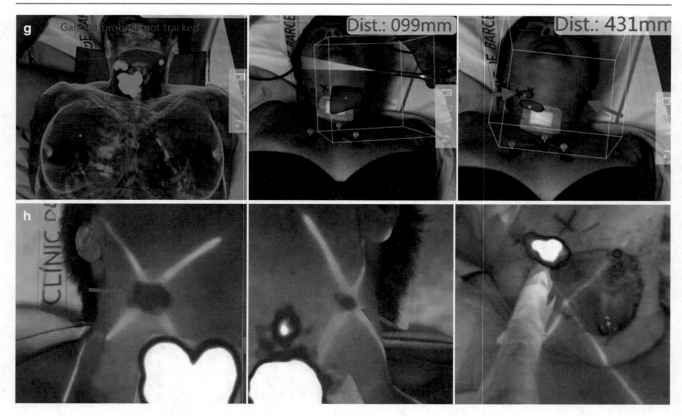

Fig. 10.23 *Upper row: Declipse freehand SPECT in cervical area (g).* 3D SPECT/CT data overlay showing the position of every SLN (left). Data collection with freehand technique using a handheld gamma probe (central). SLN depiction (arrows) after data reconstruction (right). *Lower row: Sentinella portable gamma camera in cervical area (h).* Right lateral cervical view demonstrating the uptake (arrow) cranially to the injection site corresponding to the SLNs (right). A tiny uptake (arrow) is depicted on the left-hand side, at similar level, corresponding to the left cervical level II SLN (central). Intraoperative activity (arrow) corresponding to the right cervical level II SLNs after the wide local excision of the lesion. A handheld gamma probe is used (as well as the portable gamma camera) to assess that activity (left)

Case 10.5: SLN Mapping in Melanoma of the Head and Neck: Drainage to Ipsilateral Preauricular (Parotid) and Cervical Nodes

Andrés Tapias, Agustí Toll, Carles Martí, Andrés Perissinotti, and Sergi Vidal-Sicart

Background Clinical Case

A 59-year-old man with melanoma in the right frontal region (superficial spread melanoma, 1.8 Breslow thickness, IV Clark, 2 mitoses per mm^2) was submitted to lymphoscintigraphy for radioguided SLNB.

Lymphoscintigraphy

Lymphoscintigraphy was performed 18 h before SLNB, to define the draining lymphatic basin at risk for metastasis and to locate the corresponding SLN. Four aliquots of 0.1 mL each containing 18.5 MBq of ^{99m}Tc-Tilmanocept were intradermally injected around the margins of the surgical scar, since the primary lesion had already been excised for biopsy. A single-detector gamma camera (E-Cam, Siemens, Erlangen, Germany) equipped with low-energy high-resolution (LEHR) collimators was used to obtain head-neck planar images, by early dynamic imaging (1 frame/30 s for 10 min) and delayed static imaging (anterior and lateral views at 15 min and 2 h p.i.). SPECT/CT acquisition was performed with a dual-detector gamma camera (Symbia Intevo Bold, Siemens Healthcare, Erlangen, Germany) using a step-and-shoot protocol of 30 s/3° for a total of 60 views per camera head, 128 × 128 matrix, zoom factor 1.45. CT parameters included a current of 40 mA, a voltage of 130 kV and a slice thickness of 2.75 mm slice.

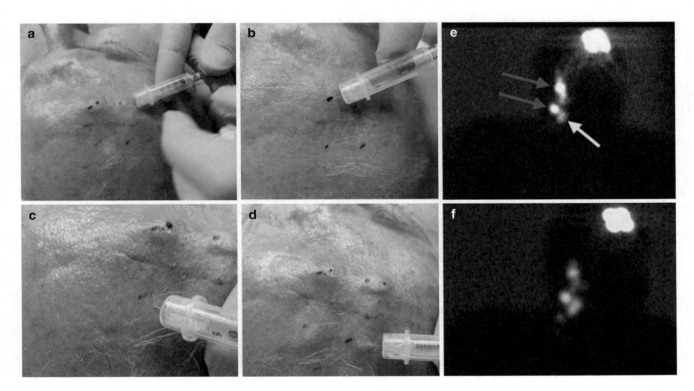

Fig. 10.24 Intradermal injections around biopsy scar located in right frontal area. In this part of the body it is not always easy to raise a wheal in the skin when injecting the radiotracer. (**a–d**) Early (15 min, **e**) planar imaging (right lateral view) shows two separate lymphatic channels leading to two separate areas of focal uptake of the tracer corresponding to two right cervical SLNs (*red arrows*), without specifying their topographic location. Two subsequent-tier nodes caudally to SLNs were also depicted (*yellow arrow*). Delayed (2 h, **f**) planar right lateral view showed the same SLNs and two more active nodes near the most caudal SLN

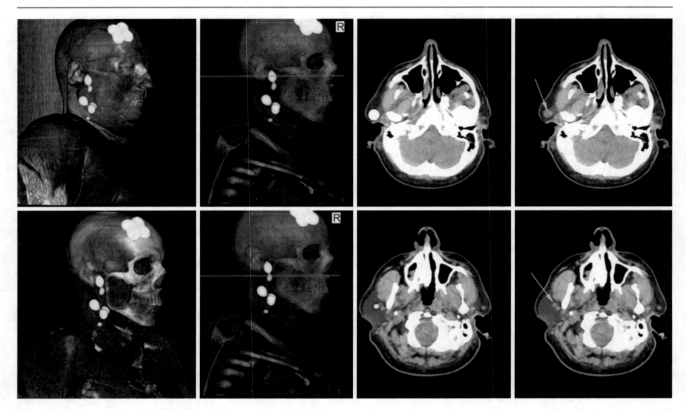

Fig. 10.25 3D volume-rendering images and SPECT/CT fused images in axial plane show that were actually two cranial SLNs, one located in right preauricular zone (upper row) and the other within the right parotid gland (lower row)

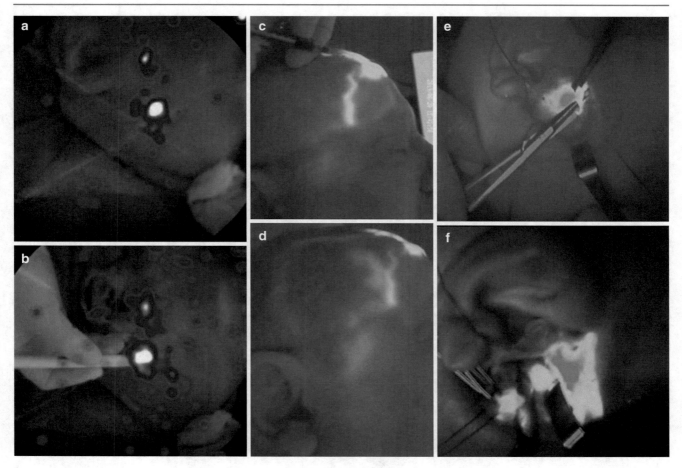

Fig. 10.26 Intraoperative images. A portable gamma camera (Sentinella, Oncovision, Valencia, Spain) was used to preoperatively demonstrate the activity of the tracer just before surgical procedure and to refine the skin marks done the day before (**a, b**). One millilitre of indocyanine green (25 mg/5 mL sterile water dilution) was preopera-tively injected. A fluorescence camera (Hamamatsu FIS-00, Hamamatsu Photonics K.K., Shizuoka, Japan) was used to visualize lymphatic mapping, showing two separate lymphatic ducts confluent to right preauricular area (**c, d**). After careful dissection, a preauricular node was clearly seen (**e, f**)

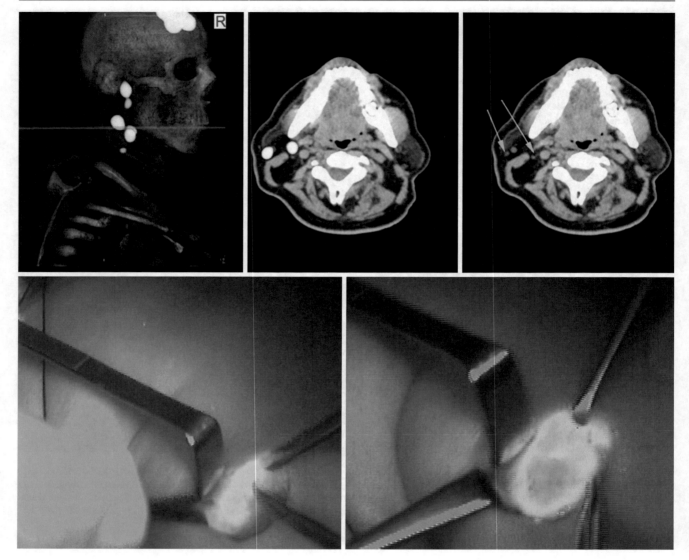

Fig. 10.27 Cervical SLNs in level IIa (green *arrows*) were easily located with the combination of radioactive signal and fluorescence signal

References

1. Siegel RL, Miller KD, Jemal A. Cancer statistics, 2019. CA Cancer J Clin. 2019;69:7–34.
2. Ferlay J, Ervik M, Lam F, et al. Global cancer observatory: cancer today. International Agency for Research on Cancer: Lyon; 2018. https://gco.iarc.fr/today. Accessed 2 Aug 2019.
3. Schadendorf DE, Fisher DE, Garbe C, et al. Melanoma. Nat Rev Dis Prim. 2015;1:1–20.
4. Nieweg OE, Uren RF, Thompson JF. Radioguided sentinel lymph node mapping and biopsy in cutaneous melanoma. In: Hermann K, Nieweg OE, Povosky SP, editors. Radioguided surgery. Basel: Springer; 2016. p. 152–63.
5. de Bree R, Nieweg OE. The history of sentinel node biopsy in head and neck cancer: from visualization of lymphatic vessels to sentinel nodes. Oral Oncol. 2015;51:819–23.
6. Nieweg OE, Uren RF, Thompson JF. The history of sentinel lymph node biopsy. Cancer J. 2015;21:3–6.
7. Wong SL, Faries MB, Kennedy EB, et al. Sentinel lymph node biopsy and management of regional lymph nodes in melanoma: American Society of Clinical Oncology and Society of Surgical Oncology clinical practice guideline update. Ann Surg Oncol. 2018;25:356–77.
8. Gangi A, Essner R, Giuliano AE. Long-term clinical impact of sentinel lymph node in breast cancer and cutaneous melanoma. Q J Nucl Med Mol Imaging. 2014;58:95–104.
9. Riquelme-Mc Loughlin C, Podlipnik S, Bosch-Amate X, et al. Diagnostic accuracy of imaging studies for initial staging of T2b-T4b melanoma patients. A cross-sectional study. J Am Acad Dermatol. 2019;81(6):1330–8. [Epub ahead of print].
10. Kretschmer L, Thoms KM, Peeters S, et al. Postoperative morbidity of lymph node excision for cutaneous melanoma-sentinel lymph-

adenectomy versus complete regional lymph node dissection. Melanoma Res. 2008;18:16–21.

11. Delgado AF, Delgado AF. Complete lymph node dissection in melanoma: a systematic review and meta-analysis. Anticancer Res. 2017;37:6825–9.

12. Nieweg OE, Tanis PJ, Kroon BB. The definition of a sentinel node. Ann Surg Oncol. 2001;8:538–41.

13. Vitali GC, Trifirò G, Zonta M, et al. Lymphoscintigraphy in clinical routine practice: reproducibility and accuracy in melanoma patients with a long-term follow-up. Eur J Surg Oncol. 2014;40:55–60.

14. van der Ploeg IM, Madu MF, van der Hage JA, et al. Blue dye can be safely omitted in most sentinel node procedures for melanoma. Melanoma Res. 2016;26:464–8.

15. Valsecchi ME, Silbermins D, de Rosa N, et al. Lymphatic mapping and sentinel node biopsy in patients with melanoma: a meta-analysis. J Clin Oncol. 2011;29:1479–87.

16. Gershenwald JE, Ross MI. Sentinel lymph node biopsy for cutaneous melanoma. N Engl J Med. 2011;364:1738–45.

17. Morton DL, Thompson JF, Cochran AJ, et al. Final trial report of sentinel-node biopsy versus nodal observation in melanoma. N Engl J Med. 2014;370:599–609.

18. Faries MB, Thompson JF, Cochran AJ, et al. Completion dissection or observation for sentinel-node metastasis in melanoma. N Engl J Med. 2017;376:2211–22.

19. Leiter U, Stadler R, Mauch C, et al. Complete lymph node dissection versus no dissection in patients with sentinel lymph node biopsy positive melanoma (DeCOG-SLT): a multicentre, randomised, phase 3 trial. Lancet Oncol. 2016;17:757–67.

20. Uren RF, Howman-Giles R, Chung D, et al. Imaging sentinel lymph nodes. Cancer J. 2015;21:25–32.

21. Thompson JF, Uren RF. Lymphatic mapping in management of patients with primary cutaneous melanoma. Lancet Oncol. 2005;6:877–85.

22. Mariani G, Erba P, Manca G, et al. Radioguided sentinel lymph node biopsy in patients with malignant cutaneous melanoma. The nuclear medicine contribution. J Surg Oncol. 2004;85:141–51.

23. Vidal M, Vidal-Sicart S, Torrents A, et al. Accuracy and reproducibility of lymphoscintigraphy for sentinel node detection in patients with cutaneous melanoma. J Nucl Med. 2012;53:1193–9.

24. Vidal M, Vidal-Sicart S, Torres F, et al. Correlation between theoretical anatomical patterns of lymphatic drainage and lymphoscintigraphy findings during sentinel node detection in head and neck melanomas. Eur J Nucl Med Mol Imaging. 2016;43:626–34.

25. Brouwer OR, Buckle T, Vermeeren L, et al. Comparing the hybrid fluorescent-radioactive tracer indocyanine green-^{99m}Tc-nanocolloid with ^{99m}Tc-nanocolloid for sentinel node identification: a validation study using lymphoscintigraphy and SPECT/CT. J Nucl Med. 2012;53:1034–40.

26. Moncayo VM, Aarsvold JN, Alazraki NP. Lymphoscintigraphy and sentinel nodes. J Nucl Med. 2015;56:901–7.

27. Moncayo VM, Alazraki AL, Alazraki NP, et al. Sentinel lymph node biopsy procedures. Semin Nucl Med. 2017;47:595–617.

28. Boada A, Tejera-Vaquerizo A, Ribero S, et al. Sentinel lymph node biopsy versus observation in thick melanoma: a multicenter propensity score matching study. Int J Cancer. 2018;142:641–8.

29. Amin MB, Edge S, Greene F, et al. AJCC cancer staging manual. 8th ed. New York: Springer; 2017.

30. Gershenwald JE, Scolyer RA, Hess KR, et al. Melanoma staging: evidence-based changes in the American Joint Committee on Cancer eighth edition cancer staging manual. CA Cancer J Clin. 2017;67:472–92.

31. Chakera AH, Hesse B, Burak Z, et al. EANM–EORTC general recommendations for sentinel node diagnostics in melanoma. Eur J Nucl Med Mol Imaging. 2009;36:1713–42.

32. Giammarile F, Alazraki N, Aarsvold JN, et al. The EANM and SNMMI practice guideline for lymphoscintigraphy and sentinel node localization in breast cancer. Eur J Nucl Med Mol Imaging. 2013;40:1932–47.

33. Xiong L, Engel H, Gazyakan E, et al. Current techniques for lymphatic imaging: state of the art and future perspectives. Eur J Surg Oncol. 2014;40:270–6.

34. Vidal-Sicart S, Vera D, Valdés-Olmos RA. Next generation of radiotracers for sentinel lymph node biopsy: what is still necessary to establish new imaging paradigms? Rev Esp Med Nucl Imagen Mol. 2018;37:373–9.

35. Leong SP, Kim J, Ross M, et al. A phase 2 study of 99mTc-tilmanocept in the detection of sentinel lymph nodes in melanoma and breast cancer. Ann Surg Oncol. 2011;18:961–9.

36. Sondak VK, King DW, Zager JS, et al. Combined analysis of phase III trials evaluating [99mTc]-tilmanocept and vital blue dye for identification of sentinel lymph nodes in clinically node-negative cutaneous melanoma. Ann Surg Oncol. 2013;20:680–8.

37. Puleo CA, Berman C, Montilla-Soler JL, et al. ^{99m}Tc-tilmanocept for lymphoscintigraphy. Imaging Med. 2013;5:119–25.

38. Bluemel C, Herrmann K, Giammarile F, et al. EANM practice guidelines for lymphoscintigraphy and sentinel lymph node biopsy in melanoma. Eur J Nucl Med Mol Imaging. 2015;42:1750–66.

39. Tardelli E, Mazzarri S, Rubello D, et al. Sentinel lymph node biopsy in cutaneous melanoma: standard and new technical procedures and clinical advances. A systematic review of the literature. Clin Nucl Med. 2016;41:e498–507.

40. Fitzgerald TL, Gronet EM, Atluri P, et al. Patterns of node mapping differ for axial and extremity primary cutaneous melanoma: a case for a more selective use of pre-operative imaging. Surgeon. 2016;14:190–5.

41. Jaukovic L, Sijan G, Rajović M, et al. Lymphoscintigraphy and sentinel lymph node biopsy, in cutaneous melanoma staging and treatment decisions. Hell J Nucl Med. 2015;18:146–51.

42. Perissinotti A, Vidal-Sicart S, Nieweg O, et al. Melanoma and nuclear medicine. Melanoma Manag. 2014;1:57–74.

43. Uren RF, Howman-Giles R, Chung D, et al. Guidelines for lymphoscintigraphy and F18 FDG PET scans in melanoma. J Surg Oncol. 2011;104:405–19.

44. Uren RF, Nieweg OE, Thompson JF. Sentinel lymph node biopsy: evolution of the technique since the original description by Morton et al. in 1992. Crit Rev Oncol. 2016;21:7–17.

45. Vidal-Sicart S, Vilalta Solsona A, Alonso Vargas MI. Sentinel node in melanoma and breast cancer. Current considerations. Rev Esp Med Nucl Imagen Mol. 2015;34:30–44.

46. Kretschmer L, Bertsch HP, Bardzik P, et al. The impact of nodal tumour burden on lymphoscintigraphic imaging in patients with melanomas. Eur J Nucl Med Mol Imaging. 2015;42:231–40.

47. Ribero S, Osella-Abate S, Pasquali S, et al. Prognostic role of multiple lymphatic basin drainage in sentinel lymph node-negative trunk melanoma patients: a multicenter study from the Italian Melanoma Intergroup. Ann Surg Oncol. 2016;23:1708–15.

48. Ahmadzadehfar H, Hinz T, Wierzbicki A, et al. Significance of multiple nodal basin drainage in patients with truncal melanoma. Q J Nucl Med Mol Imaging. 2016;60:274–9.

49. Ribero S, Osella Abate S, Pasquali S, et al. Multiple lymph node basin drainage in trunk melanoma is not associated with survival of sentinel lymph node-positive patients. Dermatology. 2017;233:205–11.

50. Vidal-Sicart S, Brouwer OR, Valdés-Olmos RA. Evaluation of the sentinel lymph node combining SPECT/CT with the planar image and its importance for the surgical act. Rev Esp Med Nucl. 2011;30:331–7.

51. Valdés Olmos RA, Rietbergen DD, Vidal-Sicart S, et al. Contribution of SPECT/CT imaging to radioguided sentinel lymph node biopsy in breast cancer, melanoma, and other solid cancers: from "open and see" to "see and open". Q J Nucl Med Mol Imaging. 2014;58:127–39.

52. Israel O, Pellet O, Biassoni L, et al. Two decades of SPECT/CT—the coming of age of a technology: an updated review of literature evidence. Eur J Nucl Med Mol Imaging. 2019;46:1990–2012.

53. Jimenez-Heffernan A, Ellmann A, Sado H, et al. Results of a prospective multicenter International Atomic Energy Agency sentinel node trial on the value of SPECT/CT over planar imaging in various malignancies. J Nucl Med. 2015;56:1338–44.

54. Stoffels I, Müller M, Geisel MH, et al. Cost-effectiveness of preoperative SPECT/CT combined with lymphoscintigraphy vs. lymphoscintigraphy for sentinel lymph node excision in patients with cutaneous malignant melanoma. Eur J Nucl Med Mol Imaging. 2014;41:1723–31.

55. Valdés Olmos RA, Rietbergen DDD, Vidal-Sicart S. SPECT/CT and sentinel node lymphoscintigraphy. Clin Transl Imaging. 2014;2:491–504.

56. Perissinotti A, Rietbergen DD, Vidal-Sicart S, et al. Melanoma & nuclear medicine: new insights & advances. Melanoma Manag. 2018;5:MMT06.

57. Stoffels I, Boy C, Pöppel T, et al. Association between sentinel lymph node excision with or without preoperative SPECT/CT and metastatic node detection and disease-free survival in melanoma. JAMA. 2012;308:1007–14.

58. Stoffels I, Herrmann K, Rekowski J, et al. Sentinel lymph node excision with or without preoperative hybrid single-photon emission computed tomography/computed tomography (SPECT/CT) in melanoma: study protocol for a multicentric randomized controlled trial. Trials. 2019;20:99.

59. Valdés Olmos RA, Vidal-Sicart S, Manca G, et al. Advances in radioguided surgery in oncology. Q J Nucl Med Mol Imaging. 2017;61:247–70.

60. Ranson JM, Pantelides NM, Pandit DG, et al. Sentinel lymph node biopsy in melanoma: which hot nodes should be harvested and is blue dye really necessary? J Plast Reconstr Aesthet Surg. 2018;71:1269–73.

61. Stebbins WG, Garibyan L, Sober AJ. Sentinel lymph node biopsy and melanoma: 2010 update, part I and II. J Am Acad Dermatol. 2010;62:723–48.

62. Trinh BB, Chapman BC, Gleisner A, et al. SPECT/CT adds distinct lymph node basins and influences radiologic findings and surgical approach for sentinel lymph node biopsy in head and neck melanoma. Ann Surg Oncol. 2018;25:1716–22.

63. Vidal-Sicart S, Rioja ME, Paredes P, et al. Contribution of perioperative imaging to radioguided surgery. Q J Nucl Med Mol Imaging. 2014;58:140–60.

64. Hellingman D, de Wit-van der Veen LJ, Klop WM, et al. Detecting near-the-injection-site sentinel nodes in head and neck melanomas with a high resolution portable gamma camera. Clin Nucl Med. 2015;40:e11–6.

65. Leong SP, Wu M, Lu Y, et al. Intraoperative imaging with a portable gamma camera may reduce the false-negative rate for melanoma sentinel lymph node surgery. Ann Surg Oncol. 2018;5:3326–33.

66. Haneishi H, Onishi Y, Shimura H, et al. Simultaneous acquisition and image synthesis of gamma cameras and optical cameras for sentinel lymph node identification during radioguided surgery. IEEE Trans Nucl Sci. 2007;54:1703–9.

67. Hellingman D, Vidal-Sicart S, de Wit-van der Veen LJ, et al. A new portable hybrid camera for fused optical and scintigraphic imaging: first clinical experiences. Clin Nucl Med. 2016;41:e39–43.

68. Ng AH, Blackshaw PE, Alqahtani MS, et al. A novel compact small field of view hybrid gamma camera: first clinical results. Nucl Med Commun. 2017;38:729–36.

69. Pouw B, de Wit-van der Veen LJ, Stokkel MP, et al. Improved accuracy and reproducibility using a training protocol for freehand-SPECT 3D mapping in radio-guided surgery. Clin Nucl Med. 2015;40:e457–60.

70. Sulzbacher L, Klinger M, Scheurecker C, et al. Clinical usefulness of a novel freehand 3D imaging device for radio-guided intraoperative sentinel lymph node detection in malignant melanoma. Clin Nucl Med. 2015;40:e436–40.

71. Stammes MA, Bugby SL, Porta T, et al. Modalities for image- and molecular-guided cancer surgery. Br J Surg. 2018;105:e69–83.

72. Rietbergen DDD, van den Berg NS, van Leeuwen FWB, et al. Hybrid techniques for intraoperative sentinel lymph node imaging: early experiences and future prospects. Imaging Med. 2013;5:147–59.

73. Klein Jan GH, van Werkhoven E, van den Berg NS, et al. The best of both worlds: a hybrid approach for optimal pre- and intraoperative identification of sentinel lymph nodes. Eur J Nucl Med Mol Imaging. 2018;45:1915–25.

74. van den Berg NS, Brouwer OR, Schaafsma BE, et al. Multimodal surgical guidance during sentinel node biopsy for melanoma: combined gamma tracing and fluorescence imaging of the sentinel node through use of the hybrid tracer indocyanine green-technetium-99m nanocolloid. Radiology. 2015;275:521–9.

75. Vidal-Sicart S, Valdés Olmos R, Nieweg OE, et al. From interventionist imaging to navigation with radio-guided surgery. Rev Esp Med Nucl Imagen Mol. 2018;37:28–40.

76. Nogareda Z, Vilalta A, Bennassar A, et al. Aberrant lymphatic drainage from a melanoma located in epigastric area. Rev Esp Med Nucl Imagen Mol. 2014;33:390–1.

77. Ortín-Pérez J, Vidal-Sicart S, Doménech B, et al. In-transit sentinel lymph nodes in malignant melanoma. What is their importance? Rev Esp Med Nucl. 2008;27:424–9.

78. Zager JS, Puleo CA, Sondak VK. What is the significance of the in transit or interval sentinel node in melanoma. Ann Surg Oncol. 2011;18:3232–4.

79. Veenstra HJ, Klop MW, Lohuis PJ, et al. Lymphatic drainage of melanomas located on the manubrium sterni to cervical lymph nodes: a case series assessed by SPECT/CT. Clin Nucl Med. 2013;38:e137–9.

80. Brammen L, Nedomansky J, Haslik W, et al. Extraordinary lymph drainage in cutaneous malignant melanoma and the value of hybrid imaging: a case report. Nucl Med Mol Imaging. 2014;48:306–8.

81. Peral Rubio F, de la Riva P, Moreno-Ramírez D, et al. Portable gamma camera guidance in sentinel lymph node biopsy: prospective observational study of consecutive cases. Actas Dermosifiliogr. 2015;106:408–14.

82. Brandão PHDM, Bertolli E, Doria-Filho E, et al. In transit sentinel node drainage as a prognostic factor for patients with cutaneous melanoma. J Surg Oncol. 2018;117:864–7.

83. Patuzzo R, Maurichi A, Camerini T, et al. Accuracy and prognostic value of sentinel lymph node biopsy in head and neck melanomas. J Surg Res. 2014;187:518–24.

84. Zender C, Guo T, Weng C, et al. Utility of SPECT/CT for periparotid sentinel lymph node mapping in the surgical management of head and neck melanoma. Am J Otolaryngol. 2014;35:12–8.

85. Borbón-Arce M, Brouwer OR, van den Berg NS, et al. An innovative multimodality approach for sentinel node mapping and biopsy in head and neck malignancies. Rev Esp Med Nucl Imagen Mol. 2014;33:274–9.

86. Verver D, van Klaveren D, van Akkooi ACJ, et al. Risk stratification of sentinel node-positive melanoma patients defines surgical management and adjuvant therapy treatment considerations. Eur J Cancer. 2018;96:25–33.

87. Franke V, van Akkooi ACJ. The extent of surgery for stage III melanoma: how much is appropriate? Lancet Oncol. 2019;20:e167–74.

88. Peach H, Board R, Cook M, et al. The current role of sentinel lymph node biopsy in the management of cutaneous melanoma—a UK consensus statement. J Plastic Reconstr Aesthet Surg. 2020;73(1):36–42. [Epub ahead of print].

Preoperative and Intraoperative Lymphatic Mapping for Radioguided Sentinel Node Biopsy in Head and Neck Cancers

Renato A. Valdés Olmos, W. Martin C. Klop, and Maarten L. Donswijk

Contents

11.1   **Introduction** 262

11.2   **The Clinical Problem** 262

11.3   **Indications for SLNB** 262

11.4   **Radiocolloids and Modalities of Injection** 264

11.5   **Preoperative SLN Imaging** 264

11.6   **Lymphatic Drainage and Lymph Node Groups of the Neck** 265

11.7   **Intraoperative SLN Detection in the Head and Neck** 267

11.8   **Intraoperative Imaging for SLNB in the Head and Neck** 267

11.9   **Contribution of SPECT/CT Imaging** 268

11.10 **Common and Rare Variants for SLN Mapping in Head and Neck Cancers** 268

11.11 **Technical Pitfalls During SLN Mapping in Head and Neck Cancers** 270

11.12 **Accuracy of Radioguided SLNB in Head and Neck Cancers** 274

11.13 **Reporting SLN Mapping** 275

Clinical Cases 277

References 289

R. A. Valdés Olmos (✉)
Department of Radiology, Section of Nuclear Medicine and Interventional Molecular Imaging Laboratory, Leiden University Medical Center, Leiden, The Netherlands
e-mail: R.A.Valdes_Olmos@lumc.nl

W. M. C. Klop
Department of Head and Neck Oncology, Netherlands Cancer Institute—Antoni van Leeuwenhoek Hospital, Amsterdam, Netherlands

M. L. Donswijk
Division of Diagnostic Oncology, Department of Nuclear Medicine, Netherlands Cancer Institute—Antoni van Leeuwenhoek Hospital, Amsterdam, Netherlands

Learning Objectives
- To acquire basic knowledge about the role of nuclear medicine imaging in the sentinel lymph node (SLN) procedure in head and neck malignancies
- To know when sentinel lymph node biopsy (SLNB) is indicated in patients with melanoma localized in head and neck
- To learn the clinical indication of SLNB in patients with oral squamous cell carcinoma
- To understand the variability in head/neck lymphatic drainage and the need to use preoperative lymphatic mapping to assess the different individual patterns

© Springer Nature Switzerland AG 2020
G. Mariani et al. (eds.), *Atlas of Lymphoscintigraphy and Sentinel Node Mapping*,
https://doi.org/10.1007/978-3-030-45296-4_11

- To know the role of lymphoscintigraphy and SPECT/CT to identify and localize SLNs
- To understand the importance of SPECT/CT to localize SLNs in the anatomical environment of the head and neck
- To preoperatively identify SLNs and to learn how this information can be transferred to head/neck surgeons for the intraoperative procedure
- To get basic knowledge about imaging report generation combining lymphoscintigraphy and SPECT/CT

11.1 Introduction

The two most important applications of SLNB in the head and neck region are melanoma and oral squamous cell cancer (OSCC). The SLN status provides relevant prognostic information in patients with melanoma and also in oral cavity cancer a positive SLN is an unfavourable prognostic factor. In general, SLN mapping is indicated for staging in patients with histologically proven melanoma or OSCC with clinically (palpation) and radiologically (ultrasound, CT or MRI) established node-negative (cN0) neck.

11.2 The Clinical Problem

SLNB in the head and neck region may be difficult due to complex anatomic relations and unpredictable lymphatic drainage. This is one of the most likely reasons for the relatively high false-negative rates found in the earlier studies on validation of the procedure in head and neck melanoma [1]. Generally, lymphatic drainage of melanomas located in the occipital region is expected to the dorsal areas of the neck, and for melanomas of the temporal region to the preauricular lymph node stations. However, in many cases unexpected lymphatic drainage is observed in multiple basins, including lower areas of the neck [2]. In OSCC, lymphatic drainage is also highly unpredictable, and contralateral drainage is often seen even in well-lateralized malignancies of the tongue or floor of the mouth (Fig. 11.1). This crossing over has been observed in up to 20% of the cases, although it is more frequent in larger tumours [3].

11.3 Indications for SLNB

In melanoma, patients with clinically and radiologically negative lymph node assessment (stage N0) are considered as good candidates for the procedure. SLNB was initially indicated for patients with intermediate Breslow thickness (>1–4 mm). However, more recently SLNB may also be considered for thin melanomas that are T1b (0.8–1 mm or <0.8 thickness with ulceration) after a thorough discussion with the patient of the potential benefits and risk of harms associated with the procedure [4]. Due to the low risk of finding lymph node metastasis in melanoma lesions that are T1a (non-ulcerated lesions <0.8 mm thickness), SLN staging can be omitted in these patients. In lesions >4 mm SLNB is currently also offered because it has proven to yield valuable prognostic information with rates of positive SLNs ranging from 30 to 40% in spite of the risk of synchronous distant metastases reported for this group of patients [5]. Especially now, in the era of immunotherapy, a positive SLN can discriminate between the indication for adjuvant immunotherapy and a wait-and-see policy [6, 7].

SLNB in OSCC is generally recommended for T1 or T2 tumours, although criteria defining tumour stage can change as it has recently been illustrated in the new edition of the TNM classification [8]. Recent surgical consensus guidelines recommend that the most important selection criteria for SLNB are that the tumour can be reliably resected with adequate margins and the defect repaired locally without requiring access to the neck. This may allow the patient to avoid adjuvant therapy to the primary site [9]. Eligibility for SLNB consists of patients with biopsy-proven OSCC with clinically and radiologically established N0 neck.

> **Key Learning Points**
> - The two most important applications of the SLN procedure in the head and neck region are melanoma and oral squamous cell cancer (OSCC).
> - The SLN status provides relevant information, as a metastatic SLN is an unfavourable prognostic factor.
> - SLNB in the head and neck region may be difficult, due to complex anatomic relations and unpredictable lymphatic drainage.
> - Eligibility for SLNB consists of patients with biopsy-proven OSCC or melanoma with clinically and radiologically established N0 neck.

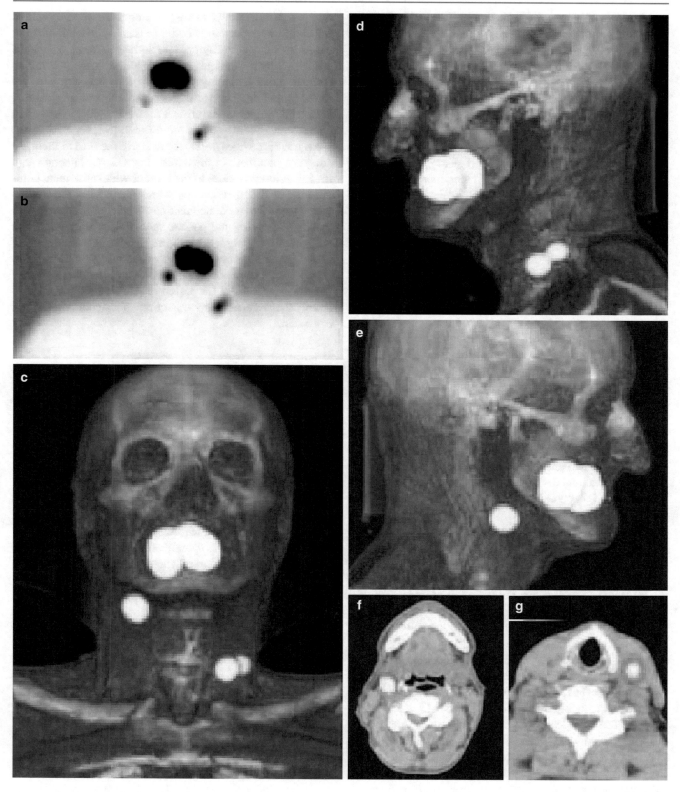

Fig. 11.1 An 81-year-old man with a T1 carcinoma on the right side of the lingual apex. After administration of 82 MBq ^{99m}Tc-nanocolloid in four injections into the mucosa around the tumour, early drainage to both sides of the neck is seen in anterior planar imaging (**a**), with sub-sequent increasing lymph node uptake in delayed images (**b**). Volume-rendering (**c–e**) and axial SPECT/CT fusion images show the SLNs in level II on the right and in level III on the left. All SLNs were tumour free at histopathology

- In melanoma, SLNB was initially indicated for patients with intermediate Breslow thickness (>1–4 mm); current indications also include thin lesions that are T1b (0.8–1 mm or <0.8 thickness with ulceration)· and tumours >4 mm (due to the high prognostic information with rates of positive SLNs ranging between 30 and 40%).
- A positive SLN in melanoma treatment (stage IIIC) indicates adjuvant immunotherapy.
- In OSCC SLNB is generally recommended for T1 or T2 tumours that can be reliably resected with adequate margins and the defect repaired locally without requiring access to the neck.

11.4 Radiocolloids and Modalities of Injection

Although a number of different radiopharmaceuticals are suitable for the SLN procedure worldwide, in Europe the standard radiotracer for lymphoscintigraphy is ^{99m}Tc-nanocolloidal albumin. In general, use of radiotracers is primarily based on the availability and different tracers are available in Australia (^{99m}Tc-antimony trisulphide) or in the United States (^{99m}Tc-sulphur colloid). More recently, the alternative radiotracer ^{99m}Tc-tilmanocept has become available in Europe and the United States; due to its small molecular size (7 nm) and the high affinity of its mannose residues for mannose receptors on the surface of macrophages, this tracer combines a rapid clearance from the injection site with increased SN uptake, which can be an advantage in the head and neck area when SLNs are located in proximity of the primary lesion [10].

For both melanoma and oral cavity cancer an activity of 60–80 MBq in a total volume of 0.4 mL is sufficient for adequate visualization of lymphatic vessels and lymph nodes. In case of a two-day protocol with surgery the following day, the activity can be increased to 120 MBq or more to compensate for the decay of ^{99m}Tc, which has a physical half-life of 6 h. Four intradermal injections are used for melanoma (11), whereas in oral cavity malignancies the radiotracer is administered into the mucosa in 3–4 sites around the primary lesion [8]. The use of a local anaesthetic for topical application (10% xylocaine spray) a few minutes before radiocolloid injection is recommended for oral cavity tumours. In patients with melanoma generally no local anaesthesia is given. However, in areas such as the scalp or ear, injections are painful, and local topical anaesthesia is recommended. In the case of melanoma, radiocolloid administration must be

applied intradermally, raising a bleb with each injection. Subcutaneous injection is easier to accomplish, but may not delineate the route of lymphatic drainage from a cutaneous site overlying the tumour. The radiocolloid must be administered in close proximity to the lesion or excision site, not farther than 1 cm from the edges of the lesion or surgical scar [11]. This factor may be critical for melanomas of the ear, in which small excision scars are difficult to recognize; in the scalp it is sometimes necessary to shave the area to facilitate adequate radiocolloid injections. For OSCC, injection into the intact mucosa close to the tumour with subsequent compression of the injection site with rolled swabs to immediately start dynamic acquisition is recommended. After dynamic scanning the patient should rinse the oral cavity without swallowing in order to reduce oral accumulation of non-injected radiotracer and to avoid saliva contamination [10]. For both melanoma and OSCC it is essential to identify the exact location of the lesion or excision site; in case of doubt the referring or operating physician should be consulted.

11.5 Preoperative SLN Imaging

The combination of planar lymphoscintigraphy and SPECT/CT imaging is crucial for lymphatic mapping and SLN localization in head and neck malignancies [10, 11].

Lymphoscintigraphy is based on sequential planar (2-dimensional) images depicting subsequent phases of lymph drainage. Due to the short distance between the injection site and the first draining lymph nodes in the head and neck region, dynamic images must be obtained as soon as possible after radiotracer administration. This approach frequently leads to the visualization of the lymphatic vessels, whereas static planar images recorded 15 min postinjection usually depict the first draining lymph nodes. Delayed static images (2–3 h after injection) enable to discriminate SLNs from second-tier nodes. Static images are based on both anterior and lateral views. For lateral views, the patient is asked to turn the head, in order to enable positioning of the gamma camera as close as possible to the area of interest.

Planar images provide a 2-dimensional overview based on which SLNs can be localized and marked on the patient's skin with the help of an external radioactive marker, such as a ^{57}Co-source pen. Anterior images must be complemented by oblique or lateral images, in order to define the location of the lymph nodes relative to the neck levels. The SLNs thus identified are marked on the skin on the basis of lateral views, in order to mimic the position of the neck during surgery.

Interpretation of planar images may be difficult, because no anatomical information is provided and the 3-dimensional surface of the structures of the head and neck area is not visualized. Moreover, the injection site on planar imaging may mask SLNs located in the proximity of or underneath the injection area. To avoid masking of a SLN, injections inferior to the lesion may be omitted. Transmission images can be used to improve anatomical orientation; to obtain these images, a ^{57}Co flood source is positioned so that the head of the patient is between the camera and the source during static imaging.

To overcome the anatomical limitations of planar images SPECT/CT was incorporated in the preoperative SLN imaging and its use is currently mandatory [8]. SPECT/CT is mostly performed after recording the delayed planar images. A SPECT/CT system consisting of a dual-head variable-angle gamma camera equipped with low-energy high-resolution collimators and a multislice spiral CT optimized for rapid rotation is generally used. SPECT acquisition is based on a 128×128 matrix and 25 s per view using $4°$- to $6°$-angle steps. CT is based on 2 mm slices, and settings are aimed at obtaining a low-dose CT (e.g. 130 KV, 40 mAs, B30s kernel), which is appropriate for both attenuation correction and anatomic mapping. The head of the patient rests on a head holder in order to avoid motion during acquisition and possible misalignment between the SPECT and the CT acquisition. After reconstruction, SPECT images are corrected for attenuation and scatter. Axial SPECT and CT slices are fused and are displayed in axial, sagittal and coronal orientations [12]. A 3-dimensional volume-rendered image may also be generated and is helpful in providing an overview of the lymphatic mapping in addition to the cross-sectional analysis.

Key Learning Points
- In Europe the standard radiotracer for lymphoscintigraphy is ^{99m}Tc-nanocolloid, in Australia ^{99m}Tc-antimony trisulphide and in the United States ^{99m}Tc-sulphur colloid.
- The alternative radiotracer ^{99m}Tc-tilmanocept, currently available in Europe and the United States, combines a rapid clearance from injection site with increased SLN uptake, which can be advantageous in the head and neck area, where SLNs are usually located in the vicinity of primary lesions.
- For melanoma and oral cavity cancer an activity of 60–80 MBq in a total volume of 0.4 mL is sufficient for adequate visualization of lymphatic vessels and lymph nodes. The activity can be increased to 120 MBq or more in case of a 2-day protocol with surgery the following day.

- Local anaesthetics for topical application a few minutes before radiocolloid injection are recommended for oral cavity tumours and in patients with scalp or ear melanomas.
- Lymphoscintigraphy is based on sequential images depicting subsequent phases of drainage to identify SLNs.
- SPECT/CT overcomes the anatomical limitations of planar images, by providing landmarks for localization of SLNs in the operating room.
- SPECT/CT is mostly performed after recording the delayed planar images.

11.6 Lymphatic Drainage and Lymph Node Groups of the Neck

The lymphatic system of the head and neck includes approximately 250–350 lymph nodes divided into various nodal groups: the occipital lymph nodes, the retroauricular or mastoid lymph nodes, the preauricular nodes and deep parotid nodes, the jugular chain nodes, the superficial and deep cervical nodes, the buccinator lymph nodes, and the submental and submandibular nodes. Lymph nodes of the spinal accessory chain are also included in the lymphatic network of the neck [13].

There are marked inter-subject variations in the lymphatic drainage of the head and neck. For instance for the scalp, drainage from the frontal zone is expected into the preauricular parotid lymph nodes, whereas the parietal zone drains to the retroauricular nodes and the occipital skin to the internal jugular or spinal accessory nodes. The face above the commissure of the lip and anterior to the pinna of the ear drains to the parotid lymph nodes, whereas the face inferior to the commissure of the lip drains to the cervical nodal basin. For the forehead, drainage is expected to the superficial parotid lymph nodes, whereas the lower lip, external nose, cheeks, upper lip and mucous membranes of the lips drain to the submandibular lymph nodes. For the central part of the lower lip, floor of the mouth and lingual apex lymphatic drainage to the submental nodes is expected [13].

Based on the classification according to Robbins et al. [14] lymph nodes in the neck have been subdivided into specific anatomic subsites and grouped into seven levels in each side of the neck to facilitate adherence to guidelines for neck dissection (Fig. 11.2). Level I includes the submental (sublevel Ia) and submandibular (sublevel Ib) lymph nodes. Level II contains the upper jugular lymph nodes that extend from the inferior border of the hyoid bone to the base of the skull; in relation to the vertical plane defined by the spinal accessory nerve, the lymph nodes located anteriorly (medial) constitute sublevel IIa, and the nodes located posteriorly

Fig. 11.2 Schematic illustration of the head and neck showing the levels for neck dissection (I–VII) and anatomical landmarks according to Robbins et al. [14]. The complementary levels utilized for radiation oncology are also displayed (circles) according to Grégoire et al. [15]

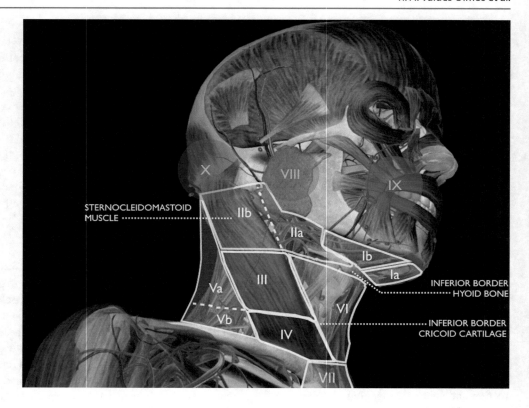

(lateral) correspond to sublevel IIb. Level III includes the middle jugular nodes, and level IV the lower jugular nodes. The posterior border of regions II, III and IV is the posterior border of the sternocleidomastoid muscle, which is the anterior border of level V. This latter group is composed of the sublevels Va (which includes the spinal accessory nodes) and sublevel Vb (which includes lymph nodes along the transverse cervical vessels) and the supraclavicular lymph nodes (with the exception of the Virchow node which is located on level IV). Level VI contains the pretracheal and paratracheal nodes, the precricoid Delphian node and the perithyroidal nodes including the lymph nodes along the recurrent laryngeal nerves. Finally, level VII includes the superior mediastinal lymph nodes above the level of the innominate artery. Levels VI and VII have recently been subdivided into sublevels VIa (anterior jugular nodes), VIb (prelaryngeal, pretracheal and paratracheal nodes), VIIa (retropharyngeal nodes) and VIIb (retro-styloid nodes) in order to facilitate the daily practice of radiation oncology [15]. This latter approach also recognizes the levels VIII (parotid group), IX (bucco-facial group) and X (posterior skull group) that is subdivided into Xa (retroauricular and subauricular nodes) and Xb (occipital nodes).

Key Learning Points

- The lymphatic system of the head and neck includes the following groups: occipital, retroauricular or mastoid, preauricular and deep parotid, jugular chain, superficial and deep cervical, buccinator, submental and submandibular as well as spinal accessory chain.

- Lymph nodes in the neck have been grouped into levels I–VII in each side of the neck in order to facilitate adherence to guidelines for neck dissection.

- Levels VI and VII have recently been subdivided into sublevels in order to facilitate the daily practice of radiation oncology. This latter approach also recognizes the additional levels VIII–X.

- Some important reference anatomical points to localize SLNs in relation to surgical levels are muscles (e.g. sternocleidomastoid, digastric, omohyoid), vessels (e.g. jugular vein), organs (e.g. parotid gland) and other structures (hyoid bone, cricoid cartilage).

11.7   Intraoperative SLN Detection in the Head and Neck

A gamma ray detection handheld probe is routinely used for intraoperative detection of the SLNs in the head and neck region. Blue dyes currently are less used because of inconsistent results in the head and neck [9]; due to the fast lymphatic migration of vital blue dyes SLNs in the head and neck region are frequently not stained blue. This limitation has led to combine radioguided detection with real-time near-infrared fluorescence imaging using hybrid tracers making blue dye unnecessary [16].

The gamma probe provides an acoustic signal when pointed straight towards the radioactive lymph node(s). Deeply located SLNs can be difficult to detect because of tissue attenuation, while the relatively large amount of radioactivity at the injection site may cause adjacent SLNs to be missed (Fig. 11.3). Checking the position of the SLN with the gamma probe is necessary prior to skin incision. This is particularly important in sites such as the submandibular region, where the skin marking guided by the gamma camera is less accurate and may be masked by the injection site. Also, after removing SLNs the activity of the injection site can complicate the measurement of the residual activity in the excision fossa.

11.8   Intraoperative Imaging for SLNB in the Head and Neck

A number of portable and handheld small-field-of-view gamma cameras have recently been developed to provide intraoperative visualization [17]. The entire lymph node excision procedure in the head and neck area can be monitored with a portable gamma camera, as these images provide an overview of all radioactive hot spots in the surgical field. SLNs located close to the injection site are easily overlooked using the gamma probe, but can be visualized with a gamma camera. If it turns out to be difficult to localize intraoperatively a SLN that had been identified during preoperative imaging, the intraoperative gamma camera may be able to show the surgeon where the node is located.

Furthermore, by detecting residual radioactivity after excision of the SLNs, the portable gamma camera can help to assess completeness of the procedure. This may replace application of the so-called 10% rule associated with the use of the gamma probe (resection of nodes with 10% of the lymph node with the highest radioactivity and/or at least tenfold background radioactivity) during surgery. Imaging after excision can also lead to finding of additional SLNs in more than 20% of the cases [18]. In some cases, intense radioactive uptake at the site of the SLN on preoperative imaging corresponds to a cluster of SLNs. Imaging after excision of the first hot node can reveal the remaining SLNs. Acquiring intraoperative images only takes a few minutes, but, if more lymph nodes are found and excised because of intraoperative imaging, the procedure is likely to be prolonged.

Although intraoperative visualization of SLNs with a portable gamma camera may optimize intraoperative detection of SLNs in the head and neck region, further improvements in the SLNB procedure can be achieved by combining the use of the intraoperative gamma camera with fluorescence cameras for simultaneous SLN signal detection using hybrid tracers such as indocyanine green (ICG)-^{99m}Tc-nanocolloid [16, 19]. The high resolution of the fluorescent signal complements the radioguided localization especially when the SLNs are located close to the injection site, for instance in patients with malignancies of the floor of mouth and submental SLNs, or in periauricular melanomas and SLNs located in the parotid region (Figs. 11.4 and 11.5).

Key Learning Points

- Handheld gamma detection probes are routinely used for intraoperative SLN detection in the head and neck region. Blue dyes are currently less used and are gradually being replaced by fluorescent agents and hybrid tracers (with combined radioactivity/fluorescence signatures).
- Checking SLN location with the gamma probe prior to surgical incision is particularly important in the submandibular region, where the skin marking guided by the gamma camera is somewhat inaccurate and may be masked by the injection site.
- Intraoperative use of a small-field-of-view gamma camera can show where SLNs are located, especially when they are close to the injection site and may be easily overlooked using the gamma counting probe only.
- Use of a portable gamma camera can also help to assess completeness of the procedure without resorting to application of the 10% rule for gamma probe counting during surgery.
- Intraoperative visualization of SLNs with a portable gamma camera can be combined with fluorescence cameras for simultaneous SLN signal detection using hybrid tracers such as ICG-^{99m}Tc-nanocolloid.
- The high resolution of the fluorescent signal complements the radioguided localization when SLNs are close to the injection site in patients with malignancies of the floor of mouth and submental SLNs, or in periauricular melanomas and SLNs in the parotid region.

11.9 Contribution of SPECT/CT Imaging

SPECT/CT can optimize SLN visualization and localization in the head and neck region. In melanoma patients SPECT/CT has been reported to visualize 29% additional SLNs in the parotid/preauricular region and 44% in level Vb in comparison with planar imaging acquired during lymphoscintigraphy [20]. These additional SLNs found on SPECT/CT imaging increase the likelihood of retrieving a tumour-positive SLN [21] and decrease the false-negative rate. Especially lymph nodes adjacent to the injection site are more frequently detected by SPECT/CT than by planar imaging. Furthermore, non-nodal radioactivity accumulation (radiocolloid leakage or contamination, possibly causing false-positive scintigraphic findings) can be more easily identified on the basis of SPECT/CT images [10].

Also in OSCC SPECT/CT has been able to identify a 22% additional SLNs in the neck, and in 20% of the patients with at least one positive SLN the only positive node was detected thanks to SPECT/CT imaging [22].

SPECT/CT is very useful for exact anatomic localization of the SLNs. In the head and neck area it is very important to identify the anatomic correlates of SLNs with the various vascular and neural structures, in order to be able to safely remove these lymph nodes without damaging such important anatomic structures. SPECT/CT can localize these SLNs with reference to anatomical structures such as the mandible, parotid gland, jugular vein and sternocleidomastoid muscle. SPECT/CT also shows whether the nodes are located superficially underneath the skin or hidden below other structures. SPECT/CT thus provides crucial anatomical reference points for planning the optimal surgical approach. The superior localization information provided by SPECT/CT frequently leads to modifying of the surgical approach, with significant shortening of operation times.

Location of a melanoma in the head and neck has been found to be a predictive factor for a false-negative SLNB, and the number of false-negative SLNBs reported for this region is higher compared to other areas [1]. This relatively high number might be reduced by optimal preoperative localization with SPECT/CT.

Another advantage is the possibility to correlate findings of fused SPECT/CT with those of the CT component, which has been significantly improved in the new generation of SPECT/CT devices, making it possible to obtain more accurate morphological information in the head and neck. In many cases radioactive SLNs correspond to single nodes. However, in some cases the radioactive signal on SPECT/CT may correspond to a cluster of lymph nodes on CT. This preoperative information may lead to more careful post-excision control after removal of the first radioactive lymph node [10].

11.10 Common and Rare Variants for SLN Mapping in Head and Neck Cancers

On lymphoscintigraphy the preauricular lymph node basin usually receives drainage from melanomas of the face, anterior and coronal midline scalp, and coronal neck. In contrast, the ipsilateral level II lymph node field can receive drainage from any region in the head and neck area [23]. More specifically, expected drainage of melanomas of the coronal and posterior scalp is to lymph nodes of neck level V and the suboccipital nodes; drainage to neck level II, the parotid area and retroauricular areas is less frequent. Anterior scalp melanomas are expected to drain to levels I–III or IV, but on lymphoscintigrams drainage to level V has been observed. In lateralized scalp melanomas unexpected contralateral drainage is also seen. Drainage from posterior scalp melanomas to high occipital scalp SLNs can also be observed. Preauricular melanomas drain usually to levels I–III or IV and to the parotid basin, while SLNs are rarely found in level V. For melanomas on the ear, drainage is expected to levels II–V, but can also occur towards occipital and parotid nodes.

Melanomas of the upper face, nose and lower face can drain to nodes of levels I–III or IV, or to the parotid region, while drainage to SLNs in level V has been more rarely observed.

Melanomas located in the neck may frequently drain to levels I–IV and, depending on the location (anterior or dorsal, lower or upper), to level V or to the parotid area. More

Fig. 11.3 A 46-year-old woman with a left infra-auricular melanoma (5 mm Breslow thickness). Planar lymphoscintigraphy and SPECT/CT performed after intradermal administration of 70 MBq ^{99m}Tc-nanocolloid divided into four injections around the excision scar. Volume rendering (**a**, **b**) and fused axial SPECT/CT (**c**) show a SLN in level II, very close to the inferior part of the injection site. This lymph node was not seen in the planar lateral (**d**) and anterior (**e**) images. The SLN localized during surgery with a portable gamma camera (**f**) was tumour free at histopathology

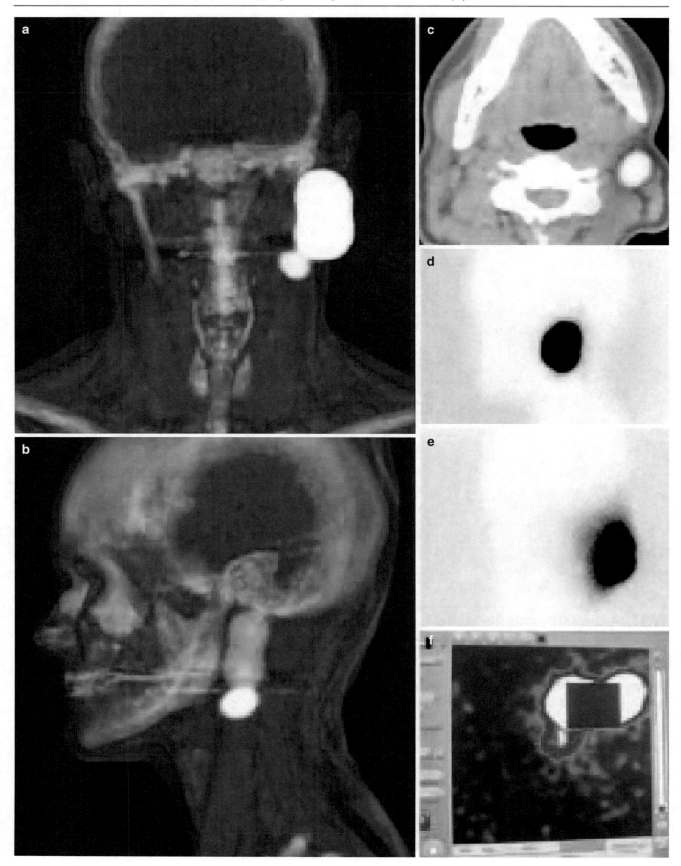

rarely occipital SLNs have been seen in melanomas of the posterior upper neck [2] (Fig. 11.6).

Oral cavity malignancies located in the lateral tongue and posterior floor of the mouth generally drain to ipsilateral neck level II nodes [24]. However, drainage to levels I and III is also possible, as well as drainage to contralateral lymph nodes (Fig. 11.7). From the anterior floor of the mouth and lingual apex drainage to level I is expected; however, not seldom bilateral drainage to level II/III can be observed.

Key Learning Points

- In melanoma and OSCC, SPECT/CT imaging visualizes significantly more SLNs than planar imaging of lymphoscintigraphy.
- SPECT/CT localizes SLNs with reference to anatomical structures such as the mandible, parotid gland, jugular vein and sternocleidomastoid muscle and also shows whether the nodes are located superficially underneath the skin or hidden below other structures.
- Sometimes the radioactive signal on SPECT/CT may correspond to a cluster of lymph nodes on the CT component. This preoperative information may lead to more careful post-excision control after removal of the first radioactive lymph node by the surgeon.
- OSCCs located in the lateral tongue and posterior floor of the mouth generally drain to ipsilateral neck level II nodes. From the anterior floor of the mouth and lingual apex drainage is expected to level I.
- Melanomas of the upper face, nose, lower face and preauricular area usually drain to levels I–III or IV and to the parotid basin.

11.11 Technical Pitfalls During SLN Mapping in Head and Neck Cancers

The most frequent pitfall is skin contamination. The high pressure of the intradermal bleb can result in leakage during injection, or after removal of the needle. This may occur more frequently on the skin of the scalp, ear and nose. The use of a surgical type light to adequately visualize the site of injection and a fenestrated drape to cover the area may help to avoid contamination.

Also in oral cavity tumours some contamination may be observed after peritumoural injections; for this reason, it is recommended to cover the injection site with rolled swabs to absorb tracer and blood after injection, in order to start as soon as possible with the dynamic phase of the acquisition. After dynamic scanning, it is mandatory to request the patient to rinse the oral cavity without swallowing in order to reduce oral uptake of non-injected radiotracer and to avoid saliva contamination.

The hot spots due to contamination may be confused with SLNs in the vicinity of the tumour, thus leading to unnecessary intraoperative pursuit. In head and neck melanomas skin decontamination following verification of contamination is crucial. Complementary SPECT/CT imaging may also help in detecting these skin artefacts and especially remnant activity in areas of the oral cavity [10].

Another pitfall may be caused by differences in patient position between the time when projection of the SLN is marked on the overlying skin in the nuclear medicine department and the time of surgery. Verifying the site of incision in the operation room using a gamma probe or the portable gamma camera helps solving this problem. A pitfall related to SPECT/CT may be caused by misalignment between acquisition of the SPECT and of the CT component, which can cause spurious results in the anatomical localization of SLNs. Immobilization of the head and, if necessary, use of manual image alignment help to prevent/correct this artefact. Another important pitfall is the "shine-through" phenomenon in the floor-of-the-mouth tumours, due to the close proximity of the injection side with the draining basin. Especially SLNs in level I are easily missed because of this occurrence.

It is recommended to analyse not only the attenuation- and scatter-corrected SPECT images but also the non-attenuation-corrected and non-scatter-corrected SPECT images and to vary the intensity levels of the displayed SPECT images during analysis, in order to detect low-uptake SLNs that may otherwise be missed.

Fig. 11.4 A 59-year-old man with a 2 mm Breslow thickness melanoma of the left ear. A total of 88 MBq of the hybrid imaging agent ^{99m}Tc/ICG-nanocolloid was injected into four sites around the lesion in the border of the ear. Planar lateral image (**a**) shows drainage to the left side of the neck. Volume rendering (**b**) and axial SPECT/CT (**c**, **d**) show the radioactive lymph nodes in level II and behind the parotid gland. After incision at the site marked on skin (**e**), two SLNs in level II and two in the parotid area were found using the radioactive (**f**) and fluorescent (**g**) signals. The SLNs were smaller than 3 mm (**h**) and were tumour free

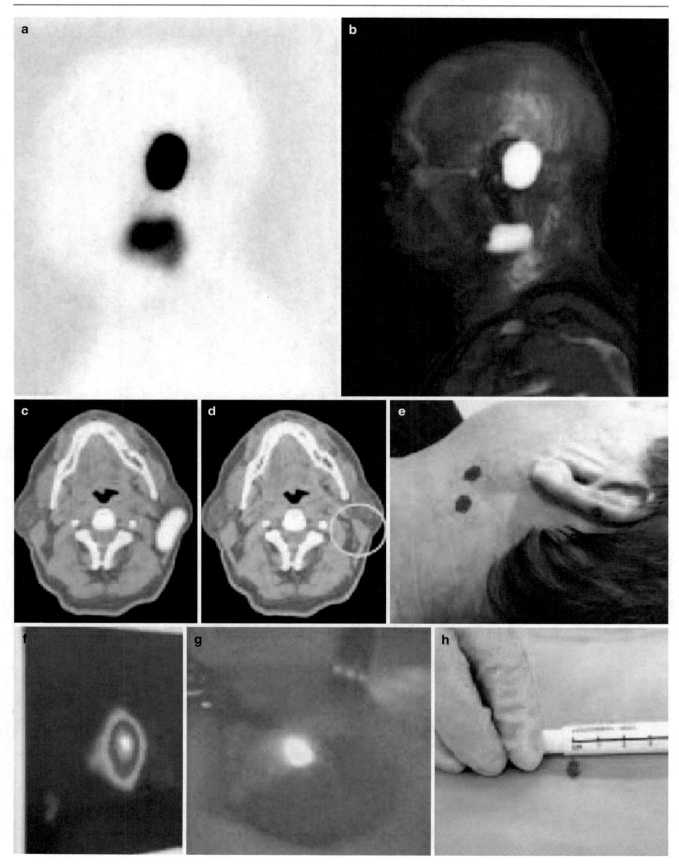

Fig. 11.5 A 64-year-old woman with a 5 mm Breslow thickness melanoma in the posterior area of scalp. Volume rendering (**a**) and fused axial SPECT/CT (**b**) show bilateral drainage to two SLNs in the occipital region. These SLNs, localized intraoperatively by detecting the radioactive (**c**) and fluorescent (**d**) signals, were free of metastasis

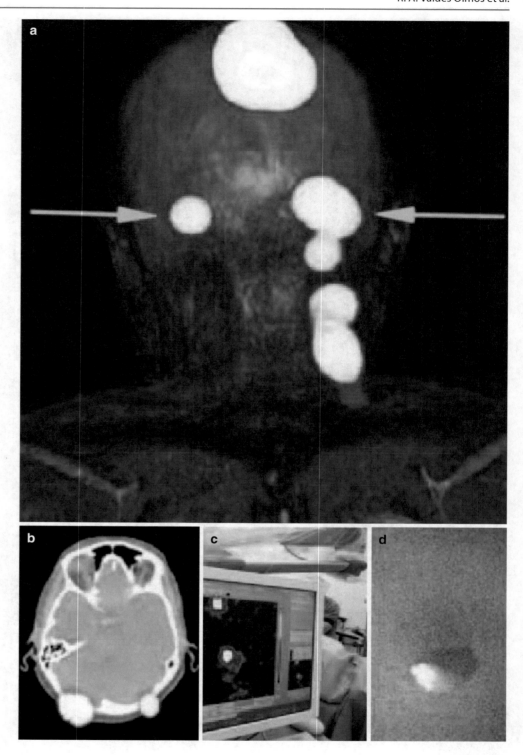

Fig. 11.6 A 64-year-old woman with a 3 mm thickness Breslow melanoma of the posterior part of the neck. Volume-rendering (**a**, **b**) and fused SPECT/CT axial images (**c**, **d**) show drainage to upper part of the left neck (with SN(s) in the occipital region and in level II) as well as to the left axilla. Note that on planar imaging (**e**) one of the neck lymph nodes is masked by the injection site. The occipital SLN was tumour positive. The SLNs in level II and in the axilla were also tumour free

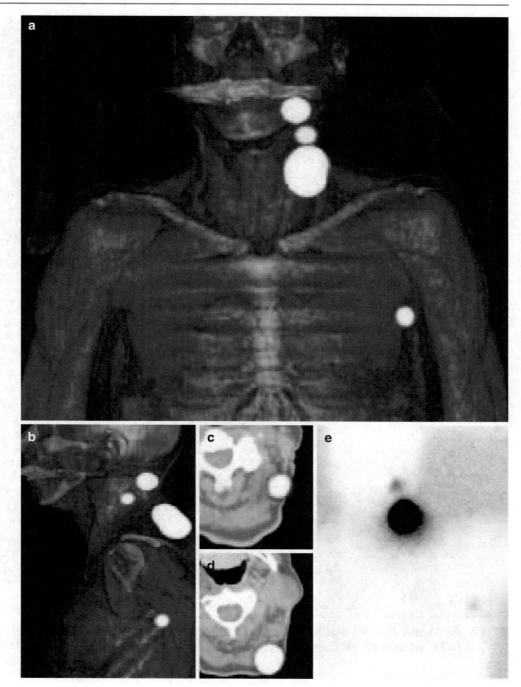

Fig. 11.7 A 60-year-old woman with a T1 carcinoma of the right border of the tongue. SPECT/CT performed 2 h after peritumoural administration of 80 MBq ^{99m}Tc-nanocolloid. Early imaging had depicted two early draining lymph nodes on the right side of the neck. Volume rendering (**a**) and axial SPECT/CT localized these SLNs in level II (**b, c**) and level III (**d, e**) of the neck. Only the SLN of level III was found to contain metastasis at histopathology

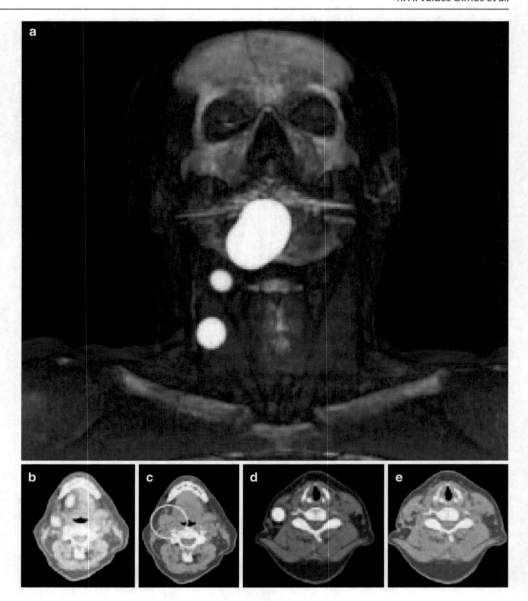

11.12 Accuracy of Radioguided SLNB in Head and Neck Cancers

In early series concerning head and neck melanomas, false-negative rates appeared to be higher (>10% in various series) than the 2–3% value commonly reported for other sites [25]. However, when performed by experienced head and neck surgeons, the SLN procedure may achieve negative predictive values close to 98%, similarly as for other cutaneous malignancies [26]. Nevertheless, head and neck localization remains a factor associated with more false-negative SLNBs in patients with melanoma compared to other anatomical locations [27].

Concerning OSCC, the negative predictive value has varied from 93 to 100% on the basis of 2–5-year follow-up studies, with reduced sensitivity for floor-of-the-mouth cancers [28]. This is one of the most important reasons in recent surgical guidelines to recommend surgical exploration in level I of the neck in this latter patient category in the case that preoperative lymphatic mapping does not detect radioactive nodes in this area. Furthermore, the use of additional portable imaging devices, fluorescence dyes, hybrid tracers (ICG-^{99m}Tc-nanocolloid) and more specific radiotracers such as ^{99m}Tc-tilmanocept is strongly recommended [9] to reduce false-negative results (Fig. 11.8).

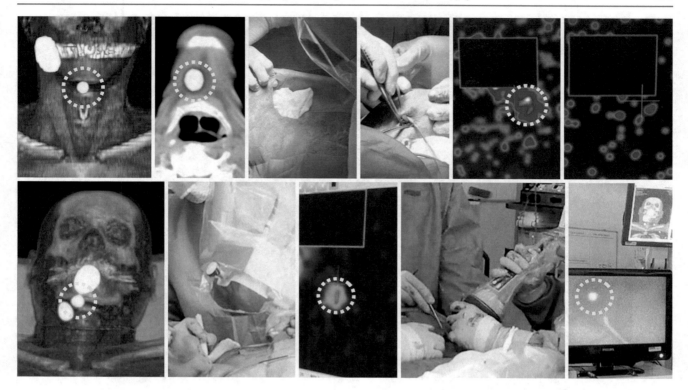

Fig. 11.8 Surgical exploration of level I of the neck. In *upper row*, a SLN (circles) in a patient with a melanoma of the lower part of the right cheek is depicted using SPECT/CT (first two images) and subsequently removed (middle images) after intraoperative detection (circle) using a portable gamma camera. In *lower row*, a SLN (circles) depicted by preoperative SPECT/CT and intraoperative portable gamma camera is subsequently removed using a fluorescence camera thanks to the peritumoral administration of the hybrid tracer ICG-^{99m}Tc-nanocolloid

---

Key Learning Points

- The most frequent pitfall in the SLN procedure for melanoma is skin contamination; the high pressure of the intradermal bleb during injection or after removal of the needle may lead to leakage.
- In OSCC, mouth contamination with non-injected radiotracer may be observed after peritumoural injections; in order to avoid this pitfall, it is mandatory to ask the patient rinse the oral cavity without swallowing.
- A general pitfall may be caused when skin marking of the SLN in the nuclear medicine department is performed with the neck positioned in a different manner than during surgery.
- In floor-of-the-mouth cancer, when SLNs are not detected in level I consensus guidelines recommend surgical exploration of the level.
- The use of additional fluorescence dyes, hybrid tracers (ICG-^{99m}Tc-nanocolloid) and specific radiotracers such as ^{99m}Tc-tilmanocept is strongly recommended to reduce false-negatives in areas close to the primary tumour.

11.13 Reporting SLN Mapping

Identification of SLNs in the nuclear medicine report is crucial to facilitate excision biopsy in the operating room. Specific practical guidelines to generate imaging report in the SLN procedure have recently been described for oral cavity cancers [10]. A similar approach must be employed for head and neck melanoma. This includes (Fig. 11.9) the description of each component of the lymphatic mapping as follows:

1. For dynamic studies: lymphatic ducts directly draining from the injection site as well as the visualization of bilateral or unilateral drainage.
2. For early and delayed static images: the number and uptake intensity of first-echelon nodes, number of second-echelon nodes and additional lymph nodes appearing on delayed images in other basins.
3. For SPECT/CT imaging: additional SLNs, localization of SLNs with reference to anatomical landmarks (vessels and muscles) and surgical levels.

In the conclusion it is necessary to specify the following:

- The skin marking in surgical position of the identified SLNs

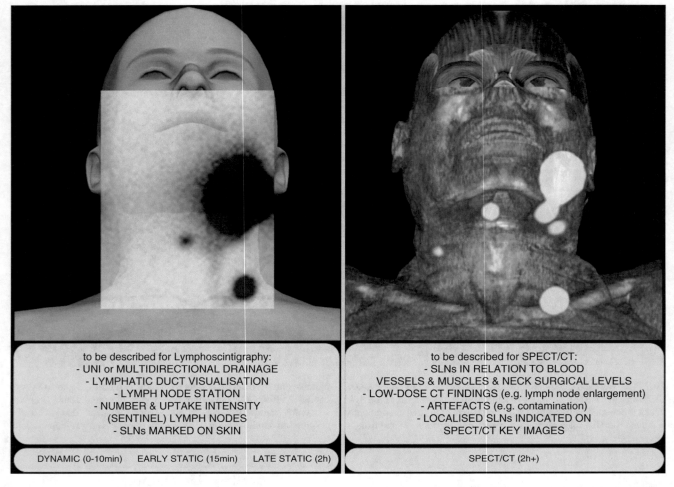

to be described for Lymphoscintigraphy:
- UNI or MULTIDIRECTIONAL DRAINAGE
- LYMPHATIC DUCT VISUALISATION
- LYMPH NODE STATION
- NUMBER & UPTAKE INTENSITY
(SENTINEL) LYMPH NODES
- SLNs MARKED ON SKIN

DYNAMIC (0-10min)   EARLY STATIC (15min)   LATE STATIC (2h)

to be described for SPECT/CT:
- SLNs IN RELATION TO BLOOD
VESSELS & MUSCLES & NECK SURGICAL LEVELS
- LOW-DOSE CT FINDINGS (e.g. lymph node enlargement)
- ARTEFACTS (e.g. contamination)
- LOCALISED SLNs INDICATED ON
SPECT/CT KEY IMAGES

SPECT/CT (2h+)

Fig. 11.9 Schematic generation of the nuclear medicine report for SLN mapping. For lymphoscintigraphy (*on the left*) an example of bilateral neck drainage from the injection site in the oral cavity as well as key aspects to be considered in the report are shown. For SPECT/CT repro- duced with volume rendering (*on the right*) various SLNs in different levels of the neck are displayed together with a summary of key aspects to be included in the report

- The anatomical localization of SLNs on SPECT/CT key images, indicating their location with reference to muscles (e.g. sternocleidomastoid, digastric, omohyoid), vessels (e.g. jugular vein), organs (e.g. parotid gland), other structures (hyoid bone, cricoid cartilage), lymph node groups and surgical levels

- Secondary findings on the low-dose non-enhanced CT component of the study, including enlarged nodes, cluster of nodes, incidental findings and other abnormalities

Clinical Cases

Case 11.1: SLN Mapping in Floor-of-the-Mouth Carcinoma with Drainage to Bilateral Cervical Lymph Nodes: What to do when the SLN Is Not Found?

Renato A. Valdés Olmos, Martin Klop, and Maarten Donswijk

Background Clinical Case

A 78-year-old woman with squamous-cell carcinoma of floor of mouth was referred for SLNB. During staging of the neck, MRI showed an enlarged lymph node in level 1b of the right side of the neck. Partly explained by the obesity of the patient, this node was not palpable on physical examination. Following MRI, the patient was referred for ultrasound-guided fine-needle aspiration cytology (FNAC) of the suspected node, which resulted negative for tumour involvement. It was decided to proceed with the SLN procedure. However, in spite of a successful preoperative mapping, the SLN in level 1b was not found in the operating

room. Sequential surveillance with ultrasound was then performed and, due to increase in size of the right cervical node, 6 weeks after the SLN procedure a repeated FNAC was performed—which demonstrated metastasis. Dissection of the right side of the neck followed, and 54 lymph nodes were removed. Metastasis was found only in the enlarged lymph node of level 1b.

Lymphoscintigraphy and SPECT/CT

In the afternoon before surgery a total of 120 MBq ICG-^{99m}Tc-nanocolloid was administered in four injections around the tumour in the intact mucosa of the right part of the floor of the mouth, following local anaesthesia with xylocaine 10% spray. Immediately after tracer administration, a dynamic study was acquired during 10 min with the patient in supine position using a dual-head gamma camera (Symbia T, Siemens, Erlangen, Germany) equipped with low-energy high-resolution collimators. Subsequently, 5-min planar static images were acquired at 15 min and 2 h post-injection. In addition, SPECT/CT was acquired at 2 h using the same gamma camera.

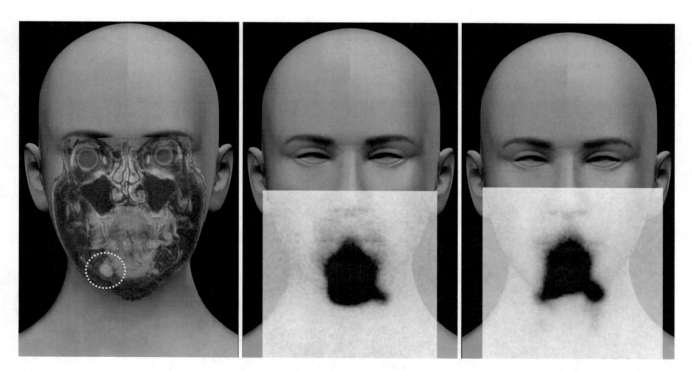

Fig. 11.10 Coronal MRI (on the left), anterior early (middle) and delayed (on the right) planar images superimposed to anatomical models. The enlarged lymph node of level 1b is seen on MRI (circle), whereas bilateral drainage to cervical lymph node stations is particularly well delineated in delayed images

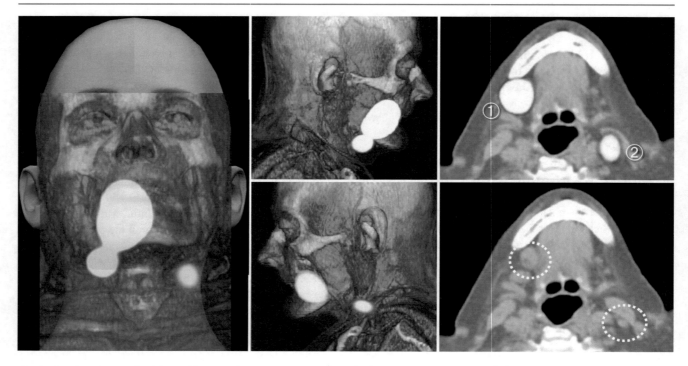

Fig. 11.11 Anterior (on the right) and lateral (middle row) SPECT/CT images displayed with volume rendering showing SLNs in level 1b of the right side and level 2b of the left side. Note in cross-sectional images (on the right) that the radioactive node in right level 1b on SPECT/CT (top) appears to correspond with the enlarged lymph node on low-dose CT (circle), whereas in level 2b of the right side the radioactivity corresponds to a lymph node with normal size (circle)

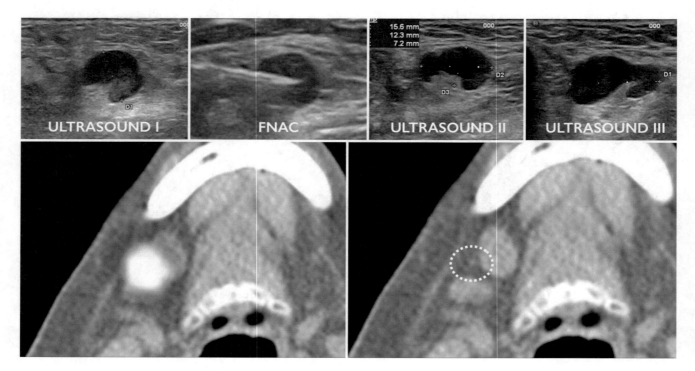

Fig. 11.12 Due to the failure of the intraoperative procedure to find the SLN on the right side of the neck, surveillance with ultrasonography was performed, showing a progressive increase in size of the suspected lymph node in level 1b; however, only the third follow-up ultrasound scan demonstrated metastasis on FNAC (upper row). A revision with magnification of the cross-sectional images showed that the radioactivity seen on SPECT/CT in level 1b corresponded to a small lymph node on low-dose CT, located in the proximity of the enlarged node (circle)

Case 11.2: SLN Mapping in Floor-of-the-Mouth Carcinoma with Drainage to Bilateral Cervical Lymph Nodes: The Complementary Role of SPECT/CT and Planar Imaging

Renato A. Valdés Olmos, Martin Klop, and Maarten Donswijk

Background Clinical Case

A 61-year-old man with squamous-cell carcinoma in the midline of the floor of mouth was referred for a SLN procedure. No lymph node abnormalities had been detected on physical and radiological examination of the neck (clinical stage T2N0M0).

Planar Lymphoscintigraphy and SPECT/CT

In the afternoon before surgery a total of 115 MBq ICG-^{99m}Tc-nanocolloid was administered in four injections in the intact mucosa around the tumour of the middle part of floor of mouth following oral preparation with xylocaine 10% spray for local anaesthesia. Immediately after tracer administration a dynamic study was acquired during 10 min with the patient in supine position using a dual-head gamma camera (Symbia T, Siemens, Erlangen, Germany) equipped with low-energy high-resolution collimators. Subsequently 5-min planar static images were acquired at 15 min and 2 h post-injection. In addition, SPECT/CT was acquired after delayed planar images using the same gamma camera.

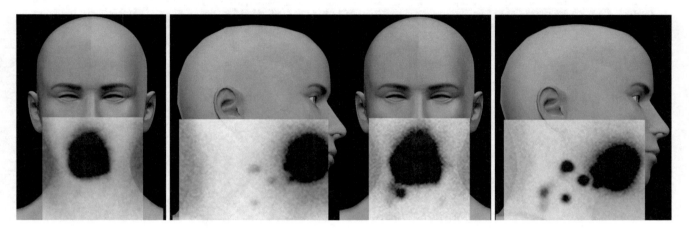

Fig. 11.13 Static planar images are displayed in superposition to anatomical models. On early anterior (first frame) and right lateral (second frame) views initial lymph node uptake is seen principally on the right side of the neck. Bilateral cervical drainage is particularly depicted in delayed anterior planar imaging (third frame), whereas in right lateral delayed image (fourth frame) multiple radioactive lymph nodes are visualized

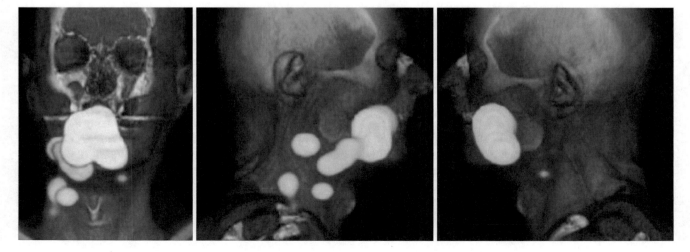

Fig. 11.14 Radioactive lymph nodes are displayed in an anatomical environment using SPECT/CT with volume rendering. Note that radioactive lymph nodes are clearer depicted in relation to the planar images showed in Fig. 11.13

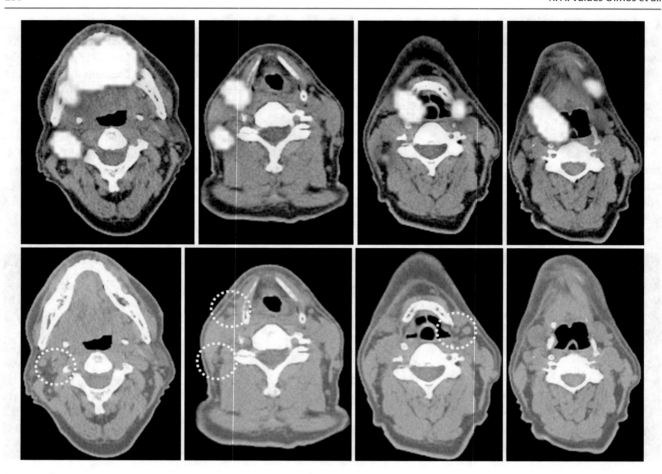

Fig. 11.15 Cross-sectional images of SPECT/CT (upper row) and low-dose CT (low row) showing distribution of ICG-^{99m}Tc-nanocolloid after injections around the tumour in the midline of floor of mouth. Note that radioactive lymph nodes seen on SPECT/CT correspond to normal-size lymph nodes on low-dose CT (circles). However, for the enlarged tracer concentration on the right part of the oral cavity (upper image in fourth column) no lymph nodes are seen on CT (bottom). This area of radioactivity accumulation was associated with internal contamination along the oropharynx, due to leakage during tracer administration

Case 11.3: SLN Mapping in Floor-of-the-Mouth Carcinoma with Drainage to Bilateral Cervical Lymph Nodes

Renato A. Valdés Olmos, Martin Klop, and Maarten Donswijk

Background Clinical Case

A 53-year-old man with squamous-cell carcinoma in the right lateral part of floor of mouth was referred for SLNB. No lymph node abnormalities had been detected on physical and radiological examination of the neck (clinical stage T2N0M0).

Planar Lymphoscintigraphy and SPECT/CT

In the afternoon before surgery a total of 120 MBq ICG-^{99m}Tc-nanocolloid was administered in four injections around the tumour in the intact mucosa of the right part of the floor of the mouth following oral preparation with xylocaine 10% spray for local anaesthesia. Immediately after tracer administration a dynamic study was acquired during 10 min with the patient in supine position using a dual-head gamma camera (Symbia T, Siemens, Erlangen, Germany) equipped with low-energy high-resolution collimators. Subsequently 5-min planar static images were acquired at 15 min and 2 h post-injection. In addition, SPECT/CT was acquired after delayed planar images using the same gamma camera.

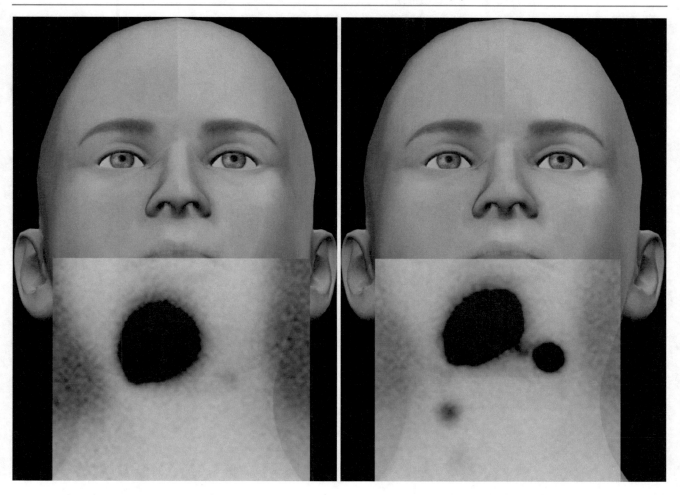

Fig. 11.16 Anterior static planar images displayed in superposition to anatomical models show initial tracer migration on early frame (on the left), and well-delineated cervical drainage on delayed anterior planar image (on the right)

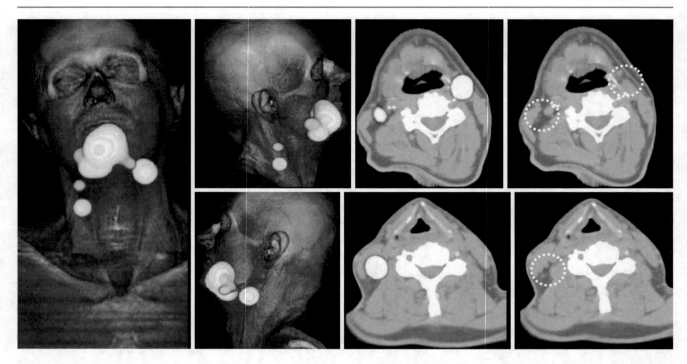

Fig. 11.17 SPECT/CT displayed with volume rendering (on the left) showing distribution of ICG-^{99m}Tc-nanocolloid to both sides of the neck. In cross-sectional images (on the right) of fused SPECT/CT (left column) and low-dose CT (right column) note that radioactive lymph nodes seen on SPECT/CT correspond to normal-size lymph nodes on low-dose CT (circles). Cervical SLNs are localized in level 2a on the left and levels 2b and 3 on the right

Case 11.4: SLN Mapping in Tongue Carcinoma with Bilateral Drainage to Various Lymph Node Neck Levels

Renato A. Valdés Olmos, Martin Klop, and Maarten Donswijk

Background Clinical Case

A 56-year-old man with squamous-cell carcinoma in the right lateral part of the tongue was referred for SLNB. No lymph node abnormalities had been detected on physical and radiological examination of the neck (clinical stage T1N0M0).

Planar Lymphoscintigraphy and SPECT/CT Imaging

In the afternoon before surgery a total of 105 MBq ICG-^{99m}Tc-nanocolloid was administered in four injections around the tumour in the right part of the mobile part of the tongue following oral preparation with xylocaine 10% spray for local anaesthesia. Following tracer administration, a dynamic study was acquired during 10 min with the patient in supine position using a dual-head gamma camera (Symbia T, Siemens, Erlangen, Germany) equipped with low-energy high-resolution collimators. Subsequently, 5-min planar static images were acquired at 15 min and 2 h post-injection. In addition, SPECT/CT imaging was acquired after delayed planar images using the same gamma camera.

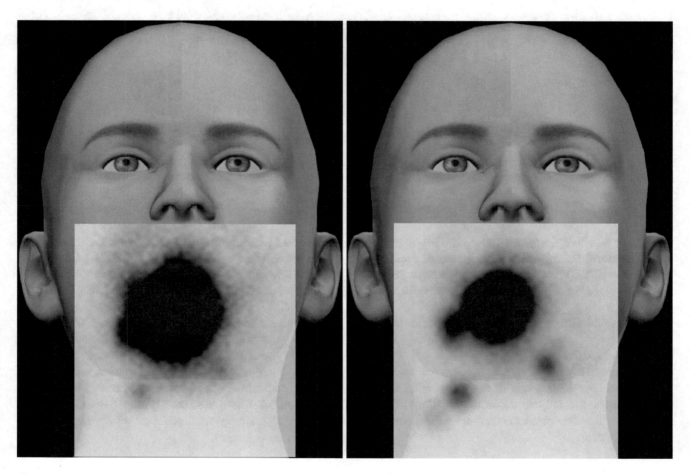

Fig. 11.18 Anterior static planar images superimposed to anatomical models show bilateral drainage to cervical lymph nodes in early (on the left) and delayed frames (on the right). Note in delayed image that a radioactive lymph node on the right side of the neck becomes better delineated in relation to the radioactivity of the injection site

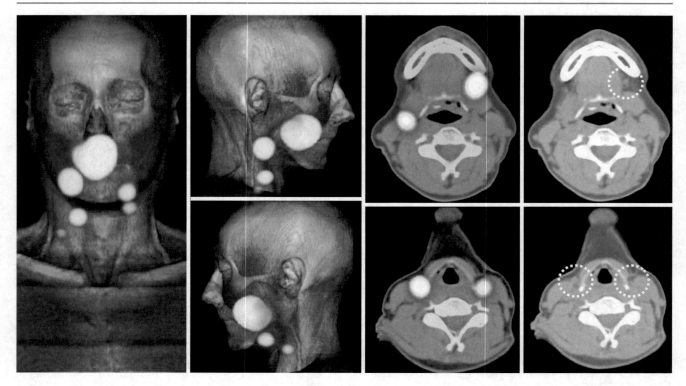

Fig. 11.19 SPECT/CT imaging displayed with volume rendering (on the left) showing bilateral migration of ICG-^{99m}Tc-nanocolloid to various lymph node levels in the neck. On the right, cross-sectional SPECT/ CT images show radioactive lymph nodes on both cervical sides corresponding to normal-size lymph nodes on low-dose CT (circles) in levels 2b and 3 on the right and levels 1b and 2b on the left

Case 11.5: SLN Mapping in Suboccipital Melanoma with Ipsilateral Drainage to Cervical Lymph Nodes on Planar and SPECT/CT Imaging: The Decisive Role of Histopathology for Avoiding a False-Negative Result

Renato A. Valdés Olmos, Martin Klop, and Maarten Donswijk

Background Clinical Case

A 59-year-old man with a 5.8 mm Breslow thick melanoma located on the left side of the suboccipital area was referred for SLNB. No lymph node abnormalities (N0 stage) had been detected on physical examination and ultrasonography of the neck.

Planar Lymphoscintigraphy and SPECT/CT Imaging

In the afternoon before surgery a total of 110 MBq ICG-^{99m}Tc-nanocolloid was administered in four intradermal injections around the primary lesion scar in the left suboccipital region. Immediately after tracer administration, dynamic frames were acquired during 10 min with the patient in supine position using a dual-head gamma camera (Symbia T, Siemens, Erlangen, Germany) equipped with low-energy high-resolution collimators. Subsequently, 5-min planar static images were acquired at 15 min and 2 h post-injection. Using the same gamma camera additional SPECT/CT imaging was acquired after acquiring the delayed planar images.

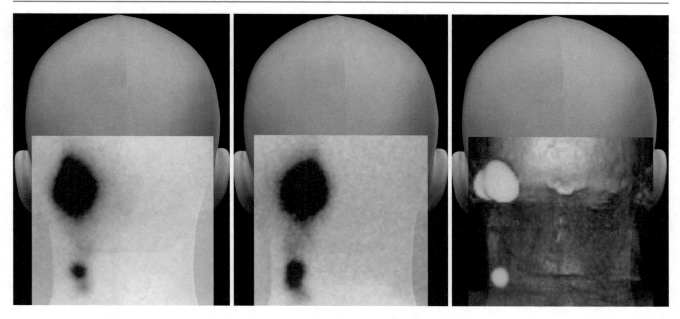

Fig. 11.20 From left to right early and delayed planar images, as well as volume-rendered SPECT/CT images in posterior view superimposed to anatomical models. Lymphatic drainage to the left side of the neck increasing in delayed planar images (middle) with no radioactive lymph nodes seen in the vicinity of the injection site on SPECT/CT (on the right)

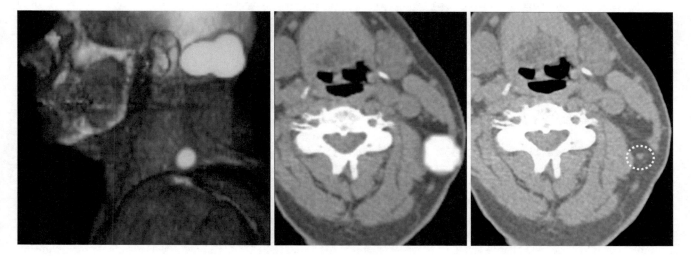

Fig. 11.21 Left lateral view of volume-rendered SPECT/CT (on the left) with a radioactive SLN in level 5b of the neck. This radioactive node is seen on cross-sectional SPECT/CT behind the posterior border of the sternocleidomastoid muscle (middle) and corresponds to a normal-size lymph node on the low-dose CT (circle)

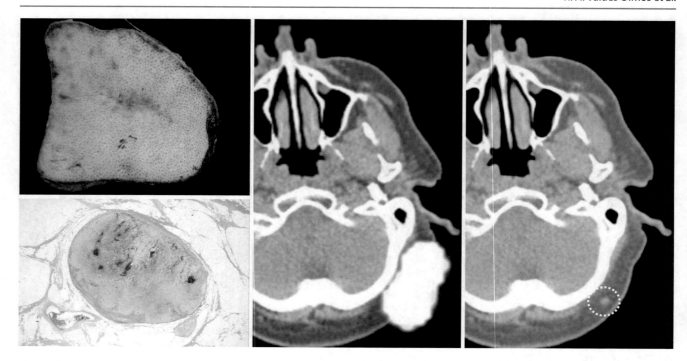

Fig. 11.22 The removed SLN of level 5b of the left neck was found to be free of tumour on histopathology. However, in the specimen corresponding to excision of the primary lesion a lymph node with a 6 mm macrometastasis was found (left column). This lymph node was not visualized in planar imaging nor on cross-sectional SPECT/CT (middle image), due to radioactivity remaining at the injection site. However, postoperative comparison of SPECT/CT with low-dose CT (right image) showed this real SLN in the area of the injection (circle)

Case 11.6: SLN Mapping in Frontal Melanoma with Drainage to Ipsilateral Cervical Lymph Nodes on Planar and SPECT/CT Imaging

Renato A. Valdés Olmos, Martin Klop, and Maarten Donswijk

Background Clinical Case

A 72-year-old woman with a 4 mm Breslow thick melanoma located on the right side of the frontal area was referred for SLNB after excision of the primary lesion. No lymph node abnormalities (N0 stage) had been detected on physical examination and ultrasonography of the neck.

Planar Lymphoscintigraphy and SPECT/CT Imaging

A total of 110 MBq ICG-^{99m}Tc-nanocolloid was administered in four intradermal injections around the excision scar in the left frontal region the afternoon before surgery. Immediately after tracer administration, dynamic frames were acquired during 10 min with the patient in supine position using a dual-head gamma camera (Symbia T, Siemens, Erlangen, Germany) equipped with low-energy high-resolution collimators. Subsequently, 5-min planar static images were acquired at 15 min and 2 h post-injection. Additional SPECT/CT imaging was acquired after acquiring the delayed planar images using the same gamma camera.

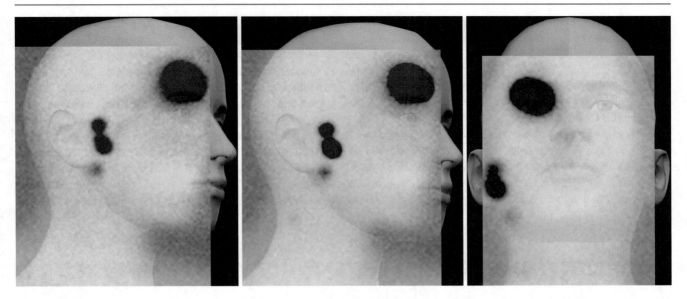

Fig. 11.23 Planar static lateral (first two frames) and anterior (third frame) images superimposed to anatomical models show unilateral drainage of ICG-^{99m}Tc-nanocolloid from the frontal injection site to cervical lymph nodes in the right preauricular area

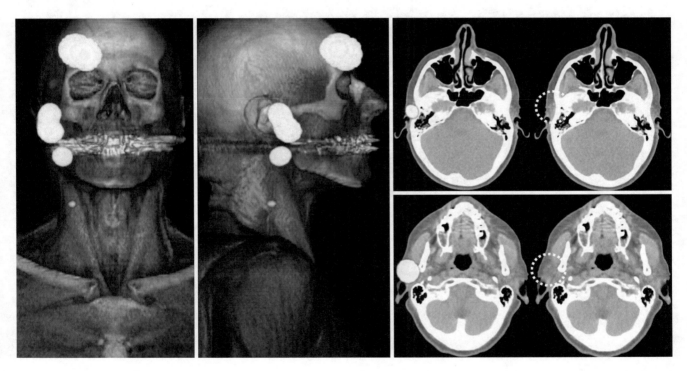

Fig. 11.24 Anterior and lateral SPECT/CT display using volume rendering (on the left) showing unilateral migration to various lymph nodes in the right preauricular area. Cross-sectional SPECT/CT on the right shows that the radioactive lymph nodes in the preauricular and superior parotid areas correspond to normal-size lymph nodes on low-dose CT (circles)

Case 11.7: SLN Mapping in Preauricular Melanoma with Drainage to Ipsilateral Cervical Lymph Nodes on Planar and SPECT/CT Imaging

Renato A. Valdés Olmos, Martin Klop, and Maarten Donswijk

Background Clinical Case

A 45-year-old man with a 3.5 mm Breslow thick melanoma located in the left preauricular area was referred for SLNB after excision of the primary lesion. No lymph node abnormalities (N0 stage) had been detected on physical examination and ultrasonography of the neck.

Planar Lymphoscintigraphy and SPECT/CT Imaging

A total of 118 MBq ICG-^{99m}Tc-nanocolloid was administered in four intradermal injections around the excision scar in the left preauricular region the afternoon before surgery. Immediately after tracer administration, dynamic frames were acquired during 10 min with the patient in supine position using a dual-head gamma camera (Symbia T, Siemens, Erlangen, Germany) equipped with low-energy high-resolution collimators. Subsequently, 5-min planar static images were acquired at 15 min and 2 h post-injection. Additional SPECT/CT imaging was acquired after acquiring the delayed planar images using the same gamma camera.

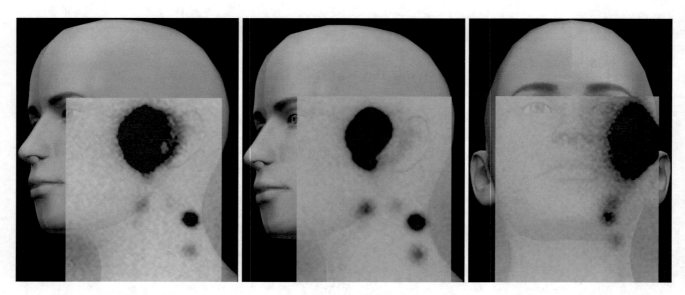

Fig. 11.25 Planar static lateral (first two frames) and delayed anterior (third frame) images superimposed to anatomical figures show unilateral drainage of ICG-^{99m}Tc-nanocolloid from the preauricular injection site to cervical lymph nodes in the right cervical area

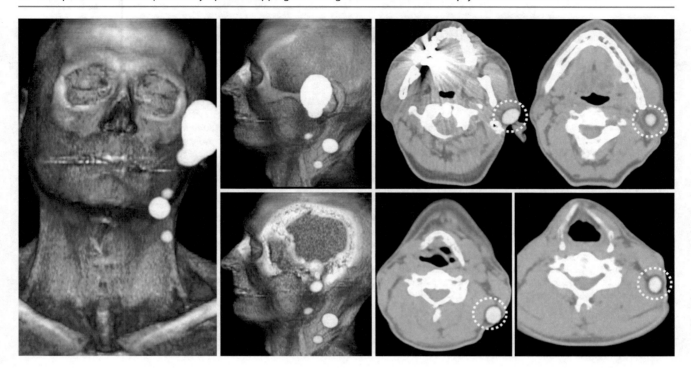

Fig. 11.26 Anterior and lateral SPECT/CT views using volume rendering (on the left) showing unilateral various radioactive lymph nodes on the left cervical side. A lymph node close to the injection site is visualized after suppression of the injection site (bottom). Cross-sectional SPECT/CT (on the right) shows the radioactive nodes in the left parotid area as well as in ipsilateral levels 2b, 5a and 3 (circles)

Acknowledgements This chapter is a revision of the original chapter written by R. A. Valdés Olmos, W. M. C. Klop and O. R. Brouwer in the previous edition of the book.

References

1. Miller MW, Vetto JT, Monroe MM, et al. False-negative sentinel lymph node biopsy in head and neck melanoma. Otolaryngol Head Neck Surg. 2011;145:606–11.
2. Klop MC, Veenstra HJ, Vermeeren L, et al. Assessment of lymphatic drainage patterns and implications for the extent of neck dissection in head and neck melanoma patients. J Surg Oncol. 2011;103:756–60.
3. de Veij Mestdagh PD, Jonker MCJ, Vogel WV, et al. SPECT/CT-guided lymph drainage mapping for the planning of unilateral elective nodal irradiation in head and neck squamous cell carcinoma. Eur Arch Otorhinolaryngol. 2018;275:2135–44.
4. Wong SL, Faries MB, Kennedy EB, et al. Sentinel lymph node biopsy and management of regional lymph nodes in melanoma: American Society of Clinical Oncology and Society of Surgical Oncology clinical practice guideline update. Ann Surg Oncol. 2018;25:356–77.
5. Gangi A, Essner R, Giuliano AE. Long-term clinical impact of sentinel lymph node in breast cancer and cutaneous melanoma. Q J Nucl Med Mol Imaging. 2014;58:95–104.
6. Eggermont AMM, Robert C, Ribas A. The new era of adjuvant therapies for melanoma. Nat Rev Clin Oncol. 2018;15:535–6.
7. Franke V, van Akkooi ACJ. The extent of surgery for stage III melanoma: how much is appropriate? Lancet Oncol. 2019;20:e167–74.
8. Lydiatt WM, Patel SG, O'Sullivan B, et al. Head and neck cancers—major changes in the American Joint Committee on Cancer eighth edition cancer staging manual. CA Cancer J Clin. 2017;67:122–37.
9. Schilling C, Stoeckli SJ, Vigili MG, et al. Surgical consensus guidelines on sentinel node biopsy (SNB) in patients with oral cancer. Head Neck. 2019;41:2655–64.
10. Giammarile F, Schilling C, Gnanasegaran G, et al. The EANM practical guidelines for sentinel lymph node localization in oral cavity squamous cell carcinoma. Eur J Nucl Med Mol Imaging. 2019;46:623–37.
11. Bluemel C, Herrmann K, Giammarile F, et al. EANM practice guidelines for lymphoscintigraphy and sentinel lymph node biopsy in melanoma. Eur J Nucl Med Mol Imaging. 2015;42:1750–66.
12. Jimenez-Hefferman A, Ellmann A, Sado H, et al. Results of a prospective multicentre International Atomic Energy Agency. Sentinel node trial on the value of SPECT/CT over planar imaging in various malignancies. J Nucl Med. 2015;56:1338–44.
13. Ananthakrishnan P, Mariani G, Moresco L, et al. The anatomy and physiology of lymphatic circulation. In: Mariani G, Giuliano AE, Strauss WH, editors. Radioguided surgery: a comprehensive team approach. New York: Springer Science; 2008. p. 57–71.
14. Robbins KT, Shaha AR, Medina JE, et al.; Committee for Neck Dissection Classification, American Head and Neck Society. Consensus statement on the classification and terminology of neck dissection. Arch Otolaryngol Head Neck Surg. 2008;134:536–538.
15. Grégoire V, Ang K, Budach W, et al. Delineation of the neck node levels for head and neck tumors: a 2013 update. DAHANCA, EORTC, HKNPCSG, NCIC CTG, NCRI, RTOG, TROG consensus guidelines. Radiother Oncol. 2014;110:172–81.

16. KleinJan GH, van Werkhoven E, van den Berg NS, et al. The best of both worlds: a hybrid approach for optimal pre- and intraoperative identification of sentinel lymph nodes. Eur J Nucl Med Mol Imaging. 2018;45:1915–25.

17. Valdés Olmos RA, Vidal-Sicart S, Manca G, et al. Advances in radioguided surgery in oncology. Q J Nucl Med Mol Imaging. 2017;61:247–70.

18. Vermeeren L, Valdés Olmos RA, Klop WM, et al. A portable gamma camera for intraoperative detection of sentinel nodes in the head and neck region. J Nucl Med. 2010;51:700–3.

19. Van den Berg NS, Brouwer OR, Schaafsma BE, et al. Multimodal surgical guidance during sentinel node biopsy for melanoma: combined gamma tracing and fluorescence imaging of the sentinel node through use of the hybrid tracer indocyanine green-^{99m}Tc-nanocolloid. Radiology. 2015;275:521–9.

20. Trinh BB, Chapman BC, Gleisner A, et al. SPECT/CT adds distinct lymph node basins and influences radiologic findings and surgical approach for sentinel lymph node biopsy in head and neck melanoma. Ann Surg Oncol. 2018;25:1716–22.

21. Chapman BC, Gleisner A, Kwak JJ, et al. SPECT/CT improves detection of metastatic sentinel lymph nodes in patients with head and neck melanoma. Ann Surg Oncol. 2016;23:2652–7.

22. Den Toom IJ, van Schie A, van Weert S, et al. The added value of SPECT/CT for the identification of sentinel lymph nodes in early stage oral cancer. Eur J Nucl Med Imaging. 2017;44:998–1004.

23. Reynolds HM, Smith NP, Uren RF, et al. Three-dimensional visualization of skin lymphatic drainage patterns of the head and neck. Head Neck. 2009;31:1316–25.

24. Calabrese L, Soutar D, Werner J, et al. Sentinel lymph node biopsy in cancer of the head and neck. In: Mariani G, Giuliano AE, Strauss WH, editors. Radioguided surgery: a comprehensive team approach. New York: Springer Science; 2008. p. 120–9.

25. Civantos FJ, Zitsch R, Bared A. Sentinel node biopsy in oral squamous cell carcinoma. J Surg Oncol. 2007;94:330–6.

26. Civantos FJ, Zitsch RP, Schuller DE, et al. Sentinel lymph node biopsy accurately stages the regional lymph nodes for T1-T2 oral squamous cell carcinomas: results of a prospective multi-institutional trial. J Clin Oncol. 2010;28:1395–400.

27. Lee DY, Huynh KT, Teng A, et al. Predictors and survival impact of false-negative sentinel nodes in melanoma. Ann Surg Oncol. 2016;23:1012–218.

28. Wu JX. Sentinel node biopsy for cancer of the oral cavity. J Surg Oncol. 2019;129:99–100.

Preoperative and Intraoperative Lymphatic Mapping for Radioguided Sentinel Node Biopsy in Non-small Cell Lung Cancer

12

Giuseppe Boni, Franca M. A. Melfi, Giampiero Manca, Federico Davini, and Giuliano Mariani

Contents

12.1   **Introduction**... 291

12.2   **The Clinical Problem**.. 292

12.3   **Indications for SLNB in NSCLC**................................ 292

12.4   **SLN Mapping Techniques in NSCLC**........................ 293

12.5   **Preoperative SLN Imaging**.. 294

12.6   **Intraoperative SLN Detection**................................... 295

12.7   **Accuracy and Perspectives of Radioguided SLNB in NSCLC**................................ 296

References.. 297

Learning Objectives

- To acquire basic knowledge on the role of lymph node staging in non-small cell lung cancer, including the benefits and risks of de novo systematic mediastinal lymph node dissection
- To acquire basic knowledge on the role of nuclear medicine imaging for sentinel lymph node (SLN) mapping in non-small cell lung cancer
- To acquire basic knowledge on the feasibility and techniques of radioguided SLN mapping in non-small cell lung cancer
- To acquire basic knowledge on the role of SLN mapping using non-radionuclide techniques in non-small cell lung cancer
- To understand the current limitations and perspectives for SLN mapping in patients with non-small cell lung cancer

G. Boni (✉) · G. Manca
Regional Center of Nuclear Medicine, University Hospital of Pisa, Pisa, Italy
e-mail: g.boni@ao-pisa.toscana.it

F. M. A. Melfi · F. Davini
Division of Thoracic Surgery, University Hospital of Pisa, Pisa, Italy

G. Mariani
Regional Center of Nuclear Medicine, Department of Translational Research and Advanced Technologies in Medicine and Surgery, University of Pisa, Pisa, Italy

12.1 Introduction

Non-small cell lung cancer (NSCLC) is the most common malignancy in the world and the major cause of cancer-related death [1]. It represents 85% of all lung cancers and usually grows and spreads at distant sites more slowly than small-cell lung cancer. Despite advances in surgery, chemotherapy, and radiation therapy over the last decades, the death rate from NSCLC has remained largely unchanged. Such poor long-term survival probably results from the fact that early-stage disease is asymptomatic and the onset of symptoms marks the presence of advanced, inoperable disease.

The presence or absence of mediastinal lymph node metastasis is a key prognostic factor in NSCLC, and lymph node dissection is an effective therapeutic procedure when carried out in patients with nodal metastasis [2, 3].

The procedure of SLN mapping has been developed in recent years and validated in a variety of solid epithelial tumors as a way to avoid the complications associated with systematic de novo lymph node dissection; the validity of sentinel lymph node biopsy (SLNB) is now well established mainly in patients with breast cancer and melanoma, as well as head and neck cancers (oral squamous cell carcinoma), penile cancer, and some gynecological malignancies. The SLNB procedure has more recently been explored also in patients with NSCLC [4–7].

12.2 The Clinical Problem

Mediastinal lymph node staging is one of the most important prognostic factors for patients with operable non-small cell lung cancers. In fact, the presence of lymph node involvement decreases the 5-year survival rate by nearly 50% as compared to similar patients without nodal metastasis [8].

Furthermore, many investigators have clearly demonstrated that more careful histopathologic evaluation of previously reported negative lymph nodes in resected lung cancer patients revealed that over 20% of patients classified as having negative lymph nodes (N0) at conventional hematoxylin and eosin staining were actually upstaged by immunohistochemistry (IHC), a procedure that is capable of identifying previously undetected micrometastatic disease [9, 10].

Preoperative staging modalities include imaging techniques (standard chest X-ray, high-resolution contrast CT, [^{18}F]FDG PET/CT, MRI, bone scan). If these tests do not reveal the presence of distant metastatic disease or unresectable local disease, then further invasive staging procedures (including bronchoscopy, mediastinoscopy, video-assisted thoracoscopic surgery, VATS) may be necessary. Moreover, invasive N-staging modalities such as complete thoracic lymphadenectomy or nodal sampling by either VATS or robotic-assisted thoracic surgery (RATS) may help to further stratify patients into appropriate therapeutic and prognostic categories.

The choice between de novo systematic mediastinal lymph node dissection and selective lymph node sampling for the staging and treatment of NSCLC is the subject of ongoing debate. Advocates of complete lymphadenectomy believe that residual cancer may remain if complete resection of nodal tissue is not performed, leading to poorer prognosis due to locoregional recurrence and to understaging of disease [11, 12]. Conversely, proponents of lymph node sampling argue that, contrary to complete lymphadenectomy, sampling does not impair the local immune response, which may reduce the potential for local recurrence; moreover, the more limited sampling procedure is not associated with increased morbidity such as increased perioperative

blood loss, recurrent nerve injury, chylothorax, or bronchopleural fistula [13]. To date, neither survival advantage nor significant differences in morbidity or mortality rates have been clearly demonstrated using either surgical procedures [14, 15].

If the prognosis of NSCLC is not affected by complete mediastinal lymph node dissection, then it can be argued that morbidity of selective mediastinal lymph node sampling and histopathologic staging of lung cancer can be improved by SLN mapping [16]. This procedure allows to detect occult micrometastatic disease in SLNs by sensitive immunohistochemistry (IHC) and/or molecular biology analysis based on the reverse transcription polymerase chain reaction (RT-PCR), thus avoiding extensive serial sectioning and IHC of all dissected lymph nodes [17, 18].

A reliable, minimally invasive lymphatic mapping procedure could improve staging and outcomes for the patients with early-stage non-small cell lung cancer, such as those identified on low-dose CT screening [19].

Key Learning Points

- Staging of mediastinal lymph nodes in non-small cell lung cancer is one of the most important prognostic factors, as the presence of metastasis decreases overall survival by nearly 50% versus nonmetastatic lymph nodes.
- A sensitive staining technique such as immunohistochemistry upstages over 20% of patients who had been classified as metastasis free at conventional hematoxylin and eosin staining.
- Preoperative staging of lymph node status by current imaging techniques is not sensitive enough to exclude with certainty the presence of metastasis in mediastinal lymph nodes.
- Current surgical protocols in patients with operable non-small cell lung cancer include either de novo systematic dissection of mediastinal lymph nodes or lymph node sampling, each of the two protocols having relative advantages and limitations.
- A reliable, minimally invasive lymphatic mapping procedure could improve staging and outcomes for the patients with early-stage non-small cell lung cancer.

12.3 Indications for SLNB in NSCLC

Patients with cT1N0M0 NSCLC are the best candidates for SLNB. The recent widespread diffusion of high-resolution computed tomography (HRCT) has resulted in the more frequent detection of this subset of NSCLC patients, in whom limited mediastinal lymph node dissection and/or segmentectomy could be as curative as lobectomy with mediastinal lymph node dissection.

12.4 SLN Mapping Techniques in NSCLC

12.4.1 Non-radionuclide Methods

Several techniques using non-radionuclide tracers for SLN mapping in patients with NSCLC have been proposed [20–22]. The first SLN mapping procedure in patients with NSCLC was performed using intratumoral injection of isosulfan blue [20]. Unfortunately, since it was difficult to detect the blue dye migrating to the anthracotic lymph nodes in the thoracic cavity, the identification rate of the SLN was too low to be clinically useful. Similar problems were encountered in the past with other dyes, such as indocyanine green (ICG) [21].

Japanese authors from a single institution have developed a novel method for SLN mapping based on the use of magnetic particles [22, 23]. In particular, colloidal ferumoxides (a superparamagnetic iron) were injected during thoracotomy at the periphery of the tumor. A highly sensitive, handheld magnetometer was then used to detect ex vivo the presence of the ferumoxides within SLNs. The in vivo SLN detection rate was 80%, and more recent results confirm the feasibility and efficacy of this technique, with 97.6% accuracy, 75% sensitivity, and false-negative rates ranging between 2.3% and 13.2% for SLN mapping in patients with NSCLC. Furthermore, Minamiva et al. have proposed to combine subpleural tracer injection with injection in the peritumoral quadrants, in order to improve identification rate and diagnostic accuracy for mediastinal SLNs [24].

More recently, the use of fluorescent-labeled agents, such as ICG, has been explored further for SLN mapping in patients with NSCLC [25–29]. This procedure provides real-time visual mapping using near-infrared (NIR) imaging of fluorescent lymphatic tracers; ICG is injected peritumorally during surgery, and its migration through lymphatic pathways is visualized using cameras based on indium gallium arsenide (InGaAs) sensors. The underlying physical principle is that, when excited with a ~780 nm laser source, ICG (as well as other fluorophores) emits light with wavelengths of 700–1000 nm that can be represented in a grayscale or color image visualizing the NIR signal in green within a thoracoscopic or robotic camera.

With the ICG-NIR technique, SLNs were identified and dissected in over 80% of the cases [25–29]. Higher rates of SLN detection were identified when ICG was mixed with a higher molecular weight carrier, such as human serum albumin (HSA) [30].

The feasibility of preoperative CT lymphography for lymphatic mapping in non-small cell lung cancer was also tested [31–35]. Peritumoral CT-guided transpleural or transbronchial injection of a water-soluble contrast agent (iopamidol or iohexol) was performed followed by serial CT images for up to 5 min after injection. SLNs were detected as nodes with increased attenuation by 30 Hounsfield units when the CT images obtained after the peritumoral injection of the contrast medium were compared to the baseline CT scan. The anatomical location of the SLNs (with respect to bronchial anatomy) was also identified by 3D reconstructions of multidetector CT scanning [31–35].

A SLN identification rate >90% has been demonstrated using this technique in these preliminary trials, conducted in a limited number of subjects. Potential pitfalls may be the identification of very small SLNs (size less than 2–3 mm) and possible artifacts or confounding effects due to the presence of lymph node calcification [31–35].

With the increasing availability of hybrid operating rooms, CT lymphography could become a diagnostic tool for improving the accuracy of preoperative mapping N2 level SLNs prior to definitive resection of a lung cancer.

> **Key Learning Points**
> - SLN mapping based on intraoperative visual guidance following intratumoral injection of isosulfan blue is not reliable in the presence of anthracotic lymph nodes.
> - Novel methods based on the use of a handheld magnetometer to detect migration to lymph nodes of ferumoxides injected peritumorally during thoracotomy have been proposed.
> - Intraoperative SLN mapping based on near-infrared imaging after injection of the fluorescent lymphatic indocyanine green is a promising novel technique.
> - Preoperative CT lymphography for lymphatic mapping after peritumoral injection of an iodinated contrast medium is also feasible in patients with non-small cell lung cancer.

12.4.2 Radiocolloids and Modalities of Injection

After the pioneering work by Liptay and colleagues in 2000, several articles have been published on the feasibility, technical aspects, and efficacy of radioguided SLNB in the surgical management of patients with NSCLC [6, 7, 35–51]. ^{99m}Tc-tin colloid, ^{99m}Tc-sulfur colloid, ^{99m}Tc-nanocolloidal human albumin, and more recently ^{99m}Tc-neomannosylated human serum albumin (MSA) have been used for radioguided SLNB in NSCLC patients [52]. The total activity administered varies from 9.25 MBq to 296 MBq, which is injected in a total volume of 0.5–2 mL.

Neomannosylated human serum albumin particles labeled with [68]Ga (^{68}Ga-MSA) have also been synthesized and used for SLN imaging by PET/CT lymphoscintigraphy in NSCLC patients [53, 54]. The activity administered through a single peritumoral injection of ^{68}Ga-MSA ranged from 6 to 122 MBq.

Three different modalities of injection of the radiocolloids have been described. Liptay et al. have advocated intraoperative radiocolloid injection into or around the primary tumor after direct visualization of the lesion, injecting the radiocolloid in a four-quadrant peritumoral fashion at the time of thoracotomy [7]. An average waiting period of 30–60 min after the injection is necessary for radiocolloid migration into the lymphatic vessels and to the SLN basin. During this time, the operation proceeds normally, taking care to avoid the peribronchial lymphatic vessels until the last phase of the resection. Some disadvantages of this modality of injection are the long intraoperative time whilst waiting for radiocolloid migration, the possible contamination of the pleural cavity after the injection, and the accumulation of the radiocolloid in the trachea, due to the absence of coughing in the anesthetized patient. Scintigraphic imaging of lymphatic drainage is virtually impossible when the procedure is based on such intraoperative radiocolloid administration.

A second modality is preoperative injection of radiocolloid into or around the primary tumor under CT guidance on the day of surgery or on the day before [6, 36].

Lymphoscintigraphy can be performed preoperatively, and the main advantage of the preoperative injection technique is that it enables intraoperative measurement of count rates in the upper mediastinal lymph node, because coughing of the patient rapidly removes radiocolloid accumulated in the trachea.

A useful alternative to CT-guided injection of the radiocolloid seems to be preoperative endobronchial injection of the radiocolloid into the directly visualized endobronchial tumor, or transbronchially at the most distal pulmonary sub-segment that can be reached endobronchially within the proximity of the primary tumor [37].

> **Key Learning Points**
> - The most widely adopted technique based on radioguidance for SLN mapping in patients with non-small cell lung cancer involves intra-tumoral or peritumoral injection of a ^{99m}Tc-labeled lymphotropic agent.
> - A more recent technique is based on preoperative PET/CT imaging after peritumoral injection of neo-
> mannosylated human serum albumin particles labeled with [68]Ga (^{68}Ga-MSA).
> - Different modalities for the injection of radiolabeled lymphatic mapping agents have been described, mostly performed during surgery.
> - The need to administer the lymphatic mapping agent during surgery precludes in most instances the possibility to acquire lymphoscintigraphic images preoperatively.

12.5 Preoperative SLN Imaging

The feasibility of preoperative SLN imaging in NSCLC has been tested by Nomori et al. [6]. On the same day or on the day before surgery, 111–296 MBq of ^{99m}Tc-tin colloid in a volume of 1–1.5 mL is injected with a single shot through a transthoracic 23-gauge needle inserted into the peritumoral region. In order to determine the optimal timing for radiocolloid injection before surgery, in a subset of patients the authors acquired planar scintigraphic images at 5 min, and then at 1, 6, 9, and 24 h after the injection. Based on this preliminary protocol, the authors then performed routine lymphoscintigraphy by acquiring planar images of the chest 5 min after the injection, and then immediately before surgery.

The early planar images usually visualize radioactivity accumulation at the site of injection and in the tracheobronchial lumen, due to physiological leakage. After about 1 h, washout of the radiocolloid from the tracheobronchial tree is observed, but migration to mediastinal lymph nodes is not yet visualized. More than 6 h after the injection, sufficient radiocolloid has been taken up by the lymph nodes, with a virtually unchanged pattern until 24 h post-administration (Fig. 12.1).

More recently, a new method for in vivo SLN detection in NSCLC by PET/CT imaging was developed and evaluated in 34 patients by Eo et al. [54]. ^{68}Ga-MSA was administered in one peritumoral injection under CT guidance approximately 1–3 h before surgery. PET/CT scanning started 15–30 min after injection and images were acquired for 10 min covering the chest volume. The distribution of the dissected lymph nodes, and lymph node metastases according to the tumor location, was compared with the PET/CT findings. A preliminary evaluation of the time course distribution of ^{68}Ga-MSA in vivo by sequential PET/CT scans showed that SLNs were well visualized between 15 and 120 min after injection, the highest tracer accumulation being observed within 60 min. The PET/CT images clearly visualize focal radioactivity at the site of injection as well as in the SLNs, and in some cases in the tracheobronchial lumen—due to physiological leakage. Furthermore, SLNs were well visualized in either metastasis-negative or

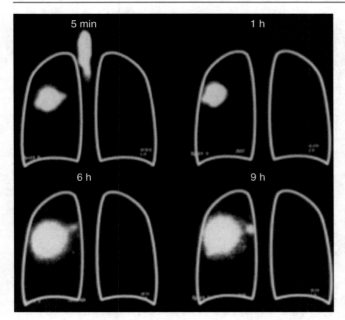

Fig. 12.1 Planar lymphoscintigraphic images acquired sequentially after injection of ^{99m}Tc-tin colloid for SLN mapping in a patient with NSCLC. The early image shows important accumulation of radioactivity at the injection site and in the trachea; the latter is cleared already at the 1-h imaging point. Migration of the radiocolloid is barely detectable at 1 h postinjection, becoming however more clear at the later imaging time points (6 h and 9 h postinjection) (reproduced with permission from Nomori H, Horio H, Naruke T, et al. Use of technetium-99m tin colloid for SLN identification in non-small cell lung cancer. J Thorac Cardiovasc Surg. 2002;124:486–492)

metastasis-positive cases (Fig. 12.2). In this initial report, SLNs were detected in vivo by PET/TC in all the studied patients. Metastatic SLNs were found in 23.5% of the patients, with no false-negative SLNs being found in patients with N1 or N2 disease [54].

Key Learning Point
- When the radiolabeled lymphatic mapping agent can be injected preoperatively under CT guidance or trans-bronchially in the nuclear medicine department, then lymphoscintigraphic imaging is feasible, by using either a gamma camera (when a ^{99m}Tc-labeled agent is employed) or a PECT/CT scanner (when the novel ^{68}Ga-MSA agent is employed).

12.6 Intraoperative SLN Detection

Intraoperative SLN detection is usually guided by a hand-held gamma-detecting probe, which can be a standard gamma probe if used during open thoracotomy. Instead, dedicated, small-diameter gamma probes must be used during VATS or RATS. During the operation radioactivity in the lymph nodes is counted before (in vivo) and after (ex vivo) dissection.

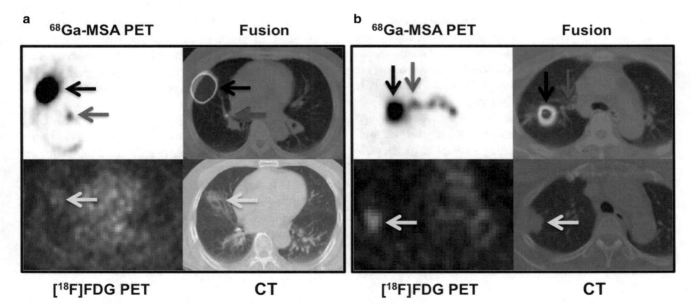

Fig. 12.2 ^{68}Ga-MSA lymphoscintigraphic PET/CT in patients with metastasis-negative (**a**) and metastasis-positive (**b**) SLN imaging. The peritumor injection site (black arrow) and SLN activity (red arrow) are shown. Tumor uptake was observed on [^{18}FDG]PET/CT (yellow arrow)

(modified from Eo JS, Kim HK, Kim S, et al. Gallium-68 neomannosylated human serum albumin-based PET/CT lymphoscintigraphy for SLN mapping in non-small cell lung cancer. Ann Surg Oncol. 2015;22:636–41)

Fig. 12.3 SLN mapping of the lung with NIR quantum dots (QD) in an animal model (adult Yorkshire pigs). Color video (left), NIR fluorescence (middle), and color-NIR merge (right) are presented. The SLN (arrow) was identified 45 s after QD injection into the right upper lobe of the lung (arrowhead) (reproduced with permission from Soltesz EG, Kim S, Laurence RG, et al. Intraoperative SLN mapping of the lung using near-infrared fluorescent quantum dots. Ann Thorac Surg. 2005;79:269–277)

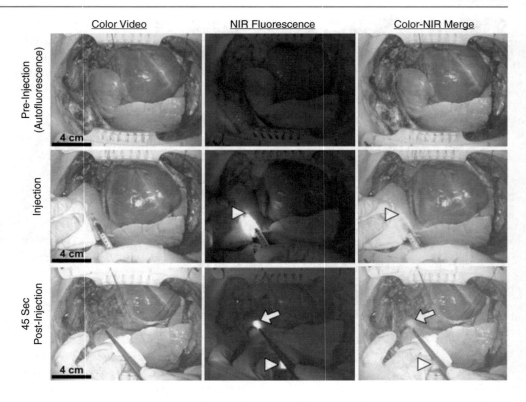

For in vivo counting, SLNs are usually identified as any lymph node with a count rate three- to tenfold higher than a preset intrathoracic background value. For ex vivo counting, the SLNs are usually defined in a similar fashion, as any lymph node with a count rate three- to tenfold the count rate of the resected lung tissue with the lowest count. The ex vivo "hot" lymph node(s) are considered to be the true SLNs, because in this condition the radioactivity measurements are not influenced by the "shine-through" effect of radioactivity retained at the site of injection [40, 42].

In case of mediastinal dissection, after lobectomy and SLN excision the mediastinal stations are also explored with the gamma probe before performing a complete lymph node dissection. Upon completion of the procedure, exploration with the gamma probe is repeated, checking for any residual activity. If indicated by high count rates, resection of the nodal stations is completed.

> **Key Learning Points**
> - Dedicated gamma-detecting probes are used during surgery for SLN detection.
> - Both in vivo and ex vivo count rates are recorded for each radioactive lymph node.
> - Gamma probe counting of the surgical field after mediastinal lymph node dissection helps to assess completeness of lymph node dissection.

12.7 Accuracy and Perspectives of Radioguided SLNB in NSCLC

In all series reporting more than 200 patients undergoing radioguided SLNB for NSCLC [40, 42, 45, 51], a SLN was identified in 70–100% of the patients, with false-negative rates generally reported as 10% or lower. However, it should be noted that a multicenter phase 2 trial investigating the use of ^{99m}Tc-tin colloid for SLNB reported an identification rate as low as 51% only [55].

A promising, relatively simple and reliable method for SLN mapping in NSCLC is the new intraoperative instrumentation that uses the invisible near-infrared (NIR) fluorescent light of ICG for imaging in vivo the lymphatic drainage and the SLNs (Fig. 12.3). This technique has been validated in human trials carried out in breast and gastric cancers, as well in patients with gynecological malignancies or with prostate cancer.

Recent data obtained in NSCLC patients shows that intraoperative NIR SLN mapping is feasible with a high detection rate (80–89%), a very low false-negative rate, and a significant percentage of patients upstaged based on the SLN mapping procedure [56].

In a report reviewing the long-term outcomes after NIR-guided SLN mapping with peritumoral ICG injection, Digesu et al. compared patients who underwent mediastinal lymph node sampling with or without SLN mapping [57]. An improved estimated overall and disease-free survival was observed in the group of patients who underwent SLN mapping who were found not to have metastatic lymph node disease at histopathology (pN0) [57].

Concerning the detection of micrometastatic involvement of mediastinal lymph nodes by RT-PCR or IHC, similar results have been obtained for SLNB with different techniques versus analysis of all metastasis-positive lymph nodes [16–18]. These reports also suggest that micrometastasis is limited to SLNs in early NSCLC, but tends to spread to lymph nodes other than the SLNs with the progression of metastasis.

In conclusion, SLNB is an effective procedure that may allow reduction in the number of lymph nodes to be examined for micrometastasis and selection of patients with micrometastatic mediastinal lymph node involvement who could benefit by postoperative adjunctive therapy. Since most of the studies published so far have adopted direct intra- or peritumoral injection of the radiocolloid in the operating theatre at the time of thoracotomy, this procedure basically precludes the possibility of imaging with large-field-of-view gamma cameras. New perspectives in this regard can be opened by the use of dedicated small-field-of-view cameras to be used also in the intraoperative setting.

Key Learning Points
- Radioguided SLNB for non-small cell lung cancer has 70–100% sensitivity and false-negative rates generally lower than 10% in studies that have reported more than 200 patients.
- SLN mapping using near-infrared imaging based on the use of indocyanine green is also characterized by satisfactory detection rates (80–89%) and very low false-negative rates.
- Analysis of the resected SLNs with sensitive techniques such as immunohistochemistry and molecular analysis with RT-PCR allows detection of micrometastases, an important parameter for therapy planning in patients with non-small cell lung cancer.

References

1. Bray F, Ferlay J, Soerjomataram I, et al. Global cancer statistics 2018: GLOBOCAN estimates of incidence and mortality worldwide for 36 cancers in 185 countries. CA Cancer J Clin. 2018;68:394–424.
2. Keller SM, Adak S, Wagner H, et al. Mediastinal lymph node dissection improves survival in patients with stages II and IIIa non-small cell lung cancer. Eastern Cooperative Oncology Group. Ann Thorac Surg. 2000;70:358–65.
3. Naruke T, Goya T, Tsuchiya R, et al. The importance of surgery to non-small cell carcinoma of lung with mediastinal lymph node metastasis. Ann Thorac Surg. 1988;46:603–10.
4. Shen J, Wallace AM, Bouvet M. The role of sentinel lymph node biopsy for melanoma. Semin Oncol. 2002;29:341–52.
5. Petrek JA, Senie RT, Peters M, et al. Lymphedema in a cohort of breast carcinoma survivors 20 years after diagnosis. Cancer. 2001;92:1368–77.
6. Nomori H, Horio H, Naruke T, et al. Use of technetium-99m tin colloid for sentinel lymph node identification in non-small cell lung cancer. J Thorac Cardiovasc Surg. 2002;124:486–92.
7. Liptay MJ, Grondin SC, Fry WA, et al. Intraoperative sentinel lymph node mapping in non-small-cell lung cancer improves detection of micrometastases. J Clin Oncol. 2002;20:1984–8.
8. Mountain CF, Dresler CM. Regional lymph node classification for lung cancer staging. Chest. 1997;111:1718–23.
9. Kubuschock B, Passlick B, Izbicki JR, et al. Disseminated tumor cells in lymph nodes as a determinant for survival in surgically resected non-small cell lung cancer. J Clin Oncol. 1999;17:19–24.
10. Riquet M, Manac'h D, Pimpec-Barthes F, et al. Prognostic significance of surgical-pathologic N1 disease in non-small cell carcinoma of the lung. Ann Thorac Surg. 1999;67:1572–6.
11. Passlick B, Kubuschock B, Sienel W, et al. Mediastinal lymphadenectomy in non-small cell lung cancer: effectiveness in patients with or without nodal micrometastases—results of a preliminary study. Eur J Cardiothorac Surg. 2002;21:520–6.
12. Naruke T, Tsuchiya R, Kondo H, et al. Lymph node sampling in lung cancer: how should it be done? Eur J Cardiothorac Surg. 1999;16:17–24.
13. Izbicki JR, Thetter O, Habekost M, et al. Radical systematic mediastinal lymphadenectomy in non-small cell lung cancer: a randomized controlled trial. Br J Surg. 1994;81:229–35.
14. Allen MS, Darling G, Pechet T, et al. Morbidity and mortality of major pulmonary resection in patients with early stage lung cancer initial results of the randomized, prospective ACOSOG Z0030 trial. Ann Thorac Surg. 2006;81:1013–9.
15. Mokhlesa S, Macbethb F, Tom Treasurec T, et al. Systematic lymphadenectomy versus sampling of ipsilateral mediastinal lymph-nodes during lobectomy for non-small-cell lung cancer: a systematic review of randomized trials and a meta-analysis. Eur J Cardiothorac Surg. 2017;51:1149–56.
16. Li SH, Wang Z, Liu XY, et al. Gene diagnosis and prognostic significance of lymph node micrometastasis after complete resection of histologically node-negative non-small cell lung cancer. World J Surg. 2008;32:1651–6.
17. Tezel C, Ersev AA, Kiral H, et al. The impact of immunohistochemical detection of positive lymph nodes in early stage lung cancer. Thorac Cardiovasc Surg. 2006;54:124–8.
18. Nosotti M, Falleni M, Palleschi A, et al. Quantitative real-time polymerase chain reaction detection of lymph node lung cancer micrometastasis using carcinoembryonic antigen marker. Chest. 2005;128:1539–44.
19. Church TR, Black WC, Aberle DR, et al. Results of initial low-dose computed tomographic screening for lung cancer. N Engl J Med. 2013;368:1980–91.
20. Little AG, DeHoyos A, Kirgan DM, et al. Intraoperative lymphatic mapping for non-small cell lung cancer: the sentinel node technique. J Thorac Cardiovasc Surg. 1999;117:220–34.
21. Sugi K, Fukuda M, Nakamura H, et al. Comparison of three tracers for detecting sentinel lymph nodes in patients with clinical N0 lung cancer. Lung Cancer. 2003;39:37–40.
22. Nakagawa T, Minamiya Y, Katayose Y, et al. A novel method for sentinel lymph node mapping using magnetite in patients with non-small cell lung cancer. J Thorac Cardiovasc Surg. 2003;126:563–7.
23. Sugi K, Kobayashi S, Yagi R, et al. Sentinel node mapping and micrometastasis in patients with clinical stage IA non-small cell lung cancer. Interact Cardiovasc Thorac Surg. 2008;7:913–5.

24. Minamiya Y, Ito M, Hosono Y, et al. Subpleural injection of tracer improves detection of mediastinal sentinel lymph nodes in non-small cell lung cancer. Eur J Cardiothorac Surg. 2007;32:770–5.

25. Khullar O, Frangioni JV, Colson Y. Image-guided sentinel lymph node mapping and nanotechnology-based nodal treatment in lung cancer using invisible near-infrared fluorescent light. Semin Thorac Cardiovasc Surg. 2009;21:309–15.

26. Gilmore DM, Khullar OV, Jaklitsch MT, et al. Identification of metastatic nodal disease in a phase 1 dose-escalation trial of intraoperative sentinel lymph node mapping in non-small cell lung cancer using near-infrared imaging. J Thorac Cardiovasc Surg. 2013;146:562–70.

27. Yamashita S, Tokuishi K, Anami K, et al. Video-assisted thoracoscopic indocyanine green fluorescence imaging system shows sentinel lymph nodes in non-small cell lung cancer. J Thorac Cardiovasc Surg. 2011;141:141–3.

28. Yamashita S, Tokuishi K, Miyawaki M, et al. Sentinel node navigation surgery by thoracoscopic fluorescence imaging system and molecular examination in non-small cell lung cancer. Ann Surg Oncol. 2012;19:728–33.

29. Moroga T, Yamashita S, Tokuishi K, et al. Thoracoscopic segmentectomy with intraoperative evaluation of sentinel nodes for stage I non-small cell lung cancer. Ann Thorac Cardiovasc Surg. 2012;18:89–94.

30. Ohnishi S, Lomnes SJ, Laurence RG, et al. Organic alternatives to quantum dots for intraoperative near-infrared fluorescent sentinel lymph node mapping. Mol Imaging. 2005;4:172–81.

31. Suga K, Yuan Y, Ueda K, et al. Computed tomography lymphography with intrapulmonary injection of iopamidol for sentinel lymph node localization. Invest Radiol. 2004;39:313–24.

32. Ueda K, Suga K, Kaneda Y, et al. Preoperative imaging of the lung sentinel lymphatic basin with computed tomographic lymphography: a preliminary study. Ann Thorac Surg. 2004;77:1033–8.

33. Sugi K, Kitada K, Yoshino M, et al. New method of visualizing lymphatics in lung cancer patients by multidetector computed tomography. J Comput Assist Tomogr. 2005;29:210–4.

34. Takizawa H, Kondo K, Toba H, et al. Computed tomography lymphography by transbronchial injection of iopamidol to identify sentinel nodes in preoperative patients with non-small cell lung cancer: a pilot study. J Thorac Cardiovasc Surg. 2012;144:94–9.

35. Schmidt FE, Woltering EA, Webb WR, et al. Sentinel nodal assessment in patients with carcinoma of the lung. Ann Thorac Surg. 2002;74:870–4.

36. Melfi FM, Chella A, Menconi GF, et al. Intraoperative radioguided sentinel lymph node biopsy in non-small cell lung cancer. Eur J Cardiothorac Surg. 2003;23:214–20.

37. Lardinois D, Brack T, Gaspert A, et al. Bronchoscopic radioisotope injection for sentinel lymph-node mapping in potentially resectable non-small-cell lung cancer. Eur J Cardiothorac Surg. 2003;23:824–7.

38. Sugi K, Kaneda Y, Sudoh M, et al. Effect of radioisotope sentinel node mapping in patients with cT1 N0 M0 lung cancer. J Thorac Cardiovasc Surg. 2003;126:568–73.

39. Sugi K, Kitada K, Murakami T, et al. Sentinel node biopsy for staging of small peripheral lung cancer. Kyobu Geka. 2004;57:14–7.

40. Liptay MJ. Sentinel node mapping in lung cancer. Ann Surg Oncol. 2004;11:271S–4S.

41. Ueda K, Suga K, Kaneda Y, et al. Radioisotope lymph node mapping in nonsmall cell lung cancer: can it be applicable for sentinel node biopsy? Ann Thorac Surg. 2004;77:426–30.

42. Nomori H, Watanabe K, Ohtsuka T, et al. In vivo identification of sentinel lymph nodes for clinical stage I non-small cell lung cancer for abbreviation of mediastinal lymph node dissection. Lung Cancer. 2004;46:49–55.

43. Tiffet O, Nicholson AG, Khaddage A, et al. Feasibility of the detection of the sentinel lymph node in peripheral non-small cell lung cancer with radioisotopic and blue dye techniques. Chest. 2005;127:443–8.

44. Atinkaya C, Ozlem Küçük N, Koparal H, et al. Mediastinal intraoperative radioisotope sentinel lymph node mapping in non-small-cell lung cancer. Nucl Med Commun. 2005;26:717–20.

45. Rzyman W, Hagen OM, Dziadziuszko R, et al. Intraoperative, radio-guided sentinel lymph node mapping in 110 nonsmall cell lung cancer patients. Ann Thorac Surg. 2006;82:237–42.

46. Nomori H, Ikeda K, Mori T, et al. Sentinel node navigation segmentectomy for clinical stage IA non-small cell lung cancer. J Thorac Cardiovasc Surg. 2007;133:780–5.

47. Nomori H, Ikeda K, Mori T, et al. Sentinel node identification in clinical stage Ia non-small cell lung cancer by a combined single photon emission computed tomography/computed tomography system. J Thorac Cardiovasc Surg. 2007;134:182–7.

48. Meyer A, Cheng C, Antonescu C, et al. Successful migration of three tracers without identification of sentinel nodes during intraoperative lymphatic mapping for non-small cell lung cancer. Interact Cardiovasc Thorac Surg. 2007;6:214–8.

49. Di Lieto E, Gallo G, Scarpati VD, et al. Lymph node sentinel detection in lung resection for non-small cell lung cancer: our experience. Recent Prog Med. 2007;98:327–8.

50. Melfi FM, Lucchi M, Davini F, et al. Intraoperative sentinel lymph node mapping in stage I non-small cell lung cancer: detection of micrometastases by polymerase chain reaction. Eur J Cardiothorac Surg. 2008;34:181–6.

51. Sugi K, Kobayashi S, Yagi R, et al. Usefulness of sentinel lymph node biopsy for the detection of lymph node micrometastasis in early lung cancer. Interact Cardiovasc Thorac Surg. 2008;7:913–5.

52. Kim S, Kim HK, Kang D-Y, et al. Intra-operative sentinel lymph node identification using a novel receptor-binding agent (technetium-99m-neomannosyl human serum albumin, ^{99m}Tc-MSA) in stage I non-small cell lung cancer. Eur J Cardiothorac Surg. 2010;37:1450–6.

53. Choi JY, Jeong JM, Yoo BC, et al. Development of ^{68}Ga-labeled mannosylated human serum albumin (MSA) as a lymph node imaging agent for positron emission tomography. Nucl Med Biol. 2011;38:371–9.

54. Eo JS, Kim HK, Kim S, et al. Gallium-68-neomannosylated human serum albumin-based PET/CT lymphoscintigraphy for sentinel lymph node mapping in non-small cell lung cancer. Ann Surg Oncol. 2015;22:636–41.

55. Liptay MJ, D'amico TA, Nwogu C, et al. Intraoperative sentinel node mapping with technetium-99m in lung cancer: results of CALGB 140203 multicenter phase II trial. J Thorac Oncol. 2009;4:198–202.

56. Hachey KJ, Digesu CS, Armstrong KW, et al. A novel technique for tumor localization and targeted lymphatic mapping in early-stage lung cancer. J Thorac Cardiovasc Surg. 2017;154:1110–8.

57. Digesu CS, Hachey KJ, Gilmore DM, et al. Long-term outcomes after near-infrared sentinel lymph node mapping in non-small cell lung cancer. J Thorac Cardiovasc Surg. 2018;155:1280–91.

Preoperative and Intraoperative Lymphatic Mapping for Sentinel Node Biopsy in Cancers of the Gastrointestinal Tract

13

Carmen Balagué and Irene Gomez

Contents

13.1   **Introduction** 299

13.2   **SLN Mapping in Esophagogastric Cancer** 300

13.3   **SLN Mapping in Colon Cancer** 303

Clinical Cases 309

References 313

Learning Objectives
- To explain the criteria for application of sentinel lymph node (SLN) detection in cancers of the gastrointestinal tract, particularly gastric and colon cancer
- To discuss the technical approach for SLN detection by intraoperative dye injection in gastric and colon cancer
- To describe the technical approach for SLN detection by endoscopic preoperative injection of a radiocolloid in gastric and colon cancer
- To compare the advantages of using the two methods (radiocolloid and dye) simultaneously

13.1 Introduction

Accurate evaluation of lymph node status is a basic requisite to predict the clinical outcome of gastrointestinal (GI) tumors and SLN mapping has become highly feasible and accurate in staging these cancers [1]. SLN identification while per-

forming surgery in patients with gastric and colorectal cancer not only has shown to be technically feasible [2], but can also identify and characterize cases with aberrant/unexpected lymphatic drainage from the primary lesion.

The increasing application of laparoscopic surgical procedures has significantly influenced GI surgery. Preliminary results indicate that SLN detection is also a valid technique to identify micrometastasis in lymph nodes during laparoscopic surgery, and can thus become an important component of minimally invasive treatment of early GI tumors. Furthermore, the combination of radiotracer and vital dye staining optimizes SLN identification. SPECT/CT imaging, as well as intraoperative imaging with dedicated gamma cameras, allows better SLN detection than planar imaging with conventional gamma cameras.

Over the last years, near-infrared (NIR) fluorescence imaging has been used to detect lymph nodes, with very good acceptance. For intraoperative purposes, the advantage of NIR light (700–900 nm) is its ability to penetrate deeper into tissue, up to 10 mm [3]. However, it requires a NIR fluorescent agent (i.e., fluorophore) combined with an imaging system that is able to both excite and detect the fluorophore. The most commonly used fluorophore is indocyanine green (ICG), approved for clinical use by the Food and Drug Administration and the European Medicines Agency. ICG is a water-soluble amphiphilic molecule with a molecular weight of 775 Dalton and a hydrodynamic diameter of 1.2 nm, making it an excellent lymphatic contrast agent if

C. Balagué (✉) · I. Gomez
Department of General and Digestive Surgery, Hospital de la Santa Creu i Sant Pau, Barcelona, Spain
e-mail: cbalague@santpau.cat

© Springer Nature Switzerland AG 2020
G. Mariani et al. (eds.), *Atlas of Lymphoscintigraphy and Sentinel Node Mapping*,
https://doi.org/10.1007/978-3-030-45296-4_13

injected into the lymphatic system (for example by subcutaneous injection) [4]. It is very safe; adverse events are reported in less than 1 in 40,000 patients and mostly comprise hypersensitivity reactions [3].

13.2 SLN Mapping in Esophagogastric Cancer

Lymph node metastasis in esophagogastric cancer patients is an established prognostic factor for survival [5], and it is widely accepted that lymph node involvement increases with tumor stage. The term "orderly progression," however, is difficult to apply when describing the pattern of lymphatic spread of esophageal and gastric cancer. Based on a retrospective analysis of patients with solitary metastasis, Sano et al. [6] reported that the perigastric nodal area, close to the primary tumor, is the first lymphatic station in only 62% of the patients with gastric cancer. Based on these clinical observations, the standard procedure is radical resection with D2 lymphadenectomy in patients with gastric cancer, and three-field lymph node dissection in esophageal cancer, regardless of the presence of lymph node metastases [7, 8]. However, since extensive (D2) lymph node dissection is associated with higher morbidity (e.g., anastomotic leakage) and mortality than D1 lymph node dissection, futile D2 lymphadenectomy in patients without metastatic lymph nodes is unfavorable [9, 10].

SLN detection can play an important role in tailoring treatment to individual patients and may lead to modifications in the surgical procedure and/or other treatments [11]. Several studies support the validity of the SLN concept in esophageal and gastric cancer [12–16]. Multiple trials analyzing different methods of SLN detection have shown accuracy rates close to 99% when detecting lymph nodes with a dual tracer consisting of radiolabeled tin colloid and blue dye [17].

Among visceral tumors, gastric cancer is currently one of the suitable targets for SLN navigation surgery. Despite the multidirectional and complicated lymphatic flow from the gastric mucosa, the anatomical situation of the stomach is relatively suitable for SLN mapping in comparison with organs embedded in closed spaces, as in the case of rectal cancers [18].

13.2.1 SLN Mapping in Gastric Cancer

SLN mapping should be considered in all patients with early-stage gastric cancer, but this procedure would not show benefit in advanced gastric cancer. Rabin et al. [19] compared SLN mapping in patients with different T-stages.

They concluded that SLN mapping in T1 and T2 tumors can indeed assist in the decision-making process regarding the extent of lymphadenectomy (100% sensitivity, 90–100% negative predictive value), while in patients with T3 tumors it will be misleading in a third of the patients and should therefore not be adopted [19]. In Japan and Korea, T1N0M0 tumors are routinely treated with endoscopic resection, which creates new opportunities for SLN mapping in selected cases [3]. Using NIR fluorescence, Bok et al. [20] showed that a combination of endoscopic submucosal dissection and SLN navigation by laparoscopy was feasible in 12 out of 13 patients.

Currently, SLN mapping can be performed using two methods based on two markers, radionuclide imaging and dye staining, respectively.

13.2.1.1 Preoperative SLN Mapping with Radiocolloid

Several types of radiocolloids can be used for lymphoscintigraphy. Those most commonly used in Japan are ^{99m}Tc-tin colloid and ^{99m}Tc-phytate. In initial pilot studies, Kitagawa et al. [2] used ^{99m}Tc-tin colloid; the particles are relatively large and migrate to lymph nodes within the first 2 h post-administration, remaining there for more than 20 h through phagocytosis by the macrophages. The use of radiolabeled particles of this size allows lymphoscintigraphic imaging to be less dependent on detection time. The particles of ^{99m}Tc-phytate are smaller and can migrate to secondary lymph nodes beyond the SLN. At present, the use of ^{99m}Tc-tin colloid for SLN mapping in gastric cancer seems preferable.

For this approach, 148 MBq (in 2 mL) ^{99m}Tc-tin colloid suspension is endoscopically injected into the gastric submucosa at four sites (0.5 mL each) around the primary tumor, using a disposable 23-gauge needle [21]. Inoculation is performed the day before surgery (or at least 3 h before surgery). Lymphoscintigraphic imaging is recommended and can be performed 2 h after endoscopic inoculation [21].

Intraoperative SLN detection is performed using a handheld gamma probe. It is crucial that the probe is not oriented towards the primary tumor. SLNs are defined as those containing tenfold more radioactivity than the surrounding tissue (background) during intraoperative gamma probe counting [22] (Fig. 13.1).

13.2.1.2 Intraoperative SLN Mapping Using Dye Staining

Several dyes have been used, such as methylene blue or patent blue. The introduction of NIR fluorescence in laparoscopy has promoted interest in the use of ICG for SLN mapping, with promising results. Use of ICG for SLN mapping has been evaluated for several applications in abdominal surgery, with a high diversity in doses used (between

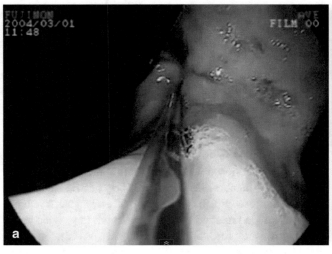 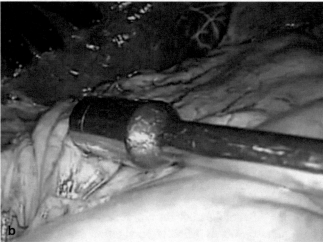

Fig. 13.1 (**a**) Blue-stained lymph nodes within 5–10 min after the dye injection (image supplied as SAGES videos by courtesy of the Division of Gastroenterologic Surgery, Kanazawa University, Kanazawa, Japan). (**b**) Gamma probe counting of the SLN containing ten times more

radioactivity than the surrounding tissue (image supplied as SAGES videos by courtesy of Hideki Hayashi, Department of Surgery II, Yamaguchi University School of Medicine, Yamaguchi, Japan)

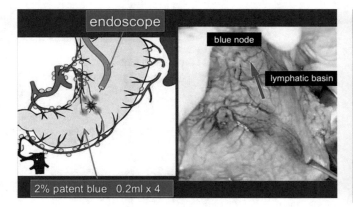 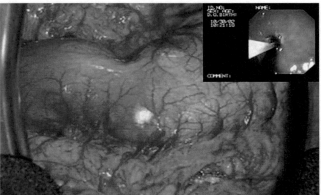

Fig. 13.2 Left panel: Schematic representation of intraoperative sub-mucosal blue dye injection during endoscopy. Right panel: Actual intra-operative submucosal blue dye injection during endoscopy (image supplied as SAGES video by courtesy of Hideki Hayashi, Department of Surgery II, Yamaguchi University School of Medicine, Yamaguchi, Japan)

Fig. 13.3 Intraoperative endoscopic submucosal injection of Patent Blue V around an antral gastric cancer, after laparotomy and opening of the lesser sac. Large image shows intra-abdominal view of injection. Small inset image shows an endoscopic view of injection (reproduced with permission from Gretschel S, Bembenek A, Ulmer Ch, et al. Prediction of gastric cancer lymph node status by SLNB and the Maruyama computer model. Eur J Surg Oncol. 2005;31:393–400)

100 μg and 25 mg), as reviewed by Van Manen et al. [3]. The authors conclude that a dose of at least 2.5 mg is recommended for good SLN visualization.

The staining method involves the submucosal or subserosal injection of dye at four points around the site of the primary tumor [16] (Fig. 13.2). As part of standard care, which consists of peritumoral blue dye injection, ICG could also be injected around the tumor.

The submucosal and the subserosal injection approaches are proven to be equivalent in SLN detection rate [23]. However, in case of the subserosal route of administration, it is difficult to identify a T1 lesion. Intraoperative subserosal inoculation is also difficult during laparoscopy, so endoscopic

submucosal injection is preferable in the case of the laparo-scopic approach (Fig. 13.3). It is important that the lymphatic drainage is not damaged before the injection of the dye.

Timing of the injection is also an important issue [3]. SLNs are defined as blue-stained nodes within 5–10 min after injection of the blue dye. Timing using ICG is also of importance but with different data. Tajima et al. [24] prefer injection (endoscopically) 1 day before surgery, but most studies have shown good results by performing injection immediately after applying general anesthesia. The SLNs can be visualized 15–30 min after injection [3].

13.2.1.3 Intraoperative SLN Mapping by Combined Radiocolloid and Staining

The dual-tracer method using both blue or green dye and radioactive colloids is considered the standard procedure in early gastric cancer patients [25]. Use of the two mapping approaches combined (radiocolloid and dye) reduces the technical errors that can occur with the use of a single SLN mapping technique.

The radioguided method confirms the complete identification and removal of SLNs with multipath distribution, while the dye-based system allows direct, real-time vision of the SLNs. Multiple trials have showed accuracy rates up to 99% when detecting lymph nodes with a dual tracer consisting of radiolabeled tin colloid and blue dye [17]. The Japanese Society of SLN Navigation Surgery Study Group completed a multicenter prospective trial of SLN mapping in gastric cancer based on the dual-tracer approach, with blue dye and radiocolloid [26]. They reported a false-negative rate of 7%, while the sensitivity of metastasis detection based on SLN status was 93% [27]. Based on these results, the combination of the two techniques seems advisable to carry out a proper and systematic mapping of SLN in gastric cancer. The irreversible hampering of the operating field by the blue dye, however, can be considered a disadvantage of this technique. In contrast, NIR fluorescence does not alter the operating field by dark staining and allows detection of deeper nodes [5] (Fig. 13.4).

Once SLNs are detected, the tissue is excised. Normally, all resected lymph nodes are examined postoperatively by routine hematoxylin and eosin (H&E) staining and resultant negative SLNs are examined further by immunohistochemistry using anti-cytokeratin antibody [22].

Based on single-institution results, SLN mapping for early gastric cancer is increasingly acceptable (Table 13.1). SLN detection rates for detecting micrometastasis based on SLN status are satisfactory both with the dye-guided method and with the radioguided method.

The results of clinical trials should provide useful perspectives on the future direction of SLN navigation surgery for gastric cancer [26]. In particular, cT1N0 gastric cancer seems to constitute a condition in which the results of SLN mapping might modify the therapeutic approach. From the data reported in the literature, micrometastases tend to be limited within the sentinel basins in cT1N0 gastric cancer. Sentinel basins are therefore good targets for selective lymphadenectomy in patients who have cT1N0 gastric cancer and a potential risk of micrometastasis. Furthermore, laparoscopic/endoscopic local resection seems feasible for curative treatment of SLN-negative early gastric cancer.

For laparoscopic SLN mapping of early gastric cancer, the radioguided method has great potential to provide a new paradigm shift for surgical management [18]. A meta-analysis by Skubleny et al. [33] concluded for encouraging results regarding the accuracy, diagnostic odds ratio, and specificity of the ICG dye method. These authors observed a suboptimal sensitivity of 87%. This percentage rose to 93% when considering only studies published after 2010, suggesting that the technique continues to improve as more experience is being gained.

Table 13.1 Methods for SLN detection in gastric cancer

Author/year	Tracer	Cases (n)	Detection rate (%)	Sensitivity (%)
Hiratsuka/2001 [12]	ICG	74	99	90
Yano/2012 [28]	ICG	130	—	100
Takahashi/2017 [29]	ICG	44	—	100
Miwa/2003 [16]	PB	211	96	89
Kim/2004 [30]	RI	46	94	85
Kitagawa/2004 [31]	RI	270	97	92
Uenosono/2011 [32]	RI	180	95	—
Arigami/2006 [21]	RI	61	100	—

RI Radionuclide, *PB* Patent blue, *ICG* Indocyanine green

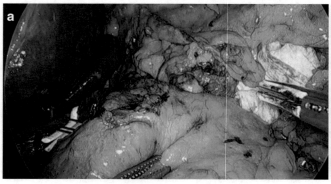 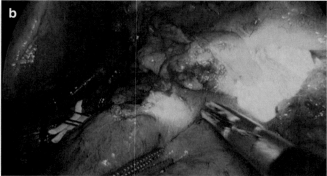

Fig. 13.4 SLN mapping with ICG dye during laparoscopic gastrectomy for gastric cancer: laparoscopic standard vision (**a**) and laparoscopic NIR vision (**b**) [images provided by courtesy of Dr. Miguel Toledano, Hospital Río Ortega, Valladolid, Spain]

13.2.2 SLN Mapping in Esophageal Cancer

SLN mapping is more complex in the case of esophageal cancer for several reasons. First, the blue dye cannot be used in this localization because lymph nodes in the region of the thoracic esophagus are frequently pigmented by anthracosis, which complicates the identification of the dye-stained lymph nodes. Moreover, in localizations such as the esophagus and rectum, prior mobilization of the primary lesion must be performed in order to achieve a proper real-time visualization of the lymphatic drainage routes by dye staining. However, such mobilization involves destruction or disruption of the lymphatic drainage patterns. The optimal method therefore is based on radiocolloid lymphoscintigraphy [15, 34]. In Western countries, the number of early-stage, newly diagnosed esophageal cancers is very low, so it is difficult to conduct clinical studies to investigate SLN mapping in these patients. In esophageal cancer, there are several SLNs, widely distributed from the cervical to the abdominal area. In over 80% of the cases, at least one SLN is located in the second or third compartment of regional lymph nodes [26]. This anatomic distribution of the SLNs is attributed to the multidirectional lymphatic drainage from the primary tumor.

The goal of SLN mapping in esophageal cancer is to reduce the need for extensive lymphadenectomy. The Kitagawa's group [1] proposed a new strategy using sentinel lymph node biopsy (SLNB) for esophageal cancer patients with clinically early-stage disease. Uenosono et al. [32] performed SLN mapping in 134 patients with newly diagnosed esophageal cancer. They concluded that SLN mapping can be applied to patients with cT1 and cN0 esophageal cancer and that the SLN concept might enable less invasive surgery and reduce unnecessary lymphadenectomies.

Several studies have evaluated the use of ICG as a NIR fluorescent marker. However, all of them were feasibility studies and no more than 20 patients were included in each study [3]. SLNs were detected in up to 95% of cases, as reported by Yuasa et al. [35]. Nevertheless, multicenter validation studies on SLN mapping in esophageal cancer are still lacking and the oncologic value of this technique is unknown [36].

13.2.2.1 SLN Harvesting

As indicated above, the technique of choice is based on radiocolloid mapping. ^{99m}Tc-tin colloid is endoscopically injected into the esophageal wall around the tumor on the day before surgery [32]. Following lymphoscintigraphy, SLNs located in the cervical area can be percutaneously identified with external gamma probe counting, and resection can be performed using less invasive procedures. Moreover, the detection and harvesting of intra-abdominal SLNs can be carried out laparoscopically following the same procedure as in gastric cancer. However, removing the mediastinal SLNs is relatively complicated and invasive, because it requires mobilization of the thoracic esophagus. Furthermore, the presence of the primary lesion (with the high activity retained at the peritumoral injection site) hampers SLN localization by gamma probe counting at this level.

Preoperative lymphoscintigraphy (usually performed 3 h after endoscopic inoculation of the radiocolloid) is useful for SLN detection in unexpected sites distant from the primary esophageal lesion.

> **Key Learning Points**
> - SLN mapping should be considered in early stages of gastric cancer since no benefit would be derived from this procedure in advanced stages of the disease.
> - Peritumoral submucosal injection by endoscopy is preferable.
> - In gastric cancer, using both mapping approaches (radiocolloid and dye) in combination reduces the technical errors that can occur with the use of a single SLN mapping technique.
> - Peritumoral injection of ICG may allow identification of SLNs during esophagectomy, although the oncologic value of this technique is unknown.

13.3 SLN Mapping in Colon Cancer

Standard treatment of colon cancer is based on surgical resection with or without adjuvant treatment. Tumor staging at diagnosis is the most important prognostic factor for predicting survival. The survival rate increases with the number of lymph nodes testing negative for metastasis and, at present, no adjuvant treatment is recommended in patients without metastatic lymph nodes (in the absence of unfavorable characteristics of the primary tumor). Thus, lymph node involvement heavily influences prognosis of patients and the decision to perform adjuvant chemotherapy [37, 38].

However, 10–25% of the patients with localized colon cancer (AJCC stages I and II) will develop disease progression and distant metastases within 5 years after completion of surgery with curative intent. Therefore, some inaccuracy must be taken into account regarding the staging methods, possibly leading to false understaging. Such understaging is considered to be around 10–20% [39], underlying the need to search for methods that can help to achieve a correct staging of the patient [40]. For histological examination of lymph nodes, these methods include serial sectioning [41], immunohistochemistry (IHC) with anti-cytokeratin antibodies [42], and molecular analysis by RT-PCR techniques. However, their implementation may be impractical for routine histology, due to the large number of lymph nodes retrieved in the surgical specimen. For this reason, SLN mapping may allow identification of a smaller number of lymph nodes that represent the tumor status of the entire nodal basin [43]. An exhaustive analysis of SLNs in order to achieve a more accurate staging of patients can influence the decision for adjuvant treatment.

Saha emphasized that SLN mapping for colorectal cancer is highly successful and accurate for predicting the presence or absence of nodal disease, with a relatively low incidence of skip metastases. Such technique provided the pathologists with the "right nodes" for detailed analysis for appropriate staging and treatment with adjuvant chemotherapy [1].

It is also interesting to consider that complete mesocolic excision (CME) has been advocated to increase the nodal yield; however, this approach is still controversial. Performing a more focused lymphadenectomy and resection may be a better option for overall patient outcomes [44].

SLN mapping in colorectal cancer is not widely employed, however, even though its potential benefit has been shown in two meta-analyses [45, 46]. One reason may be the variability in the reported sensitivity (ranging from 33 to 100%) [4]. A high variability rate has also been observed when using NIR fluorescence [3].

13.3.1 Methods for SLN Mapping in Colorectal Cancer

Initially, the most frequently used marker for visual SLN mapping was isosulfan blue 1%, injected in a volume of 1–2 mL. However, several reports described anaphylactic reactions [47–49] and possible interference with pulse oximetry monitoring [50, 51]. Moreover, in some countries isosulfan blue is not readily available or is prohibitively expensive.

In a prospective study, Soni et al. [52] compared 1% lymphazurin (L) versus 1% methylene blue (MB) as a dye for SLN mapping in GI tumors (the majority were colon cancer). They concluded that the success rate, nodal positivity, average SLNs per patient, and overall accuracy were similar between L and MB. Absence of anaphylaxis and lower cost made MB more desirable than L for SLN mapping in GI tumors.

Fluorescein (at 10% dilution) is more widely available and much cheaper, and moreover, it has not been associated with known allergic reactions. Its application is comparable to that described for isosulfan blue in terms of both administration and the quantity administered. Saha et al. [39] used

fluorescein SLN mapping in 120 patients, with results comparable to those obtained with isosulfan blue. The agent migrates quickly to the SLNs that then turn fluorescent and can be identified with Wood's light as bright yellow lymph nodes.

NIR fluorescent imaging with other available dyes, such as ICG, has been used in several clinical studies during laparoscopic or open surgery. Detection rates range between 65.5 and 100%, the differences likely being related to the experience at each center [3].

The use of ^{99m}Tc-tin colloid has also been described for SLN mapping in colorectal cancer, with similar results [15].

There are therefore two methods for SLN mapping in patients with colorectal cancer, the dye staining method and the radioguidance method, respectively.

13.3.1.1 Dye Staining Method
With this approach, SLN mapping can be performed in vivo and ex vivo.

In vivo studies. One of the advantages observed with in vivo studies is the detection of aberrant lymph nodes, those outside the expected drainage basins, thus allowing excision of the more appropriate lymphatic territories.

The staining method involves the intraoperative injection of dye (2 mL of 1% blue dye or 2 mL of sterile water containing 0.5 mg/mL of ICG) into the subserosal layer at four points around the site of the primary tumor [39] (Fig. 13.5). Endoscopic submucosal inoculation is also possible, whenever adequate. The submucosal and subserosal injection routes are equivalent in terms of detection rate. However, in case of the subserosal approach, it is difficult to identify the T1 lesions. Intraoperative subserosal inoculation is also dif-

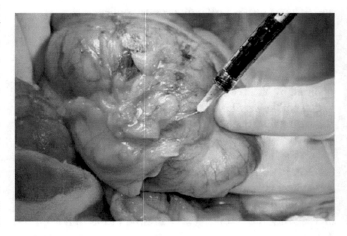

Fig. 13.5 Intraoperative injection of blue dye into the subserosal layer at four points around the site of the primary tumor (reproduced with permission from Saha S, Dan AG, Viehl CT, Zuber M, Wiese D. Selective sentinel lymphadenectomy for human solid cancer. In: Leong SPL, Kitagawa Y, Kitajima M, Eds. SLN Mapping in Colon and Rectal Cancer: Its Impact on Staging Limitations and Pitfalls. Springer; 2005:105–122)

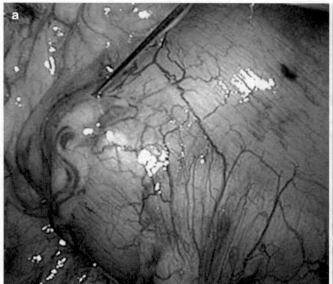 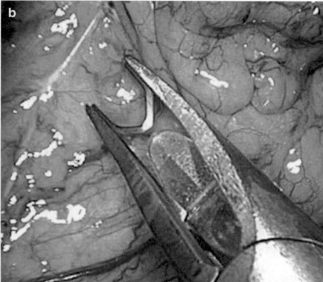

Fig. 13.6 (a) Intraoperative injection of blue dye into the subserosa layer during laparoscopy. (b) Blue-stained lymph nodes within 5–10 min after dye injection during laparoscopy (reproduced with per-

mission from Bianchi PP, Petz W, Casali L. Laparoscopic lymphatic roadmapping with blue dye and radioisotope in colon cancer. Colorectal Dis. 2011;13 (Suppl 7):67–69)

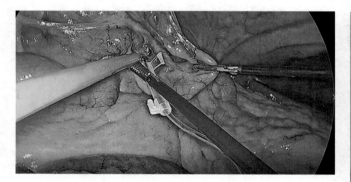 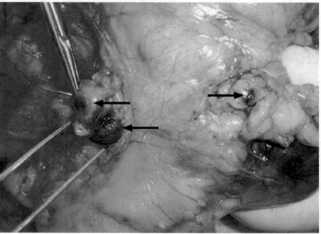

Fig. 13.7 Intraoperative injection of ICG into the subserosa layer of right colon cancer during laparoscopy (image provided by courtesy of Dr. Salvador Morales, Hospital Virgen del Rocío, Seville, Spain)

Fig. 13.8 The blue-stained lymph nodes are marked with a surgical clip in order to be identified for separate extensive histopathologic analysis (reproduced with permission from Saha S, Dan AG, Viehl CT, Zuber M, Wiese D. Selective sentinel lymphadenectomy for human solid cancer. In: Leong SPL, Kitagawa Y, Kitajima M, Eds. SLN Mapping in Colon and Rectal Cancer: Its Impact on Staging, Limitations, and Pitfalls. Springer; 2005:105–122)

ficult during laparoscopy, even though this technical approach has been described (Figs. 13.6 and 13.7).

Approximately 5–10 min after blue-dye inoculation, or some minutes later with the ICG dye, the first lymph node begins to stain, and the first 1–4 stained nodes are marked for detailed histologic analysis (Fig. 13.8). Using this method, Saha reported a 100% detection rate, 89% sensitivity, 100% specificity, and 93.5% negative predictive value. Using the same technical approach, Waters et al. [53] obtained a 100% detection rate. In 5% of patients, the SLN was the only node with metastasis. The same technical approach is feasible in cases of rectal cancer with intraperitoneal location above the peritoneal reflection. In patients with medium or low rectal cancer, a total mesorectal excision is necessary. In vivo submucosal inoculation during

proctoscopy is feasible [39], as is the submucosal ex vivo inoculation of dye. Adopting this approach in patients with rectal cancer, Saha [39] achieved a 90.6% detection rate, with 100% negative predictive value.

Ex vivo studies. This staining method involves the ex vivo injection of dye (2 mL of 1% blue dye or 2 mL of sterile water containing 0.5 mg/mL of ICG) into the subserosa or

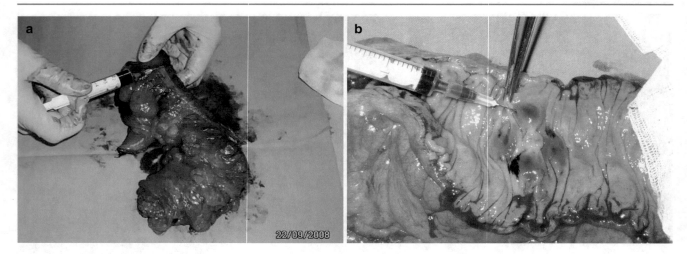

Fig. 13.9 "Ex vivo" injection of 2 mL of 1% blue dye (methylene blue) into the subserosal layer (**a**) and submucosal layer (**b**)

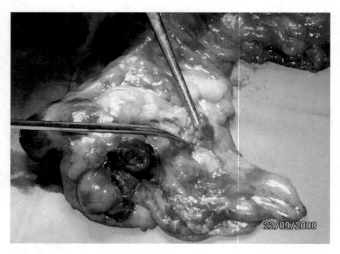

Fig. 13.10 The blue-stained SLNs after "ex vivo" subserosal injection are resected

Table 13.2 Results of "ex vivo" and "in vivo" staining methods for SLN mapping in colon cancer

Author	In vivo	Ex vivo	Detection rate (%)	Negative predictive value (%)
Saha [39]	X		100	93
Wong [54]		X	92.3	—
Fitzgerald [55]		X	88	—
Waters [53]	X		100	100
Bianchi [56]	X		100	94
Quadros[a]	X		91	67
Gretschel[b]	X		85	80
Balagué[a]		X	91	87

[a]Unpublished data
[b]Gretschel S, Bembenek A, Ulmer Ch, et al. Prediction of gastric cancer lymph node status by SLNB and the Maruyama computer model. Eur J Surg Oncol. 2005;31:393–400

submucosal layer at four points around the site of the primary tumor immediately after resection of the surgical specimen en bloc including the primary tumor (Fig. 13.9). Previous longitudinal section of the specimen through the antimesenteric border is necessary to perform submucosal injection. Once the dye has been injected, massage of the inoculated area for 5 min is necessary. Stained nodes are designated as SLNs and harvested for analysis (Fig. 13.10). Comparable results have been obtained between the ex vivo and the in vivo staining methods (Table 13.2). Wong et al. [54] achieved a 92.3% detection rate, with a mean number of three SLNs obtained per patient, while Fitzgerald et al. [55] identified the SLN in 88% of their patients. Similar detection rates (94–100%) have been reported by other authors using the same ex vivo method [57, 58].

Liberale et al. [59] compared ex vivo intraserosal peritumoral injection of ICG with blue dye in patients with colon cancer. The detection rate was 95% and sensitivity of the blue dye and ICG techniques was 43% and 57%, respectively. The two techniques were complementary and had a global 83% sensitivity. The sensitivity of ICG was higher than that for the blue dye technique in patients with a body mass index >25 [59].

13.3.1.2 Radioguided Method
In case of SLN mapping with radiocolloid lymphoscintigraphy, the study is performed following the same criteria as in gastric cancer: ^{99m}Tc-tin colloid is endoscopically injected into the colonic submucosa at four sites (0.5 mL each) around the primary tumor using a disposable 23-gauge needle (Fig. 13.11). Radiocolloid administration is generally performed the day before the operation (or at least 3 h before surgery).

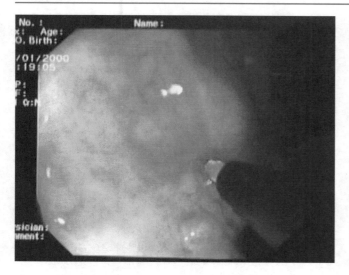

Fig. 13.11 Endoscopic injection of ^{99m}Tc-tin colloid into the colonic submucosa

Lymphoscintigraphy is recommended, and can be performed 2 h after endoscopic inoculation. SPECT/CT imaging is useful for accurate preoperative evaluation, and can be helpful to establish the most adequate surgical strategy (Fig. 13.12).

The preliminary results of intraoperative lymphoscintigraphy obtained in a well-selected small group of patients are promising, with high sensitivity and specificity, although further prospective studies are necessary.

As the best technique for SLN mapping in patients with colorectal cancer, Bilchik [1] recommended a combination of radiocolloid and blue dye, emphasizing that this technique will become increasingly popular for improving the accuracy of lymph node staging. In particular, this procedure offers the potential for significant upstaging of GI cancer [1].

SLN mapping in colon cancer has also been described with the use of laparoscopic techniques. Wood et al. [60] reported 100% SLN detection rate, with 100% accuracy in a series of nine patients submitted to laparoscopy. In surgical

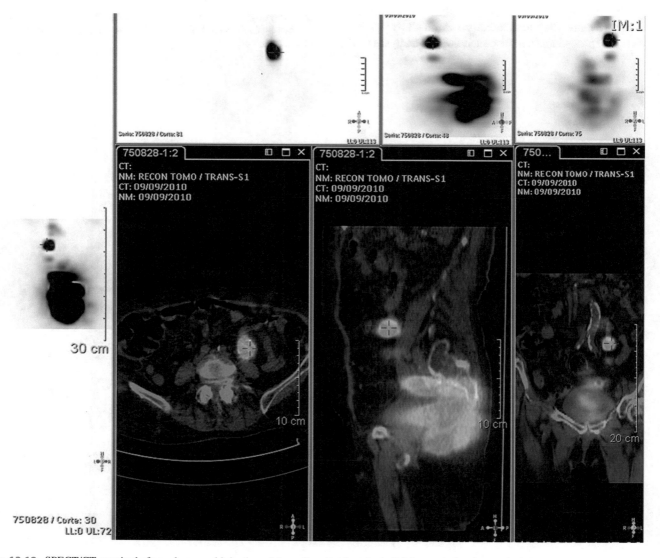

Fig. 13.12   SPECT/CT acquired after submucosal injection of the radiocolloid can be helpful to optimize the surgical strategy

laparoscopy, the marker can be inoculated ex vivo or in vivo, with either dye or radiocolloid. The dye can be injected in vivo at the submucosal level (by endoscopy), or subserosally (by laparoscopy) as described by Bianchi et al. [56] (Fig. 13.6). The laparoscopic approach makes it difficult to mark the lesion.

Kitagawa et al. [15] described correct SLN localization using a laparoscopic gamma probe. During minimally invasive surgery, Bianchi et al. [56] identified the SLNs with good specificity using the blue dye, but sensitivity was still low (78%). According to these authors, these results have limited more widespread diffusion of the method, although it is possible to improve such performance using an intraoperative gamma camera.

It is important to consider the elevated heterogeneity between the reported studies in terms such as laparoscopic versus open surgery, in vivo versus ex vivo, submucosal versus subserosal injection, volume of the injectate, type of dye used, and histopathological analyses. These heterogeneities make it difficult to analyze the benefits of the technique. It is therefore mandatory to standardize as much as possible the technical procedures and histopathological analyses used [4].

Key Learning Points
- More accurate staging of colon cancer using SLN mapping can influence the decision for adjuvant treatment.
- Results with ex vivo and in vivo staining methods are comparable.
- One advantage of the in vivo method is that it can detect aberrant lymph nodes, that is, nodes outside the expected drainage basins, thus allowing excision of the most appropriate lymphatic territories.
- The heterogeneity of study findings hinders evaluation of the benefit of the technique.
- Therefore, it is mandatory to standardize as much as possible the technical procedures and histopathological analyses used.

Acknowledgements This chapter is a revision of the original chapter written by C. Balagué and J. L. Pallarés in the previous edition of the book.

Clinical Cases

Case 13.1: SLN Mapping in Cancer of Ascending Colon: Drainage to Lumbo-Aortic Nodes After Submucosal Peritumoral Injection (SPECT/CT Imaging)

Joan Duch

Background Clinical Case

A woman (age lost in follow-up) with ascending colon cancer underwent lymphoscintigraphy for radioguided SLNB.

Lymphoscintigraphy

The afternoon before surgery, lymphoscintigraphy was performed following submucosal injections of 0.5 mL of 74 MBq 99mTc-albumin nanocolloid (divided into two aliquots) around the tumor under endoscopic guidance. A dual-detector SPECT gamma camera (Millennium MG, GE Healthcare, Milwaukee, WI) equipped with low-energy high-resolution (LEHR) collimators was used to obtain early abdominal dynamic images and subsequent planar acquisitions in anterior and posterior projection at 30 min and 60 min after radiopharmaceutical injection. Dynamic images (1 frame 60 s/30 frames) were acquired in anterior and posterior projection with a 256 × 256 matrix and zoom factor 1.00, while static images were acquired in anterior and posterior projection with a 128 × 128 matrix and zoom factor 1.00.

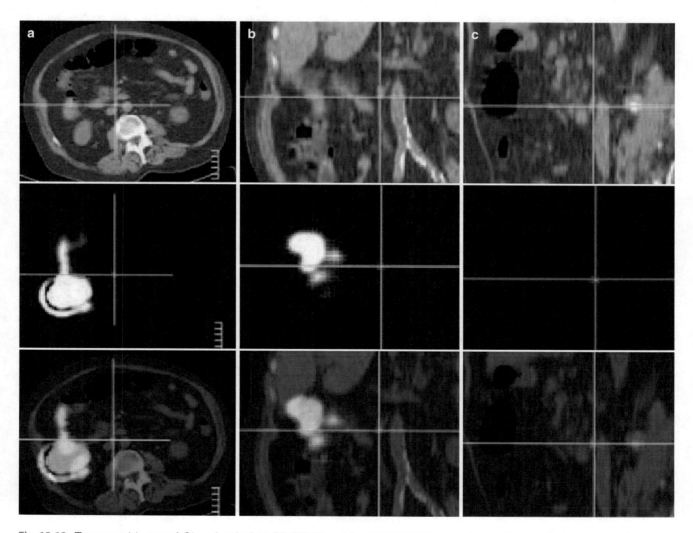

Fig. 13.13 Transverse (**a**), coronal (**b**), and sagittal (**c**) CT, SPECT, and fused SPECT/CT images show drainage to the interaortocaval region

Case 13.2: SLN Mapping in Rectal Cancer: Drainage to Lumbo-Aortic Nodes After Submucosal Peritumoral Injection (Planar, SPECT/CT, and Intraoperative Imaging)

Carmen Balagué and José Luis Pallarés

Background Clinical Case

An 85-year-old woman with rectal bleeding underwent colonoscopy, which revealed a rectal lesion 8 cm from the anal verge. Histopathology: adenocarcinoma. Local evaluation with MR: T2N0. Further evaluation with CT scan for distant metastasis: M0. Neoadjuvant chemo-radiotherapy was not accepted by the patient. Before surgery (low anterior rectal resection) the patient was submitted to SLNB.

Anatomical location of primary malignancy: large bowel, rectum, 8 cm from anal verge.

Technical Background Acquisition

SLN detected by in vivo study, using radiocolloid.

Staining method:

Endoscopic inoculation of 37 MBq of 99mTc-albumin nanocolloid at each of the quadrants around the site of the primary tumor the day before surgery. This was done in three quadrants given the difficulty to perform endoscopic inoculation behind the lesion. Two hours later, a planar lymphoscintigraphy was acquired using a Philips Brightview SPECT/CT, during 600 s and with an acquisition matrix of 256 × 256. SPECT/CT was also acquired in a Philips Brightview SPECT/CT, with an acquisition matrix of 64 × 64, with 64 projections (10 s/projection). CT was done with a Kv of 120 and a mA of 20. SPECT/CT lymphoscintigraphy demonstrated physiological uptake in left aortoiliac region, due to colonic uptake, and showed also a high mesorectal uptake, with no identification of SLNs. Low anterior resection (LAR) was performed. The pelvic study was completed by gamma probe assisted by portable gamma camera imaging (Sentinella), and no activity of nodal iliac territory was detected. Histopathological results: pT2N0M0. Total lymph nodes detected: 22 (negative).

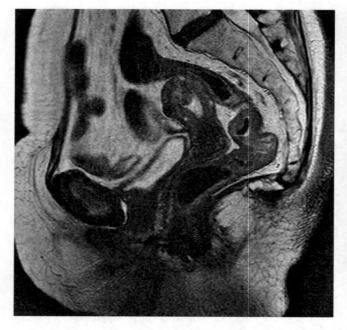

Fig. 13.14 MR for local evaluation of tumor. Rectal cancer 8 cm from anal verge

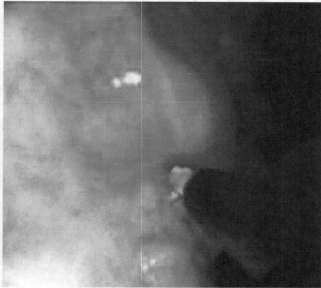

Fig. 13.15 Endoscopic submucosal inoculation of radiocolloid

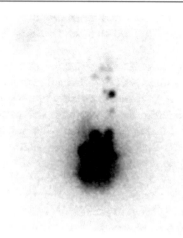

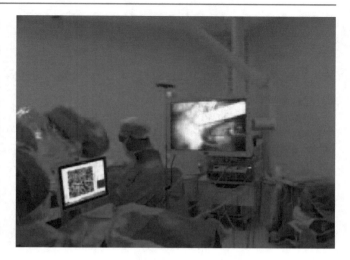

Fig. 13.18 Detection with gamma probe assisted by Sentinella gamma camera

Fig. 13.16 Planar lymphoscintigraphy showed high uptake in the mesorectal region and in the left aortoiliac region

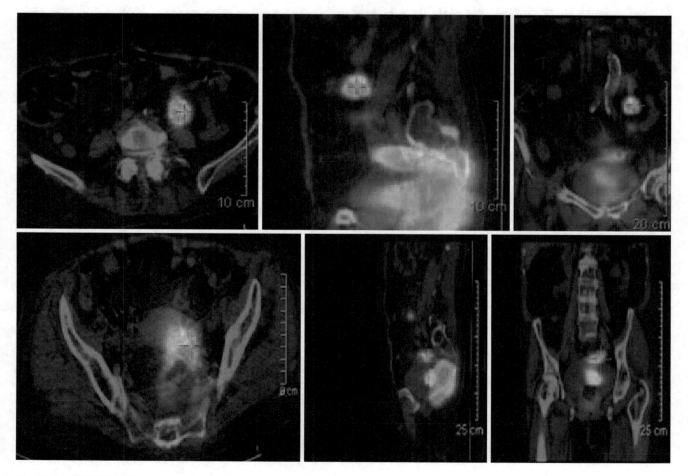

Fig. 13.17 SPECT/CT. *Upper panel*: SPECT/CT lymphoscintigraphy demonstrated that radioactivity apparently representing lymph node uptake in the left aortoiliac region was actually due to nonspecific colonic accumulation. *Lower panel*: SPECT/CT also showed a high mesorectal uptake, with no clear identification of SLNs

Case 13.3: SLN Mapping in Cancer of Ascending Colon: "Ex Vivo" Technique with Peritumoral Blue Dye and Radiocolloid Injection

José Luis Pallarés, Joan Duch, and Carmen Balagué

Background Clinical Case

An 86-year-old woman with anemia. Colonoscopy showed a 5–6 cm ulcerated lesion in the right colon. Histopathologic examination revealed an adenocarcinoma. Staging with CT scan demonstrated no distant metastasis (T2-3N0M0). Before surgery (laparoscopic right hemicolectomy) the patient was submitted to radioguided SLNB.

Anatomical location of primary malignancy: large bowel, right colon.

Technical Background Acquisition

SLN detected by ex vivo study using blue dye and radiocolloid.

Staining method: Ex vivo injection of 2 mL of 1% blue dye into the subserosa layer (0.5 mL at each of the four points around the site of the primary tumor). The radiocolloid is inoculated in the same points (37 MBq of 99mTc-nanocolloid). Massage for 5 min of the inoculated area is necessary. After that, gamma probe (Gamma Finder II) is used in order to detect the SLNs. Two SLNs are detected through the blue dye, and three by the radiocolloid. Only one SLN has been detected combining the two methods.

Histopathological results: T2N0M0. Total lymph nodes detected: 19 (all negative). SLNs were all negative.

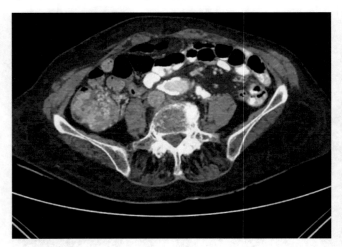

Fig. 13.19 Scanner: image of tumor. Large bowel: right colon

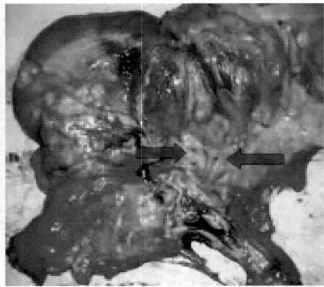

Fig. 13.21 Ex vivo SLN detection marked with blue dye

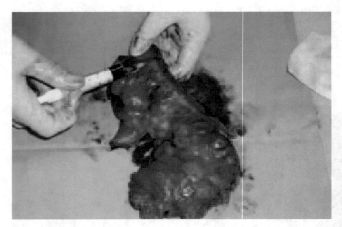

Fig. 13.20 Subserosal inoculation of blue dye and radiocolloid

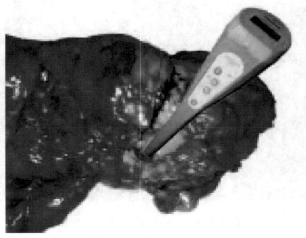

Fig. 13.22 SLN identification after radiopharmaceutical injection

References

1. Aikou T, Kitagawa Y, Kitajima M, et al. Sentinel lymph node mapping with GI cancer. Cancer Metastasis Rev. 2006;25:269–77.
2. Kitagawa Y, Ohgami M, Fujii H, et al. Laparoscopic detection of sentinel lymph nodes in gastrointestinal cancer: a novel and minimally invasive approach. Ann Surg Oncol. 2001;8(Suppl 9):86S–9S.
3. Van Manen L, Handgraaf HJM, Diana M, et al. A practical guide for the use of indocyanine green and methylene blue in fluorescence-guided abdominal surgery. J Surg Oncol. 2008;118:283–300.
4. Liberale G, Bohlok A, Bormans A. Indocyanine green fluorescence imaging for sentinel lymph node detection in colorectal cancer: a systematic review. EJSO. 2018;44:1301–6.
5. Vuijk FA, Hilling DE, Mieog JSD, et al. Fluorescent guided surgery for sentinel lymph node detection in gastric cancer and carcinoembryonic antigen targeted fluorescent guided surgery in colorectal and pancreatic cancer. J Surg Oncol. 2018;118:315–23.
6. Sano T, Katai H, Sasako M, et al. Gastric lymphadenectomy and detection of sentinel nodes. Recent Results Cancer Res. 2000;157:253–8.
7. Akiyama H, Tsurumaru M, Udagawa H, et al. Radical lymph node dissection for cancer of the thoracic oesophagus. Ann Surg. 1994;220:364–73.
8. Maruyama K, Gunven P, Okabayashi K, et al. Lymph node metastases of gastric cancer. General pattern in 1931 patients. Ann Surg. 1989;210:596–602.
9. Bonenkamp JJ, Hermans J, Sasako M, et al. Extended lymph-node dissection for gastric cancer. Dutch Gastric Cancer Group. N Engl J Med. 1999;340:908–14.
10. Hulsher JBF, Van Sandick JW, de Boer AGEM, et al. Extended transthoracic resection compared with limited transhiatal resection for adenocarcinoma of the oesophagus. N Engl J Med. 2002;347:1662–9.
11. Thompson JF, Uren RF, Scolyer RA, et al. Selective sentinel lymphadenectomy: progress to date and prospects for the future. Cancer Treat Res. 2005;127:269–87.
12. Hiratsuka M, Miyashiro I, Ishikawa O, et al. Application of sentinel node biopsy to gastric cancer surgery. Surgery. 2001;129:335–40.
13. Kitagawa Y, Fujii H, Mukai M, et al. Radio-guided sentinel node detection for gastric cancer. Br J Surg. 2002;89:604–8.
14. Kitagawa Y, Fujii H, Mukai M, et al. Intraoperative lymphatic mapping and sentinel lymph node sampling in oesophageal and gastric cancer. Surg Oncol Clin N Am. 2002;11:293–304.
15. Kitagawa Y, Fujii H, Mukai M, et al. The role of sentinel lymph node in gastrointestinal cancer. Surg Clin North Am. 2000;80:1799–809.
16. Miwa K, Kinami S, Taniguchi K, et al. Mapping sentinel nodes in patients with early-stage gastric carcinoma. Br J Surg. 2003;90:178–82.
17. Kitagawa Y, Takeuchi H, Takagi Y, et al. Sentinel node mapping for gastric cancer: a prospective multicenter trial in Japan. J Clin Oncol. 2013;31:3704–10.
18. Kitagawa Y, Kitajima M. Diagnostic validity of radio-guided sentinel node mapping for gastric cancer: a review of current status and future direction. Surg Technol Int. 2006;15:32–6.
19. Rabin I, Chikman B, Lavy R, et al. The accuracy of sentinel node mapping according to T stage in patients with gastric cancer. Gastric Cancer. 2010;13:30–5.
20. Bok GH, Kim YJ, Jin SY, et al. Endoscopic submucosal dissection with sentinel node navigation surgery for early gastric cancer. Endoscopy. 2012;44:953–6.
21. Arigami T, Natsugoe S, Uenosono Y, et al. Evaluation of sentinel node concept in gastric cancer based on lymph node micrometastasis determined by reverse transcription-polymerase chain reaction. Ann Surg. 2006;243:341–7.
22. Cheng LY, Chen XD, Zhang YX, et al. Clinical significance of sentinel lymph node detection by combining the dye-directed and radioguided methods in gastric cancer. Zhonghua Wai Ke Za Zhi. 2005;43:569–72.
23. Toth D, Kathy S, Csoban T, et al. Prospective comparative study of sentinel lymph node mapping in gastric cancer—submucosal versus subserosal marking method. Magy Seb. 2012;65:3–8.
24. Tajima Y, Yamazaki K, Masuda Y, et al. Sentinel node mapping guided by indocyanine green fluorescence imaging in gastric cancer. Ann Surg. 2009;249:58–62.
25. Hiramatsu Y, Takeuchi H, Goto O, et al. Invasive function-preserving gastrectomy with sentinel node biopsy for early gastric cancer. Digestion. 2019;99:14–20.
26. Kitagawa Y, Kubota T, Kumai K. Recent studies of sentinel lymph node. Multicenter prospective clinical trials of SN biopsy for gastric cancer. Gan To Kagaku Ryoho. 2005;32:695–8.
27. Asakum M, Cahill RA, Lee SWB. NOTES: the question for minimal resection and sentinel node in early gastric cancer. World J Gastrointest Surg. 2010;27(2):203–6.
28. Yano K, Nimura H, Mitsumori N, et al. The efficiency of micrometastasis by sentinel node navigation surgery using indocyanine green and infrared ray laparoscopy system for gastric cancer. Gastric Cancer. 2012;15:287–91.
29. Takahashi N, Nimura H, Fujita T, et al. Laparoscopic sentinel node navigation surgery for early gastric cancer: a prospective multicenter trial. Langenbecks Arch Surg. 2017;402:27–32.
30. Kim MC, Kim HH, Jung GC, et al. Lymphatic mapping and sentinel node biopsy using ^{99m}Tc tin colloid in gastric cancer. Ann Surg. 2004;239:383–7.
31. Kitagawa Y, Kitajima M. Diagnostic validity of radio-guided sentinel node mapping for gastric cancer. Surg Technol Int. 2004.
32. Uenosono Y, Arigami T, Yanagita S. Sentinel node navigation surgery is acceptable for clinical T1 and N0 esophageal cancer. Ann Surg Oncol. 2011;18:2003–9.
33. Skubleny D, Dang JT, Skulsky S, et al. Diagnostic evaluation of sentinel lymph node biopsy using indocyanine green and infrared or fluorescent imaging in gastric cancer: a systematic review and meta-analysis. Surg Endosc. 2018;32:2620–31.
34. Yasuda S, Shimada H, Chino O, et al. Sentinel lymph node detection with Tc-99m-tin colloids in patients with esophagogastric cancer. Jpn J Clin Oncol. 2003;33:68–72.
35. Yuasa Y, Seike J, Yoshida T, et al. Sentinel lymph node biopsy using intraoperative indocyanine green fluorescence imaging navigated with preoperative CT lymphography for superficial esophageal cancer. Ann Surg Oncol. 2012;19:486–93.
36. Turner SR, Molen DR. The role of intraoperative fluorescence imaging during esophagectomy. Thorac Surg Clin. 2018;28:567–71.
37. Cohen AM, Kelsen D, Saltz L, et al. Adjuvant therapy for colorectal cancer. Curr Probl Cancer. 1998;22:5–65.
38. Wolmark N, Rockette H, Fisher B, et al. The benefit of leucovorin-modulated fluorouracil as postoperative adjuvant therapy for primary colon cancer: results from National Surgical Adjuvant Breast and Bowel Protocol C-03. J Clin Oncol. 1993;11:1879–87.
39. Saha S, Dan AG, Viehl CT, et al. Selective sentinel lymphadenectomy for human solid cancer. In: SPL L, Kitagawa Y, Kitajima M, editors. Sentinel lymph node mapping in colon and rectal cancer: its impact on staging, limitations, and pitfalls. Boston: Springer; 2005. p. 105–22.
40. Mulsow J, Winter DC, O'Keane JC, et al. Sentinel lymph node mapping in colorectal cancer. Br J Surg. 2003;90:659–67.
41. Pickreen JW. Significance of occult metastases, a study of breast cancer. Cancer. 1961;14:1261–71.
42. Greenson JK, Isenhart CE, Rice R, et al. Identification of occult micrometastases in pericolic lymph nodes of Dukes B colorectal cancer patients using monoclonal antibodies against cytokeratin and CC49; correlation with long-term survival. Cancer. 1994;73:563–9.

43. Thörn M. Lymphatic mapping and sentinel node biopsy: is the method applicable to patients with colorectal and gastric cancer? Eur J Surg. 2000;166:755–8.

44. Chand M, Keller DS, Joshi HM, et al. Feasibility of fluorescence lymph node imaging in colon cancer: FLICC. Tech Coloproctol. 2018;22:271–7.

45. Des Guetz G, Uzzan B, Nicolas P, et al. Sentinel lymph node mapping in colorectal cancer—a future prognostic factor? A meta-analysis. World J Surg. 2007;31:1304–12.

46. Van der Pas MHGM, Meijer S, Hoekstra OS, et al. Sentinel-lymph-node procedure in colon and rectal cancer: a systematic review and meta-analysis. Lancet Oncol. 2011;12:540–50.

47. Kuerer HM, Wayne JD, Ross MI. Anaphylaxis during breast cancer lymphatic mapping. Surgery. 2001;129:119–20.

48. Leong SP, Donegan E, Hefferson W, et al. Adverse reactions to isosulfan blue during selective sentinel lymph node dissection in melanoma. Ann Surg Oncol. 2000;7:361–6.

49. Longnecker SM, Guzzardo MM, Van Voris LP. Life-threatening anaphylaxis following subcutaneous administration of isosulfan blue 1%. Clin Pharmacol. 1985;4:219–21.

50. Coleman RL, Whitten CW, O'Boyle J, et al. Unexplained decrease in measured oxygen saturation by pulse oximetry following injection of lymphazurin 1% (isosulfan blue) during a lymphatic mapping procedure. J Surg Oncol. 1999;70:126–9.

51. Larsen VH, Freudendal A, Fogh-Andersen N. The influence of patent blue V on pulse oximetry and haemoximetry. Acta Anaesthesiol Scand. 1995;107(Suppl):53–5.

52. Soni M, Saha S, Korant A, et al. A prospective trial comparing 1% lymphazurin vs 1% methylene blue in sentinel lymph node mapping of gastrointestinal tumors. Ann Surg Oncol. 2009;6:2224–30.

53. Waters GS, Geisenger KR, Garske DD, et al. Sentinel lymph node mapping for carcinoma of the colon: a pilot study. Am Surg. 2000;66:943–5.

54. Wong JH, Steineman S, Calderia C, et al. Ex vivo sentinel node mapping in carcinoma of the colon and rectum. Ann Surg. 2001;233:515–21.

55. Fitzgerald TL, Khalifa MA, Al Zahrani M, et al. Ex vivo sentinel lymph node biopsy in colorectal cancer: a feasibility study. J Surg Oncol. 2002;80:27–32.

56. Bianchi PP, Petz W, Casali L. Laparoscopic lymphatic roadmapping with blue dye and radioisotope in colon cancer. Color Dis. 2011;13(Suppl 7):67–9.

57. Cox ED, Kellicut D, Adair C, et al. Sentinel lymph node evaluation is technically feasible and may improve staging in colorectal cancer. Curr Surg. 2002;59:301–6.

58. Wood TF, Tsioulias GJ, Rangel D, et al. Focused examination of sentinel lymph nodes upstages early colorectal carcinoma. Am Surg. 2000;66:998–1003.

59. Liberale G, Vankerckhove S, Galdon MG, et al. Sentinel lymph node detection by blue dye versus indocyanine green fluorescence imaging in colon cancer. Anticancer Res. 2016;36:4853–8.

60. Wood T, Saha S, Morton D, et al. Validation of lymphatic mapping in colorectal cancer: in vivo, ex vivo, and laparoscopic techniques. Dis Colon Rectum. 2016;8:150–7.

Preoperative and Intraoperative Lymphatic Mapping for Radioguided Sentinel Node Biopsy in Cancers of the Female Reproductive System

14

Angela Collarino, Annalisa Zurru, and Sergi Vidal-Sicart

Contents

14.1	**Introduction**	315
14.2	**The Clinical Problem**	316
14.3	**Lymphatic Drainage of Gynecological Tumors**	317
14.4	**Indications and Contraindications of SLN Mapping**	318
14.5	**Modalities of Radiocolloid Injection**	318
14.6	**Preoperative SLN Imaging**	319
14.7	**Added Value of SPECT/CT Imaging**	321
14.8	**Intraoperative SLN Detection**	323
14.9	**Technical Pitfalls in SLN Mapping**	324
	Clinical Cases	325
	References	329

Learning Objectives
- To understand the rationale of the sentinel lymph node biopsy (SLNB) in patients with early-stage vulvar cancer, cervical cancer, and endometrial cancer.
- To acquire basic knowledge on the clinical applications of SLNB in gynecological cancers.
- To become familiar with preoperative and intraoperative procedures for sentinel lymph node (SLN) mapping in gynecological cancers.

A. Collarino (✉)
Nuclear Medicine Unit, Fondazione Policlinico Universitario
A. Gemelli IRCCS, Rome, Italy
e-mail: angela.collarino@policlinicogemelli.it

A. Zurru
Institute of Nuclear Medicine, Università Cattolica del Sacro Cuore, Rome, Italy

S. Vidal-Sicart
Nuclear Medicine Department, Hospital Clinic Barcelona, Barcelona, Catalonia, Spain

Institut d'Investigacions Biomèdiques August Pi Sunyer (IDIBAPS), Barcelona, Catalonia, Spain

14.1 Introduction

SLNB is a minimally invasive surgical approach for staging the lymph node status. The rationale is that the SLN represents the first lymph node(s) with direct lymphatic drainage from the primary tumor. Hence, when the histopathological evaluation of SLN reveals the absence of metastases the other lymph nodes should in principle be negative, and radical lymphadenectomy should be omitted. So far, SLNB is the standard of care in well-selected patients with vulvar cancer, cervical cancer, and endometrial cancer [1–5]. In 1994, Levenback and co-workers published the first study on SLNB for vulvar cancer. They used isosulfan blue as a

© Springer Nature Switzerland AG 2020
G. Mariani et al. (eds.), *Atlas of Lymphoscintigraphy and Sentinel Node Mapping*,
https://doi.org/10.1007/978-3-030-45296-4_14

marker for visual guidance, and identified the SLN in 7 of 9 patients (7 of 12 groins) without false-negative SLN (i.e., no metastatic SLN but metastatic non-SLN) [6]. In 1996, Burke et al. introduced the SLNB in high-risk endometrial cancer, similarly using isosulfan blue for visual guidance. The authors identified the SLN in 10 of 15 patients [7]. In 2002, Levenback et al. described the first study on preoperative and intraoperative SLN mapping for invasive cervical cancer. They identified at least one SLN in 33 patients with preoperative imaging, and detected intraoperatively at least one SLN in all 39 patients; 1 patient had a false-negative SLN [8]. Blue dye has been the first lymphatic tracer for intraoperative SLN mapping in gynecological cancers [6, 7]. However, this visual marker has a low tissue penetration, and thus is not applicable in obese patients. Moreover, it is contraindicated in women during pregnancy and lactation or with possible anaphylactic allergic reactions (favism). ^{99m}Tc-labeled colloids are currently the lymphatic mapping radiotracers widely used for gynecological cancers [8, 9]. In particular, ^{99m}Tc emits gamma rays with a relatively short half-life (6 h), and so is safe for both patients and medical personnel. Nevertheless, the combination of ^{99m}Tc-labeled colloid and blue dye is the most appropriate technique for SLN mapping, because it is associated with a greater SLN detection rate than blue dye or the radiocolloid alone, especially for cervical cancer [10]. Recently, the fluorescence guidance with a marker like indocyanine green (ICG) has been introduced for the SLN mapping in gynecological cancers [11, 12]. This marker emits a light signal in the near-infrared band after excitation, thereby offering a real-time intraoperative guidance with higher tissue penetration than the blue dye. However, the rapid lymphatic diffusion of ICG causes the visualization of more lymph nodes than SLNs. Even more recently, a hybrid tracer, known as ICG-^{99m}Tc-nanocolloid, has been used for SLNB in vulvar cancer and cervical cancer [13–15]. This radiotracer combines both radioactive (^{99m}Tc-nanocolloid) and fluorescent (ICG) guidance in a single injection, thereby allowing both a preoperative and intraoperative lymphatic mapping.

Key Learning Points
- SLNB is a minimally invasive surgical approach for lymph node staging in gynecological cancers.
- In 1994, Levenback et al. published the first study on SLNB for vulvar cancer, using visual guidance with a blue dye.

- The combination of radiotracer and blue dye is the most appropriate technique for SLN mapping, especially for cervical cancer.
- A dual-signature hybrid tracer, ICG-^{99m}Tc-nanocolloid, has been recently used for vulvar cancer and cervical cancer. It combines both radioactive and fluorescent guidance in a single injection, thereby allowing both preoperative and intraoperative lymphatic mapping.

14.2 The Clinical Problem

Vulvar cancer is a rare disease in the Western world, with an incidence rate of 2.4 per 100,000 women per year in the United States [16]. In younger patients vulvar cancer is mostly associated with infection from the human papillomavirus, whereas vulvar cancer occurring in elderly women is rarely associated with the human papillomavirus [17]. Squamous cell carcinoma constitutes about 90% of vulvar cancers [18]. The pattern of metastatic spread is mainly lymphatic, while hematogenous metastasis is uncommon. The key prognostic factor is the presence of lymph node metastasis. Indeed, the 5-year overall survival rate decreases from 95% in the absence of groin metastasis to 62% in the presence of groin metastasis [19]. Only 25–35% of women with early-stage vulvar squamous cell carcinoma have groin lymph node metastasis [19]. Therefore, the majority of these women undergo unnecessary inguino-femoral lymphadenectomy with a high risk of postoperative short- and long-term morbidity, such as infection and breakdown of the surgical wound, lymphocyst formation, and lymphedema of the legs [20]. These postoperative complications may severely impact the patient's quality of life, and delay the inguinal-pelvic adjuvant radiation if indicated. To minimize these complications, SLNB is recommended in well-selected women with early-stage vulvar cancer [2, 3]. Furthermore, preoperative SLN mapping enables to define lymphatic drainage of the tumor, which is useful for planning a more personalized surgery. Lymphatic drainage of a lateral tumor is mainly ipsilateral, while lymphatic drainage of a midline tumor is bilateral. Thus, when a unilateral drainage in a midline lesion is present, the lymphatic basins of both sides should be explored [2, 3]. Finding SLN metastasis guides for a more extensive lymphadenectomy, or adjuvant radiotherapy. Instead, nonmetastatic SLNB avoids extensive lymphadenectomy, and is associated with a low incidence of relapse (2.5%) [21], a low incidence of postoperative complications [9], and good survival [21]. Finally, SLNB involves a shorter operation time and length of hospital stay, lower costs, and improved pathological examination than lymphadenectomy [22].

Cervical cancer is the third most common female cancer worldwide, with an incidence rate of 7.4 cases per 100,000 women per year in the United States [16]. It occurs mainly in younger women, and is frequently associated with the human papillomavirus infection. Squamous cell carcinoma is the most common cancer of the uterine cervix. The key prognostic factor is the presence of pelvic lymph node metastasis. Indeed, the 5-year overall survival rate decreases from 95–88% in the absence of lymph node metastasis to 78–51% in presence of lymph node metastasis in early stages IB and IIA [23]. Pelvic lymphadenectomy is an overtreatment in early-stage cervical cancer, due to the low incidence (21%) of metastatic lymph nodes [24]. Moreover, it is associated with short- and long-term morbidities such as lymphocyst formation, nerve injury, venous thromboembolism, and lower extremity lymphedema. In an attempt to reduce these morbidities, SLNB is recommended in well-selected women with early cervical cancer [4]. Furthermore, SLNB enables to identify unusual lymphatic drainage patterns, such as those towards the para-aortic, common iliac, internal iliac, and parametrium areas [25], known as Marnitz areas 1, 2, 5, and 6, respectively [26]. In particular, Bats et al. showed that 3/23 patients with SLN metastases (13%) had a single metastatic lymph node located only in unexpected areas and detected only by SLNB [25]. Additionally, SLNB increases the identification of micrometastases (>0.2 but ≤2 mm) and isolated tumor cells (≤0.2 mm) through SLN ultrastaging with immunohistochemistry [25]. The lymphatic spread of cervical tumor (midline organ) is mainly bilateral; thus, if only ipsilateral is observed during SLN mapping, a contralateral pelvic lymphadenectomy is necessary [4, 27].

Endometrial cancer is the most common female cancer worldwide, with an incidence rate of 24.9 per 100,000 women per year in the United States [16]. It occurs principally in older women and adenocarcinoma is the most common histologic type. Lymph node status is the major prognostic factor in endometrial cancers. Indeed, the 5-year survival rate varies from 52 to 44% in women with metastatic pelvic or para-aortic lymph nodes [28]. Systematic pelvic and para-aortic lymphadenectomy was traditionally advised for all patients. Although lymphadenectomy provides an accurate lymph node staging for guiding adjuvant therapy, it has a high risk of postoperative complications without benefit in terms of overall survival and recurrence-free survival [29]. SLNB, as a more selective and tailored lymphadenectomy, is currently recommended in well-selected women with endometrial cancer [5]. In particular,

SLNB with ultrastaging may increase the detection of lymph node metastasis (micrometastasis and isolated tumor cells) with low false-negative rates [30], and thus avoids unnecessary surgical complications in women with negative lymph nodes.

> **Key Learning Points**
> - In all gynecological cancers the key prognostic factor is the presence of lymph node metastases.
> - Preoperative SLN mapping enables to define the lymphatic drainage of gynecological tumors, which is useful for planning a more personalized surgery.
> - SLNB increases the identification of lymph node metastases (micrometastases and isolated tumor cells) through ultrastaging.

14.3   Lymphatic Drainage of Gynecological Tumors

In vulvar cancer, the lymphatic spread is principally to the superficial inguinal nodes, then to the deep inguinal nodes, and to the pelvic lymph nodes. However, clitoris and perineum cancers can drain directly to the deep lymph nodes or to the pelvic lymph nodes. Nevertheless, it is unlikely to find pelvic metastases without groin metastasis [9]. The presence of pelvic metastasis is considered as distant metastasis [31]. Lateral tumors of the vulva (more than 1–2 cm from the midline) most likely spread to the ipsilateral lymph nodes, while midline tumors (within 1–2 cm from midline) drain to both groins. The most common localization of metastatic lymph nodes is the groin, especially in the medial superior of Daseler's zones [32].

In cervical cancer, the lymphatic drainage is bilateral owing to the midline location of the uterine cervix in the pelvis. There are three different lymphatic pathways: (a) laterally to the external iliac lymph nodes; (b) posterolaterally to the internal iliac lymph nodes; and (c) posteriorly to the presacral lymph nodes. The most common locations of pelvic lymph nodes are the obturator region and the external iliac basin [24].

In endometrial cancer, the lymphatic drainage is bilateral due to the midline position of corpus uteri in the pelvis. There are two different lymphatic routes: the upper segment of corpus uteri drains to the para-aortic region, while the lower segment of corpus uteri drains to the pelvic lymph nodes. The most common location of metastatic lymph nodes is in the pelvic area [7].

14.4 Indications and Contraindications of SLN Mapping

In women with squamous cell carcinoma of the vulva, SLNB is indicated in case of unifocal primary tumor smaller than 4 cm in diameter, with more than 1 mm depth of stromal invasion and clinically at N0 stage (2009 FIGO Stages IB and II) [2] (Table 14.1). In women with vulvar melanoma, SLNB is indicated in tumor with Breslow thickness between 1 and 4 mm (Table 14.1).

SLNB is recommended in women with early-stage cervical cancer who have a primary tumor ≤4 cm in diameter, with depth of stromal invasion >3 mm, and clinically at N0 stage (stage IA1 with lymphovascular invasion [LVI], stages IA2, IB1, and IIA1) (Table 14.1) [4]. However, the best detection rates and mapping results are in tumors <2 cm in diameter [33].

SLNB is advised in women with early-stage (stages IB and II) endometrial cancer who have uterine-confined disease, grading G3 (poorly differentiated or undifferentiated), one half or more of myometrial invasion, and high-risk histologies (papillary serous, carcinosarcoma, or clear-cell cancer) (Table 14.1) [5].

For all gynecological cancers, SLNB is not indicated in the following cases: (a) presence of metastatic lymph nodes on clinical examination; (b) prior surgery of the tumor or previous lymphadenectomy; (c) prior radiotherapy of the inguino-pelvic area; and (d) contraindication to surgical treatment (Table 14.1) [1].

Table 14.1 Indication and contraindication for SLNB in gynecological cancers

Gynecological tumor	Indications	Contraindications (for all gynecological cancers)
Vulvar cancer	– Squamous cell carcinoma – Tumors <4 cm – Stages IB and II	– Clinical N+ – Prior surgery – Prior radiotherapy of inguinal-pelvic area – Contraindication to surgical treatment
Vulvar melanoma	– Breslow thickness 1–4 mm	
Cervical cancer	– Squamous cell carcinoma – Tumors ≤4 cm (better results if <2 cm) – Stages: IA1 with LVI, IA2, IB1, IIA1	
Endometrial cancer	– Uterine-confined tumor – Myometrial invasion ≥50% – Grade G3 – High-risk histological subtype – Stages IB and II	

14.5 Modalities of Radiocolloid Injection

As a first step, a local anesthetic such as lidocaine is applied on the primary vulvar cancer or scar for pain relief. After 5–10 min from application of the anesthetic, the radiotracer (^{99m}Tc-nanocolloid or ICG-^{99m}Tc-nanocolloid) is injected intradermally into the four quadrants around the tumor edge or scar using a 25-gauge needle [1].

In cervical cancer, the speculum is used for helping to expose the cervical orifice. Afterwards, the radiotracer (^{99m}Tc-nanocolloid or ICG-^{99m}Tc-nanocolloid) is injected into the subserosa in four divided quadrants around the primary tumor or cervical orifice, using a 20- or 22-gauge spinal needle. In case of prior conization, the injection should be around the scar. In case of small tumors, the submucosal injection would be preferred, while the injection into the necrotic part of the tumor should be carefully avoided, especially in the presence of large tumors [1].

In endometrial cancer, there are three different modalities of injection. The first is cervical injection. The radiotracer is injected in the four cardinal points of the cervical orifice before surgery, enabling to obtain the preoperative SLN mapping. The second is endometrial injection: the radiotracer is injected around the primary tumor through a hysteroscope at the beginning of surgery, therefore without preoperative SLN mapping. The third is myometrial injection: the radiotracer is injected in the myometrium during surgery. An alternative modality is myometrial injection guided by transvaginal ultrasonography [1].

14.6 Preoperative SLN Imaging

Scintigraphic images are obtained using a dual-head gamma camera equipped with low-energy, high-resolution collimators. The energy window should be ±15% centered over the 140 Kev photopeak of ^{99m}Tc. The acquisition protocol includes four steps (Fig. 14.1).

In the case of vulvar cancer, the first step is the dynamic acquisition. Five minutes after radiotracer injection, dynamic images of the pelvis in the anterior and posterior views are recorded by acquiring 30 frames of 30-s duration, with a 128×128 matrix and zoom 1 (a dynamic study is not acquired for cervical and endometrial cancers). Dynamic images enable to visualize the lymphatic ducts directly draining from the injection site (the primary lesion) to the lymph nodes, thus identifying bilateral or unilateral lymphatic drainage from the tumor and the first-draining lymph nodes.

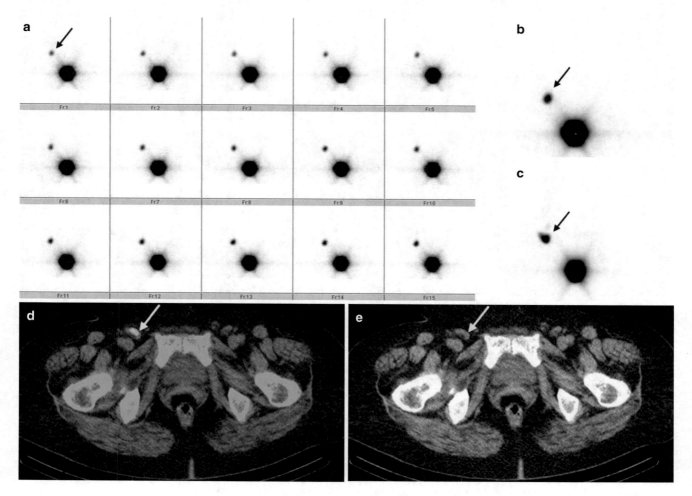

Fig. 14.1 A 75-year-old woman with invasive vulvar squamous cell carcinoma of the right labia majora. Anterior dynamic (**a**), early (**b**), and late (**c**) planar images show unilateral lymphatic drainage with visualization of a single SLN (black arrow) in the right groin, corresponding to a focal uptake (yellow arrow) in the transaxial fused SPECT/CT image (**d**) and normal-sized lymph node located in the medial superior inguinal zone on transaxial low-dose CT (**e**)

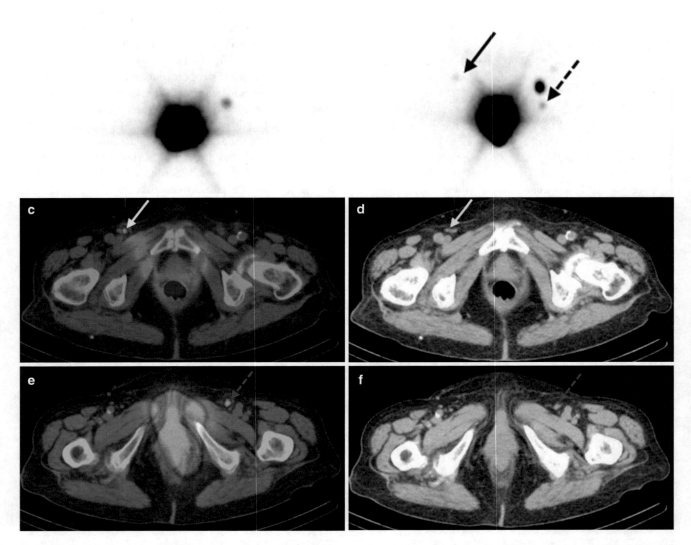

Fig. 14.2 An 85-year-old woman with squamous cell carcinoma of the clitoris. Anterior dynamic and early (**a**) images show unilateral lymphatic drainage with visualization of a single SLN in left groin. Anterior late image (**b**) shows bilateral lymphatic drainage with visualization of one additional SLN (arrow) in right groin corresponding to a single focal uptake (yellow arrow) in transaxial fused SPECT/CT image (**c**) and normal-sized lymph node (yellow arrow) located in the medial superior inguinal zone on transaxial low-dose CT (**d**), plus another additional SLN in left groin (dashed arrow, **b**) corresponding to a focal uptake (red dashed arrow) in transaxial fused SPECT/CT images (**e**) and normal-sized lymph node (red dashed arrow) localized in the medial inferior inguinal zone on transaxial low-dose CT (**f**)

The second step is acquisition on an early planar scan. Immediately after the dynamic study (or about 20–25 min after radiocolloid injection), early planar images in anterior and lateral views are acquired for 3–5 min, with a 128 × 128 matrix and zoom 1. In cervical and endometrial cancers, the early planar images are acquired 30 min after radiotracer injection. The early images allow identification of the number of higher echelon node(s), that is, the lymph node(s) draining from the SLNs.

The third step is acquisition of a late planar scan. About 120 min after radiotracer injection, late planar images in anterior and lateral views are acquired using the same parameters as for the early planar scan. These images permit to identify additional SLNs and higher echelon nodes that appear later (Fig. 14.2).

Afterwards, a reference source (such as ^{57}Co-penmarker) is used for SLN localization on the overlying groin skin in women with vulvar cancer. The site of SLN is then skin-

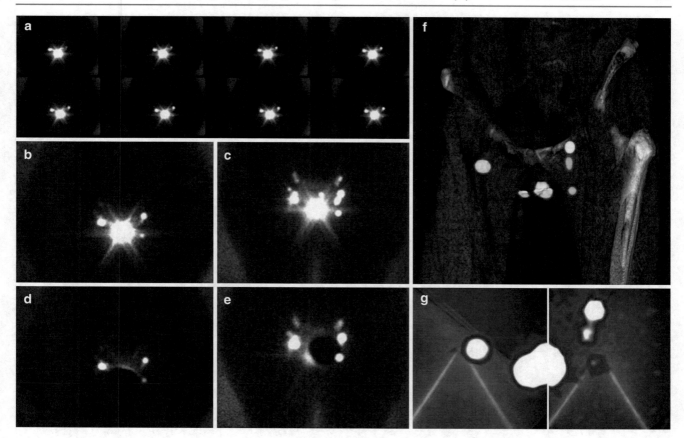

Fig. 14.3 A 53-year-old woman with squamous cell carcinoma of clitoris. After injection of ^{99m}Tc-nanocolloid into four depots surrounding the tumor, a dynamic study of the pelvis (**a**) was acquired. Early (**b**) and late (**c**) planar images show bilateral lymphatic drainage and a star artifact at the site of injection. The use of lead pieces as a shield may improve the early (**d**) and late (**e**) images, but much care must be taken in order to avoid covering SLNs close to the site of injection. Coronal CT image with 3D volume rendering (**f**) in variable angles enables to clearly separate the injection activity from the draining lymph nodes. The use of a portable gamma camera can help the precise marking of SLNs on the groin skin (**g**), and to assess intraoperatively complete removal of SLNs

marked with indelible ink in the anterior and lateral static views, so allowing a small and selective incision in vulvar cancers. On the other hand, a mark on the skin is not a useful guide in cervical and endometrial tumors, due to overdistension of the abdominal wall during surgery.

The fourth step is acquisition of a SPECT/CT scan. After acquiring the late planar scan, SPECT/CT images are obtained using 20 s per frame, 3° angular views, with a 128 × 128 matrix and zoom 1. Reinjection of the radiocolloid is recommended when no lymphatic drainage is visualized on the SPECT/CT scan [1].

14.7 Added Value of SPECT/CT Imaging

In gynecological tumors, especially cervical and endometrial cancers, lymphatic drainage to deep lymph nodes is difficult to localize on planar images. Hence, SPECT/CT plays a relevant role for preoperative SLN mapping. In particular, SPECT/CT imaging provides an exact anatomical location of SLNs (Figs. 14.3, 14.4, and 14.5) [32, 34–39], and allows detection of a greater number of SLNs than planar images [32, 37], and detection of SLNs close to the injection site (especially for cervical cancer in which the deep location of corpus uteri hides the parametrial SLNs [36, 37, 40]), or lymphatic drainage to unusual locations [34]. Furthermore, SPECT/CT images decrease false-positive findings due to external contamination [41], or presence of radioactivity in enlarged lymphatic vessels [39]. SPECT/CT images also help in the visualization of bilateral drainage from endometrial cancer, especially in obese patients (Fig. 14.5). A novel approach to SLN mapping in patients with gynecological cancers is the fusion of ultrasound and 3D SPECT/CT images, as shown by the encouraging results of a feasibility study reported by Garganese et al. in five patients with vulvar cancer [42].

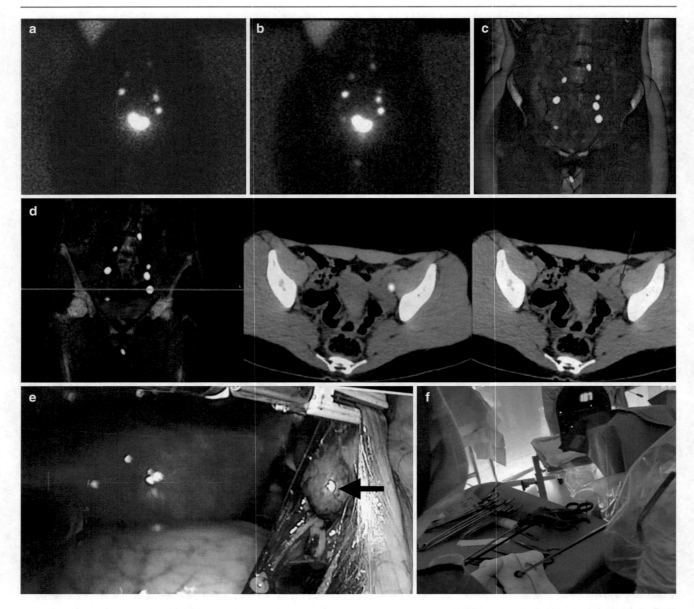

Fig. 14.4 A 28-year-old woman with early-stage cervical cancer (stage IB1). The hybrid tracer, ICG-^{99m}Tc-nanocolloid, was preoperatively injected into four depots around the tumor. Early (**a**) and late (**b**) planar images of the pelvis show the bilateral drainage with some asymmetry in lymph node distribution. Coronal CT images with 3D volume rendering (**c**, **d**) and their corresponding transaxial CT images (**d**) show the correct anatomical position of SLNs (red arrow). Intraoperatively, 2 mL of methylene blue dye was injected in the same site as the hybrid tracer. During laparoscopic approach (**e**), a blue-stained and fluorescent SLN (black arrow) was clearly depicted in the external iliac area. This SLN shows radioactivity (187 counts/s, **f**) during the ex vivo counting with laparoscopy-adapted gamma probe

Key Learning Points

- Firstly, the dynamic images of the pelvis in anterior and posterior projections are acquired 5 min after the radiotracer injection. This step is not used for cervical cancers and endometrial cancers.
- Secondly, early planar images and late planar images in anterior and lateral projections are acquired for identifying additional SLN and the higher echelon nodes.
- Thirdly, SPECT/CT images are acquired for providing an exact anatomical localization of SLN, detecting deep SLN or close to the injection site, and helping the visualization of bilateral SLNs, especially in obese patients.

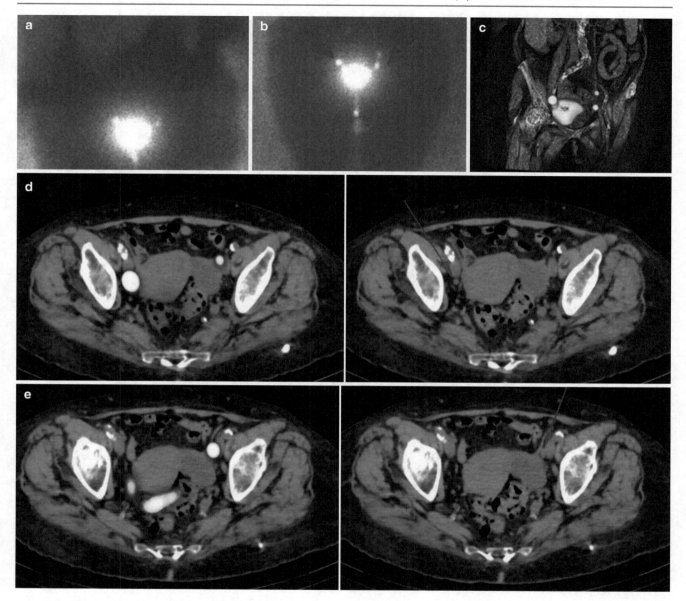

Fig. 14.5 A 36-year-old woman with high-risk endometrial cancer. The day before surgery the hybrid tracer, ICG-^{99m}Tc-nanocolloid, was injected in the four cardinal points of the cervical orifice. Early (**a**) and late (**b**) planar images show bilateral drainage (red arrows) in the pelvic area. Coronal CT image with 3D volume rendering (**c**) shows the depicted SLNs with the surrounding anatomical structures. Transaxial fused SPECT/CT images and their corresponding transaxial CT images (**d, e**) help to better define the position of these SLNs in the right and left external iliac vessels

14.8   Intraoperative SLN Detection

Prior to surgery and after starting the general anesthesia, blue dye or ICG is injected around the tumor or scar, in the same site as the radiotracer had been injected. A volume of 0.5–1 mL of blue dye is used in vulvar cancer, whereas larger volumes (2–4 mL) are required for cervical cancer and endometrial cancer [1]. While the blue dye is directly visible, a fluorescence probe and gamma probe (both with a sterile cover) are used for the intraoperative detection of fluorescent SLNs and radioactive SLNs, respectively. In particular, hand-held probes are used for vulvar cancer, whereas laparoscopy-adapted probes are used in cervical cancer and endometrial cancer. In vulvar cancer, the gamma probe is placed near the mark on the groin skin for identifying the area of greatest radioactivity (preoperative counting), thus guiding the skin incision. In cervical cancer and endometrial cancer, preoperative gamma counting is not possible due to the deep locations of SLNs. The probe is used intraoperatively for localizing the SLNs (intraoperative counting). During surgery, the gamma probe should not be directed towards the injection site. Shortly after excision of the radioactive SLNs, the probe is used to measure ex vivo SLN radioactivity (ex vivo counting), and background radioactivity in order to confirm the correct removal of all radioactive SLNs (at least 10% of the ex vivo counting of the hottest SLN) according to the previous lymphoscintigraphy results. Finally, all excised SLNs are sent for pathological examination. The SLNs are submitted to routine hematoxylin and eosin staining and, when no metastases are detected, ultrastaging is to be performed with immunohistochemistry. Patients with metastatic SLNs are scheduled for lymphadenectomy.

Recently, a small-field-of view, dedicated portable gamma cameras have been used for increasing the intraoperative detection rate (Fig. 14.3) [13, 15]. Acquisition time for intraoperative imaging is only 1 min, so the procedure might take 5–10 min in total. Comparison of the intraoperative images acquired before and after SLNB provides several benefits: (1) better localization of SLNs, especially for the parametrial SLNs that are close to the site of injections; (2) possibility to remove gamma counts due to liver's interference during resection of the para-aortic lymph nodes; and (3) assessment of completeness of SLN excision in the surgical bed.

The intraoperative SLN detection rate is high using the combined technique of radiocolloid and blue dye, especially in cervical cancer (Fig. 14.4) [10]. The majority of patients with endometrial cancer are obese, so the fat tissue located around the lymphatic ducts hampers visualization of the blue-stained lymph nodes. For this reason the combined technique has a limited value in endometrial cancer compared to the use of radiotracer alone [43]. Conversely, ICG is commonly used in the clinical routine because it provides a higher SLN detection rate than the blue dye [30, 43].

In cervical and endometrial tumors, it is important to consider the SLN detection separately in both sides of the pelvis. Thus, if there is no SLN visualization in one side, a side-specific node dissection is needed.

> **Key Learning Points**
> - During surgery, blue dye or ICG is injected around the tumor or scar in the same site as the radiotracer.
> - Only in vulvar cancer, the gamma probe is placed near the mark on the groin skin for identifying the area of greatest radioactivity (preoperative counting) and thus guiding the skin incision.
> - The gamma probe is used intraoperatively for localizing the SLNs (intraoperative counting) and postoperatively to measure ex vivo radioactivity of the excised SLNs (ex vivo counting).
> - All excised SLNs are processed for routine hematoxylin and eosin staining; when no metastases are detected, ultrastaging with immunohistochemistry is to be performed for revealing small metastases.
> - Every patient with metastatic SLNs is scheduled for lymphadenectomy.

14.9 Technical Pitfalls in SLN Mapping

Several technical pitfalls can interfere with the SLN procedure in gynecological tumors. One typical pitfall is represented by the false-positive SLN. One possible cause is radioactive contamination during injection of the radiocolloid [41]. In cervical or endometrial cancer, the retrograde radioactive leakage during the injection in the vagina can contaminate the gamma camera. For this reason, the use of an absorbent sheet during the injection is recommended, to be changed before imaging. Otherwise, hot spots produced by contamination can be easily identified in the lateral view of planar images or with SPECT/CT imaging. Another possible case of false-positive SLN is when the true SLN is totally replaced by tumor cells causing a lymphatic stasis, and consequently a bypass of lymphatic flow to another lymph node [44].

Another typical pitfall is represented by the non-visualization of SLNs. Possible causes for such occurrence include technical problems during radiocolloid injection, such as an injection too deep, or loss of injection fluid, or in case of overweight patients [45]. Another possible cause is the lymph node damage due to chemotherapy or radiotherapy, which can lead to lymphatic stasis. Moreover, gamma probe exploration of the surgical bed can be affected by pathophysiological uptake such as (1) the site of injection, especially in cervical cancer where hysterectomy is performed only after excluding lymph node metastasis node; (2) ^{99m}Tc activity accumulated in the ureters because of physiologic kidney excretion; or (3) liver activity due to radiocolloid uptake in the reticuloendothelial system [1].

To minimize these pitfalls, it is crucial to include well-selected women with clinically negative lymph node status, to standardize the procedure including SPECT/CT images in the clinical workup, to use both tracers for intraoperative guidance (blue/ICG and radiotracer), and to perform the procedure in experienced tertiary referral centers.

> **Key Learning Points**
> - Technical pitfalls are the contamination during the radioactive injection, the lymphatic stasis due to a metastatic SLN, and consequently a bypass of lymphatic flow to another lymph node as well as too deep injection or loss of injection fluid with non-visualization of SLN.
> - To minimize these pitfalls, it is crucial to include SPECT/CT imaging in the clinical workup, to use both tracers (blue/ICG and radiotracer), and to perform the procedure in experienced tertiary referral centers.

Acknowledgements This chapter is a revision of the original chapter written by P. Paredes and S. Vidal-Sicart in the previous edition of the book.

Clinical Cases

Case 14.1 SLN Mapping in Vulvar Carcinoma: False-Positive Finding Due to Lymphatic Duct

Alberto Fragano, Danilo Fortini, and Luca Zagaria

Background Clinical Case

A 73-year-old woman with two foci of invasive vulvar squamous cell carcinoma located in both left and right labia minora. She was scheduled for radical vulvectomy and bilateral SLNB.

Lymphoscintigraphy

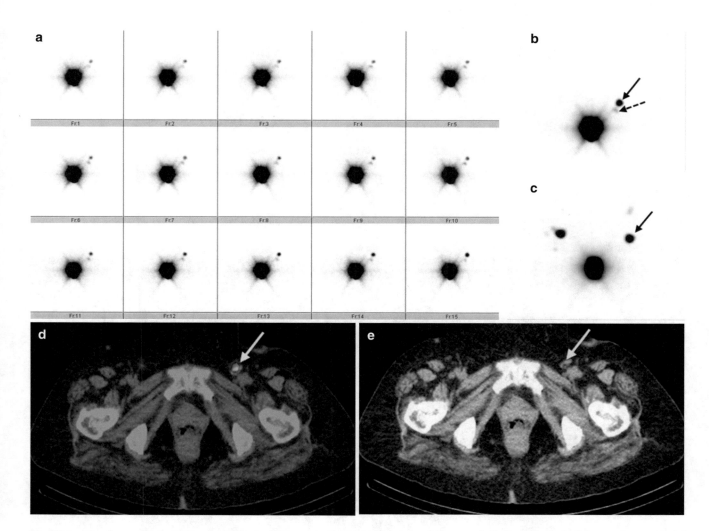

Fig. 14.6 After the application of local anesthesia, ⁹⁹ᵐTc-nanocolloid (four aliquots of 74 MBq in 0.2 mL) was injected around the two lesions the day before the surgery (2-day protocol). The anterior dynamic (**a**) and early (**b**) images show unilateral lymphatic drainage with visualization of two SLNs (arrows, **b**) in the left groin. The anterior late image (**c**) shows bilateral lymphatic drainage with only one SLN (arrow) in the left groin corresponding to a single focal uptake (yellow arrow) on transaxial SPECT/CT image (**d**) and a non-enlarged lymph node (yellow arrow) located in the medial superior inguinal zone on transaxial low-dose CT (**e**). In conclusion, the two foci of uptake defined as SLNs in the left groin at dynamic and early planar images correspond to one SLN and to its lymphatic vessel on transaxial fused SPECT/CT image, respectively

Case 14.2 SLN Mapping in Vulvar Carcinoma: Visualization of Pelvic SLN

Alberto Fragano, Danilo Fortini, and Germano Perotti

Background Clinical Case

An 82-year-old woman who had a vulvar squamous cell carcinoma of clitoris. She was scheduled for radical vulvectomy and bilateral SLNB.

Lymphoscintigraphy

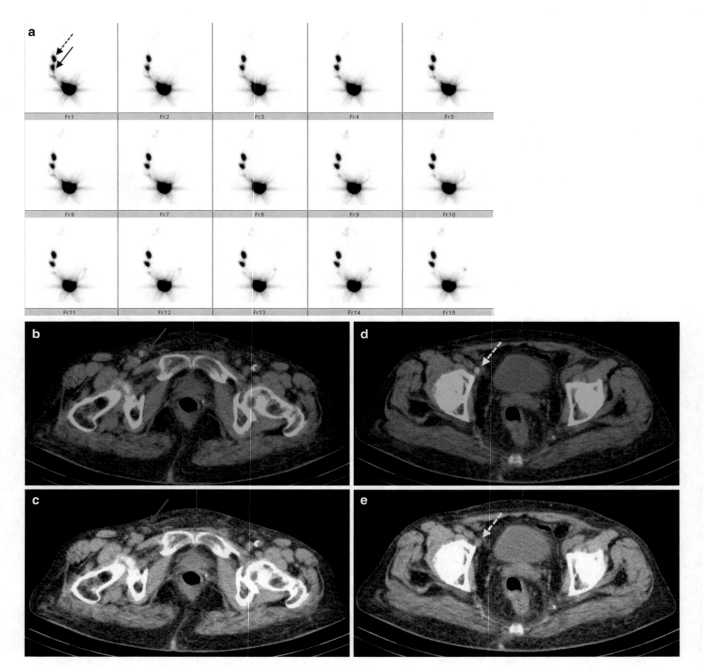

Fig. 14.7 After the application of local anesthesia, ^{99m}Tc-nanocolloid (four aliquots of 37 MBq in 0.1 mL) was injected around the tumor the same day of the surgery (1-day protocol). The anterior dynamic images (**a**) show bilateral lymphatic drainage with one SLN in the right groin (arrow) corresponding to one focal uptake (red arrow) on transaxial SPECT/CT image (**b**) and non-enlarged lymph node (red arrow) in the medial superior zone on transaxial low-dose CT (**c**), plus another focal uptake in the pelvic area (yellow dashed arrow, **d**) corresponding to a non-enlarged lymph node (yellow dashed arrow) located in the external iliac zone on transaxial low-dose CT (**e**)

Case 14.3 SLN Mapping in Cervical Cancer: Visualization of Para-aortic SLN

Sergi   Vidal-Sicart,   Andrés   Perissinotti,   and
Sebastian Casanueva

Background Clinical Case

A 34-year-old woman who had early-stage cervical cancer (stage IB1).

Lymphoscintigraphy

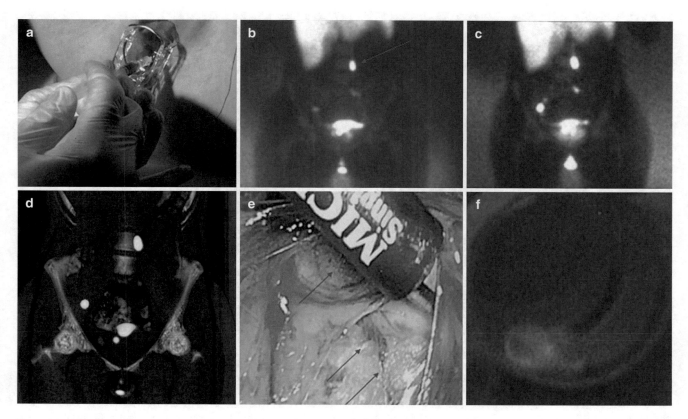

Fig. 14.8 After peritumoral injection of 111 MBq of ICG-^{99m}Tc-nanocolloid in four deposits of 0.5 mL each (**a**), anterior planar images were obtained at 30 min (early imaging, **b**) and 120 min (late imaging, **c**). A focal uptake in the para-aortic area (red arrow) was clearly seen in the early image (**b**), and was considered as para-aortic SLN. Coronal CT image with 3D volume rendering (**d**) shows the depicted SLN with the surrounding anatomical structures. It is unusual to find para-aortic SLNs after radiotracer injection into the uterine cervix. Para-aortic nodal spread occurs usually orderly, with progressive involvement of the pelvic and common iliac lymph nodes before para-aortic lymph nodes. However, cervical cancer can occasionally metastasize directly to the para-aortic lymph nodes by embolization of the posterior lymphatic pathway (presacral area). Just before surgery, 2 mL of methylene blue dye was injected in the same site as the radiotracer. During laparoscopy (**e**), a net of blue-stained lymphatic channels (blue arrows) were depicted running upwards to the para-aortic SLN. This SLN was excised and exhibited radioactivity (150 cps/s), fluorescence (**f**), and blue color. Histopathology did not show metastatic involvement in this, nor in two additional SLNs located in the pelvis

Case 14.4 SLN Mapping in Endometrial Cancer

Sergi Vidal-Sicart, Andrés Tapias, and Sebastian Casanueva

Background Clinical Case

A 70-year-old woman who had endometrial carcinoma with myometrial involvement >50% of the uterine wall thickness.

Lymphoscintigraphy

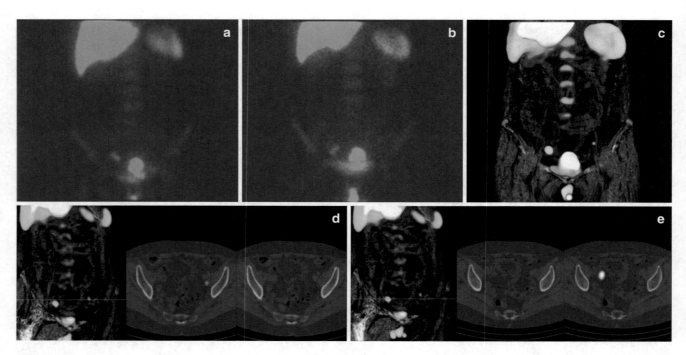

Fig. 14.9 After injection of 185 MBq of hybrid tracer (ICG-99mTc-nanocolloid) in the myometrial tissue guided by transvaginal ultrasound, early (at 30 min, **a**) and late (at 120 min, **b**) images were obtained. The deep injection in the myometrial area results in fast diffusion into the bloodstream with ensuing early visualization of the bone marrow that can hinder visualization of lymph nodes. Only one area of focal uptake in the right pelvic area was seen at early (**a**) and late (**b**) planar imaging, and was considered as a pelvic SLN. Coronal CT images with 3D volume rendering (**c**) and their corresponding transaxial CT images (**d**, **e**) show a second focal uptake in the left pelvic side (red arrow, **d**) corresponding to a second SLN in the left obturator fossae. During surgery, only the left SLN was resected. No activity was observed with the laparoscopic adapted gamma probe nor fluorescence was detected in the right pelvic area. Histopathology revealed metastasis of the resected left SLN. Pelvic lymphadenectomy resulted in harvesting of 12 negative lymph nodes and 1 positive node in the left side, and only 5 negative lymph nodes in the right pelvis

References

1. Giammarile F, Bozkurt MF, Cibula D, et al. The EANM clinical and technical guidelines for lymphoscintigraphy and sentinel node localization in gynaecological cancers. Eur J Nucl Med Mol Imaging. 2014;41(7):1463–77.
2. Koh WJ, Abu-Rustum NR, Bean S, et al. NCCN clinical practice guidelines in oncology (NCCN guidelines), vulvar cancer (squamous cell carcinoma): version 2.2019. 2018. https://www.nccn.org/professionals/physician_gls/pdf/vulvar.pdf. Accessed 6 Aug 2019.
3. Oonk MHM, Planchamp F, Baldwin P, et al. European Society of Gynaecological Oncology guidelines for the management of patients with vulvar cancer. Int J Gynecol Cancer. 2017;27(4):832–7.
4. Koh WJ, Abu-Rustum NR, Bean S, et al. Cervical cancer, version 3.2019, NCCN clinical practice guidelines in oncology. J Natl Compr Cancer Netw. 2019;17(1):64–84.
5. Koh WJ, Abu-Rustum NR, Bean S, et al. NCCN clinical practice guidelines in oncology (NCCN guidelines), uterine neoplasms: version 3.2019. 2019. https://www.nccn.org/professionals/physician_gls/pdf/uterine.pdf. Accessed 6 Aug 2019.
6. Levenback C, Burke TW, Gershenson DM, et al. Intraoperative lymphatic mapping for vulvar cancer. Obstet Gynecol. 1994;84(2):163–7.
7. Burke TW, Levenback C, Tornos C, et al. Intra-abdominal lymphatic mapping to direct selective pelvic and paraaortic lymphadenectomy in women with high-risk endometrial cancer: results of a pilot study. Gynecol Oncol. 1996;62(2):169–73.
8. Levenback C, Coleman RL, Burke TW, et al. Lymphatic mapping and sentinel node identification in patients with cervix cancer undergoing radical hysterectomy and pelvic lymphadenectomy. J Clin Oncol. 2002;20:688–93.
9. Van der Zee AG, Oonk MH, De Hullu JA, et al. Sentinel node dissection is safe in the treatment of early-stage vulvar cancer. J Clin Oncol. 2008;26(6):884–9.
10. Lécuru F, Mathevet P, Querleu D, et al. Bilateral negative sentinel nodes accurately predict absence of lymph node metastasis in early cervical cancer: results of the SENTICOL study. J Clin Oncol. 2011;29(13):1686–91.
11. Crane LM, Themelis G, Arts HJ, et al. Intraoperative near-infrared fluorescence imaging for sentinel lymph node detection in vulvar cancer: first clinical results. Gynecol Oncol. 2011;120(2):291–5.
12. Rossi EC, Ivanova A, Boggess JF. Robotically assisted fluorescence-guided lymph node mapping with ICG for gynecologic malignancies: a feasibility study. Gynecol Oncol. 2012;124(1):78–82.
13. Mathéron HM, van den Berg NS, Brouwer OR, et al. Multimodal surgical guidance towards the sentinel node in vulvar cancer. Gynecol Oncol. 2013;131(3):720–5.
14. Verbeek FP, Tummers QR, Rietbergen DD, et al. Sentinel lymph node biopsy in vulvar cancer using combined radioactive and fluorescence guidance. Int J Gynecol Cancer. 2015;25(6):1086–93.
15. Paredes P, Vidal-Sicart S, Campos F, et al. Role of ICG-^{99m}Tc-nanocolloid for sentinel lymph node detection in cervical cancer: a pilot study. Eur J Nucl Med Mol Imaging. 2017;44(11):1853–61.
16. Howlader N, Noone AM, Krapcho M, et al. SEER cancer statistics review, 1975–2014. Bethesda: National Cancer Institute; 2017. https://seer.cancer.gov/csr/1975_2014/, based on November 2016 SEER data submission, posted to the SEER web site, April 2017.
17. Del Pino M, Rodriguez-Carunchio L, Ordi J. Pathways of vulvar intraepithelial neoplasia and squamous cell carcinoma. Histopathology. 2013;62(1):161–75.
18. Hacker NF, Eifel PJ, van der Velden J. Cancer of the vulva. Int J Gynaecol Obstet. 2012;119(2):S90–6.
19. Burger MP, Hollema H, Emanuels AG, et al. The importance of the groin node status for the survival of T1 and T2 vulval carcinoma patients. Gynecol Oncol. 1995;57(3):327–34.
20. Gaarenstroom KN, Kenter GG, Trimbos JB, et al. Postoperative complications after vulvectomy and inguinofemoral lymphadenectomy using separate groin incisions. Int J Gynecol Cancer. 2003;13(4):522–7.
21. Te Grootenhuis NC, van der Zee AG, van Doorn HC, et al. Sentinel nodes in vulvar cancer: long-term follow-up of the GROningen INternational study on sentinel nodes in vulvar cancer (GROINSS-V) I. Gynecol Oncol. 2016;140(1):8–14.
22. McCann GA, Cohn DE, Jewell EL, et al. Lymphatic mapping and sentinel lymph node dissection compared to complete lymphadenectomy in the management of early-stage vulvar cancer: a cost-utility analysis. Gynecol Oncol. 2015;136(2):300–4.
23. Kim SM, Choi HS, Byun JS. Overall 5-year survival rate and prognostic factors in patients with stage IB and IIA cervical cancer treated by radical hysterectomy and pelvic lymph node dissection. Int J Gynecol Cancer. 2000;10(4):305–12.
24. Benedetti-Panici P, Maneschi F, Scambia G, et al. Lymphatic spread of cervical cancer: an anatomical and pathological study based on 225 radical hysterectomies with systematic pelvic and aortic lymphadenectomy. Gynecol Oncol. 1996;62(1):19–24.
25. Bats AS, Mathevet P, Buenerd A, et al. The sentinel node technique detects unexpected drainage pathways and allows nodal ultrastaging in early cervical cancer: insights from the multicenter prospective SENTICOL study. Ann Surg Oncol. 2013;20(2):413–22.
26. Marnitz S, Köhler C, Bongardt S, et al. Topographic distribution of sentinel lymph nodes in patients with cervical cancer. Gynecol Oncol. 2006;103(1):35–44.
27. Cormier B, Diaz JP, Shih K, et al. Establishing a sentinel lymph node mapping algorithm for the treatment of early cervical cancer. Gynecol Oncol. 2011;122(2):275–80.
28. Partridge EE, Shingleton HM, Menck HR. The national cancer data base report on endometrial cancer. J Surg Oncol. 1996;61(2):111–23.
29. ASTEC Study Group, Kitchener H, Swart AM, Qian Q, et al. Efficacy of systematic pelvic lymphadenectomy in endometrial cancer (MRC ASTEC trial): a randomised study. Lancet. 2009;373(9658):125–36.
30. Rossi EC, Kowalski LD, Scalici J, et al. A comparison of sentinel lymph node biopsy to lymphadenectomy for endometrial cancer staging (FIRES trial): a multicentre, prospective, cohort study. Lancet Oncol. 2017;18(3):384–92.
31. Tan J, Chetty N, Kondalsamy-Chennakesavan S, et al. Validation of the FIGO 2009 staging system for carcinoma of the vulva. Int J Gynecol Cancer. 2012;22(3):498–502.

32. Collarino A, Donswijk ML, van Driel WJ, et al. The use of SPECT/CT for anatomical mapping of lymphatic drainage in vulvar cancer: possible implications for the extent of inguinal lymph node dissection. Eur J Nucl Med Mol Imaging. 2015;42(13):2064–71.

33. Altgassen C, Hertel H, Brandstädt A, et al. Multicenter validation study of the sentinel lymph node concept in cervical cancer: AGO Study Group. J Clin Oncol. 2008;26(18):2943–51.

34. Klapdor R, Länger F, Gratz KF, et al. SPECT/CT for SLN dissection in vulvar cancer: improved SLN detection and dissection by preoperative three-dimensional anatomical localisation. Gynecol Oncol. 2015;138(3):590–6.

35. Beneder C, Fuechsel FG, Krause T, et al. The role of 3D fusion imaging in sentinel lymphadenectomy for vulvar cancer. Gynecol Oncol. 2008;109(1):76–80.

36. Martínez A, Zerdoud S, Mery E, et al. Hybrid imaging by SPECT/CT for sentinel lymph node detection in patients with cancer of the uterine cervix. Gynecol Oncol. 2010;119(3):431–5.

37. Pandit-Taskar N, Gemignani ML, Lyall A, et al. Single photon emission computed tomography SPECT-CT improves sentinel node detection and localization in cervical and uterine malignancy. Gynecol Oncol. 2010;117(1):59–64.

38. Díaz-Feijoo B, Pérez-Benavente MA, Cabrera-Diaz S, et al. Change in clinical management of sentinel lymph node location in early stage cervical cancer: the role of SPECT/CT. Gynecol Oncol. 2011;120(3):353–7.

39. Kraft O, Havel M. Detection of sentinel lymph nodes in gynecologic tumours by planar scintigraphy and SPECT/CT. Mol Imaging Radionucl Ther. 2012;21(2):47–55.

40. Belhocine TZ, Prefontaine M, Lanvin D, et al. Added-value of SPECT/CT to lymphatic mapping and sentinel lymphadenectomy in gynaecological cancers. Am J Nucl Med Mol Imaging. 2013;3(2):182–93.

41. Collarino A, Perotti G, Giordano A. Pitfall detected by SPECT/CT in vulvar cancer sentinel lymph node mapping. Case reports. In: Herrmann K, Nieweg OE, Povoski SP, Stephen P, editors. Radioguided current applications and innovative directions in clinical practice. Basel: Springer; 2016. p. 483–94.

42. Garganese G, Bove S, Zagaria L, et al. Ultrasound and 3D SPECT/CT fusion to identify sentinel lymph nodes in vulvar cancer: a feasibility study. Ultrasound Obstet Gynecol. 2019;54(4):545–51. https://doi.org/10.1002/uog.20364. [Epub ahead of print].

43. Sinno AK, Fader AN, Roche KL, et al. A comparison of colorimetric versus fluorometric sentinel lymph node mapping during robotic surgery for endometrial cancer. Gynecol Oncol. 2014;134(2):281–6.

44. de Hullu JA, Oonk MH, Ansink AC, et al. Pitfalls in the sentinel lymph node procedure in vulvar cancer. Gynecol Oncol. 2004;94(1):10–5.

45. Fons G, ter Rahe B, Sloof G, et al. Failure in the detection of the sentinel lymph node with a combined technique of radioactive tracer and blue dye in a patient with cancer of the vulva and a single positive lymph node. Gynecol Oncol. 2004;92(3):981–4.

Preoperative and Intraoperative Lymphatic Mapping for Radioguided Sentinel Node Biopsy in Cancers of the Male Reproductive System

15

Hielke Martijn de Vries, Joost M. Blok, Hans N. Veerman, Florian van Beurden, Henk G. van der Poel, Renato A. Valdés Olmos, and Oscar R. Brouwer

Contents

15.1   **Introduction** 331

15.2   **Penile Cancer** 332

15.3   **Prostate Cancer** 337

15.4   **Testicular Cancer** 343

Clinical Cases 347

References 354

Learning Objectives
- To learn indications and clinical rationale for the sentinel lymph node (SLN) procedure in penile, prostate, and testicular cancer
- To acquire knowledge on the different techniques to use for lymphatic mapping and SLN visualization in urological malignancies
- To broaden the knowledge about the dissemination routes in cancer of the male reproductive system
- To understand the techniques used to reduce the SLN false-negative rates in penile, prostate, and testicular cancer
- To acquire knowledge about the practical execution and implications of the SLN procedure in penile, prostate, and testicular cancer
- To understand the role of preoperative and intraoperative imaging in the SLN procedure in penile, prostate, and testicular cancer

H. M. de Vries · J. M. Blok · H. N. Veerman · F. van Beurden
H. G. van der Poel · O. R. Brouwer (✉)
Department of Urology, Netherlands Cancer Institute,
Amsterdam, Netherlands
e-mail: hm.d.vries@nki.nl; j.blok@nki.nl; h.veerman@nki.nl;
f.van.beurden@nki.nl; h.vd.poel@nki.nl; o.brouwer@nki.nl

R. A. Valdés Olmos
Department of Radiology, Section of Nuclear Medicine and
Interventional Molecular Imaging Laboratory, Leiden University
Medical Center, Leiden, The Netherlands
e-mail: r.a.valdes_olmos@lumc.nl

15.1 Introduction

The SLN procedure, including preoperative lymphatic mapping, has become an essential component of lymph node staging in penile cancer. The extensive experience with sentinel lymph node biopsy (SLNB) in this cancer has led to an increasing application of the procedure for other urological malignancies. Although both preoperative lymphatic mapping and intraoperative SLN detection are common parts of the urological applications, injection techniques for tracer administration and lymphatic drainage patterns may differ for the different cancers. In penile cancer, lymphatic drainage is mainly superficial, the first draining lymph nodes are usually located in the groin, and the biopsy is performed by means of open surgery. In con-

© Springer Nature Switzerland AG 2020
G. Mariani et al. (eds.), *Atlas of Lymphoscintigraphy and Sentinel Node Mapping*,
https://doi.org/10.1007/978-3-030-45296-4_15

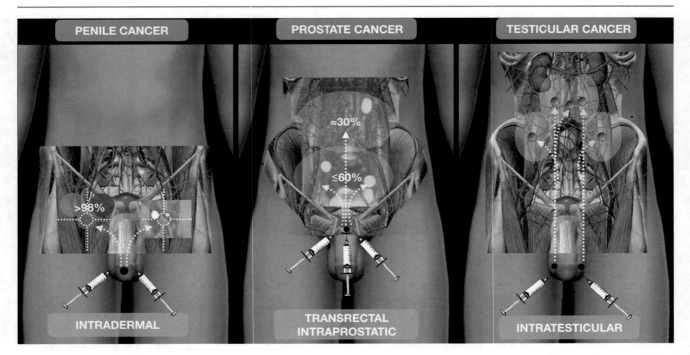

Fig. 15.1 Schematic illustration of tracer injection and areas of SLN drainage in urological malignancies. For penile cancer (on the left) radiotracer is superficially injected and drainage is mostly bilateral with >98% SLNs located in the upper and central inguinal Daseler's areas, especially the inner superior quadrant (dark green circle) [28]; this is illustrated by a superimposed coronal SPEC/CT in the left groin. For prostate cancer (middle) after deep tracer injection drainage is multidirectional with approximately 60% of the SLNs along the internal iliac vessels, obturator fossa, and external iliac vessels; in almost 19% there is direct drainage to lymph nodes above the common iliac bifurcation and 10% above the aorta bifurcation [52, 53]; this is illustrated by a superimposed coronal volume-rendered SPECT/CT. In testicular cancer (on the right) following injection in the left testicle drainage to retroperitoneal para-aortic SLNs is mostly seen whereas after injection in the right testicle both paracaval and interaortocaval lymphatic drainage is expected; less frequently, SLNs are observed along the testicular vessels [71]

trast, in prostate cancer radiotracer migration from the injection site mostly concerns SLNs along the iliac vessels, and other deep-located lymphatic areas, which are resected by (robot-assisted) laparoscopy. In testicular cancer the most frequent drainage route is retroperitoneal along the aorta or vena cava inferior and SLNs are removed using laparoscopy. Some differences in radiotracer administration and lymphatic drainage for penile cancer, prostate cancer, and testicular cancer are illustrated in Fig. 15.1 and further in this chapter the principles of lymphatic mapping and SLNB for these urological malignancies are described.

15.1.1 Tracer Development: Hybrid Radio- and Fluorescence-Guided Approaches

Among other advances in recent years, combined fluorescence- and radioguided approaches such as the hybrid tracer indocyanine green (ICG)-^{99m}Tc-nanocolloid have been introduced during SLN procedures for penile and prostate cancer [1] in the Netherlands and other European countries. This hybrid nanocolloid has both fluorescence and radio-

logic properties. Adding the fluorescent moieties does not alter the biological properties of the parental radiocolloid, and it enables intraoperative near-infrared fluorescence imaging of the exact same (radioactive) lymph nodes which are preoperatively identified by lymphoscintigraphy and SPECT/CT [2]. ICG absorbs light in the near-infrared spectrum, mainly between 600 and 900 nm, and emits fluorescence between 750 and 950 nm, which can be detected by a fluorescence camera allowing real-time visual guidance during surgery [1]. It is prepared by adding pertechnetate to a vial of nanocolloid (GE Healthcare, Eindhoven, The Netherlands). ICG (PULSION Medical, Feldkirchen, Germany) is added and the content of the vial is subtracted in a syringe after which saline is added to reach a specified volume [3].

15.2 Penile Cancer

Penile cancer is a relatively rare disease in the Western world, with an incidence of approximately 1 per 100,000 [4]. Nearly all penile malignancies are squamous cell carcinomas. The presence of lymph node involvement is the single most important prognostic factor for cancer-specific death and warrants a poor cancer-specific survival of 80%, 66%, or 37%, respectively, for N1, N2, or N3 disease [5, 6]. Likewise, distant metastases without lymph node metastases are extremely rare. Since the introduction of an anatomically based SLN procedure in penile carcinoma by Cabañas et al. in 1977, the procedure has evolved into a reliable dynamic staging technique, with a low complication rate (7.6–21.4%) compared to (prophylactic) inguinal lymphadenectomy (ILND) (24–58%) [7–13].

15.2.1 The Clinical Problem

Penile cancer patients are divided into two subgroups: patients with (cN+) or without (cN0) palpable inguinal nodes. Patients that are staged cN+ have nodal metastases in 60–80% of cases [14], while cN0 patients have nodal metastases in 13–16% [14]. Initially, for the best chance of cure, ILND was performed directly in all patients [15]. However, this leads to an overtreatment in more than 80% of the cN0 patients. Furthermore, the morbidity (such as lymphedema and infection) of ILND had decreased in the past years but remains, nevertheless, substantial. As currently available noninvasive staging techniques lack sufficient accuracy, minimally invasive staging remains necessary for the time being. Initially, the SLN procedure for penile cancer had a high false-negative rate after its clinical introduction in 1994. After analysis of false-negative cases, several modifications were made to the dynamic SLNB procedure, which increased its sensitivity from 79 to 94% [7, 9, 16, 17]. For these reasons, the EAU and NCCN guidelines of 2018 both recommend the SLN procedure (in expert centers) for cN0 patients [18, 19].

15.2.2 Indications and Contraindications for SLNB

According to the guidelines patients with ≥T1G2 tumors and cN0 groins defined by palpation are eligible for SLNB. However, a preoperative negative ultrasound with fine-needle cytology of suspicious nodes (US ± FNAC) is strongly advised to reduce false negatives due to, e.g., tumor blockage [20]. Studies have also safely included cN+ patients with a negative US ± FNAC or cN+ patients where the suspicious nodes on ultrasound were also removed [21, 22]. Repeat SLNB after tumor recurrence is also a validated procedure [11, 23, 24]. If the SLN is tumor positive, radical ipsilateral lymphadenectomy is performed. In 80% of patients, no additional metastases are found at ILND after a positive SLNB [25]. However, currently no other treatment options are available for this group. Groins with tumor-free SLNs are managed with close surveillance, thereby avoiding the morbidity associated with lymphadenectomy.

15.2.3 Radiocolloid and Modalities of Injection

The tracer (^{99m}Tc-nanocolloid in most European countries) is injected intradermally. In fact, subcutaneous administration is easier to accomplish, but may not accurately identify the route of drainage from an overlying cutaneous site. Furthermore, lymphatic drainage from the dermis is much faster than drainage from subcutaneous tissue. Application of a spray containing xylocaine 10% 30 min before tracer administration is recommended. As an alternative, a lidocaine/prilocaine-based crème can be used. This local anesthesia ensures that the radiocolloid injections are well tolerated and relatively easy to perform. A volume of 0.2–0.4 mL containing 50–90 MBq divided into three depots (0.1 mL each) is subsequently administered intradermally. Each depot is injected raising a bleb. The radiocolloid is injected proximally from the tumor. For large tumors not restricted to the glans, the radiocolloid can be injected in the prepuce. Injection margins within 1 cm from the primary tumor are recommended. A reproducibility rate of 100% for penile lymphoscintigraphy has been reported with an injection distance of 5 mm [26]. In patients with a previous excision biopsy scar, a secondary SLN procedure can be performed by administrating injections using similar margins. Recently, Winter et al. reported the first application of superparamagnetic iron oxide nanoparticles in a patient using MRI for preoperative SLN mapping and a handheld magnetometer for the intraoperative procedure [27].

15.2.4 Preoperative Imaging of SLNs

Lymphoscintigraphy after radiocolloid injection consists of two phases: (a) Dynamic scintigraphy, performed during the first 10 min after radiocolloid injection, preferably in both the anterior and lateral views: The dynamic study is helpful to identify lymphatic ducts and the first directly draining lymph nodes. (b) Static planar imaging at 20–30 min and at 2 h: The early planar images visualize the first draining lymph nodes in about 77–95% of the cases [8, 21, 22, 28]. On SPECT/CT visualization is seen in 90–97% of groins [21, 22, 28]. Immediate or delayed (a few weeks later) radiocolloid reinjection or additional images at 4 h are recommended when no SLNs are visualized [8]. If still no visualization is seen exploration of the groin is an option and in low-risk patients (<pT1G3) close clinical surveillance with ultrasound can be considered [29]. Generally, the lymph nodes draining directly from the injection site are classified as SLNs. The first node appearing in a basin is considered to be the SLN in case of multiple visible nodes without visible afferent vessels.

15.2.5 Lymphatic Drainage

The most frequently visualized lymphatic drainage pattern is bilateral drainage to both groins (80%) (Fig. 15.2). This pattern is, however, asynchronous in two-thirds of cases, and often visualization of the contralateral lymph nodes is only possible on delayed imaging [30]. Drainage from the injection site mostly occurs through one or two visualized afferent lymphatic ducts leading to one or two SLNs in each groin. In some cases a cluster of inguinal lymph nodes is observed. After drainage to both groins, drainage through the node of Rossemüller-Cloquet, on the interface of the groin and pelvis, into the iliacal and obturator nodes is seen. These are almost always second-echelon nodes. Crossover drainage from the groin to the contralateral pelvis has never been seen.

15.2.6 Intraoperative Detection of SLNs

It is safe to perform surgery on the day or the day after injection and nodal imaging [11]. There are indications that the 1-day protocol has higher radioactive count, more nodes, and more morbidity [11].

As is customary for SLNB in melanoma and breast cancer, intraoperative SLN detection is guided by a gamma ray detection probe and blue dye or indocyanine

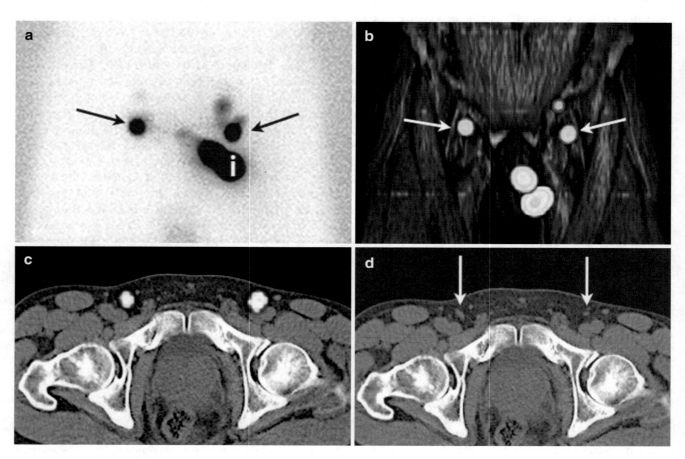

Fig. 15.2 A 49-year-old patient with penile squamous cell carcinoma scheduled for partial penectomy and SLNB. (**a**) Lymphoscintigraphy 2 h after injection of 81 MBq ^{99m}Tc-nanocolloid (i) shows drainage to a SLN in both groins (arrows) and bilateral higher echelon drainage. (**b**) 3D volume-rendered SPECT/CT image revealing that both SLNs are located in the central zone of Daseler. (**c**, **d**) Axial fused SPECT/CT images depicting both radioactive SLNs with the corresponding lymph nodes on CT (arrows)

green (ICG). After excision of all preoperatively defined SLNs, it is important to carefully search for any residual radioactivity using the probe and if available a portable gamma camera, to prevent that any remaining/additional SLNs are left behind [31, 32]. Furthermore, intraoperative palpation of the wound should take place to identify suspicious lymph nodes that failed to pick up any radiocolloid [33].

15.2.7 Contribution of SPECT/CT

SPECT/CT images are usually acquired after the 2-h planar images, and contribute to a better understanding of the location of the SLNs in penile carcinoma (Figs. 15.2 and 15.3). SPECT/CT enables the anatomical localization of the SLNs that were previously identified by lymphoscintigraphy. For instance, the modality can differentiate inguinal from iliac (most frequently second-echelon) lymph nodes. Moreover, SPECT/CT enables visualization of the SLNs in the so-called Daseler's superior and central inguinal zones that are superior to and directly overlying the saphenofemoral junction, respectively. SPECT/CT has confirmed that in the majority of patients SLNs are found in the superior medial (30–73%), in the superior lateral (9–37%), and in the central zones (18–32%) [28]. Lymphatic drainage to the inferior quadrants is rare (inferior medial 1.6%, inferior lateral 0%) [28]. SPECT/CT identifies SLNs in groins which

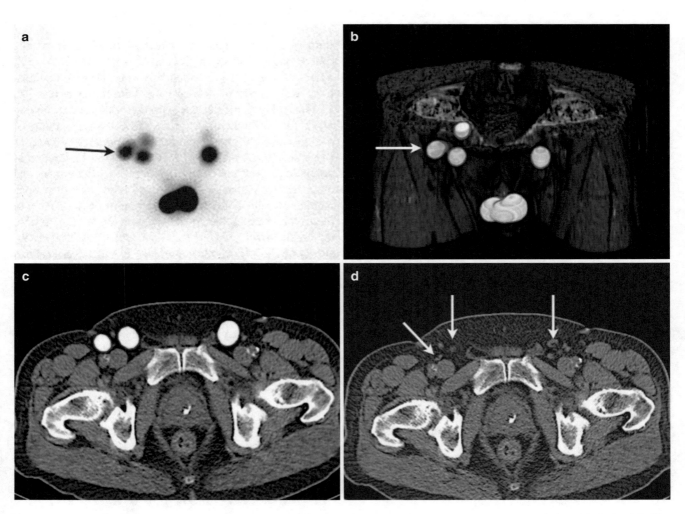

Fig. 15.3 (**a**) Intradermal injection of 82.92 MBq ^{99m}Tc-nanocolloid in a 71-year-old male resulting in visualization of a SLN in both groins with a second more laterally localized SLN on the right side (arrow) on delayed planar lymphoscintigraphy. (**b**) 3D volume-rendered SPECT/CT images revealing a SLN in the superior medial quadrant on both sides, and a SLN in the superior lateral quadrant on the right side (arrow). The image also shows a second-echelon node in the right iliac area. (**c**, **d**) Axial fused SPECT/CT images depicting both radioactive SLNs with the corresponding lymph nodes on CT (arrows). Histopathological examination revealed micrometastases in the left excised SLN

would have had non-visualization if only conventional lymphoscintigraphy had been used [34, 35]. Finally, SPECT/CT is able to identify contamination of the skin with the radiocolloid, an occurrence which can sometimes be erroneously interpreted as lymph nodes on planar lymphoscintigrams.

15.2.8 Intraoperative Imaging

Accurate staging with SLNB can be achieved only if all nodes on a direct drainage pathway from the tumor are harvested. If SLNs are left behind, this constitutes one of the potential causes for false-negative results. The integration of a portable gamma camera in the intraoperative procedure may increase the detection sensitivity, as it provides an intraoperative overview image of the radioactive SLNs and enables post-excision confirmation of complete removal of the SLNs in the operating room. For optical visualization of the SLN, vital blue dyes are traditionally used to stain 43–56% of nodes [8, 32, 36]. To increase intraoperative visualization rate, ICG-^{99m}Tc-nanocolloid can be utilized as mentioned in the second paragraph [37]. With this combined tracer, 95–97% of the removed SLNs were fluorescent in vivo [32, 36]. These developments may help to further refine intraoperative retrieval of SLNs.

15.2.9 Common and Rare Variants

One of the advantages of lymphatic mapping is its ability to identify SLNs outside the usual nodal basins. In penile cancer, direct drainage to prepubic SLNs has been described [38]. In particular, dynamic lymphoscintigraphy often shows one or two lymphatic vessels leading to the SLNs. Such vessels have also been observed to directly lead to deep inguinal and even to iliac SLNs.

Blockage of the lymph flow by tumor metastasis in the lymph node may cause non-visualization and lymph rerouting with occasionally retrograde or contralateral flow of the ^{99m}Tc-nanocolloid. This occurrence has been visualized by SPECT/CT imaging [33].

15.2.10 Technical Pitfalls

The most frequent pitfall is skin contamination. The high pressure of the intradermal bleb can result in leakage during injection or after removal of the needle. The use of (surgical) lights to adequately visualize the site of injection and of a

fenestrated drape to cover the area may help to avoid skin contamination. Furthermore, voiding of radioactive urine between the early and delayed scintigraphy may also cause skin contamination. The hot spots due to skin contamination may be confused with SLNs, thus leading to an unnecessary intraoperative pursuit. In these cases skin decontamination is mandatory. Complementary SPECT/CT may also be helpful in detecting these artifacts. Another possible pitfall is accidental injection into the corpus cavernosum, an occurrence that will cause no visualization of lymphatic flow. Furthermore, in some cases the injection site (penis) may obscure visualization of the more inferiorly located SLNs on anterior planar imaging.

15.2.11 Accuracy of Radioguided SLNB

Initially, the most significant drawback of SLNB for penile cancer was a relatively high false-negative rate (22%) [39]. After analysis of the false-negative cases, several modifications were made to decrease the false-negative rate [9]. Histopathologic analysis was expanded with serial sectioning of the SLNs. Furthermore, preoperative ultrasonography of cN0 groins with fine-needle aspiration cytology (FNAC) of suspicious lymph nodes was added, as well as exploration of groins in case of non-visualization during scintigraphy and intraoperative palpation of the wound to identify suspicious lymph nodes that failed to pick up any radiocolloid. Thanks to these modifications, the procedure has evolved into a reliable minimally invasive staging technique with an associated sensitivity of 93–95% with low morbidity in experienced centers [9, 40]. At the same time the SLN procedure has also increased survival of penile cancer patients significantly [6, 41]. However, a recent multicenter meta-analysis reported pooled sensitivity rates of 88% [17, 42]. One explanation for such lower sensitivity may be represented by differences in protocols (that is, screening with ultrasound and FNAC to detect lymph node metastases that fail to pick up radioactivity), low-volume centers, and/or possibly different phases of the learning curve.

Key Learning Objectives Penile Cancer
- The SLN procedure in penile cancer has helped increase survival and prevents unnecessary lymphadenectomy in patients with a tumor-negative SLN.
- The SLN procedure in penile cancer can be performed in a 1- or 2-day protocol.

- SLNB after primary tumor excision is also possible and can be performed in a similar fashion.
- Repeat SLNB for penile cancer recurrence is safe.
- SPECT/CT provides anatomical information giving specific landmarks for SLN localization during the surgical act.

15.3 Prostate Cancer

In prostate cancer, lymph node staging is important for both prognosis and therapeutic management. The presence of lymph node metastases may lead to adjuvant treatment in case of prostatectomy, such as hormonal therapy with or without radiotherapy, or extension of the radiotherapeutic field [43]. To date, none of the available noninvasive diagnostic imaging modalities provide a reliable assessment of lymph node (micro)metastases. Positron-emission tomography (PET) with prostate-specific membrane antigen (PSMA) labeled with ^{68}Ga or ^{18}F is an emerging imaging modality; however, the sensitivity for detection of lymph node metastases is still limited to 64% in the case of ^{68}Ga-PSMA PET/CT. Moreover, ^{68}Ga-PSMA PET/CT has been found not to detect lymph node metastases smaller than 2 mm [44, 45]. Therefore, surgical staging by extended pelvic lymph node dissection (ePLND) is still the current standard of care. However, SLNB is emerging as an alternative staging method, with a lower incidence of complications and with the potential to identify relevant lymph nodes outside the standard ePLND field [46, 47].

15.3.1 The Clinical Problem

Current international guidelines recommend that a pelvic lymph node dissection (PLND) should be performed at the time of a radical prostatectomy (RP) in all men with intermediate- or high-risk prostate cancer, if the estimated risk of lymph node metastases exceeds 5% in the current EAU guidelines or 2% with NCCN guideline nomograms (grade recommendation: "B"). Despite this, 25–35% of the PC patients who are treated with curative intent with RP and extended PLND will develop clinically significant biochemical recurrence with local and/or distant disease. An extended dissection (ePLND) is preferred over limited PLND. However, even with an extended dissection template including external iliac, hypogastric, and obturator nodes, 35% of lymph nodes potentially containing PC will not be removed at surgery,

either being located out of the standard surgical field or being missed within.

The advantages of SLN dissection are the possibility to identify tumor draining lymph nodes outside the field of an ePLND and lower the incidence of complications compared to ePLND [46]. However, accurate localization of SLNs in the pelvis can be challenging, especially when SLNs are located near the prostatic injection site (because of the high radioactive background signal), or in case of aberrantly located SLNs (e.g., para-aortic) [48].

15.3.2 Indications and Contraindications for SLNB

The probability of having lymph node metastasis from prostate cancer increases with the serum level of prostate-specific antigen (PSA), biopsy grade (Gleason score), and clinical T stage. Like the indications for an ePLND, SLNB could be performed in all men with intermediate- and high-risk prostate cancer, if the estimated risk of lymph node metastases exceeds 5% with EAU guidelines or 2% with NCCN guideline nomograms and PSMA PET/CT or any other conventional imaging modality showed no evidence of lymph node metastases. However, according to the guidelines, due to lack of reliable evidence regarding oncological effectiveness, SLNB is still an experimental nodal staging procedure. A tumor-bearing SLN may influence the boundaries of the radiotherapy field and duration of hormonal (androgen deprivation) therapy. Another possible indication is to select patients who are eligible for salvage treatment of the prostate, as the usual parameters to stratify patients in risk groups do not apply to patients with intraprostatic recurrence [49]. Since salvage treatment of the prostate may result in serious complications, it is considered when the prostate is actually the only tumor-bearing site.

15.3.3 Radiocolloid and Modalities of Injection

Most of the experience in the SLN procedure for prostate cancer has been acquired in European countries and the most frequently used radiopharmaceutical has been ^{99m}Tc-nanocolloid. Transrectal intraprostatic injection is guided by (transrectal) ultrasound, injecting the radiocolloid under continuous monitoring using a needle of 0.5 × 150 mm (Fig. 15.4). Prostate cancer may be multifocal; therefore injections are performed in both lobes. An activity of about 240 MBq in 0.4 mL is recommended. The lymph node visu-

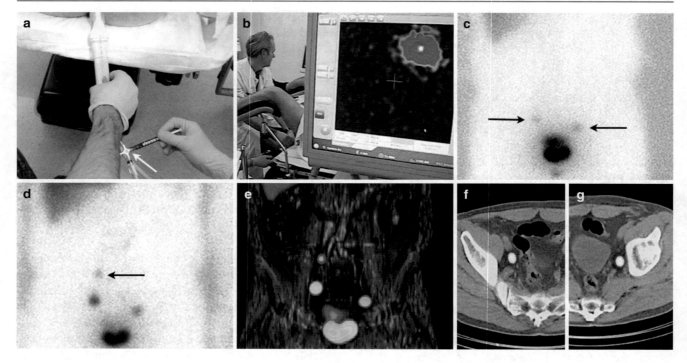

Fig. 15.4 Preoperative SLN mapping in a 65-year-old patient with intermediate-risk prostate cancer. (**a**) Tracer administration guided by transrectal ultrasound guidance using a long needle and a three-way system. (**b**) The radioactive dose is divided into 2–4 injections. The procedure is monitored using a portable gamma camera to verify adequate tracer retention within the prostate. (**c**) Early planar lymphoscintigram showing two SLNs with direct drainage from the prostate (arrows). (**d**) The delayed lymphoscintigram enables differentiation of the SLNs and a higher echelon lymph node (arrow). (**e**) 3D volume-rendered SPECT/CT image displaying the location of the SLNs in more detail. (**f**) Axial fused SPECT/CT image showing the SLN on the right side along the external iliac veins and the SLN on the left side (**g**) in the obturator fossa

alization rate tends to be less optimal when lower activities are used. The particle concentration also appears to be important, and the use of a reduced labeling dilution volume (0.4 mL ^{99m}Tc per 0.2 mg nanocolloid) yields more visualized SLNs with higher radioactivity count rates [50]. The radiocolloid is divided into 2–4 injections depending on the prostate volume. A three-way system is recommended, and after each depot saline is used for flushing the residual radioactivity in the needle. When using ICG-^{99m}Tc-nanocolloid a similar injection scheme is applied with a volume of 2.0 mL and an activity of 300 MBq (Fig. 15.5).

15.3.4 Preoperative Imaging of SLNs

In the pelvis, lymphatic ducts are seldom visualized and the relatively slower deep lymphatic drainage renders dynamic lymphoscintigraphy less useful. Early planar images of lymphoscintigraphy acquired 15 min after radiocolloid administration can visualize the first draining lymph nodes in almost 88% of the cases [51]. Delayed imaging may be performed 2–4 h after injection. On delayed imaging the lymph node visualization rate increases to more than 95%. Comparing the early and delayed images enables to differentiate second-echelon lymph nodes from the first draining nodes. This discrimination is based on the anatomical lymph node basins of the pelvis. As a rule, late-appearing lymph nodes located higher in the same basin are considered as second-echelon lymph nodes. Late-appearing lymph nodes in distal or more ventral and dorsal basins suggest direct draining from the prostate. These lymph nodes may also be considered as SLNs. If no SPECT/CT is available, lateral planar images can differentiate between dorsal and more ventral located SLNs.

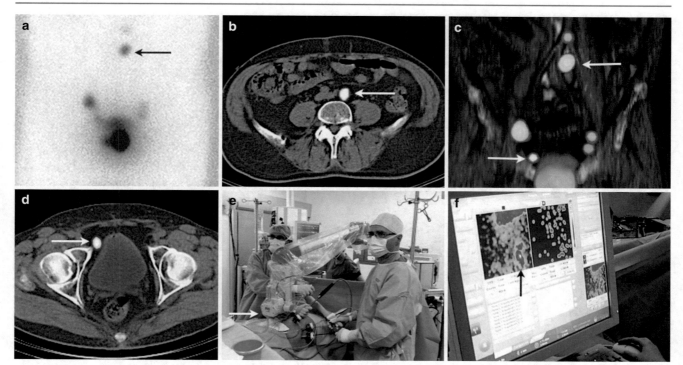

Fig. 15.5 (a) Early lymphoscintigraphy after transrectal intraprostatic injection of ^{99m}Tc-nanocolloid (170 MBq) in a 70-year-old male scheduled for SLNB resulted in visualization of bilateral lymphatic drainage with an early-appearing SLN along the great abdominal vessels (arrow). (b) Axial SPECT/CT image showing the exact location of this SLN next to the common iliac artery. (c) The 3D volume-rendered SPECT/CT image providing an overview of all SLNs: the upper SLN next to the common iliac artery (upper arrow), two along the external iliac vessels on the left side, one along the external iliac artery on the right side, but also an additional SLN located more mediocaudally (lower arrow). (d) The axial image shows that this SLN is located paravesically. (e) All SLNs were harvested laparoscopically aided by a portable gamma camera (arrow) and a laparoscopic gamma probe. (f) Intraoperative visualization of a SLN (arrow) using a portable gamma camera allowing post-excision confirmation that the SLN has been removed completely. After excision (right on screen), no significant remaining activity is seen

15.3.5 Lymphatic Drainage

The lymphatic drainage pathways of the prostate are highly variable in individual patients. Lymph node mapping studies [52, 53] using SPECT/CT, lymphoscintigraphy, SLN procedures, and lymph node dissections improved our understanding of lymphatic drainage. Main drainage pathways include the internal iliac nodes, obturator nodes, and external iliac nodes (Fig. 15.1). These regions are included in the extended pelvic lymph node dissection (ePLND). The borders of the internal iliac nodes are the bifurcation of the internal and external iliac arteries, pelvic floor, bladder wall, and medial to obturator nerve. The obturator region is found lateral to obturator nerve and medial to external iliac artery. The external iliac nodes are found cranial to inguinal ligament, medial to genitofemoral nerve, medial to psoas muscle, and caudal to ureter and bifurcation of internal and external iliac arteries. Less frequently, metastasis is found in the distal or proximal (divided by the ureteric crossing) common iliac artery nodes with the following borders: bifurcation of the aorta (cranial), bifurcation of the internal and external iliac nodes (caudal), internal iliac artery (medial), and genitofemoral nerve and psoas muscle (lateral). The borders of the presacral regions are the common iliac arteries (cranial/lateral), bifurcation of the internal and external iliac arteries (caudal), and promontorium and proximal sacrum (dorsal). These regions are included in the "super-extended PLND." Other rare variants are discussed below.

15.3.6 Intraoperative Detection of SLNs

Initial validation of SLNB in prostate cancer is based on open surgery and use of a gamma ray detection probe to guide detection of the radioactive SLNs. Performing SLNB

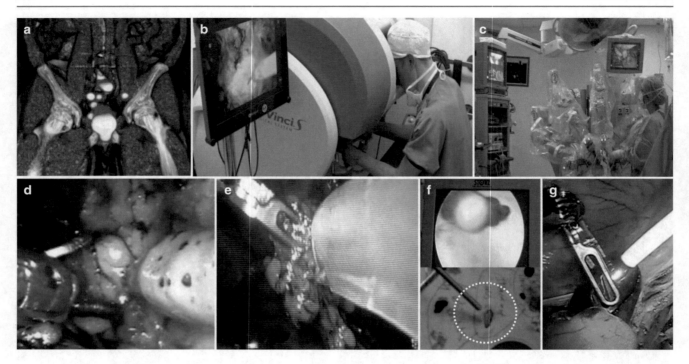

Fig. 15.6 Following administration of the hybrid tracer ICG-^{99m}Tc-nanocolloid, volume-rendered SPECT/CT (**a**) is able to anatomically localize the SLNs in the pelvis. Based on this information, urological surgeons can remove the nodes by means of robot-assisted laparoscopy (**b**, **c**). Thanks to the fluorescence signature of the tracer the SLNs are localized (**d**) and subsequently removed and measured with a rigid laparoscopy gamma probe (**e**). Due to the dual signature of the tracer both fluorescence (top) and radioactivity (circle bottom) can successively be measured (**f**). The replacement of the standard rigid probe by a flexible drop-in gamma probe (**g**) will optimize the procedure in the future

in a robot-assisted laparoscopic setting can be challenging because of the limited maneuverability of gamma ray detection probes. Especially SLNs that lie in close proximity to the injection site are easily missed, because the relatively high background signal from the injection site hinders the localization of the low-intensity signal from the SLN. The introduction of several new technologies has made the incorporation of SLNB in robot-assisted surgery possible [54, 55]. The hybrid tracer ICG-^{99m}Tc-nanocolloid aids in the intraoperative detection of SLNs. However, 14.3–19.6% of SLNs cannot be visualized due to the limited tissue penetration of the ICG fluorescent signal [55]. Those SLNs missed using fluorescence imaging can be localized using preoperatively obtained lymphoscintigraphy and SPECT/CT images and per-operatively with the use of a gamma ray detection probe [54]. Additionally, fluorescence imaging has been incorporated in robotic assisted surgery using a da Vinci Si system with an integrated Firefly fluorescence laparoscope [55]. During the procedure, the urologist can switch between white light imaging and fluorescence imaging using the controllers of the console (Fig. 15.6).

In open surgery, the use of a portable gamma probe aids the detection of SLNs. Current portable gamma cameras are capable of detecting two different signals: the signal of ^{99m}Tc-nanocolloid for SKLN visualization, plus the signal of a ^{125}I seed pointer placed on the tip of the laparoscopic gamma ray detection probe [56]. During surgery the signal of ^{99m}TC, which indicates the location of the SLN, and the signal of ^{125}I seed pointer are both displayed on a screen. The signal of the ^{125}I seed pointer is depicted as a yellow circle, guiding the surgeon spatially to the signal of the SLN. The ^{125}I seed additionally aids in quantifying the amount of radioactivity in the nodes, thus allowing more reliable discrimination between SLNs and second-echelon nodes. After removal of all SLNs, the portable gamma camera can show whether there are any remaining SLNs that have to be removed or a second-echelon node that can confidently be left in place (see Fig. 15.6). This approach provides certainty about completeness of the surgical procedure. The excised lymph nodes are checked for radioactivity with the gamma probe ex vivo.

The use of a drop-in gamma probe in robot-assisted surgery has recently been investigated to overcome the limited maneuverability of laparoscopic gamma ray detection probes (Fig. 15.6). The drop-in probe is inserted via a trocar and can be maneuvered with laparoscopic surgical tools [57]. This allows placing the drop-in gamma probe in between low-intensity objects (e.g., SN) and high-background objectives like the injection site (e.g., prostate), therewith being able to distinguish signals from low-intensity objects from high-background objectives with a relative intensity ratio of 1:100 [57]. The drop-in probe can remain in the abdominal cavity during the nodal resection and is picked up for placement with the ProGrasp® forceps whenever necessary. A feasibility study showed that the wide scanning range of the drop-in probe allowed the surgeon to remove 35 SLNs in 10 prostate cancer patients. In total, 45% of the SLNs identified with the drop-in probe were considered difficult to trace using the traditional laparoscopic gamma probe [58].

15.3.7 Contribution of SPECT/CT

Hybrid imaging with SPECT/CT enables anatomical localization of SLNs. A 98–99% SLN visualization rate has been reported for SPECT/CT (versus 91% for planar imaging) [52, 53, 59]. Moreover, in 56% of the cases SLNs are localized inside the area of ePLND [52, 53]; there is a considerable number of SLNs in regions not routinely excised when performing an ePLND (see below: accuracy of radioguided SLNB) [47]. SPECT/CT is mostly performed after the delayed planar imaging, and must be interpreted in combination with lymphoscintigraphy. Sequential planar images are able to identify the lymph nodes draining directly from the tumor site, but give only limited information about their anatomical location. With SPECT/CT it is possible to better localize SLNs both inside and outside the pelvis. In many cases early-appearing lymph nodes seen as a single hot spot on planar imaging are displayed as separate lymph nodes in different basins by SPECT/CT, and all of them must be considered as SLNs. In other cases, intense lymph node uptake seen on fused images may correspond to a cluster of SLNs as depicted on the CT component of the SPECT/CT acquisition. As such, SPECT/CT provides valuable information for the urologist, which may lead to a significant shortening of the operation time, as less extensive exploration might be required. Furthermore, SPECT/CT may also provide important information for planning radiotherapy, concerning especially treatment volume and optimization of irradiation fields in the pelvis.

15.3.8 Common and Rare Variants

In prostate cancer, lymphoscintigraphy and SPECT/CT may identify SLNs outside the ePLND in 16–44% of the cases [51–53]. These aberrantly located SLNs can be located in the following regions: common iliac (19%), para-aortic (10%), presacral (7%), aortic bifurcation (4%), pararectal (3%), paravesical (<1%), mesenteric fat (<1%), and inguinal (<1%) [52, 53].

15.3.9 Technical Pitfalls

The relatively complicated radiocolloid injection procedure for prostate cancer is probably the most frequent cause of pitfalls. One must be careful to avoid tracer leakage during injection, possibly resulting in subsequent contamination of the floor or of the ultrasound probe. It is therefore recommended to check for contamination of the room after injection using a Geiger counter.

During injection, incorrect needle placement may result in passage of the radiocolloid directly to the bladder or bloodstream, which in turn may cause non-visualization during scintigraphy. By monitoring the injection procedure with a portable gamma camera, one can ensure adequate radiocolloid retention in the prostate. As the injection is performed transrectally, a possible pitfall is visualization of lymphatic drainage from the rectum, leading to, e.g., visualization of inguinal lymph nodes on SPECT/CT imaging (Fig. 15.7). Furthermore, accidental funicular administration can also occur, possibly leading to retrograde drainage toward the scrotum (Fig. 15.8).

15.3.10 Accuracy of Radioguided SLNB

Original validation of SLNB for prostate cancer was based on open surgery and on the use of a gamma probe to guide detection of the radioactive SLNs. Out of more than 2000 patients evaluated, only 11 false-negative cases (5.5%) were reported [60]. More recently, SLNB has been validated using a laparoscopic gamma probe during minimally invasive surgery [61].

The combined diagnostic accuracy of open, laparoscopic, and robot-assisted SLNB with ePLND as reference standard has been described in a recent systematic review including 2509 patients and showed a 95.2% (81.8–100%) sensitivity, 100% (95.0–100%) specificity, 100% (IQR 87.0–100%) positive predictive value, and 98% (94.3–100%) negative predictive value. In 4.8% (0–18.2%) of cases a metastasis

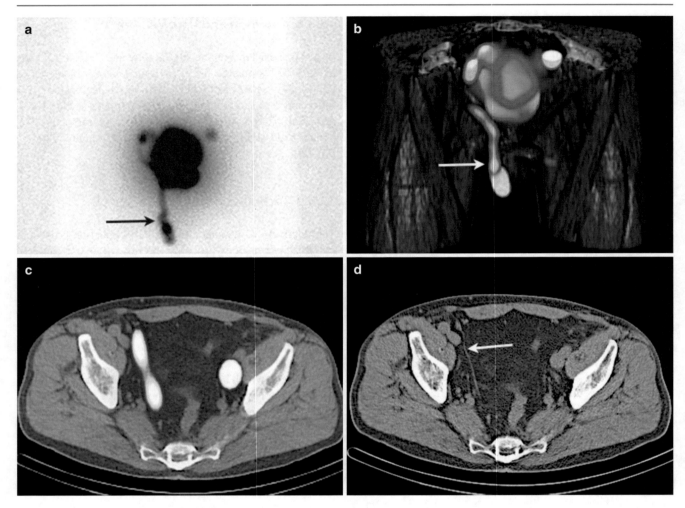

Fig. 15.7 (**a**) Planar lymphoscintigraphy after intraprostatic injection of 180 MBq ^{99m}Tc-nanocolloid in a 60-year-old patient showing bilateral drainage with a single hot spot on both sides, but also with drainage on the right side in caudal direction (arrow). (**b**) 3D volume-rendered SPECT/CT image showing that the caudal drainage on the right side is directed toward the right testicle (arrow). (**c, d**) Axial images showing elongated drainage along the funiculus (arrow). The drainage toward the testicle thus reflects retrograde drainage after accidental funicular administration, one of the possible pitfalls of this procedure

was found in the SLN outside the ePLND template without metastasis inside the ePLND template (false positive), suggesting diagnostic advantage and a higher yield of tumor-positive nodes when combining the procedures [47].

Key Learning Points: Prostate Cancer
- Indications for SLN procedure of the prostate are to determine lymph node metastasis in patients with intermediate- and high-risk prostate cancer eligible for radiotherapy with hormonal therapy or patients with prostate cancer eligible for salvage treatment of the prostate.
- With the (new) hybrid tracer ICG-^{99m}Tc-nanocolloid it is possible to perform preoperative imaging with lymphoscintigraphy and SPECT/CT as well as intraoperative imaging with a fluorescence camera and a gamma ray detection probe.
- SLN mapping enables the identification of lymph node metastasis outside the template of extended pelvic lymph node dissection.
- The introduction of drop-in gamma probes may help to overcome the limited maneuverability of rigid laparoscopic gamma probes with advantages especially for robot-assisted SLNB during laparoscopy.

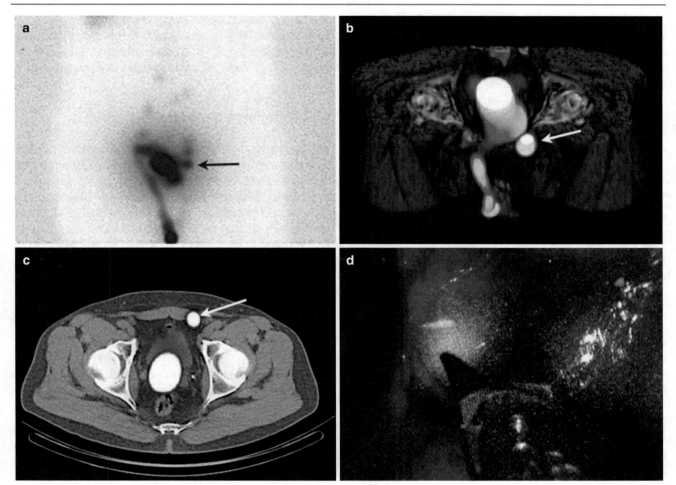

Fig. 15.8 A similar situation arose after transrectal intraprostatic injection (211 MBq) of hybrid radioactive and fluorescent ICG-^{99m}Tc-nanocolloid in a 59-year-old male with intermediate-risk prostate cancer. (**a**) Delayed planar lymphoscintigram showing retrograde drainage toward the scrotum on the right side due to partial funicular tracer administration as well as drainage to SLNs on both sides (obturator fossa); and a SLN located more caudally on the left side (arrow). (**b, c**) The 3D volume-rendered and axial SPECT/CT images reveal that the most caudal SLN on the left side reflects aberrant drainage ventrally against the abdominal wall (arrow). The SLNs were harvested during robot-assisted laparoscopy guided by a laparoscopic gamma probe and fluorescence endoscope. (**d**) Fluorescence endoscope image showing the SLN against the abdominal wall along the umbilical ligament (green). This SLN (and an iliac SLN on the right side) contained metastases at histopathology

15.4   Testicular Cancer

Testicular germ cell tumor (TGCT) is the most frequent solid malignancy in young men and affects up to 10 in 10,000 men [62, 63]. Depending on the histologic subtype (seminoma or nonseminomatous germ cell tumor), the peak incidence is between 25 and 35 years old [62]. Incidence rates are rising and increases as high as 4.9% per year have been reported [64]. The prognosis is favorable and cancer-specific survival rates up to 100% have been reported [65–67]. The majority of patients have clinical stage I disease at first presentation [68]. The optimal management of these patients remains controversial. A surveillance policy requires intensive, frequent follow-up visits with costly examinations and defers detection and treatment of lymph node metastases to a later stage. Up to 30% of patients with clinical stage I disease will relapse under surveillance and have to be treated with multiple cycles of toxic chemotherapy. Therefore, there is a need for diagnostic techniques that enable the identification and treatment of patients with occult lymph node metastasis at an earlier stage. In this respect, the SLN procedure is of potential high value [69–71].

15.4.1   The Clinical Problem

Approximately two-thirds of patients present with clinical stage I [68]. The predominant management strategy for these patients is inguinal orchiectomy followed by active surveillance for 5 years [72]. However, 20–30% of patients with clinical stage I will relapse under surveillance [73, 74]. These patients had occult metastatic disease in their lymph nodes at the time of first presentation, undetectable by current imaging protocols or biomarkers.

Patients who suffer from relapse are treated with multiple cycles of platinum-based chemotherapy. These regimens cause serious short- and long-term side effects [75]. For example, the risk of cardiovascular disease or a second malignancy is ~2 times higher after chemotherapy [76]. As a consequence, the relative survival of these patients continues to decline even beyond 30 years of follow-up [77]. For intermediate/poor-risk patients, the treatment-related mortality is even higher than the disease-related mortality.

To overcome the high relapse rate, several risk-adapted strategies have been introduced [78–80]. Risk stratification is based on the outcome of the orchiectomy specimen and high-risk patients receive one cycle of chemotherapy. Approximately 52–68.5% of high-risk patients, however, do not relapse if followed with active surveillance [78, 79, 81]. Thus, treating all high-risk patients with chemotherapy would lead to serious overtreatment. Conversely, 12–14% of low-risk patients will relapse [78, 79, 81]. These patients would have benefitted from adjuvant treatment, but did not receive it.

Thus, the high relapse rate in clinical stage I testicular cancer, the high rate of over- and undertreatment, and the serious morbidity associated with the toxic treatment of relapsed patients urge for a better and earlier identification of patients with occult metastatic disease. The SLN procedure could lead to less intensive follow-up protocols for node-negative patients and reduction of systemic treatment. In one study with a median follow-up of more than 5 years, none of the patients with a negative SLN suffered from relapse [69].

15.4.2 Indications and Contraindications for SLNB

SLN visualization is feasible in patients with clinical stage I disease [69, 70, 82, 83]. Clinical stage I is defined by the absence of enlarged (>1 cm) lymph nodes on abdomino-thoracic computed tomography (CT) scan plus normal or normalizing serum values of alpha-fetoprotein (AFP), human chorionic gonadotropin (HCG), and lactate dehydrogenase (LDH).

15.4.3 Radiocolloid and Modalities of Injection

The route of administration of ^{99m}Tc-nanocolloid has been evaluated in multiple feasibility studies. While funicular administration showed only lymph node uptake in the inguinal region (which does not reflect the actual testicular tumor drainage pattern), intratesticular administration resulted in visualization of retroperitoneal SLNs, in accordance with known drainage patterns. No side effects were observed using the latter method, which proved to be easy to perform and

was well tolerated under local anesthesia (funicular block with lidocaine 2%). Generally, a single aliquot of radioactivity (approximately 100 MBq) in a volume of 0.1–0.2 mL is injected with a fine needle into the testicular parenchyma.

15.4.4 Preoperative Imaging of SLNs

The fast lymphatic drainage from the testicle requires dynamic gamma camera acquisition to facilitate differentiation between first- and second-echelon lymph nodes in the retroperitoneum. Immediately following radiocolloid injection, anterior and lateral dynamic images are obtained with a dual-head gamma camera to visualize the lymphatic flow and early-draining lymph nodes. Static planar images are obtained immediately after the dynamic study. Two hours after tracer injection, additional static images are obtained to identify slower draining SLNs and unexpected drainage patterns.

15.4.5 Lymphatic Drainage

Left-sided testicular tumors primarily drain to the para-aortic retroperitoneal region [84]. Right-sided tumors show a less uniform pattern of dissemination and drain to the paracaval, precaval, and interaortocaval region [84, 85].

15.4.6 Intraoperative Detection of SLNs

SLNB in testicular cancer was introduced in a laparoscopic setting, and can also be performed robot assisted. Intraoperative SLN localization is guided by a laparoscopic gamma probe or a portable gamma camera [69, 71].

15.4.7 Contribution of SPECT/CT

In the initial feasibility study, preoperative lymphatic mapping was performed using planar lymphoscintigraphy only [70]. However, this technique can provide two-dimensional information only, and exact preoperative anatomical SLN localization is not possible. SPECT/CT provides not only useful anatomic information about the location of SLNs but its improved sensitivity and the added third dimension may also lead to the detection of additional SLNs (Fig. 15.8). Sequential planar imaging will remain important for the preoperative identification of early-appearing lymph nodes as SLNs.

15.4.8 Intraoperative Imaging

Since the lymphatic drainage of the testes is directed to retroperitoneal areas deeply within the abdomen that can often

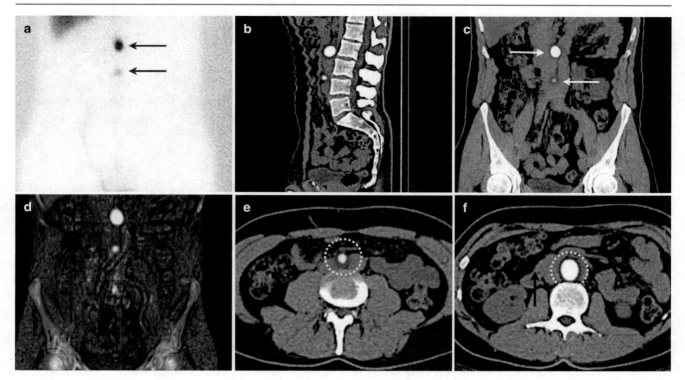

Fig. 15.9 A 42-year-old male with a seminoma in the right testicle was injected with ^{99m}Tc-nanocolloid (87.32 MBq) followed by SLN mapping. (**a**) Early planar anterior image showing drainage to two abdominal SLNs (arrows) and radioactivity along the lymphatic channel, which decreased in time, indicating lymphatic tract visualization. (**b**) Sagittal SPECT/CT image fusion showing the injection site and both SLNs along the great abdominal vessels. (**c**, **d**) The coronal SPECT/CT image fusion and 3D volume-rendered image reveal that both SLNs are located interaortocavally (arrows). (**e**, **f**) Axial SPECT/CT images providing additional anatomical information about the location of both SLNs (dotted circles). Both SLNs were harvested laparoscopically and were tumor free at histopathology

be complex, preoperative anatomical information about the location of the SLNs is important for planning the surgical procedure. For this reason, the SPECT/CT images should be displayed in the operating room. Urological surgery has shifted from the open approach toward minimally invasive laparoscopic and robot-assisted techniques. During laparoscopic surgery, the urologist localizes a SLN under guidance by the sound pitch from the laparoscopic gamma probe. However, intraoperative spatial orientation using this device can be difficult, as a laparoscopic probe does not provide visual information. The use of a portable gamma camera helps to intraoperatively guide laparoscopic SLN localization as described above (see section *Intraoperative detection of SLNs: prostate cancer*). This approach provides certainty about completeness of the surgical procedure and complements the laparoscopic probe. Currently, intraoperative navigation approaches that are based on the preoperative (SPECT/CT) images are being developed [86].

15.4.9 Common and Rare Variants

Although drainage from the testes is usually directed to paracaval, interaortocaval, and para-aortic SLNs, in some patients SLNs may also be seen along the testicular vessels (Fig. 15.9) [71].

15.4.10 Technical Pitfalls

The route of administration of ^{99m}Tc-nanocolloid may cause pitfalls. For instance, funicular administration may result in lymph node uptake in the inguinal region, which does not reflect testicular tumor drainage. Intratesticular administration in the parenchyma results in retroperitoneal SLN visualization, in accordance with known drainage patterns (Fig. 15.10).

15.4.11 Accuracy of Radioguided SLNB

To date, no studies have been published other than the aforementioned feasibility studies limited by small size of the study populations (~25 patients per study). Although refinement of the SLN procedure may enable better selection of patients who would benefit from adjuvant treatment after orchidectomy, further studies are required to substantiate the clinical value of the SLNs procedure in this disease.

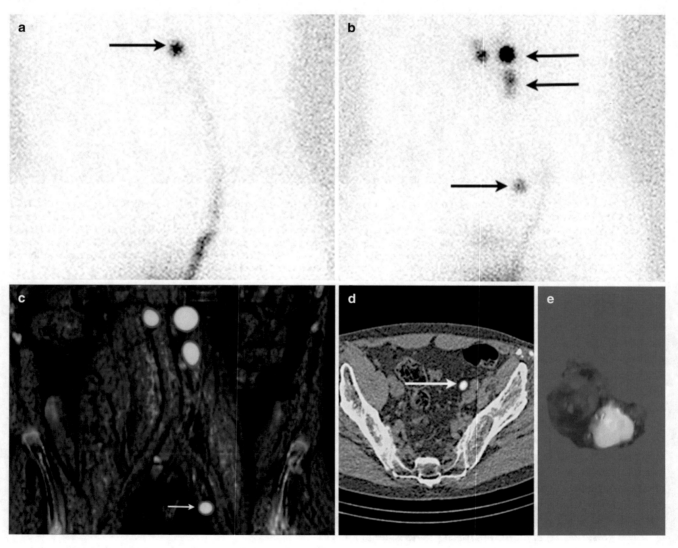

Fig. 15.10 Intratesticular injection of hybrid ICG-^{99m}Tc-nanocolloid (67.7 MBq) in a 52-year-old male with a seminoma in his left testicle followed by lymphoscintigraphy and SPECT/CT. (**a**) Early planar anterior image showing drainage from the left testicle toward an abdominal SLN (arrow). (**b**) The delayed lymphoscintigram reveals an additional SLN just below the SLN which was visualized on the early image (upper arrows), a second-echelon node to the right, and an additional hot spot located more caudally (lower arrow) which was therefore also defined as SLN. (**c**) Fused SPECT/CT image displayed with 3D volume rendering showing the cranial two SLNs alongside the aorta, the inter-aortocaval second-echelon node, and the more caudal SLN (arrow) next to the funiculus. (**d**) Axial fused SPECT/CT image depicting the caudal SLN along the external iliac vessels next to the funiculus. All SLNs were excised during laparoscopy guided by a laparoscopic gamma probe and fluorescence endoscope. (**e**) Ex vivo fluorescence image of a para-aortal SLN revealing the location of the node within the excised tissue specimen

Clinical Cases

Case 15.1: SLN Mapping in Penile Cancer with Bilateral Drainage to Both Groins

Renato A. Valdés Olmos, Henk G. van der Poel, and Oscar R. Brouwer

Background Clinical Case

A 78-year-old man with penile carcinoma was referred for SLNB. During staging of both groins no lymph node abnormalities had been detected on physical examination and ultrasonography (clinical stage T1N0).

Planar Lymphoscintigraphy and SPECT/CT Imaging

In the afternoon before surgery a total of 110 MBq ICG-^{99m}Tc-nanocolloid was administered in three intradermal injections proximal to the primary tumor into the glans. Immediately after tracer administration, a dynamic study was acquired during 10 min with the patient in supine position using a dual-head gamma camera (Symbia T, Siemens, Erlangen, Germany) equipped with low-energy high-resolution collimators. Subsequently, 5-min planar static images were acquired at 15 min and 2 h postinjection. In addition, SPECT/CT imaging was acquired after the 2-h delayed planar imaging using the same gamma camera.

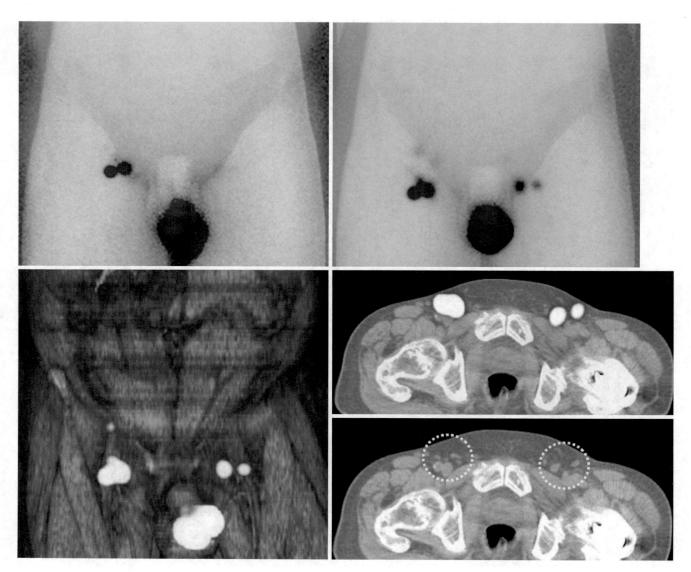

Fig. 15.11 Anterior early (on the left) and delayed (on the right) planar images, displayed in superposition to anatomical models, showing bilateral drainage to both groins. Inguinal SLNs in the left groin become clear only on delayed images. On SPECT/CT (bottom) radioactive SLNs in both groins are located above the saphenofemoral junction corresponding on low-dose CT to normal-size lymph nodes in the so-called upper inguinal zones of Daseler (circles)

Case 15.2: SLN Mapping in Recurrent Penile Carcinoma with Drainage to Iliac and Inguinal Lymph Nodes

Renato A. Valdés Olmos, Henk G. van der Poel, and Oscar R. Brouwer

Background Clinical Case

A 57-year-old man with a squamous-cell penile carcinoma recurrence was referred for SLNB. The patient had undergone partial penis amputation 13 years earlier because of a primary penile carcinoma (cT2N0) with subsequent lymph node dissection of the right groin due to SLN metastases (pT2N1). The SLN of the left groin at that time was free of tumor and no further surgical intervention had been performed. Following confirmation of the recurrence, no lymph node abnormalities had been detected on palpation and ultrasonography.

Planar Lymphoscintigraphy and SPECT/CT Imaging

In the afternoon before surgery a total of 100 MBq ICG-^{99m}Tc-nanocolloid was administered in three intradermal injections around the tumor recurrence following preparation with xylocaine 10% spray for local anesthesia. Immediately after tracer administration, a dynamic study was acquired during 10 min with the patient in supine position using a dual-head gamma camera (Symbia T, Siemens, Erlangen, Germany) equipped with low-energy high-resolution collimators. Subsequently, 5-min planar static images were acquired at 15 min and 2 h postinjection. In addition, SPECT/CT imaging was acquired after acquiring the delayed planar images using the same gamma camera.

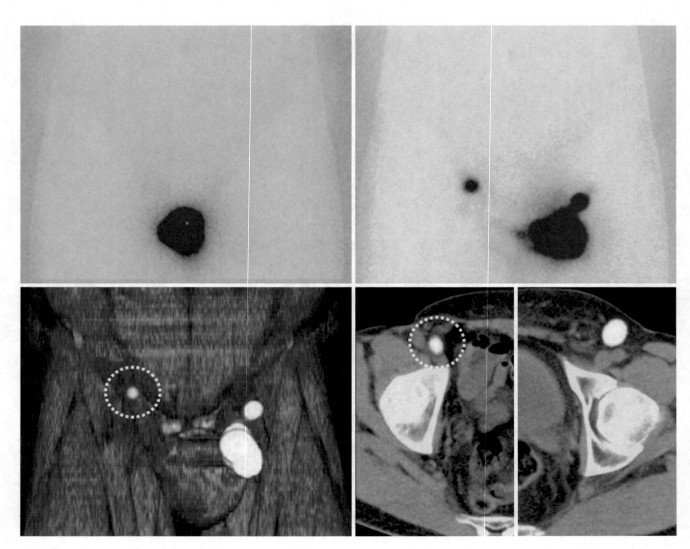

Fig. 15.12 Anterior static planar images displayed in superposition to anatomical models (upper row). Bilateral tracer migration to lymph nodes is only seen on delayed image (on the right) with a radioactive left lymph node near the penile injection site and a higher located node with a visible lymphatic duct in the right side. Note on SPECT/CT imaging (lower row) that the SLN in the right side is located in the vicinity of the external iliac artery (circles), whereas the SLN in the left side is located in the groin

Case 15.3: SLN Mapping in Prostate Carcinoma with Bilateral Drainage to Pelvic Lymph Nodes

Renato A. Valdés Olmos, Henk G. van der Poel, and Oscar R. Brouwer

Background Clinical Case

A 70-year-old man with confirmed carcinoma in the right lobe of the prostate on histopathology and Gleason 7 was referred for a SLN procedure with robot-assisted surgery. No lymph node abnormalities had been detected on radiological examination (clinical stage T2N0).

Planar Lymphoscintigraphy and SPECT/CT Imaging

The patient was planned for a 1-day SLN procedure. Early in the morning a total of 125 MBq ICG-^{99m}Tc-nanocolloid was administered in both lobes of the prostate by means of four injections guided by transrectal ultrasonography. Immediately after tracer administration, the patient was transferred to the department of nuclear medicine and a static image was acquired during 5 min with the patient in supine position using a dual-head gamma camera (Symbia T, Siemens, Erlangen, Germany) equipped with low-energy high-resolution collimators. Subsequently, delayed static images were acquired at 2 h postinjection. In addition, SPECT/CT imaging was acquired after acquiring the delayed planar images using the same gamma camera.

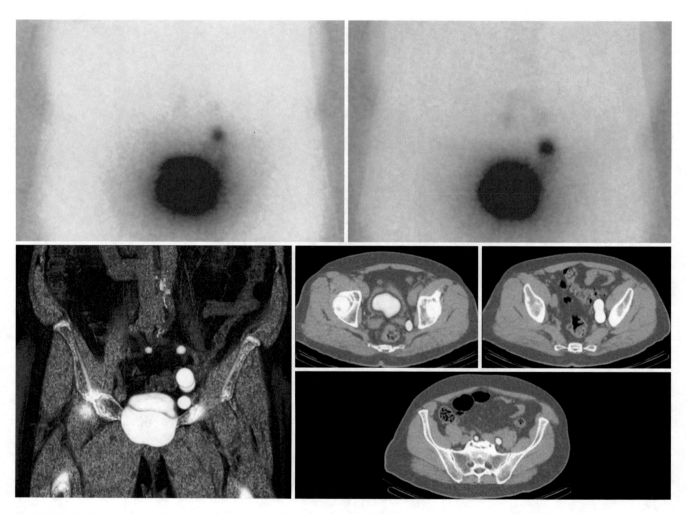

Fig. 15.13 Static planar images (upper row) are displayed in superposition to anatomical models. On early anterior (first frame) and right lateral (second frame) views bilateral lymph node uptake is seen principally on the left side of the pelvis. Volume-rendering and cross-sectional SPECT/CT images (lower row) show four SLNs along the left internal and common iliac arteries, whereas on the right side of the pelvis the SLN is located medially from the right common iliac vessels

Case 15.4: SLN Mapping in Prostate Carcinoma with Unilateral Drainage to a Pelvic Lymph Node

Renato A. Valdés Olmos, Henk G. van der Poel, and Oscar R. Brouwer

Background Clinical Case

A 70-year-old man with confirmed carcinoma in both lobes of the prostate on histopathology was referred for a SLN procedure with robot-assisted surgery. No lymph node abnormalities had been detected on radiological examination (clinical stage T2N0).

Planar Lymphoscintigraphy and SPECT/CT Imaging

Since a 1-day SLN procedure had been planned, the patient received in the morning a total of 115 MBq ICG-^{99m}Tc-nanocolloid by means of four injections in both lobes of the prostate guided by transrectal ultrasonography. Immediately after tracer administration, the patient was moved to the department of nuclear medicine and static 5-min images were acquired at 15 min and 2 h postinjection with the patient in supine position using a dual-head gamma camera (Symbia T, Siemens, Erlangen, Germany) equipped with low-energy high-resolution collimators. Subsequently to delayed static images, SPECT/CT imaging was acquired using the same gamma camera.

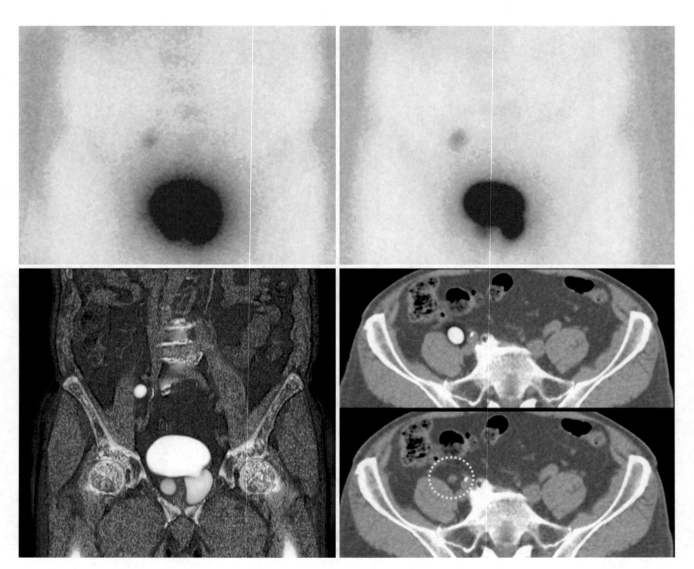

Fig. 15.14 Both early and delayed planar images (upper row), displayed in superposition to anatomical models, show migration of the tracer to the right side of the pelvis. Volume-rendering and cross-sectional SPECT/CT images (lower row) show one single SLN located laterally from the right common iliac vessels. The corresponding lymph node on low-dose CT (circle) is not enlarged

Case 15.5: SLN Mapping in Prostate Carcinoma with Drainage to Presacral and Mesorectal Lymph Nodes

Renato A. Valdés Olmos, Henk G. van der Poel, and Oscar R. Brouwer

Background Clinical Case

A 67-year-old man with carcinoma in both lobes of the prostate was referred for SLN procedure with robot-assisted surgery. No lymph node abnormalities had been detected on radiological examination (clinical stage T2N0).

Planar Lymphoscintigraphy and SPECT/CT Imaging

The procedure was based on a 1-day SLN procedure. Early in the morning the patient received a total of 120 MBq ICG-^{99m}Tc-nanocolloid by means of four injections in both lobes of the prostate guided by transrectal ultrasonography. Immediately after tracer administration, the patient was moved to the department of nuclear medicine and static 5-min images were acquired at 15 min and 2 h postinjection with the patient in supine position using a dual-head gamma camera (Symbia T, Siemens, Erlangen, Germany) equipped with low-energy high-resolution collimators. Subsequently to delayed static imaging, SPECT/CT imaging was acquired using the same gamma camera.

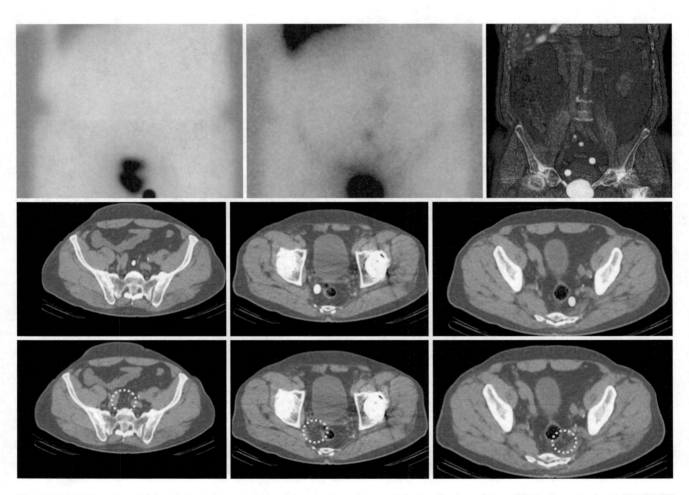

Fig. 15.15 Both early and delayed planar images (first two images in upper row), displayed in superposition to anatomical models, show delayed migration of the tracer to both sides of the pelvis. On volume-rendering SPECT/CT (last frame in upper row) the drainage becomes clearer, with visualization of three SLNs. Cross-sectional SPECT/CT images (lower row) show presacral and mesorectal SLNs. These radioactive nodes correspond to normal-size lymph nodes on low-dose CT (circles)

Case 15.6: SLN Mapping in Left Testicular Cancer with Unilateral Drainage to Para-aortic, Funicular, Iliac, and Inguinal Lymph Nodes

Renato A. Valdés Olmos, Henk G. van der Poel, and Oscar R. Brouwer

Background Clinical Case

A 35-year-old man with left testicle cancer was referred for SLN procedure. No lymph node abnormalities had been detected on radiological examination (clinical stage I).

Planar Lymphoscintigraphy and SPECT/CT Imaging

The day before surgery the patient received a total of 100 MBq ICG-^{99m}Tc-nanocolloid by means of a single injection in the left testicle in the proximity of the primary tumor following funicular block with 2% lidocaine. Immediately after tracer administration, a dynamic study was started during 10 min. Subsequently, static 5-min images were acquired at 15 min and 2 h postinjection with the patient in supine position using a dual-head gamma camera (Symbia T, Siemens, Erlangen, Germany) equipped with low-energy high-resolution collimators. Subsequently to delayed static images, SPECT/CT imaging was acquired using the same gamma camera.

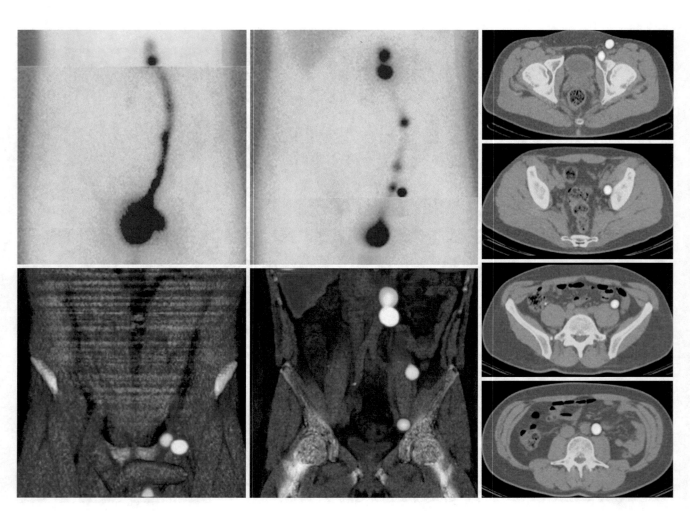

Fig. 15.16 Anterior planar images (first two images in upper row) are displayed in superposition to anatomical figures. Early static image (on the left) shows migration of the tracer from the left testicle through a long lymphatic vessel whereas delayed lymph node uptake is observed (second image) at various levels of pelvis and abdomen. On volume-rendering SPECT/CT (lower row) superficial (left image) and deep (second image) are displayed. Cross-sectional SPECT/CT images (right column) show inguinal and external iliac (top) as well as obturator and funicular SLNs (middle images) whereas the most cranial located lymph node is para-aortic (bottom)

Case 15.7: SLN Mapping in Right Testicular Cancer with Unilateral Drainage to Lymph Nodes Along the Vena Cava Inferior

Renato A. Valdés Olmos, Henk G. van der Poel, and Oscar R. Brouwer

Background Clinical Case

A 46-year-old man with right testicular cancer was referred for SLN procedure. No lymph node abnormalities had been detected on radiological examination (clinical stage I).

Planar Lymphoscintigraphy and SPECT/CT Imaging

The day before surgery the patient received a total of 90 MBq ^{99m}Tc-nanocolloid by means of a single injection in the right testicle in the vicinity of the primary tumor following funicular block with 2% lidocaine. Immediately after tracer administration a dynamic study was started during 10 min. Subsequently, static 5-min images were acquired at 15 min and 2 h postinjection with the patient in supine position using a dual-head gamma camera (Symbia T, Siemens, Erlangen, Germany) equipped with low-energy high-resolution collimators. Subsequently to delayed static images, SPECT/CT imaging was acquired using the same gamma camera.

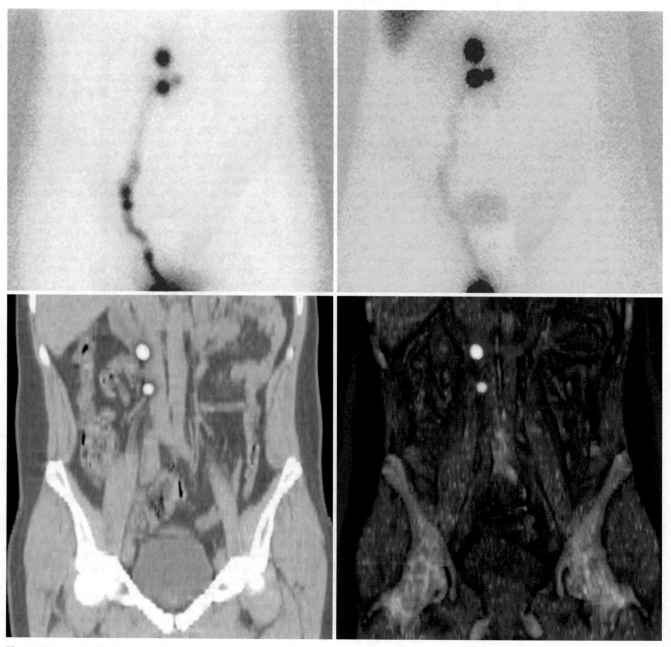

Fig. 15.17 Anterior planar images (upper row) are displayed in superposition to anatomical models. Early static image (on the left) shows migration of the tracer from the right testicle through a long lymphatic vessel with uptake in two lymph nodes. Delayed planar image (on the right) shows increasing uptake in the first draining lymph nodes and in a second echelon more medially located. On SPECT/CT imaging (lower row) both SLNs are seen laterally from the vena cava inferior

References

1. Van Den Berg NS, Van Leeuwen FWB, Van Der Poel HG. Fluorescence guidance in urologic surgery. Curr Opin Urol. 2012;22:109–20.
2. Brouwer OR, Buckle T, Vermeeren L, et al. Comparing the hybrid fluorescent-radioactive tracer indocyanine green-99mTc-nanocolloid with 99mTc-nanocolloid for sentinel node identification: a validation study using lymphoscintigraphy and SPECT/CT. J Nucl Med. 2012;53:1034–40.
3. Kleinjan GH, Van Den Berg NS, Brouwer OR, et al. Optimisation of fluorescence guidance during robot-assisted laparoscopic sentinel node biopsy for prostate cancer. Eur Urol. 2014;66:991–8.
4. Hernandez BY, Barnholtz-Sloan J, German RR, et al. Burden of invasive squamous cell carcinoma of the penis in the United States, 1998-2003. Cancer. 2008;113:2883–91.
5. Horenblas S, van Tinteren H. Squamous cell carcinoma of the penis. IV. Prognostic factors of survival: analysis of tumor, nodes and metastasis classification system. J Urol. 1994;151:1239–43.
6. Djajadiningrat RS, Graafland NM, van Werkhoven E, et al. Contemporary management of regional nodes in penile cancer-improvement of survival? J Urol. 2014;191:68–73.
7. Leijte JAP, Hughes B, Graafland NM, et al. Two-center evaluation of dynamic sentinel node biopsy for squamous cell carcinoma of the penis. J Clin Oncol. 2009;27:3325–9.
8. Kirrander P, Andrén O, Windahl T. Dynamic sentinel node biopsy in penile cancer: initial experiences at a Swedish Referral Centre. BJU Int. 2013;111:E48–53.
9. Lam W, Alnajjar HM, La-Touche S, et al. Dynamic sentinel lymph node biopsy in patients with invasive squamous cell carcinoma of the penis: a prospective study of the long-term outcome of 500 inguinal basins assessed at a single institution. Eur Urol. 2013;63:657–63.
10. Jakobsen JK, Krarup KP, Sommer P, et al. DaPeCa-1: diagnostic accuracy of sentinel lymph node biopsy in 222 patients with penile cancer at four tertiary referral centres - a national study from Denmark. BJU Int. 2016;117:235–43.
11. Dimopoulos P, Christopoulos P, Shilito S, et al. Dynamic sentinel lymph node biopsy for penile cancer: a comparison between 1- and 2-day protocols. BJU Int. 2016;117:890–6.
12. Stuiver MM, Djajadiningrat RS, Graafland NM, et al. Early wound complications after inguinal lymphadenectomy in penile cancer: a historical cohort study and risk-factor analysis. Eur Urol. 2013;64:486–92.
13. Spiess PE, Hernandez MS, Pettaway CA. Contemporary inguinal lymph node dissection: minimizing complications. World J Urol. 2009;27:205–12.
14. Hughes B, Leijte J, Shabbir M, et al. Non-invasive and minimally invasive staging of regional lymph nodes in penile cancer. World J Urol. 2009;27:197–203.
15. Woldu SL, Ci B, Hutchinson RC, et al. Usage and survival implications of surgical staging of inguinal lymph nodes in intermediate- to high-risk, clinical localized penile cancer: a propensity-score matched analysis. Urol Oncol. 2018;36:159.e7–159.e17.
16. Kroon BK, Horenblas S, Meinhardt W, et al. Dynamic sentinel node biopsy in penile carcinoma: evaluation of 10 years experience. Eur Urol. 2005;47:601–6.
17. Sadeghi R, Gholami H, Zakavi SR, et al. Accuracy of sentinel lymph node biopsy for inguinal lymph node staging of penile squamous cell carcinoma: systematic review and meta-analysis of the literature. J Urol. 2012;187:25–31.
18. TW Flaig PES. NCCN penile cancer 2018; 2018.
19. Hakenberg OW, Comperat E, Minhas S, et al. EAU guidelines penile cancer 2018; 2018.

20. Kroon BK, Horenblas S, Deurloo EE, et al. Ultrasonography-guided fine-needle aspiration cytology before sentinel node biopsy in patients with penile carcinoma. BJU Int. 2005;95:517–20.
21. Jakobsen JK, Alslev L, Ipsen P, et al. DaPeCa-3: promising results of sentinel node biopsy combined with (18) F-fluorodeoxyglucose positron emission tomography/computed tomography in clinically lymph node-negative patients with penile cancer—a national study from Denmark. BJU Int. 2016;118:102–11.
22. Lutzen U, Zuhayra M, Marx M, et al. Value and efficiency of sentinel lymph node diagnostics in patients with penile carcinoma with palpable inguinal lymph nodes as a new multimodal, minimally invasive approach. Eur J Nucl Med Mol Imaging. 2016;43:2313–23.
23. Graafland NM, Leijte JAP, Valdés Olmos RA, et al. Repeat dynamic sentinel node biopsy in locally recurrent penile carcinoma. BJU Int. 2010;105:1121–4.
24. Omorphos S, Saad Z, Arya M, et al. Feasibility of performing dynamic sentinel lymph node biopsy as a delayed procedure in penile cancer. World J Urol. 2016;34:329–35.
25. Kroon BK, Nieweg OE, van Boven H, et al. Size of metastasis in the sentinel node predicts additional nodal involvement in penile carcinoma. J Urol. 2006;176:105–8.
26. Kroon BK, Valdés Olmos RA, van Tinteren H, et al. Reproducibility of lymphoscintigraphy for lymphatic mapping in patients with penile carcinoma. J Urol. 2005;174:2214–7.
27. Winter A, Kowald T, Engels S, et al. Magnetic resonance sentinel lymph node imaging and magnetometer-guided intraoperative detection in penile cancer, using superparamagnetic iron oxide nanoparticles: first results. Urol Int. 2019:1–4.
28. Omorphos S, Saad Z, Kirkham A, et al. Zonal mapping of sentinel lymph nodes in penile cancer patients using fused SPECT/CT imaging and lymphoscintigraphy. Urol Oncol. 2018;36:530.e1–6.
29. Sahdev V, Albersen M, Christodoulidou M, et al. The management of non-visualisation following dynamic sentinel lymph node biopsy for squamous cell carcinoma of the penis. BJU Int. 2016;119:573–8.
30. Valdés Olmos RA, Tanis PJ, Hoefnagel CA, et al. Penile lymphoscintigraphy for sentinel node identification. Eur J Nucl Med. 2001;28:581–5.
31. Brouwer OR, van der Poel HG, Bevers RF, et al. Beyond penile cancer, is there a role for sentinel node biopsy in urological malignancies? Clin Transl Imaging. 2016;4:395–410.
32. Brouwer OR, Van Den Berg NS, Mathéron HM, et al. A hybrid radioactive and fluorescent tracer for sentinel node biopsy in penile carcinoma as a potential replacement for blue dye. Eur Urol. 2014;65:600–9.
33. Leijte JAP, van der Ploeg IMC, Valdés Olmos RA, et al. Visualization of tumor blockage and rerouting of lymphatic drainage in penile cancer patients by use of SPECT/CT. J Nucl Med. 2009;50:364–7.
34. Naumann CM, Colberg C, Jüptner M, et al. Evaluation of the diagnostic value of preoperative sentinel lymph node (SLN) imaging in penile carcinoma patients without palpable inguinal lymph nodes via single photon emission computed tomography/computed tomography (SPECT/CT) as compared to planar sci. Urol Oncol Semin Orig Investig. 2018;36:92.e17–24.
35. Saad ZZ, Omorphos S, Michopoulou S, et al. Investigating the role of SPECT/CT in dynamic sentinel lymph node biopsy for penile cancers. Eur J Nucl Med Mol Imaging. 2017;44:1176–84.
36. KleinJan GH, van Werkhoven E, van den Berg NS, et al. The best of both worlds: a hybrid approach for optimal pre- and intraoperative identification of sentinel lymph nodes. Eur J Nucl Med Mol Imaging. 2018;45:1915–25.
37. van Leeuwen AC, Buckle T, Bendle G, et al. Tracer-cocktail injections for combined pre- and intraoperative multimodal imaging of lymph nodes in a spontaneous mouse prostate tumor model. J Biomed Opt. 2011;16:016004.

38. Kroon BK, Valdés Olmos RA, van der Poel HG, et al. Prepubic sentinel node location in penile carcinoma. Clin Nucl Med. 2005;30:649–50.
39. Tanis PJ, Lont AP, Meinhardt W, et al. Dynamic sentinel node biopsy for penile cancer: reliability of a staging technique. J Urol. 2002;168:76–80.
40. Leijte JAP, Kroon BK, Valdés Olmos RA, et al. Reliability and safety of current dynamic sentinel node biopsy for penile carcinoma. Eur Urol. 2007;52:170–7.
41. Lont AP, Horenblas S, Tanis PJ, et al. Management of clinically node negative penile carcinoma: improved survival after the introduction of dynamic sentinel node biopsy. J Urol. 2003;170:783–6.
42. Zou Z-J, Liu Z-H, Tang L-Y, et al. Radiocolloid-based dynamic sentinel lymph node biopsy in penile cancer with clinically negative inguinal lymph node: an updated systematic review and meta-analysis. Int Urol Nephrol. 2016;48:2001–13.
43. Mottet N, Bellmunt J, Bolla M, et al. EAU-ESTRO-SIOG guidelines on prostate cancer. Part 1: screening, diagnosis, and local treatment with curative intent. Eur Urol. 2017;71(4):618–29.
44. Perera M, Papa N, Roberts M, et al. Gallium-68 prostate-specific membrane antigen positron emission tomography in advanced prostate cancer—updated diagnostic utility, sensitivity, specificity, and distribution of prostate-specific membrane antigen-avid lesions: a systematic review and meta-analysis. Eur Urol. 2020;77(4):403–17.
45. van Leeuwen PJ, Emmett L, Ho B, et al. Prospective evaluation of 68Gallium-prostate-specific membrane antigen positron emission tomography/computed tomography for preoperative lymph node staging in prostate cancer. BJU Int. 2017;119:209–15.
46. Meinhardt W, van der Poel HG, Valdés Olmos RA, et al. Laparoscopic sentinel lymph node biopsy for prostate cancer: the relevance of locations outside the extended dissection area. Prostate Cancer. 2012;2012:1–4.
47. Wit EMK, Acar C, Grivas N, et al. Sentinel node procedure in prostate cancer: a systematic review to assess diagnostic accuracy. Eur Urol. 2017;71:596–605.
48. Vermeeren L, Valdes Olmos RA, Meinhardt W, et al. Intraoperative imaging for sentinel node identification in prostate carcinoma: its use in combination with other techniques. J Nucl Med. 2011;52:741–4.
49. Meinhardt W. Sentinel node evaluation in prostate cancer. EAU-EBU Update Series. 2007;5:223–31.
50. Vermeeren L, Muller SH, Meinhardt W, et al. Optimizing the colloid particle concentration for improved preoperative and intraoperative image-guided detection of sentinel nodes in prostate cancer. Eur J Nucl Med Mol Imaging. 2010;37:1328–34.
51. de Bonilla-Damiá A, Roberto Brouwer O, Meinhardt W, et al. Lymphatic drainage in prostate carcinoma assessed by lymphoscintigraphy and SPECT/CT: its importance for the sentinel node procedure. Rev Esp Med Nucl Imagen Mol. 2012;31:66–70.
52. Joniau S, Van Den Bergh L, Lerut E, et al. Mapping of pelvic lymph node metastases in prostate cancer. Eur Urol. 2013;63:450–8
53. Van Den Bergh L, Joniau S, Haustermans K, et al. Reliability of sentinel node procedure for lymph node staging in prostate cancer patients at high risk for lymph node involvement. Acta Oncol (Madr). 2015;54:896–902.
54. van der Poel HG, Buckle T, Brouwer OR, et al. Intraoperative laparoscopic fluorescence guidance to the sentinel lymph node in prostate cancer patients: clinical proof of concept of an integrated functional imaging approach using a multimodal tracer. Eur Urol. 2011;60:826–33.
55. KleinJan GH, van den Berg NS, de Jong J, et al. Multimodal hybrid imaging agents for sentinel node mapping as a means to (re)connect nuclear medicine to advances made in robot-assisted surgery. Eur J Nucl Med Mol Imaging. 2016;43:1278–87.
56. Vermeeren L, Valdés Olmos RA, Meinhardt W, et al. Intraoperative radioguidance with a portable gamma camera: a novel technique for laparoscopic sentinel node localisation in urological malignancies. Eur J Nucl Med Mol Imaging. 2009;36:1029–36.
57. van Oosterom MN, Simon H, Mengus L, et al. Revolutionizing (robot-assisted) laparoscopic gamma tracing using a drop-in gamma probe technology. Am J Nucl Med Mol Imaging. 2016;6:1–17.
58. Meershoek P, van Oosterom MN, Simon H, et al. Robot-assisted laparoscopic surgery using DROP-IN radioguidance: first-in-human translation. Eur J Nucl Med Mol Imaging. 2019;46:49–53.
59. Vermeeren L, Valdés Olmos RA, Meinhardt W, et al. Value of SPECT/CT for detection and anatomic localization of sentinel lymph nodes before laparoscopic sentinel node lymphadenectomy in prostate carcinoma. J Nucl Med. 2009;50:865–70.
60. Holl G, Dorn R, Wengenmair H, et al. Validation of sentinel lymph node dissection in prostate cancer: experience in more than 2,000 patients. Eur J Nucl Med Mol Imaging. 2009;36:1377–82.
61. Meinhardt W, Valdés Olmos RA, Van Der Poel HG, et al. Laparoscopic sentinel lymph node dissection for prostate carcinoma: technical and anatomical observations. BJU Int. 2008;102:714–7.
62. Rajpert-De Meyts E, McGlynn KA, Okamoto K, et al. Testicular germ cell tumours. Lancet. 2016;387:1762–74.
63. Nallu A, Mannuel HD, Hussain A. Testicular germ cell tumors. Curr Opin Oncol. 2013;25:266–72.
64. Trabert B, Chen J, Devesa SS, et al. International patterns and trends in testicular cancer incidence, overall and by histologic subtype, 1973-2007. Andrology. 2015;3:4–12.
65. Tandstad T, Smaaland R, Solberg A, et al. Management of seminomatous testicular cancer: a binational prospective population-based study from the Swedish Norwegian Testicular Cancer Study Group. J Clin Oncol. 2011;29:719–25.
66. Aparicio J, García del Muro X, Maroto P, et al. Multicenter study evaluating a dual policy of postorchiectomy surveillance and selective adjuvant single-agent carboplatin for patients with clinical stage I seminoma. Ann Oncol. 2003;14:867–72.
67. Kollmannsberger C, Moore C, Chi KN, et al. Non-risk-adapted surveillance for patients with stage I nonseminomatous testicular germ-cell tumors: diminishing treatment-related morbidity while maintaining efficacy. Ann Oncol. 2010;21:1296–301.
68. Powles TB, Bhardwa J, Shamash J, et al. The changing presentation of germ cell tumours of the testis between 1983 and 2002. BJU Int. 2005;95:1197–200.
69. Blok JM, Kerst JM, Vegt E, et al. Sentinel node biopsy in clinical stage I testicular cancer enables early detection of occult metastatic disease. BJU Int. 2019;124(3):424–30.
70. Tanis PJ, Horenblas S, Valdés Olmos RA, et al. Feasibility of sentinel node lymphoscintigraphy in stage I testicular cancer. Eur J Nucl Med. 2002;29:670–3.
71. Brouwer OR, Valdes Olmos RA, Vermeeren L, et al. SPECT/CT and a portable camera for image-guided laparoscopic sentinel node biopsy in testicular cancer. J Nucl Med. 2011;52:551–4.
72. Albers P, Albrecht W, Algaba F, et al. Guidelines on testicular cancer: 2015 update. Eur Urol. 2015;68:1054–68.
73. Kollmannsberger C, Tandstad T, Bedard PL, et al. Patterns of relapse in patients with clinical stage I testicular cancer managed with active surveillance. J Clin Oncol. 2015;33:51–7.
74. Pierorazio PM, Albers P, Black PC, et al. Non-risk-adapted surveillance for stage I testicular cancer: critical review and summary. Eur Urol. 2018;73:899–907.
75. Kerns SL, Fung C, Monahan PO, et al. Cumulative burden of morbidity among testicular cancer survivors after standard cisplatin-based chemotherapy: a multi-institutional study. J Clin Oncol. 2018;36:1505–12.
76. van den Belt-Dusebout AW, de Wit R, Gietema JA, et al. Treatment-specific risks of second malignancies and cardiovascular disease in 5-year survivors of testicular cancer. J Clin Oncol. 2007;25:4370–8.

77. Kvammen O, Myklebust TA, Solberg A, et al. Long-term relative survival after diagnosis of testicular germ cell tumor. Cancer
Epidemiol Biomark Prev. 2016;25:773–9.

78. Warde P, Specht L, Horwich A, et al. Prognostic factors for relapse
in stage I seminoma managed by surveillance: a pooled analysis. J
Clin Oncol. 2002;20:4448–52.

79. Albers P, Siener R, Kliesch S, et al. Risk factors for relapse in clinical stage I nonseminomatous testicular germ cell tumors: results
of the German Testicular Cancer Study Group Trial. J Clin Oncol.
2003;21:1505–12.

80. Lago-Hernandez CA, Feldman H, O'Donnell E, et al. A refined risk
stratification scheme for clinical stage 1 NSGCT based on evaluation of both embryonal predominance and lymphovascular invasion. Ann Oncol. 2015;26:1396–401.

81. Klepp O, Dahl O, Flodgren P, et al. Risk-adapted treatment
of clinical stage 1 non-seminoma testis cancer. Eur J Cancer.
1997;33:1038–44.

82. Ohyama C, Chiba Y, Yamazaki T, et al. Lymphatic mapping and
gamma probe guided laparoscopic biopsy of sentinel lymph
node in patients with clinical stage I testicular tumor. J Urol.
2002;168:1390–5.

83. Satoh M, Ito A, Kaiho Y, et al. Intraoperative, radio-guided sentinel lymph node mapping in laparoscopic lymph node dissection for stage I testicular carcinoma. Cancer. 2005;103:2067–72.

84. Weissbach L, Boedefeld EA. Localization of solitary and multiple metastases in stage II nonseminomatous testis tumor as basis
for a modified staging lymph node dissection in stage I. J Urol.
1987;138:77–83.

85. Ray B, Hajdu SI, Whitmore WF. Distribution of retroperitoneal
lymph node metastases in testicular germinal tumors. Cancer.
1974;33:340–8.

86. Brouwer OR, Buckle T, Bunschoten A, et al. Image navigation as
a means to expand the boundaries of fluorescence-guided surgery.
Phys Med Biol. 2012;57:3123–36.

Preoperative and Intraoperative Lymphatic Mapping for Radioguided Sentinel Lymph Node Biopsy in Kidney and Bladder Cancers

Axel Bex, Teele Kuusk, Oscar R. Brouwer, and Renato A. Valdés Olmos

Contents

16.1   **Introduction** 358

16.2   **The Clinical Problem** 358

16.3   **Lymphatic Drainage and Nodal Groups in Renal Cancer** 359

16.4   **Lymphatic Drainage and Nodal Groups in Bladder Cancer** 360

16.5   **Radiocolloid Administration in Renal and Bladder Cancers** 362

16.6   **Preoperative Imaging of SLNs in Renal and Bladder Cancer** 362

16.7   **Intraoperative SLN Detection Nodes in Renal and Bladder Cancer** ... 362

16.8   **Contribution of SPECT/CT Imaging for SLN Mapping in Renal and Bladder Cancers** 364

16.9   **Intraoperative SLN Imaging in Renal and Bladder Cancers** 364

16.10   **Accuracy of Radioguided SLNB in Renal or Bladder Cancer** 365

Clinical Cases 368

References 371

Learning Objectives

- To acquire basic knowledge about the role of nuclear medicine imaging in the sentinel lymph node (SLN) procedure in renal or bladder cancer
- To know when sentinel lymph node biopsy (SLNB) is indicated in patients with renal or bladder cancer
- To learn the status of investigations to validate clinical indication of SLNB in patients with renal or bladder cancer
- To understand the variability in lymphatic drainage in the pelvis and the need to use preoperative lymphatic mapping to assess the different individual patterns
- To know the role of lymphoscintigraphy and SPECT/CT to identify and localize SLNs in patients with renal or bladder cancer
- To understand the importance of SPECT/CT to identify and localize SLNs in the anatomical areas of retroperitoneum and pelvis

A. Bex (✉) · O. R. Brouwer
Division of Surgical Oncology, Department of Urology,
Netherlands Cancer Institute—Antoni van Leeuwenhoek Hospital,
Amsterdam, Netherlands
e-mail: a.bex@nki.nl

T. Kuusk
Department of Urology, Royal Free Hospital, London, UK

R. A. Valdés Olmos
Department of Radiology, Section of Nuclear Medicine and
Interventional Molecular Imaging Laboratory, Leiden University
Medical Center, Leiden, The Netherlands

© Springer Nature Switzerland AG 2020
G. Mariani et al. (eds.), *Atlas of Lymphoscintigraphy and Sentinel Node Mapping*,
https://doi.org/10.1007/978-3-030-45296-4_16

- To preoperatively identify SLNs and to learn how this information can be transferred to urology surgeons for the intraoperative procedure
- To understand that the SLN procedure does not yet constitute the standard of care in patients with kidney or bladder cancer, but is rather the object of ongoing validation clinical trials

16.1 Introduction

Renal cell cancer (RCC) is the tenth most common malignancy in Europe and the United States. In 2018, estimated 136,500 new cases were diagnosed in the European Union and an estimated 54,700 people died from the disease [1]. However, RCC accounts for only 3–5% of cancers and is therefore relatively uncommon when compared to breast, bowel and lung cancers [2]. Histologically, several subtypes can be identified, of which clear-cell carcinoma is predominant representing up to 70–80% of the cases [3].

The management of early-stage RCC has traditionally been surgical, and nephrectomy and/or nephron-sparing strategies are often curative at this stage of the disease [4]. Even when patients present with metastases, nephrectomy and metastasectomy may be beneficial in selected cases [5, 6]. In this regard, the widespread use of ultrasound examination of the abdomen has led to renal tumours being diagnosed when they are of smaller size [7]. Stage shift may result in an increasing number of patients with early lymph node (LN) metastases only, who, in contrast to historical data, may benefit from removal of these lesions. In addition, the introduction of targeted therapy agents has revived interest in adjuvant treatment concepts [8]. Accurate LN staging is warranted to determine the risk of recurrence or progression.

Bladder cancer is more common than RCC and is related to carcinogens in the environment and/or lifestyle habits (such as tobacco smoking) [9]. The most prominent subtype is transitional cell carcinoma, representing about 90% of the cases. In the United States, bladder cancer is the fourth most common type of cancer in men and the ninth most common cancer in women [10]. Estimated number of bladder cancers in Europe in 2018 is 197,100 and mortality 65,000 [1]. Approximately 50% of bladder cancer incidence is related to cigarette smoking. In addition, further occupational hazards play a role.

Lymph node metastases are common in patients with bladder cancer and the risk of LN involvement is highly associated with the depth of invasion of the primary tumour [11]. Presence of LN metastases, their number and the vol- ume of involved nodes are strongly associated with survival [12]. Five-year survival rates up to 57% have been observed in patients with pathologically confirmed but occult N1 disease on imaging prior to surgery. The 5-year survival drops down to 0–27% for patients with N2-N3 disease. In the majority of patients with muscle invasive bladder cancer, local treatment fails due to occult systemic disease, but extensive pelvic lymph node dissection (PLND) confers a survival benefit [11]. In addition to extensive PLND, survival can be increased by using systemic chemotherapy, either in the neoadjuvant or in the adjuvant setting [13]. As for renal cancer, improving detection and successful removal of early lymph node metastasis may lead to a survival benefit.

16.2 The Clinical Problem

Generally, the clinical problem in renal and bladder cancer is a consequence of the fact that LN metastases may occur outside known and expected lymphatic basins.

Specifically for RCC, the role of lymph node dissection (LND) remains controversial despite a randomized study with a median follow-up of 12.6 years [14]. This may be due to the unpredictability of lymphatic drainage of RCC, which undergoes mainly haematogenous spread. A potential reason for the lack of evidence supporting locoregional retroperitoneal LND and the low detection of LN metastases in CT-negative locoregional nodes may simply be the fact that lymphatic landing sites of RCC are located outside the expected LND templates in a relevant fraction of the cases. In addition, in the majority of patients with RCC, LN involvement is associated with haematogenous metastases [15], and is a significant indicator of systemic disease and adverse prognosis [16]. The likelihood of identifying LN metastasis only seems to be low, given the high proportion of concurrent systemic disease.

However, there is evidence that patients with very early LN metastases and no distant disease can potentially be cured by LND [17, 18]. The true incidence of LN-only involvement is unknown, but seems to correlate with tumour size. In retrospective nephrectomy and autopsy studies, microscopic LN metastases were mainly observed in smaller tumours [18–20]. On autopsy, patients with renal tumours <3 cm revealed LN metastases in 3.5%, which increased to 21% in tumours 4–5 cm in size [21]. In nephrectomy series, this was 2.5% and 4% for tumours ≤4 cm [22, 23]. Therefore, the predominant clinical problem in early-stage RCC is the detection and subsequent removal of early metastatic disease. In addition, detection of occult LN metastases is important to assess the prognosis of the patients, which may gain more significance if ongoing trials with adjuvant immune checkpoint inhibitors yield positive results.

In bladder cancer, the value of PLND is undisputed for muscle invasive bladder cancer. Dhar et al. reported a LN metastasis rate of 13% versus 26% for limited versus extended pelvic lymph node dissection [24]. These results as well as anatomical and functional studies underline the need for elective PLND at radical cystectomy to accurately stage these cases. The total number of resected lymph nodes is generally regarded as an indicator of surgical quality [25]. Other lymph node parameters have been introduced as prognostic factors, such as the total number of tumour-positive LNs and lymph node density, that is, the number of tumour-positive LNs divided by the total number of resected LNs [26]. Although these parameters are widely accepted in clinical practice, they depend on pathologist's evaluation. It was recently demonstrated that, despite equal anatomical clearance by the same experienced surgeons, a statistically significant difference between two pathology departments was found, where the number of LNs was evaluated after extended bilateral PLND for bladder cancer [27]. With the currently poorly standardized methods, the number of reported LNs as an indicator of surgical quality and lymph node density as a prognostic factor are probably not reliable.

Key Learning Points
- Both in renal cancers and in bladder cancers the presence of lymph node metastasis is one of the key prognostic factors and its incidence seems to be correlated with tumour size.
- Other prognostic factors include the total number of tumour-positive lymph nodes and lymph node density (ratio of tumour-positive lymph nodes relative to the total number of resected lymph nodes at pelvic lymph node dissection).
- Lymphoscintigraphy (including both planar imaging and SPECT/CT imaging) has recently been explored for lymph node mapping in patients with renal or bladder cancers.

16.3 Lymphatic Drainage and Nodal Groups in Renal Cancer

The lymphatic drainage pattern in RCC has not been accurately ascertained till 2018, when a lymphatic drainage study with SLN mapping and SPECT/CT imaging was published. The drainage differs from the anatomical studies performed in non-tumour-bearing kidneys, possibly because of multiple lymphatic tumour-draining vessels [28]. Lymphatic drainage from renal tumours may be outside the proposed retroperitoneal templates.

A general notion is that the draining LNs are in the hilar region, branching off into the paracaval, interaortocaval, or para-aortal retroperitoneal LNs, depending on the tumour side. The lymphatic drainage of renal tumours may however not always follow the known pattern, as has frequently been found for other tumour entities. As back as 1935, Parker found extreme variations of lymphatic drainage between individuals by injecting blue dye at high pressure into normal cadaveric kidneys [29].

Lymphatic mapping, including planar lymphoscintigraphy and SPECT/CT imaging, of kidney tumours has been described in two pilot studies, and in a phase II study with 40 patients [30–32]. The more recent study showed that 35% of lymphatic drainage is outside the suggested lymph node dissection templates, and that 20% of lymph flow drains directly to the thoracic area [32] (Fig. 16.1). However, most of the drainage from the right side was to interaortocaval, retrocaval areas, although there was simultaneous drainage into left preaortic or para-aortic and left supraclavicular lymph nodes. Only three patients with right-sided tumours had SLNs in the right paracaval and renal hilar region, and none had drainage to precaval LNs [32]. The main lymph drainage for left-side tumours was to para-aortal LNs with simultaneous drainage to hilar, mediastinal, left supraclavicular, retrocrural, left common iliac, renal fossa and interaortocaval SLNs [32]. The other important issue to distinguish the distribution of lymphatic drainage and first landing sites is the location of single LN metastases. The drainage patterns were previously assessed by considering lymphatic metastasis in lymphadenectomy (LND) specimens, or at autopsy. In nephrectomy series, metastases are generally detected in "regional" lymphadenectomies, and often the extent of LND is poorly defined. The accuracy of detecting LN metastases increases with the number of sampled LNs, irrespective of the extent of LND [33].

In an autopsy study involving 1828 cases of RCC, a broad variation of the localization of LN metastases was observed [34]. Since most patients had multiple lymphatic metastases, it could not be concluded which LN was involved first. Interestingly, ipsilateral renal hilar LN metastases were found in only 7% of the cases, while pulmonary hilar LN metastases were found in 66.2%, retroperitoneal in 36%, para-aortal in 26.8% and supraclavicular in 20.7% of the patients [34]. Single, isolated LN metastases have been described by Hulten et al. in a supraclavicular LN in one patient and in an iliac LN in two patients, without any further metastasis [35]. Furthermore, Johnsen et al. detected single LN metastases in ten patients, with a single mediastinal, supraclavicular and axillary node in, respectively, eight, one and one patients [21]. Those single-node metastases may chronologically be the first site of metastasis.

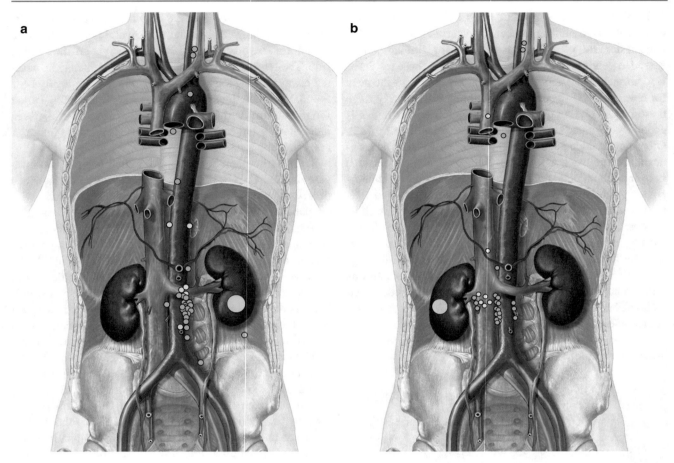

Fig. 16.1 (**a**) Distribution of 29 SLNs from 18 right kidney tumours at SPECT/CT. Green SLNs locate ventrally to blood vessels, yellow SLNs dorsally. (**b**) Distribution of 34 SLNs from 22 left kidney tumours. Green SLNs locate ventrally to blood vessels, yellow SLNs dorsally (image printed with permission of A.D.A.M. Images)

Interestingly, lymphatics from the kidney drain directly into the thoracic duct (TD), without any interposed LN. This latter situation has been described by Assouad and co-workers, who injected normal kidneys of 16 cadavers with a blue modified Gerota mass and dissected lymph vessels until their termination [36]. Renal lymphatics reached distant lymph nodes (e.g. aortic bifurcation, celiac, mesenteric and contralateral nodes). Furthermore, lymphatic vessels were always connecting to the origin of the TD, in several cases (38% on the right and 15% on the left) even directly without involving any LN (Fig. 16.2) [37]. Also in a SLN mapping study early lymphatic drainage following the course of the thoracic duct on lymphoscintigraphy and SPECT/CT images was seen. In one patient, this was observed without any retroperitoneal LN interposition [38]. Clinically, drainage through the TD may explain the isolated mediastinal LN metastasis with synchronous pulmonary metastasis that are frequently observed in RCC [19–22, 39–41].

16.4 Lymphatic Drainage and Nodal Groups in Bladder Cancer

In contrast to renal cancer, lymphatic drainage in bladder cancer is more predictable. However, autopsy and pathological postcystectomy studies have failed to accurately map the landing sites of lymphatic drainage from the urinary bladder. Contrary to renal cancer, the value of lymphoscintigraphy and intraoperative SLN mapping has been evaluated and demonstrated in large series. However, the most recent studies assume that SLNB is not a reliable technique for perioperative localization of LN metastases during cystectomy [41, 42]. In well-lateralized bladder cancer a 100% ipsilateral radiocolloid drainage rate has been observed, including drainage to the external iliac, obturator fossa and common iliac stations [43]. In 40% of the cases, additional lymphatic drainage to the contralateral side was seen.

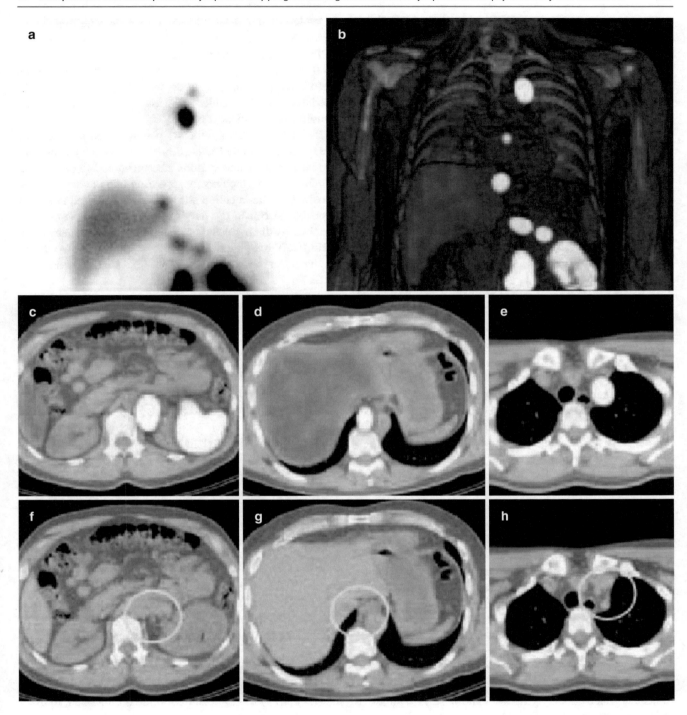

Fig. 16.2 A 39-year-old man with a T1 (5 cm) papillary renal cell carcinoma in the lateral part of the left kidney. Lymphoscintigraphy and SPECT/CT were acquired after ultrasound-guided injection of 209 MBq ^{99m}Tc-nanocolloid into the tumour. Planar anterior image (**a**) and SPECT/CT volume rendering (**b**) show drainage to lymph nodes in the abdomen and in the thorax. Axial SPECT/CT images show para-aortic SLNs (**c**) as well as retrocrural (**d**) and mediastinal lymph nodes (**e**). None of these lymph nodes were enlarged on CT (**f–h**). At histopathology two para-aortic SLNs were found to contain metastases. The *yellow circles* refer to the location of corresponding LNs on conventional CT that may represent the SLNs

Key Learning Points
- Although somewhat unpredictable, in general lymphatic drainage from renal cancers is initially to hilar lymph nodes, and then to the paracaval, inter-aortocaval or para-aortal retroperitoneal LNs, depending on the side of the tumour.
- In about 20% of the cases lymph from the kidney drains directly to the thoracic area without any interposition lymph node.
- Lymphatic drainage from the bladder is more predictable; in well-lateralized bladder cancers radiocolloid drainage occurs almost invariably to the ipsilateral LNs, including to external iliac, obturator fossa and common iliac stations, although additional contralateral drainage can also be observed.

16.5 Radiocolloid Administration in Renal and Bladder Cancers

In kidney cancer, in a study with 40 patients, ^{99m}Tc-nanocolloid was injected percutaneously (0.4 mL, 225 MBq) into the primary renal lesion under ultrasound or CT guidance the day before surgery (Fig. 16.3). Using a spinal needle, primary tumours ≤4 cm were injected centrally with a single 0.4 mL aliquot. Tumours 4–10 cm in size received in total 2–3 × 0.4 mL aliquots, injected around the centre into solid parts and avoiding areas of necrosis [30].

In bladder cancer, the radiocolloid is in most studies injected under cystoscopy guidance using an endoscopic needle (Fig. 16.4) [44]. An amount of 240 MBq of the radiocolloid is administered into the detrusor muscle in four sites around the tumour following a transurethral approach, with the patient in the lithotomy position.

16.6 Preoperative Imaging of SLNs in Renal and Bladder Cancer

In renal cancer, planar lymphoscintigraphy in a phase II study was acquired 20 min and 2–4 h post-administration, acquiring anterior and lateral planar images. Since radiocolloid administration was performed in the department of radiology, dynamic scanning with a standard gamma camera was not possible. The use of a portable gamma camera may assist radiocolloid injection and help to modify/repeat the injection procedure in case radioactivity is detected outside the tumour and the kidney. SPECT/CT imaging was usually acquired following the acquisition of delayed planar images. For this

procedure a low-dose CT was obtained, acquiring 2 mm slices for attenuation correction and for generation of SPECT/CT fusion images (Fig. 16.5).

A similar procedure is performed for bladder cancer. Before lymphoscintigraphy an indwelling catheter can be used to empty the bladder and wash out excess of the radiocolloid from the bladder cavity.

The LNs appearing on early planar lymphoscintigraphy are considered to be SLNs (Fig. 16.6), while those appearing later in the same stations are considered to be second-echelon LNs. Lymph nodes appearing late in other stations proximal to the injection site are also considered as highly probable SLNs. In the pelvis, planar images often cannot specifically distinguish the nodal groups, and in many cases SPECT/CT imaging depicts radioactive LNs in two different basins at the same level. These LNs are also considered as SLNs.

Key Learning Points
- For lymphatic mapping in patients with renal cancers, the radiocolloid can be injected intratumourally under ultrasound or CT guidance.
- In patients with bladder cancers the radiocolloid can be injected into the detrusor muscle in four sites around the tumour during transurethral cystoscopy.
- In renal cancer planar lymphoscintigraphy is acquired early (20 min) and late (2–4 h) post-radiocolloid administration; SPECT/CT imaging is usually acquired after the delayed planar scan.
- Similar protocols are adopted for lymphatic mapping in patients with bladder cancers.

16.7 Intraoperative SLN Detection Nodes in Renal and Bladder Cancer

The optimal approach for renal surgery depends on the size and location of the tumour. As a result, intraoperative SLN detection in RCC has been performed during open, transabdominal nephrectomies, open retroperitoneal partial nephrectomies and laparoscopic transperitoneal nephrectomies as well as robotic assisted laparoscopic nephron-sparing surgery. For both open and laparoscopic approaches the same method is used.

For intraoperative SLN detection during open surgery, a standard gamma probe is used, whereas for laparoscopy a special laparoscopic gamma probe is necessary. Patent blue is rarely used, due to its limited contribution.

Fig. 16.3 A 47-year-old woman with a T2 (8.8 cm) renal cell carcinoma in the lower pole of the right kidney. Following CT-guided needle placement into the tumour, 206 MBq ^{99m}Tc-nanocolloid was administered under continuous monitoring with a portable gamma camera (**a**) showing initial tumour retention of the tracer (**b**). Planar posterior image (**c**), SPECT/CT volume rendering (**d**) and axial SPECT/CT (**e, f**) show drainage to a SLN between the aorta and the vena cava. This SLN was tumour negative at histopathology. The *yellow circle* refers to the location of corresponding LNs on conventional CT that may represent the SLNs

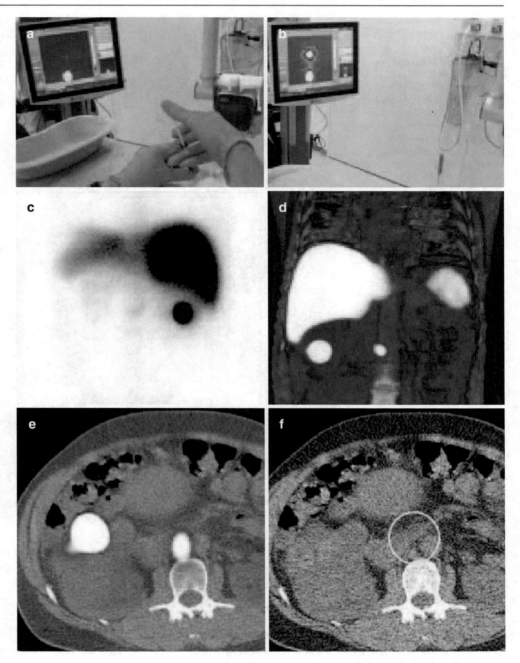

SLNs are separately excised, followed by LND (hilar, paracaval and interaortocaval on the right or hilar, para-aortal and interaortocaval on the left side). As the preliminary trials have so far investigated feasibility and drainage patterns with a yet unproven clinical benefit, only SLNs that could be approached through the access for renal surgery are removed in current study protocols.

Intraoperative SLN identification and sampling can be combined with the most common surgical approaches for renal tumours, with a median extra time of 30 min and without additional early or late complications [41]. Most of the additional time is due to the locoregional LND, especially during laparoscopic nephrectomy. If future investigations prove that additional locoregional LN metastases are not missed in case of pathologically negative SLNs, then LND may be abandoned.

In bladder cancer intraoperative SLN identification is often performed in conjunction with open surgery and

Fig. 16.4 A 46-year-old woman with bladder carcinoma. Planar lymphoscintigraphy and SPECT/CT acquired after administering an activity of 216 MBq ^{99m}Tc-nanocolloid in four injections around the tumour into the detrusor muscle under cystoscopy guidance using an endoscopic needle (**a, b**). On planar anterior image (**c**) a SLN with faint uptake is seen above the bladder radioactivity on the right. This SLN, localized at the bifurcation of the left common iliac artery as seen on volume rendering (**d**) and axial SPECT/CT (**e, f**), was tumour free at histopathology

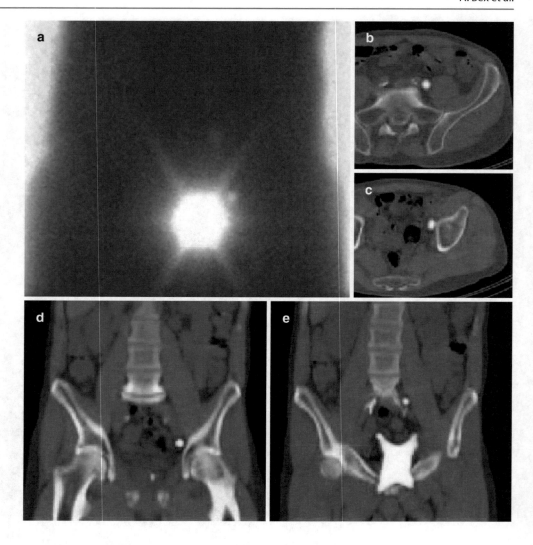

extended PLND [44, 45]. However, with the advent of laparoscopic cystectomy techniques, including robot-assisted laparoscopic cystectomies, laparoscopic gamma probes are used—as described above.

16.8 Contribution of SPECT/CT Imaging for SLN Mapping in Renal and Bladder Cancers

For both renal cell cancer and bladder cancer, use of SPECT/CT imaging is mandatory. In fact, SPECT/CT is able to detect/identify SLNs in the vicinity of the iliac vessel or aorta, thus providing a useful road map to guide urologists during surgery. In bladder cancer SPECT/CT is able to localize SLNs in the lymphatic basins of the pelvis. In many cases early-appearing LNs seen as a single hot spot on planar images are displayed as separate LNs in different basins by SPECT/CT imaging; in this case, all nodes are considered as

SLNs. In other cases intense LN uptake seen on fused images may correspond to a cluster of SLNs as depicted on the CT component of the SPECT/CT.

16.9 Intraoperative SLN Imaging in Renal and Bladder Cancers

The intraoperative SLN search may be facilitated using the gamma probe in combination with a portable gamma camera [46], which can detect both the ^{99m}Tc signals for SLN visualisation and a ^{125}I seed placed on the laparoscopic probe tip to indicate its position in relation to the SLNs.

In addition, all removed SLNs can be examined ex situ with the portable gamma camera. The use of a portable gamma camera also enables a better post-excision control and the identification of significant remaining radioactivity at the site of the SLNs as anatomically identified by SPECT/CT.

Fig. 16.5 A 43-year-old woman with a T1 (5 cm) renal cell carcinoma in the left kidney. SPECT/CT was acquired 2 h after ultrasound-guided injection of 183 MBq ^{99m}Tc-nanocolloid into the tumour. Coronal (**a**) and axial (**b–e**) SPECT/CT show two SLNs along the aorta. Both SLNs were tumour free at histopathology

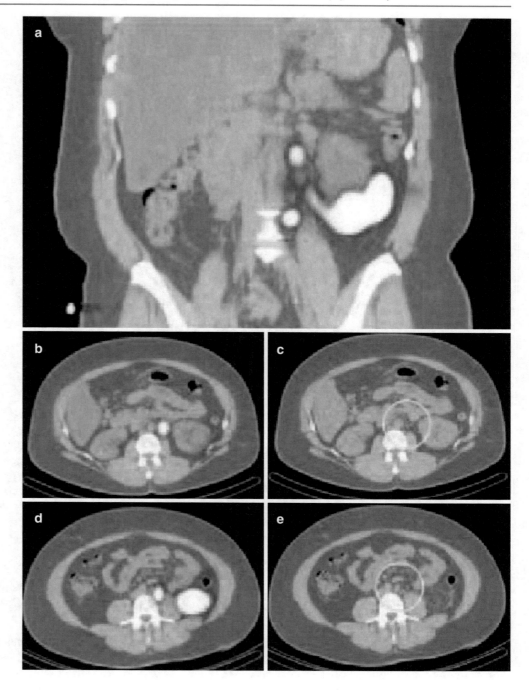

16.10 Accuracy of Radioguided SLNB in Renal or Bladder Cancer

The absence of lymphatic drainage on imaging in 37% of patients is of concern, regarding the potential clinical application of this technique [47]. No SLN could be identified, although SPECT/CT demonstrated technically correct intratumoural tracer deposition. This may be caused by lack of drainage of the radiocolloid through the lymphatic vessels. Alternatively, the radiocolloid may have drained directly into the thoracic duct (TD) without any LN interposition, as has been described by Assouad et al. [36]. Direct drainage into the TD may be rapid and difficult to detect in vivo, since the earliest planar images are acquired 20 min post-injection. We were not able to visualize the presence of lymphatic vessels on lymphoscintigraphy in

Fig. 16.6 A 50-year-old man with a carcinoma in the left dorsal wall of the bladder. On planar anterior image (**a**) drainage to the left iliac area is observed. On axial (**b**, **c**) and coronal (**d**, **e**) SPECT/CT fusion images SLNs are seen along the left external iliac artery and in the upper part of the left iliac common artery. Only the external iliac node was found to contain metastases at histopathology

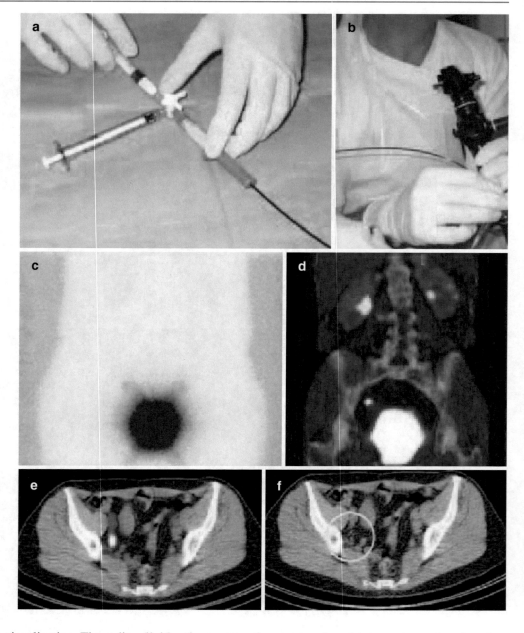

any of the patients with non-visualization. The radiocolloid was injected at the department of radiology and dynamic lymphoscintigraphy could not be performed. In four patients, radiocolloid injection was monitored with the portable gamma camera, but drainage through lymphatic vessels was not detected. SLN identification and sampling after preoperative detection on SPECT/CT are surgically feasible and safe in patients with RCC [4]. Preliminary data suggest that SLNs from the kidney are mainly located in the para-aortic, paracaval and interaortocaval region, but aberrant LNs might receive direct drainage through the TD, as was observed in 13–20% of our cases. Additional studies are required to demonstrate whether accurate mapping of lymphatic drainage and SLN sampling may lead to early detection of LN metastasis in clinically node-negative and non-metastatic RCC. In addition, it will be of interest to ascertain whether or not LND can be abandoned in patients with pathologically negative SLNs.

With regard to bladder cancer, a recent systematic review and meta-analysis [48] based on eight eligible studies published up until April 2018 included a total of 336 patients with muscle-invasive bladder cancer who underwent SLN mapping with different methods and tracers (radiocolloid, indocyanine green, blue dye—occasionally combined). The lowest SLN detection rate (21%) was found for studies employing visual guidance with the blue dye (95% CI 2–75%), while the pooled detection rate for all studies combined was 91% (95% CI 87–93%). Pooled sensitivity was 79% (95% CI 69–86%).

At the conclusion of this chapter, it must be recognized that the SLN procedure does not yet constitute the standard of care in patients with kidney or bladder cancer, but is rather the object of ongoing validation clinical trials.

Key Learning Points
- In patients with RCC, intraoperative SLN detection can be performed during open or laparoscopic transabdominal nephrectomies, open retroperitoneal partial nephrectomies and robot-assisted laparoscopic nephron-sparing surgery, depending on the size and location of the tumour.
- Standard handheld gamma probes are used during open surgery, whereas special laparoscopic gamma probes are used during laparoscopic surgery.
- In patients with bladder cancer, intraoperative SLN detection is most often performed during open surgery and extended pelvic lymph node dissection, whereas special laparoscopic gamma probes are used during laparoscopic cystectomies, including robot-assisted laparoscopic surgery.
- For both RCC and bladder cancer the use of preoperative SPECT/CT imaging is mandatory.
- Intraoperative imaging with dedicated small-field-of-view portable gamma cameras facilitates the intraoperative SLN search, as well as the post-excision control to assess completeness of SLN removal.
- Although the feasibility of SLN mapping in patients with kidney or bladder cancer has been satisfactorily demonstrated, additional studies are required to ascertain the overall accuracy of radioguided SLN mapping/biopsy.
- It must be recognized that the SLN procedure does not yet constitute the standard of care in patients with kidney or bladder cancer, but is rather the object of ongoing validation clinical trials.

Clinical Cases

Case 16.1: SLN Mapping in Renal Cell Cancer with Drainage to a Lymph Node Between Vena Cava and Aorta

Renato A. Valdés Olmos, Teele Kuusk, Oscar R. Brouwer, and Axel Bex

Background Clinical Case

A 56-year-old woman with renal cell cancer in the right kidney was referred for a SLN procedure. No lymph node abnormalities had been detected on radiological examination (clinical stage T1N0).

Planar Lymphoscintigraphy and SPECT/CT

The day before surgery the patient received 110 MBq ^{99m}Tc-nanocolloid, administered as a single intratumoural, ultrasound-guided injection in the right kidney. After moving the patient to the nuclear medicine department, static 5-min images were acquired at 15 min and 2 h post-injection with the patient in supine position using a dual-head gamma camera (Symbia T, Siemens, Erlangen, Germany) equipped with low-energy high-resolution collimators. Subsequently to the delayed static images, SPECT/CT imaging was performed using the same gamma camera.

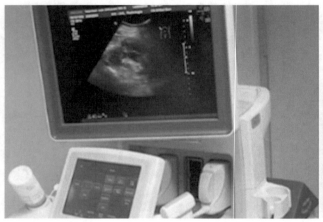
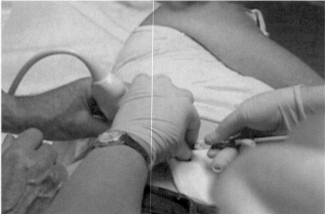
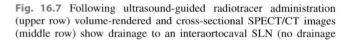

Fig. 16.7 Following ultrasound-guided radiotracer administration (upper row) volume-rendered and cross-sectional SPECT/CT images (middle row) show drainage to an interaortocaval SLN (no drainage was observed in planar images). This lymph node was subsequently localized during laparoscopy and its activity was measured ex vivo with a gamma probe (lower row)

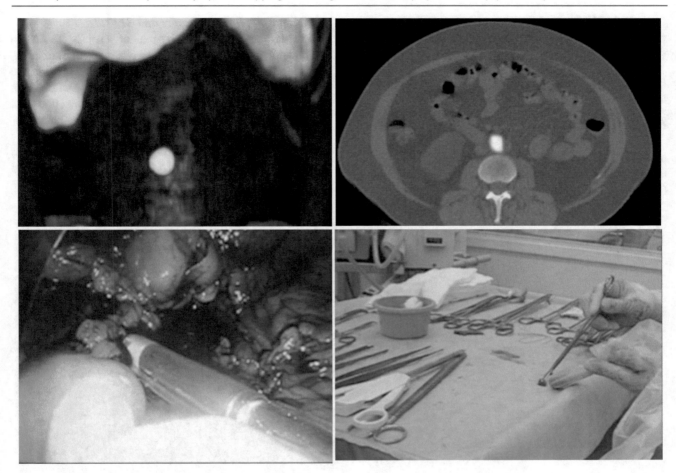

Fig. 16.7 (continued)

Case 16.2: SLN mapping in renal cell cancer with drainage to a lymph node along the vena cava

Renato A. Valdés Olmos, Teele Kuusk, Oscar R. Brouwer, and Axel Bex

Background Clinical Case

A 57-year-old male with renal cell cancer in the right kidney was referred for a SLN procedure. No lymph node abnormalities had been detected on radiological examination (clinical stage T1N0).

Planar Lymphoscintigraphy and SPECT/CT

The day before surgery the patient received 130 MBq ^{99m}Tc-nanocolloid, administered as a single intratumoural, CT-guided injection in the right kidney. After moving the patient to the nuclear medicine department, static 5-min images were acquired at 15 min and 2 h post-injection with the patient in supine position using a dual-head gamma camera (Symbia T, Siemens, Erlangen, Germany) equipped with low-energy high-resolution collimators. Subsequently to delayed static images, SPECT/CT imaging was performed using the same gamma camera.

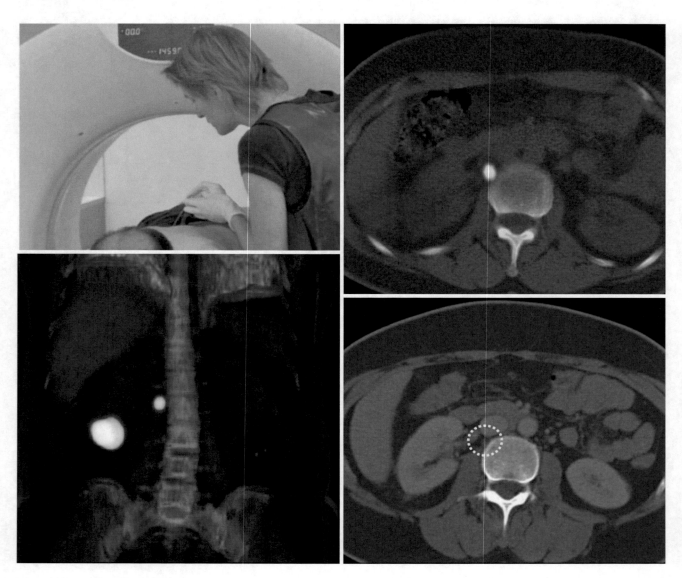

Fig. 16.8 Following CT-guided radiotracer administration (upper left image) in the lower pole of the right kidney, volume-rendered (lower image on the left) and cross-sectional SPECT/CT images (upper image on the right) show drainage to a SLN located posterolateral to the vena cava, corresponding to a normal-sized lymph node (circle) on low-dose CT (lower right image). On planar images (not displayed), no lymphatic drainage was depicted

References

1. Ferlay J, Colombet M, Soerjomataram I, et al. Cancer incidence and mortality patterns in Europe: estimates for 40 countries and 25 major cancers in 2018. Eur J Cancer. 2018;103:356–87.
2. Siegel RL, Miller KD, Jemal A. Cancer statistics, 2019. CA Cancer J Clin. 2019;69:7–34.
3. Ebele JN, Sauter G, Epstein JI, et al. Pathology and genetics of tumours of the urinary system and male genital organs. World Health Organization classification of tumours. Lyon: International Agency of Research on Cancer; 2004.
4. Ljungberg B, Albiges L, Abu-Ghanem Y, et al. European Association of Urology guidelines on renal cell carcinoma: the 2019 update. Eur Urol. 2019;75:799–810.
5. Alt AL, Boorjian SA, Lohse CM, et al. Survival after complete surgical resection of multiple metastases from renal cell carcinoma. Cancer. 2011;117:2873–82.
6. Aben KK, Heskamp S, Janssen-Heijnen ML, et al. Better survival in patients with metastasised kidney cancer after nephrectomy: a population-based study in the Netherlands. Eur J Cancer. 2011;47:2023–32.
7. Volpe A, Mattar K, Finelli A, et al. Contemporary results of percutaneous biopsy of 100 small renal masses: a single center experience. J Urol. 2008;180:2333–7.
8. Porta C, Cosmai L, Leibovich BC, et al. The adjuvant treatment of kidney cancer: a multidisciplinary outlook. Nat Rev Nephrol. 2019;15:423–33.
9. David KA, Mallin K, Milowsky MI, et al. Surveillance of urothelial carcinoma: stage and grade migration, 1993-2005 and survival trends, 1993-2000. Cancer. 2009;115:1435–47.
10. Mallin K, David KA, Carroll PR, et al. Transitional cell carcinoma of the bladder: racial and gender disparities in survival (1993 to 2002), stage and grade (1993 to 2007). J Urol. 2011;185:1631–6.
11. Herr HW, Donat SM. Outcome of patients with grossly node positive bladder cancer after pelvic lymph node dissection and radical cystectomy. J Urol. 2001;165:62–4.
12. Stenzl A, Cowan NC, De Santis M, et al. Treatment of muscle-invasive and metastatic bladder cancer: update of the EAU guidelines. Actas Urol Esp. 2012;36:449–60.
13. Wosnitzer MS, Hruby GW, Murphy AM, et al. A comparison of the outcomes of neoadjuvant and adjuvant chemotherapy for clinical T2-T4aN0-N2M0 bladder cancer. Cancer. 2012;118:358–64.
14. Blom JH, Van Poppel H, Marechal JM, et al. Radical nephrectomy with and without lymph-node dissection: final results of European Organization for Research and Treatment of Cancer (EORTC) randomized phase 3 trial 30881. Eur Urol. 2009;55:28–34.
15. Freedland SJ, de Kernion JB. Role of lymphadenectomy for patients undergoing radical nephrectomy for renal cell carcinoma. Rev Urol. 2003;5:191–5.
16. Pantuck AJ, Zisman A, Dorey F, et al. Renal cell carcinoma with retroperitoneal lymph nodes. Impact on survival and benefits of immunotherapy. Cancer. 2003;97:2995–3002.
17. Delacroix SE Jr, Chapin BF, Chen JJ, et al. Can a durable disease-free survival be achieved with surgical resection in patients with pathological node positive renal cell carcinoma? J Urol. 2011;186:1236–41.
18. Gershman B, Moreira DM, Thompson RH, et al. Renal cell carcinoma with isolated lymph node involvement: long-term natural history and predictors of oncologic outcomes following surgical resection. Eur Urol. 2017;72:300–6.
19. Hellsten S, Berge T, Linell F. Clinically unrecognised renal carcinoma: aspects of tumor morphology, lymphatic and haematogenous metastatic spread. Br J Urol. 1983;55:166–70.
20. Pantuck AJ, Zisman A, Dorey F, et al. Renal cell carcinoma with retroperitoneal lymph nodes: role of lymph node dissection. J Urol. 2003;169:2076–83.
21. Johnsen JA, Hellsten S. Lymphatogenous spread of renal cell carcinoma: an autopsy study. J Urol. 1997;157:450–3.
22. Hashimoto K, Hisasue S, Yanase M, et al. Tumor size and regional lymph node metastasis in patients with M0 renal cell carcinoma: analysis in those having regional lymph node dissection. Hinyokika Kiyo. 2005;51:621–5.
23. Matsuyama H, Hirata H, Korenaga Y, et al. Clinical significance of lymph node dissection in renal cell carcinoma. Scand J Urol Nephrol. 2005;39:30–5.
24. Dhar NB, Campbell SC, Zippe CD, et al. Outcomes in patients with urothelial carcinoma of the bladder with limited pelvic lymph node dissection. BJU Int. 2006;98:1172–5.
25. Shariat SF, Ehdaie B, Rink M, et al. Clinical nodal staging scores for bladder cancer: a proposal for preoperative risk assessment. Eur Urol. 2012;61:237–42.
26. Jensen JB, Ulhoi BP, Jensen KM. Evaluation of different lymph node (LN) variables as prognostic markers in patients undergoing radical cystectomy and extended LN dissection to the level of the inferior mesenteric artery. BJU Int. 2012;109:388–93.
27. Meijer RP, Nunnink CJ, Wassenaar AE, et al. Standard lymph node dissection for bladder cancer: significant variability in the number of reported lymph nodes. J Urol. 2012;187:446–50.
28. Hadley DA, Stephenson RA, Samlowski WE, et al. Patterns of enlarged lymph nodes in patients with metastatic renal cell carcinoma. Urol Oncol. 2011;29:751–5.
29. Parker AE. Studies on the main posterior lymph channels of the abdomen and their connections with the lymphatics of the genitourinary system. Am J Anat. 1935;56:409.
30. Bex A, Vermeeren L, de Windt G, et al. Feasibility of sentinel node detection in renal cell carcinoma: a pilot study. Eur J Nucl Med Mol Imaging. 2010;37:1117–23.
31. Sherif AM, Eriksson E, Thorn M, et al. Sentinel node detection in renal cell carcinoma. A feasibility study for detection of tumour-draining lymph nodes. BJU Int. 2012;109:1134–9.
32. Kuusk T, De Bruijn R, Brouwer OR, et al. Lymphatic drainage from renal tumors in vivo: a prospective sentinel node study using SPECT/CT imaging. J Urol. 2018;199:1426–32.
33. Terrone C, Guercio S, de Luca S. The number of lymph nodes examined and staging accuracy in renal cell carcinoma. BJU Int. 2003;91:37–40.
34. Saitoh H, Nakayama M, Nakamura K, et al. Distant metastasis of renal adenocarcinoma in nephrectomized cases. J Urol. 1982;127:1092–5.
35. Hulten L, Rosencrantz M, Seeman T, et al. Occurrence and localization of lymph node metastases in renal carcinoma. Scand J Urol Nephrol. 1969;3:129–33.
36. Assouad J, Riquet M, Foucault C, et al. Renal lymphatic drainage and thoracic duct connections: implications for cancer spread. Lymphology. 2006;39:26–32.
37. Assouad J, Riquet M, Berna P, et al. Intrapulmonary lymph node metastasis and renal cell carcinoma. Eur J Cardiothorac Surg. 2007;31:132–4.
38. Brouwer OR, Noe A, Olmos RA, et al. Lymphatic drainage from renal cell carcinoma along the thoracic duct visualized with SPECT/CT. Lymphat Res Biol. 2013;11:233–8.
39. Mahon TG, Libshitz HI. Mediastinal metastases of infradiaphragmatic malignancies. Eur J Radiol. 1992;15:130–4.
40. Riquet M, Le Pimpec Barthes F, Souilamas R, et al. Thoracic duct tributaries from intrathoracic organs. Ann Thorac Surg. 2002;73:892–8.

41. Kuusk T, Brouwer O, Graafland N, et al. Sentinel lymph node biopsy in renal tumors: surgical technique and safety. Urology. 2019;130:186–90.
42. Wright FW. Enlarged hilar and mediastinal nodes (and especially lower right hilar node enlargement) as a sign of metastasis of a renal tumour. Clin Radiol. 1977;28:431–6.
43. Aljabery F, Shabo I, Olsson H, et al. Radio-guided sentinel lymph node detection and lymph node mapping in invasive urinary bladder cancer: a prospective clinical study. BJU Int. 2017;120:329–36.
44. Roth B, Wissmeyer MP, Zehnder P, et al. A new multimodality technique accurately maps the primary lymphatic landing sites of the bladder. Eur Urol. 2010;57:205–11.
45. Roth B, Zehnder P, Birkhauser FD, et al. Is bilateral extended pelvic lymphadenectomy necessary for strictly unilateral invasive bladder cancer? J Urol. 2012;187:1577–82.
46. Vermeeren L, Valdés Olmos RA, Meinhardt W, et al. Intraoperative radioguidance with a portable gamma camera: a novel technique for laparoscopic sentinel node localisation in urological malignancies. Eur J Nucl Med Mol Imaging. 2009;36:1029–36.
47. Kuusk T, Donswijk ML, Valdés Olmos RA, et al. An analysis of SPECT/CT non-visualization of sentinel lymph nodes in renal tumors. EJNMMI Res. 2018 Dec 3;8(1):105. https://doi.org/10.1186/s13550-018-0460-y.
48. Zarifmahmoudi L, Ghorbani H, Sadri K, et al. Sentinel node biopsy in urothelial carcinoma of the bladder: systematic review and meta-analysis. Urol Int. 2019;103:373–82.

Index

A

Active trans-endothelial transport, 54
Albumin-Gd-DTPA, 29
Ambiguity, 4
Anaphylactic reactions, 304
Anatomical landmarks, 172
Anatomical localization, sentinel lymph nodes
    maximum intensity projection, 173
    multiplanar reconstruction, 173
    three-dimensional display, 173
Anti-cytokeratin antibody, 302
Arterial hypertension, 17
Atherosclerosis, 17
Autologous lymph vessel transplantation, 86
Autopsy study, 359
Axilla, 3, 4
Axillary lymph node status
    axillary lymph node dissection, 186
    ductal carcinoma in-situ, 186
    internal mammary nodes, 186
    lymph node staging, 186
    neoadjuvant chemotherapy, 186
    sentinel lymph node biopsy, 186

B

Blood-born metastases
    lymphatic mapping, 145
    tumor status, 145
Blue dye, 144, 267, 316, 334, 336
Body contour, 154
Breast cancer, 143, 147, 148
    clinical impact of SLNB, 200
    indications and controversies for sentinel lymph
        node mapping, 196
    intraoperative sentinel lymph node detection in patients, 195
    recurrent disease and sentinel lymph node mapping, 198, 199

C

CdZnTe detectors, 160
Cervical cancer, 315
Chromophore, 34
Chronic venous insufficiency, 81, 82
^{57}Co flood source, 154
^{57}Co or ^{99m}Tc point source
    maximum intensity projection, 155
    multiplanar reconstruction, 155
    SPECT/CT imaging, 154
    volume rendering for three-dimensional display, 155
Colloidal gold, 22

Colorectal cancer, methods for sentinel lymph node mapping in, 304
Contrast enhancement at CT, 28
Contrast-enhanced magnetic resonance lymphography, 68
Contrast-enhanced ultrasound (CEUS), 33
CsI(Na) scintillation crystal, 160
CT imaging
    for lymph node assessment, 66
    of lymph nodes and lymphatic circulation, 66
CT lymphography (CT-LG), 66

D

Deep lymphatic circulation, 55, 56, 59
Definitely sentinel lymph node, 174
Denatured ^{99m}Tc-collagen colloid, 22
Dendrimers for lymphatic mapping, 32
Dermal back flow, 58
Diaminobutane-core poly-propylimine, 32
Draining lymph node stations, 187
D2 lymphadenectomy, 300
Dual-tracer, 302
Ductal carcinoma in situ (DCIS), 197
Dynamic acquisition, 154
Dynamic contrast-enhanced MRI of lymph nodes, 68

E

Early gastric cancer, 302
Early metastatic disease, 358
En bloc axillary lymph node dissection, 143
Endometrial cancer, 315
Energy resolution, 158
Epifascial, 54
Expected lymph node dissection templates, 358

F

False positive finding, 321
False positive sentinel lymph node, 324
False-negative rates, 262
[^{18}F]FDG, 26
[^{18}F]FDG PET lymphography
    [18F]AlF-NEB, 26
    68Ga-NEB, 26
Fluorescence guidance, 316
Fluorescein, 304
Fluorescence imaging, 267, 299
Fluorescence probe, 323
Fluorescent light, 34
Fluorescent tracers, 5
Fluorophore, 34

FOXC2-gene
    breast-cancer-related lymphedema, 14
    chylopericardium, 15
    chylothorax, 15
    chylous ascites, 15
    intracavitary lymphedema, 15
    lipedema, 14
    lymphedema tarda, 14
    parasitic lymphedema, 15
    podoconiosis, 15
    post-thrombotic syndrome, 14
    secondary lymphedemas, 14
Free-hand SPECT, 164, 195

G
Gd^{3+}-based complexes, 29
Gadolinium-based contrast agent, 68
Gamma camera, 57, 335, 336, 340, 341
Gamma probe, 39, 323
    crystal scintillation, 158
    portable gamma cameras, 324
    semiconductor probes, 158
Gastric cancer, SLN navigation surgery for, 302
Gland sentinel, 144
Groin lymph nodes, 4
Gynecological cancers, 316

H
Hand-held gamma-detecting probe, 300
    gamma probe, 296
    shine-through effect, 296
Head and neck cancer, 262
    accuracy of radioguided SLN biopsy in, 274
    common and rare variants for SLN mapping, 268
    intraoperative imaging for SLN biopsy, 267
    intraoperative SLN detection, 267
    technical pitfalls during SLN mapping, 270
Head and neck location, 244
Hematoxylin and eosin, 302
High-energy handheld gamma probe, 63
    ^{68}Ga-labeled NOTA-Evans Blue (68Ga-NEB), 63
    ^{68}Ga-NEB, 63
Highly probable sentinel lymph node, 174
Human papillomavirus, 316
    sentinel lymph node ultrastaging, 317
Human serum albumin, 189
Hyaluronic receptor 1, 7
Hybrid SPECT/CT, 192
Hybrid tracers, 267, 316
    gamma probe, 267

I
ICG-^{99m}Tc-nanocolloid, 316
Immunohistochemistry (IHC), 292, 297, 302
Incidence rate, 316
Indocyanine green (ICG), 34, 299, 316, 332
    colloidal ferumoxides, 293
    fluorescent labeled agents, 293
    hand-held magnetometer, 293
    indium gallium arsenide (InGaAs) sensors, 293
    lymphography, 5, 72
    pre-operative CT lymphography, 293
Infrared positioning technology, 164

Integral podoplanin glycoprotein, 7
Internal mammary chain, 197
    level I lymph nodes, 188
    Level II lymph nodes, 188
    Level III, 188
    Rotter's lymph nodes, 188
Internal mammary nodal chain, 3
International Society of Lymphology (ISL), 80
Interpectoral (Rotter) lymph nodes
    axillary reverse lymphatic mapping, 3
    axillary vein lymph nodes, 3
    central lymph nodes, 3
    external mammary lymph nodes, 3
    lymphoscintigraphic data, 3
    scapular lymph nodes, 3
    subclavicular lymph nodes, 3
Interstitial fluid, 2
Interstitial injection, 54, 64
Intestinal villi, 2
    circulating cancer cells, 2
Intracavitary lymph effusions, 57
Intradermal, 54, 61
Intramuscular, 54
In-transit, aberrant, or ectopic lymph nodes, 243, 244
Intraoperative and multimodality imaging
    intraoperative imaging probes, 160
    portable gamma cameras, 160
Intraoperative gamma camera
    (ICG)-^{99m}Tc-nanocolloid, 267
    10% rule, 267
    portable gamma camera, 267
Intraoperative gamma-probe guidance, 157–159
Intraoperative imaging
    fluorescein, 241
    fluorescent agents for lymphatic mapping, 241
    free-hand SPECT technology, 241
    indocyanine green (ICG), 241
    intraoperative 3D navigation, 241
Intraoperative sentinel lymph node mapping using
    dye staining, 300, 301
Intraoperative sentinel lymph node detection, 295, 300, 323
intratumoral or peritumoral radiocolloid injection, 187
Invisible near-infrared (NIR) fluorescent light, 296
Iodine-Based CT Contrast Agents for
    Lymphatic Mapping, 27
Ionic iodinated contrast agents, 27
Iopamidol, 28
Iopamidol-CT, 66
Isosulfan blue, 293, 304

K
Kaposi's sarcoma, 16
Kaposi-Stemmer sign, 80
Klippel-Trenaunay syndrome
    lymphoangiogenesis, 12
    transcriptional factor Prox 1, 12
    vascular endothelial growth factor, 12
    VEGFR-2, 12
    VEGFR-3, 12

L
Laparoscopic gamma probe, 308
Large and multifocal/multicentric breast cancers, 197
Less probable sentinel lymph node, 175

Leukotrienes and inflammation, 11
  leukotriene B4, 11
Linearity of counting, blue dye, 158, 159
Lipiodol, 28
Lower extremity lymphedema, 79
Lymphangio-leiomyomatosis, 16
Lymphangiosarcoma, 16, 80
Lymphangiothrombosis, 16
  erysipela, 16
Lymphatic(s), 360
  of breast, 3
Lymphatic capillaries, 2, 5
Lymphatic circulation and lipid absorption, 9, 54, 55
  chylomicrons
    chylomicron-rich lymph, 9
    cisterna chili, 10
    thoracic duct, 10
  pathophysiology of, 16
Lymphatic drainage, 262, 265, 359
  of gynecological tumors, 317
  and nodal groups in bladder cancer, 360
  and nodal groups in renal cancer, 359
  predictability of, 223
  of RCC, 358
  of skin and lymph nodal groups
Lymphatic drainage patterns, 3, 4, 331
Lymphatic malignancies, 16
Lymphatic mapping
  factors affecting radiocolloid uptake during, 26
  injected volume and activity for, 25
  instrumentations for, 39
  MR, MRL and PET/MRI contrast agents, 29, 32
  multimodal tracers for, 36
  optical imaging agents fo, 34
  PET radiopharmaceuticals for, 26
Lymphatic markers, 7
Lymphatic system, 2, 3, 5
  anatomy of, 2
  breast, 187
  lymphatic circulation, 8
  physiology, peripheral cardiovascular system
    blind-ended capillaries, 8
    collecting lymphatic vessels, 8
    immunological roles, 8
    jugular and subclavian veins, 8
    pre-collecting lymphatic vessels, 8
    primary lymphatic valves, 8
    secondary collecting lymphatic vessels, 8
    thoracic duct, 8
Lymphatic vessels, 7–9, 11, 12, 15, 17, 18
  aging of, 11
Lymphazurin, 304
Lymphedema, 12–15, 17
  management of
    chylous reflux syndromes, 85
    Liposuction, 86
    lympho-venous anastomoses, 86
    Vascularized Lymph Node Transplantation, 86
Lymphedema-Distichiasis (LD) syndrome, 13
Lymph flow, physiology of, 2
Lymph node density, 359
Lymph node dissection (LND), 358
Lymph node staging, 358
Lymph drainage, failure of, 12
Lymph node groups of neck
  classification according to Robbins, 265

seven levels, 265
Lymph node metastases, 145, 358
Lymph node neck dissection
  gamma ray detection probe, 144
  hypothesis of Morton and Cochran, 144
  immunohistochemistry staining, 144
  lymphatic mapping with sentinel lymph node biopsy, 144
  lymphoscintigraphy, 144
  melanoma, 144
  penile cancer, 144
Lymph node tumor status, 299, 301
  breast cancer, 22
  cutaneous melanoma, 22
  radioguided surgery, 22
  sentinel lymph node mapping, 22
Lymphoscintigraphy, 22, 24, 25, 39, 40, 54, 56, 83, 87, 171, 172, 174, 175, 182, 187, 336, 338–341, 344, 359
  for differential diagnosis of lymphedema, 87
  imaging for, 57
  in lipedema, 88
  in management of lymphedema, 87
  methodology of, 54
  physical and/or surgical treatments, assessing efficacy, 89
    ^{68}Ga-labeled NOTA Blue Evans, 89
    ^{68}Ga-NEB, 89
  for predicting the risk to develop lymphedema, 88
  qualitative visual interpretation of, 58
  SPECT/CT, 171
  with stress test, 59
Lymphoseek®, 24, 25
Lymphostatic elephantiasis, 80
  Clinical, Etiologic, Anatomic, and Pathophysiologic (CEAP) classification, 81

M
Magnetic resonance imaging of lymph nodes and lymphatic circulation, 68
Mannose receptors, 5
Meige's syndrome, 12
Melanoma, 262, 334
  ^{99m}Tc-Tilmanocept, 220
  ambiguous SPECT/CT imaging, 220
  ambiguous zones of lymphatic drainage, 220
  hand-held gamma probe for SLN biopsy, 233
    SLN-to-background ratios, 236
  hybrid tracer, 220
  ICG-^{99m}Tc-Nanocoll, 220
  incidence, 220
  indications and contraindications, sentinel lymph node biopsy
    AJCC/UICC Cancer Staging Manual, 224
      in-transit metastases, 224
      mitosis, 224
      thickness, 224
      ulceration, 224
  lymphoscintigraphy, 220
  metastatic involvement of lymph nodes, 220
  planar images, 220
  prognosis, 220
  Sappey's lines, 220
  sentinel lymph node (SLN) biopsy, 220
Methylene blue, 300
Microbubbles, 33
Milroy's disease, 12
Modalities of injection, 264
Modalities of radiocolloid injection, 318

Molecular analysis by RT-PCR, 304
Multimodality functional imaging probes, 36
Myocardial infarction, 18

N
Near-infrared (NIR) imaging, 5, 299
    fluorescence, 300
    for lymphatic mapping, 44
Nephrectomy, 358
Nonionic contrast media, 27
Non-radionuclide methods, 293
Non-small-cell lung cancer (NSCLC)
    accuracy and perspectives of radioguided SLNB in, 296
    complete mediastinal lymph node dissection, 292
    immunohistochemistry (IHC), 292
    indications for sentinel lymph node biopsy, 293
    mediastinal lymph node metastasis, 291
    micrometastasic disease, 292
    robotic thoracic surgery (RATS), 292
    selective mediastinal lymph node sampling, 292
    sentinel lymph node, 292
    video-assisted thoracoscopic surgery, 292
Non-visualization of sentinel lymph node, 324
Noonan's syndromes, 12

O
Obesity, 17
Obturator lymph nodes, 4
    lymphoscintigraphy, 4
Oral squamous cell cancer (OSCC), 262
Osmotic pressure gradient
    active propulsion, 2
    bicuspid semilunar valves, 2
    collecting lymphatic vessels, 2
    germinal centres, 2
    immune system, 2
    large lymphatic trunks, 2
    lymphatic peristalsis, 2
    marginal sinus of lymph nodes, 2
Overlapping lymphatic drainage patterns, 5

P
Para-iliac, 4
Patent blue, 300
Pathophysiology of lymph drainage failure, 10
    edema, 10
Pelvic lymph node dissection, 358
Peripheral edema, 22
PET-based lymphoscintigraphy, imaging interpretation of, 66
PET/CT and PET/MR Lymphoscintigraphy, 63
PET/CT imaging protocol of lymphatic circulation, 64
PET/MR imaging protocol of lymphatic circulation, 65
Planar lymphoscintigraphy and SPECT/CT, 180, 182
Phagocytosis, 54
Physiological conditions in living human beings, 5
Poly-amidoamine, 32
Portable gamma cameras for lymphatic mapping, 42
Portable small-field-of-view gamma cameras, 240
Posterior lymphatic network of the breast, 3
Pregnancy, 196
Preoperative imaging, 153, 227
    dynamic lymphoscintigraphy, 229
    for sentinel lymph node mapping in patients with breast cancer,
        planar static images, 191

of sentinel lymph nodes in renal and bladder cancer, 362
Preoperative sentinel lymph node imaging, 294
    dynamic acquisition, 319
    early planar scan, 320
    late planar scan, 320
    SPECT/CT scan, 321
Preoperative sentinel lymph node mapping with radiocolloid, 300, 301
Primary lymphedema, 12
Prosperous homeobox 1, 7

Q
Quantitative lymphoscintigraphy
    depot activity transported to inguinal lymph nodes, 61
    liver-to-nodal ratio (L/N ratio), 62
    lymphatic drainage efficiency (LDE), 61
    mean transit time (MTT), 61
    removal rate constant (RRC), 61
    tracer appearance time (TAT), 61
    transit time (TT), 59
    transport capacity (TC), 61
    Transport Index (TI), 59
    uptake index of the left inguinal (UIL) to the right inguinal lymph
        nodes (UIR)., 62
    washout rate constant and depot half-life, 62
Quantum dots (QDs), 5, 35

R
Radical local-regional surgery, 144
Radiocolloid, 5, 54, 55, 57, 59, 62, 189, 264, 333
    albumin nanocolloid, 225
    and modalities of injection, 293, 294
    molecular imaging of CD206 manose-receptor, 226
    sentinel lymph node mapping, 22–26
Radiocolloid injection
    site of, 54
    for sentinel lymph node mapping in patients with breast cancer
        intratumoral injection, 189
        periareolar/subareolar radiocolloid injection, 190
        peritumoral administration, 189
        Sappey subareolar plexus, 190
        subdermal/intradermal injection, 189
Radiocolloid lymphoscintigraphy, 303, 306
Radioguided method, 306, 308
Radioguided surgery
    [198]Au-colloid, 152
    colloid particles, 152
    gamma probe, 153
    Haematoxylin & Eosin staining, 152
    hybrid SPECT/CT tomograph, 152
    immunohistochemistry, 152
    interstitial administration, 152
    intra-operative probes for, 39
    isolated tumor cells, 152
    lymphatic drainage, 152
    lymphoscintigraphy, 152
    macrophages, 152
    micrometastases, 152
    molecular analysis, 152
    occult lymph node metastases, 151
    post-surgical complications, 152
    radiocolloids, 152
    receptor-targeted radiopharmaceutical, 152
    ^{99m}Tc-albumin nanocolloid, 152
    ^{99m}Tc-antimony sulfur, 152
    ^{99m}Tc-rhenium sulfur, 152

^{99m}Tc-stannous fluoride, 152
^{99m}Tc-sulfur colloid, 152
^{99m}Tc-Tilmanocept, 152
Radiopharmaceutical, 54, 57, 61, 62
    for lymphatic mapping, 5, 22, 24
Radiotracer injection, 227
Regional lymph node dissection, 143–145
Renal/bladder cancer, accuracy of radioguided SLN biopsy in, 365, 366
    intraoperative SLN detection nodes in, 362, 364
    radiocolloid administration in, 362
Renal cell cancer, 358
Reporting sentinel lymph node mapping, 275
RT-PCR, 297

S

Sappey's lines, 4
Scintillation detectors, 39
Secondary lymphedema
    armchair legs, 82
    lipedema, 82
See and open approach, 172
    preoperative imaging, 172
Semiconductor, 39
Sensitivity, 158
Sentinel lymph node (SLN), 144, 173, 175, 177, 359
    criteria for identification, preoperative images, 174
    dedicated gamma cameras, 299
    definition of
        gamma camera, 146
        physiology of lymph drainage, 146
    intraoperative imaging, 299
    laparoscopic surgical procedures, 299
    SPECT/CT imaging, 299
Sentinel lymph node (SLN) biopsy, 151, 262, 315
    indications for, 262
    as node with a direct lymphatic drainage pathway from primary tumor, 222
    regional lymphadenectomy, 221
    stepwise spreading of melanoma through the lymphatic system, 221
    surgical complications, 221
Sentinel lymph node harvesting, 303
Sentinel lymph node mapping, 300, 316, 333, 338
    with breast cancer, hybrid tracers, 195
    in colon cancer, 303
    in esophageal cancer, 303
    in esophagogastric cancer, 300
    in gastric cancer, 300
    indications and contraindications of, 318
    interpretation of preoperative, 174
    technical pitfalls, 324
    techniques in NSCLC, 293
Sentinel lymph node navigation, 300
Sentinel lymph node-negative breast cancer, 201
Sentinel lymph node-positive breast cancer, 201, 202
Skip metastases, 304
Small-field-of-view gamma cameras, 267
Spatial resolution, 158
SPECT, 57
SPECT/CT imaging, 62, 264, 265, 268, 307, 332, 341, 359
    added value of, 321
    contribution, 231, 232
    indications for, 173
    as roadmap for intraoperative SLN detection, 179

sentinel lymph node mapping with breast cancer, 192
sentinel lymph node mapping in renal and bladder cancers, 364
Stage O lymphedema, 80
Stage I lymphedema, 80
Stage II lymphedema, 80
Stage III lymphedema, 80
Staging, 151, 331, 333, 336
Stemmer sign
    bioimpedance spectroscopy, 82
    direct lymphangiography, 83
    dual-energy X-ray absorptiometry, 83
    filariasis, 83
    high resolution cutaneous ultrasonography, 83
    measurement of limb swelling, 82
Stewart-Treves syndrome, 80
Subareolar plexus, 3, 187
Subcutaneous, 54, 57
Subfascial, 54
Suction force, 54
Superficial lymphoscintigraphy, 56, 57
Superparamagnetic iron oxide nanoparticles (SPIONs), 32
Synthetic monodispersed polymers, 32

T

^{99m}Tc-albumin nanocolloid, 22, 54
^{99m}Tc-antimony trisulfide, 264
    ^{99m}Tc-Tilmanocept, 189
    Lymphoseek®, 189
^{99m}Tc-human serum albumin, 54
^{99m}Tc-labeled colloids, 316
^{99m}Tc-labeled dextran 70
    Df-Bz-NCS-nanocolloidal albumin, 25
    lymph nodes, 23
    lymphatic circulation, 23
    peripheral lymphoscintigraphy, 24
    phagocytosis, 23
    radiocolloids, 23
    sentinel lymph node mapping, 24
^{99m}Tc-mannosyl-DTPA-dextran, 24
^{99m}Tc-nanocolloid, 189, 318
^{99m}Tc-nanocolloidal albumin, 264, 293
^{99m}Tc-neomannosylated human serum albumin (MSA)
    ^{68}Ga-MSA, 294
    lymphoscintigraphy, 294
    modalities of injection of the radiocolloids, 294
    thoracotomy, 294
^{99m}Tc-rhenium sulphide, 22
^{99m}Tc-stannous fluoride, 22
^{99m}Tc-stannous phytate, 22
^{99m}Tc-sulphur colloid, 22, 189, 264, 293
^{99m}Tc-tilmanocept, 264
^{99m}Tc-Tilmanocept, 5, 24
^{99m}Tc-tin colloid, 293
3D information, 164
Three-field lymph node dissection, 300
Transcription factor, 7, 14
Tumour
    DeCOG-SLT, 222
    hand-held gamma probe, 222
    intraoperative SLN detection, 222
    MSLT-II, 222
    Multicenter Selective Lymphadenectomy Trial-1 (MSLT-1), 222
    vital blue dye, 222
Turner's syndrome, 12
Two-compartment lymphoscintigraphy, 54, 58

U
Ultra-small particles of iron oxide (USPIO), 70
Unexpected lymphatic drainage, 262
    routes, 4
USPIO-contrast enhanced MRI, 70

V
Varicose bulges, 11
Vascular endothelial growth factor, 7
Virtual reality for preoperative planning, 99
    with lymphoscintigraphy, 62
Visual guidance, 316
Visualization of lymphatics and new developments, 5
Vital dyes, 5

isosulfan blue, 236
methylene blue, 236
patent Blue, 236
Vulvar cancer, 315

X
X-ray computed tomography (CT) scanning/magnetic resonance
        imaging (MRI)
    CT-lymphography, 92
    magnetic resonance lymphangiography, 93

Z
^{89}Zr-nanocolloidal albumin, 63

Printed in the United States
by Baker & Taylor Publisher Services